Cardiac Pacing for the Clinician

Second Edition

Cardiac Pacing for the Clinician

Second Edition

Edited by

Fred M. Kusumoto, M.D.
Associate Professor of Medicine
Director Electrophysiology and Pacing Service
Division of Cardiovascular Diseases
Department of Medicine
Mayo Clinic
Jacksonville, Florida

and

Nora F. Goldschlager, M.D.
Professor of Clinical Medicine
Co-Director Cardiology Division
Director, Pacemaker Clinic
ECG Laboratory and Coronary Care Unit
San Francisco General Hospital
University of California San Francisco School of Medicine
San Francisco, California

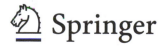 Springer

Fred M. Kusumoto, M.D.
Associate Professor of Medicine
Director Electrophysiology and Pacing Service
Division of Cardiovascular Diseases
Department of Medicine
Mayo Clinic
Jacksonville, Florida
USA

Nora F. Goldschlager, M.D.
Professor of Clinical Medicine
Co-Director Cardiology Division
Director, Pacemaker Clinic
ECG Laboratory and Coronary Care Unit
San Francisco General Hospital
University of California San Francisco
  Medical School
San Francisco, California
USA

ISBN-13: 978-0-387-72762-2   e-ISBN-13: 978-0-387-72763-9

Library of Congress Control Number: 2007927249

Printed on acid-free paper.

9 8 7 6 5 4 3 2 1

springer.com

To my wife, Laura, and my children, Miya, Hana, and Aya
Fred Kusumoto

To my husband, Arnie, and my children, Nina and Hilary
Nora Goldschlager

Preface

As early as the late 1700s, Physicians speculated that electrical current could be used to stimulate the heart. In 1882, von Ziemssen used electrical current to directly stimulate the heart of a woman whose anterior chest wall had been removed after resection of a chest tumor. In 1952, Zoll used transthoracic current to pace the heart, and in 1958 the first implantable pacemaker was placed by Ake Senning and Rune Elmquist. At the same time, Furman and Robinson demonstrated the feasibility of transvenous cardiac pacing. In the late 1960s, Mirowski and colleagues pioneered the concept of an implantable device that could be used to defibrillate the heart. Over the last 50 years, implantable cardiac devices have become the primary treatment for bradyarrhythmias and ventricular tachyarrhythmias and have emerged as an important adjunctive therapy for patients with heart failure. It is currently estimated that almost 400,000 pacemakers and defibrillators are implanted annually in the United States.

With exponential expansion of the use of implanted cardiac devices, it has become critical for all physicians to become knowledgeable about them, as they continue to increase in complexity. The second edition of Cardiac Pacing for the Clinician has the same goal as the first edition: To provide a succinct yet comprehensive reference for the implantation and follow-up of implantable cardiac rhythm devices. The book is intended to be a practical guide for the day-to-day management of these increasingly complex devices, and is intended for all physicians caring for patients with devices. We also hope that the emphasis on clinical care will be useful for implanting surgeons, nonphysician medical associates, and clinical members of industry.

The book is divided into four sections. The first section describes pacing leads and pacemaker function. The second section focuses on device implantation. New to this edition is a chapter on implantation of left ventricular leads, used in the biventricular pacing systems intended to treat patients with heart failure. Purposely we have asked two experienced implanters to discuss their personal methods for placing leads in the cardiac venous systems to illustrate the diversity of techniques and "tricks of the trade." The third section reviews the use of implantable cardiac devices in particular clinical situations. All of the chapters from the first edition have been extensively revised; new to this edition are chapters on device use for patients with atrial fibrillation, heart failure, and syncope, providing further evidence for the expanding indications for implantable devices. The final section is devoted to device follow-up. It is our belief that the greatest impact for device therapy on patient outcomes is in follow-up. Important topics such as avoiding inappropriate therapies in patients with defibrillators, ensuring optimal and individualized device function for patients, and techniques for minimizing the risks of environmental electromagnetic interference are extensively reviewed.

The last 6 years have shown rapid evolution of cardiac implanted devices that can provide not only therapy but also information on the clinical status of a patient. While beneficial, this increasing complexity also means that all clinicians must be knowledgeable about device function, indications for device use, and device follow-up. We believe that the second edition of Cardiac Pacing for the Clinician will provide the essential clinical information necessary for treating patients with implanted cardiac devices.

Acknowledgments

All books require the concerted effort of a number of people. We wish to thank our contributors for providing their expertise and taking time out of their busy schedules to write chapters for this project. We would like to thank Melissa Ramondetta from Springer Publishing for providing the enthusiasm and resources for making the second edition of Cardiac Pacing for the Clinician a reality. We also would like to thank Dianne Wuori of Springer Publishing for providing editorial and organizational support. Candy Richards provided invaluable administrative support for the second edition. Finally we wish to thank our families for the missed soccer tournaments, late dinners, and "working weekends" that a project like this requires.

Contents

Contributors

Ejigayehu Abate, MD
Department of Medicine
Mayo Clinic
Jacksonville, FL 32224

Amin Al-Ahmad, MD
Division of Cardiovascular Medicine
Stanford University Medical Center
Stanford, CA

Nitish Badhwar, MBBS, FACC
Cardiac Electrophysiology and Arrhythmia Service
Division of Cardiology
University of California
San Francisco, CA

S. Serge Barold, MD, FRACP, FACP, FACC, FESC, FHRS
Clinical Professor of Medicine
University of South Florida College of Medicine
And Division of Cardiology
Tampa, FL 33615

Peter H. Belott, MD
Sharp Grossmont Hospital
El Cajon, CA

Jane Chen, MD
Assistant Professor of Medicine
Washington University School of Medicine
St. Louis, MO

Louise Cohan
Electrophysiology and Pacing Service
Division of Cardiovascular Diseases

Department of Medicine
Mayo Clinic
Jacksonville, FL 32224

Robert E. Eckart, MD
Tripler Army Medical Center
Honolulu, Hawaii

Ehab A. Eltahawy, MD
Fellow in Cardiology
Division of Cardiology
Department of Medicine
Health Science Campus
University of Toledo
Toledo, OH

Laurence M. Epstein, MD
Chief, Arrhythmia Service
Brigham and Women's Hospital
Boston, MA

Westby G. Fisher, MD
Associate Professor, Division of Cardiology
Northwestern University
Evanston, IL

Anne M. Gillis MD, FRCPC
Professor of Medicine
Department of Cardiac Sciences
Health Sciences Centre
Calgary, AB T2N 4N1

Nora F. Goldschlager, MD
Professor of Clinical Medicine
Co-Director Cardiology Division
Director, Pacemaker Clinic
ECG Laboratory and Coronary Care Unit
San Francisco General Hospital
University of California San Francisco Medical School
San Francisco, CA

Blair P. Grubb, MD
Professor of Medicine and Pediatrics
Division of Cardiovascular Medicine
Department of Medicine
Health Science Campus
University of Toledo
Toledo, OH

David L. Hayes, MD
Professor of Medicine
Division of Cardiovascular Diseases
Mayo Clinic College of Medicine
Rochester, MN

Bengt Herweg, MD
Associate Professor of Medicine
Director Cardiac Electrophysiology and
Arrhythmia Service
University of South Florida College of Medicine and
Tampa General Hospital
Tampa, FL

Richard H. Hongo, MD
ECG Clinic and Coronary Care Unit
San Francisco General Hospital
University of California School of Medicine
San Francisco, CA

Henry H. Hsia, MD
Associate Professor
Division of Cardiovascular Medicine
Stanford University Medical Center
Stanford, CA

Dale M. Isaeff, MD, FACC
Professor of Medicine
Loma Linda University School of Medicine
Director of Pacemaker Surveillance Program
Loma Linda University Medical School
Loma Linda, CA

Jonathan M. Kalman, PhD
Royal Melbourne Hospital
Melbourne, Victoria
Australia

Fred M. Kusumoto, MD
Associate Professor of Medicine
Director, Electrophysiology and Pacing Service
Division of Cardiovascular Diseases
Department of Medicine
Mayo Clinic
Jacksonville, FL 32224

Byron K. Lee, MD
University of California at San Francisco
San Francisco, CA

Paul A. Levine, MD
St. Jude Medical Center
Sylmar, CA

Harry G. Mond, MD, FRACP, FACC, FHRS, FCSANZ
The Royal Melbourne Hospital
Cardiology Department
Melbourne, Victoria 3050
Australia

Brian Olshansky, MD
Professor of Medicine
University of Iowa Hospital
Iowa City, IA 52242

Michael A. Platonov, MD
Electrophysiology Fellow
University of Calgary
Cardiac Sciences
Calgary, Alberta
Canada

Richard S. Sanders
VP Sales and Marketing
Cameron Health, Inc.
San Clemente, CA

Salam Sbaity, MD
University of Iowa Hospitals and Clinics
Department of Internal Medicine
Iowa City, IA

Paul B. Sparks, MD, PhD
Royal Melbourne Hospital
Melbourne, Victoria 3050
Australia

Irene H. Stevenson, MD
Royal Melbourne Hospital
Melbourne, Victoria 3050
Australia

George F. Van Hare, MD
Director of the Pediatric Arrhythmia Center
University of California San Francisco
Stanford University
Pediatric Cardiology
Palo Alto, CA

Paul J. Wang, MD
Stanford University Medical Center
Stanford, CA

Paul C. Xei, MD
Instructor of Medicine
Division of Cardiovascular Medicine
Stanford University Medical Center
Stanford, CA

Section I

Pacing Leads and Modes of Function

1

Pacing Leads

Harry G. Mond

Introduction

The cardiac pacemaker lead is a relatively fragile cable of insulated conductor wire implanted into the hostile environment of the human body. Its function is to interface the power source and sophisticated electronics of the pulse generator with the heart. The pacemaker lead plays a critical role in delivering both the output pulse from the pulse generator to the myocardium and the intracardiac electrogram from the myocardium to the sensing circuit of the pulse generator.

A pacemaker lead consists of one or two electrodes at the distal end and a connector at the proximal end for attachment to the pulse generator. In comparison with the marked advances in pulse generator and sensor technology, concomitant advances in pacing leads have occurred relatively slowly. This chapter addresses the cellular electrophysiology and physics of pacing as well as reviews the engineering concepts and clinical application of lead design.

History

By modern standards, the original pacing leads were simple and very unreliable. They were epicardial or epimyocardial and implanted by exposing the heart at thoracotomy. The electrode was part of the uninsulated conductor attached directly to the myocardium. The lead, which emerged from the pulse generator casing, was directly attached to the pulse generator electronics. Failure of either the lead or pulse generator required replacement of both components, thus necessitating a further thoracotomy. It soon became apparent that a separate lead and pulse generator were required as well as a dedicated electrode. With time, the electrode became an epicardial plate or a sharp epimyocardial probe. These early leads frequently developed very high stimulation thresholds and because of continual cardiac and diaphragmatic movements, the lead body was subjected to extraordinary pressures, resulting in conductor fracture or insulation breakdown.

The necessity for repeated thoracotomies to repair or replace pacing leads stimulated an interest in insertion of pacing leads by the transvenous route.

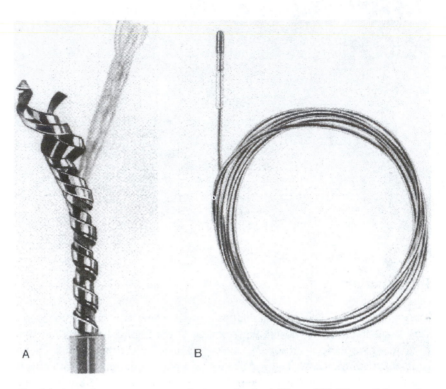

A   B

Fig. 1.1 An early transvenous ventricular pacing lead: Elema 588 (Elema-Schonander, Solna, Sweden, later Siemens Elema, and now St Jude Medical). *Left*: Central Terylene core, at least three stainless steel ribbon conductors and polyethylene insulation. *Right*: The electrode was very large and there were no fixation devices. The lead was over 100 cm long to allow tunneling from the subclavicular region to the abdomen, where a connector was attached and the pulse generator buried. (Permission for use: St Jude.)

Early transvenous leads were constructed with a Terylene or Teflon core (DuPont, Wilmington, DE) surrounded by a stainless steel ribbon conductor. They were insulated with polyethylene and had no fixation device (Fig. 1.1). The cathode electrode had a very large stimulating surface area up to 100 mm^2 and thus had a very low pacing impedance and high current drain. Because there was no provision for a central stylet for lead stiffening, these leads were very difficult to be inserted. During implantation the lead remained floppy, and positioning at the apex of the right ventricle presented a significant challenge. Once implanted, the absence of a fixation device commonly resulted in lead dislodgment. The lead was inserted via the cephalic or external jugular vein and burrowed subcutaneously down the chest wall into the abdomen where the large pulse generator was attached. At the proximal end, the lead connector was prepared at the time of surgery, simply by inserting bare conductor wire into a receiving port of the pulse generator. Insulation was achieved by using rubber O-rings and T-piece around the lead and covering with a plastic cap (Fig. 1.2). Not surprisingly, this connection was very unreliable.

Early pacing leads were either unipolar or bipolar. A bipolar epicardial or epimyocardial system required two leads whereas, a bipolar transvenous system could be achieved using a single lead composed of two parallel insulation tubes containing the anode and cathode conductors. By the late

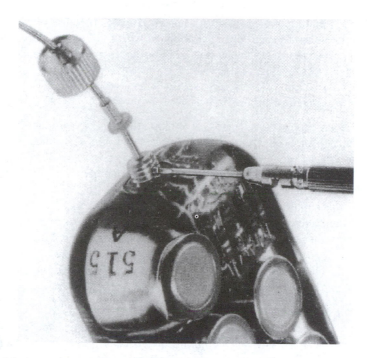

Fig. 1.2 An early lead connector (Elema-Schonander). The distal insulation was stripped and bare conductor inserted into the pulse generator receiving port and secured with a small setscrew. The area was insulated with an O-ring against the pulse generator, a piece of T-tubing to cover the conductor and a plastic cap. (Permission for use: St Jude.)

1970s, most pacing leads were thin and unipolar and the cathode electrode had surface areas in the range of 8–12 mm². The conductor was a hollow helically coiled wire, which allowed a stylet to pass to the distal end to allow easier positioning in the heart. The earliest fixation device was a wedge, later replaced by tines positioned immediately behind the electrode. With smaller pulse generators, the implant site became the subclavicular region and because no subcutaneous burrowing was required, leads were designed with sealed reliable connectors attached.

Cellular Electrophysiology and Physics of Pacing

Cardiac Depolarization

As with the normal cardiac conducting system and its propagation of impulses through the His Purkinje network, electrostimulation by an artificial cardiac pacemaker depends on the depolarization of a single or a group of myocyte cell membranes which can then act as pacemaker cells. In order for these cells to depolarize, the electric field of the applied artificial pacemaker stimulus must exceed a threshold voltage. This initiates a complex cascade of ionic currents both in and out of the cell membrane referred to as the action potential. The impulse or wave of depolarization then propagates away from the site of stimulation from cell to cell across gap junctions or intercalated disks, which with normal cells provide very low resistance to depolarization.

In this way, the impulse penetrates all areas of either the atria or ventricles and thus initiates contraction. In pathological situations, such as myocardial ischemia, propagation may slow down because of a rise in resistance in the intercalated disks.

Lead or System Impedance

Whenever electricity flows across a circuit, there is a resistance to flow encountered by the electrons. For pacing systems, the resistance is determined by the complex interaction of multiple components. Because some of these components are also characterized by the ability to retain charge or capacitance, the term impedance is preferred. At the time of lead implantation, it is this complicated series of resistance and capacitance factors that are measured and are referred to as system impedance. For a pacing circuit, the system impedance has five basic components: a low, purely resistive *conductor impedance*, a high *cathode electrode impedance*, complex *polarization effects* at the electrode–tissue interface, a low *tissue impedance*, and the *anode electrode impedance* (Fig. 1.3).

Conductor Impedance

Within a pacemaker lead, the flow of electrons from the connector lead pin to the cathode electrode is relatively unimpeded, because the materials used for modern lead conductors have a very low resistance of the order of 5–50 Ω. This is necessary to prevent wastage in delivery of energy to the cathode. For instance, a very high resistance conductor would act like a radiator generating heat in the conductor; thus, the current or number of electrons eventually delivered to the cathode would be markedly attenuated. Similarly, partial lead fractures or complete lead fractures with the fractured ends in contact with each other will result in very high resistances. In both of these cases, despite the production of an adequate voltage, the current or electron density reaching the distal end of the conductor may be inadequate for the stimulation of the myocardium. This situation can be explained by Ohm's Law:

$$\text{Voltage}\,(V) = \text{Current}\,(I) \times \text{Resistance}\,(R).$$

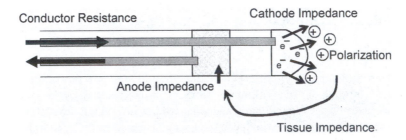

Fig. 1.3 Schematic of a bipolar lead illustrating the factors involved in determining system impedance. The arrows denote current flow. Resistance to current flow occurs at the lead conductor (conductor resistance), at the cathode–tissue interface (cathode impedance and polarization), in the myocardium (tissue impedance) and at the anode (anode impedance). The largest contributors to system impedance are the cathode impedance and polarization effects.

For a given voltage, as the resistance rises, current flow is impeded and insufficient electrons reach the cathode and surrounding tissues to allow depolarization.

Cathode Electrode Impedance

Despite the necessity for a very low resistance in the conductor, the cathode electrode should be the opposite. A small, high-resistance electrode concentrates the current flow, resulting in a high current density, which allows a low voltage to depolarize the myocytes beyond the electrode–tissue interface. Conversely a large electrode would have a low resistance and allows considerable current loss.

Polarization

There is an impedance factor or capacitance effect at the electrode–tissue interface referred to as polarization. An explanation of polarization requires an understanding of the complex electrochemical events that occur at the electrode–tissue interface. Electricity within metal conductors is ohmic, or simply the flow of electrons. However, in body tissues, current flow is due to the movement of charged molecules such as Cl^- ions. When current flows from the electrode to the tissues, there is a transfer of ohmic energy to ionic energy at the electrode–tissue interface. This involves an intense chemical reaction. The result is flowing away of the negatively charged ions leaving behind an alignment of oppositely charged particles attracted by the emerging electrons (Fig. 1.4).

The capacitance effect of these positively charged ions acts as a deterrent or resistance to ion flow and is the basis of polarization. It explains the change in impedance that occurs during the delivery of the pacing stimulus. The capacitance is zero at the leading edge of the constant-voltage stimulus. During the stimulus, the capacitance increases to reach its maximum at the trailing edge of the stimulus (Fig. 1.5). The capacitance gradually decreases after the stimulus,

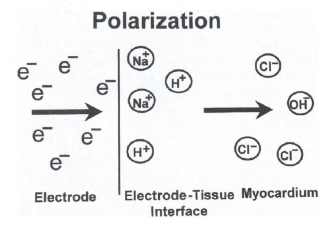

Polarization

Electrode | Electrode-Tissue Myocardium
Interface

Fig. 1.4 Polarization effect at the electrode–tissue interface. Within the electrode, current flow is due to movement of electrons (e^-). At the electrode–tissue interface, the current flow becomes ionic. The negatively charged ions (Cl^-, OH^-) flow into the tissues toward the anode leaving behind oppositely charged particles attracted by the emerging electrons. It is this capacitance effect at the electrode–tissue interface, that is the basis of polarization.

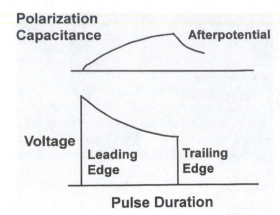

Fig. 1.5 The changes in polarization at the electrode–tissue interface with delivery of a constant voltage pulse generator stimulus. At the leading edge of the stimulus, the polarization capacitance is zero. As the resistance builds during the pulse duration, this capacitance effect acts as a barrier to current flow. At the end of the stimulus is the trailing edge and here the resistance to flow is maximum. Following this, the capacitance effect falls exponentially as positive ions dissipate. This is referred to as the afterpotential.

owing to the dissipation of positive ions and the return of the electrode-tissue interface to electrical neutrality. The accumulation of these ions in the myocardium constitutes the afterpotential that is typically recorded following a pacing stimulus.

Like the cathode electrode impedance, the electrochemical polarization effect increases as the geometric electrode surface area is reduced. For this reason, although a small electrode with a high cathode electrode impedance is desirable to allow increased current density, these small electrodes are usually associated with a high polarization effect, which is energy expensive. In addition to electrode size, polarization is also dependent on the time that has elapsed following lead implantation, the electrode materials, the electrode surface structure, the current delivered (increases with low current), the pulse duration (increases with extended pulse duration), the tissue chemistry and the stimulation polarity. The polarization effect can represent 30–40% of the total pacing impedance, but this contribution may be as high as 70% for some smooth surface, small surface area electrodes. For these reasons, polarization effects have become very important in cathode electrode design.

Tissue Impedance

After leaving the electrode-tissue interface, current flows toward the anode. The resistance of all tissues between the cathode and anode is termed the tissue impedance. For a bipolar system in which the anode is a ring electrode located within the paced chamber at a short distance from the cathode, the tissue impedance is determined by the endomyocardium with its myocytes and extracellular components including fluids (Fig. 1.6). For a unipolar system, where a section or all of the pulse generator housing serves as the anode, both cardiac and noncardiac tissues contribute to the tissue impedance. In general, most of these tissues have a high concentration of water and electrolytes, resulting in similar low tissue impedance for both unipolar and bipolar pacing systems.

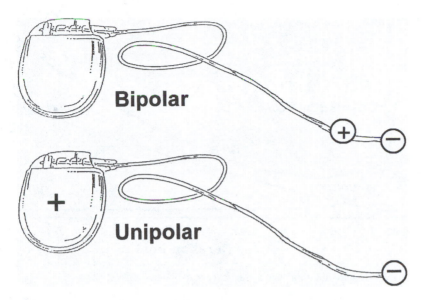

Fig. 1.6 Diagram demonstrating differences between unipolar and bipolar lead systems. Note the bipolar lead has both poles; anode and cathode on the lead, whereas the unipolar lead has only the cathode. The anode lies on the can of the pulse generator.

Anode Electrode Impedance

A final consideration is the impedance of the anode electrode. Because of the complex impedance characteristics of polarization, it makes sense that the anode is large so as not to impede current flow in order to complete the electrical circuit. However, in modern lead systems, whether they are bipolar or unipolar, the anode electrode impedance contributes very little to the overall system impedance.

Stimulation Threshold and Strength–Duration Relationships

By definition, the stimulation threshold is the lowest voltage or current necessary to consistently evoke cardiac depolarization outside the refractory period of the heart. By convention the term "consistently" refers to at least five consecutive beats. Although in clinical practice only voltage (volts = V) and pulse duration (milliseconds = ms) are used, nevertheless, a number of derived parameters are often described in lead studies but are of little value in day-to-day management. These include current (milliamperes = mA), energy (microjoules = μJ) and charge (microcoulombs = μC). These parameters are discussed later in this chapter.

The stimulation threshold is measured at lead implantation and should be remeasured at any reoperation whether it is suspected or proven malfunction or routine pulse generator replacement. Modern pulse generators also have algorithms that allow the voltage or pulse duration stimulation thresholds to be determined noninvasively. Depending on the method used to measure the stimulation threshold, the voltage output is generally programmed to at least two times greater than the voltage threshold (2:1 safety margin) or the pulse duration to at least three times greater than the pulse duration threshold (3:1 safety margin). More recently, ventricular voltage threshold stimulation

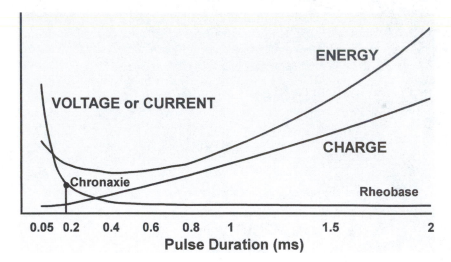

Fig. 1.7 Strength–duration curves. See text for explanation.

algorithms have been introduced that repeatedly measure the ventricular stimulation threshold and then automatically reprogram the voltage output to a value just above this threshold. This has the advantage of allowing even lower voltage outputs to conserve the power source.

A number of factors determine the stimulation threshold at implantation and in the follow-up period. Most of these are discussed in detail later in this chapter. However, apart from the cathode electrode, a relevant factor is the tissue characteristics, including ischemic or fibrous tissue, which results in higher stimulation thresholds. Interestingly, the stimulation threshold of single myocytes has been shown to be dependent on the orientation of the cell to the electric field. A cell that lies parallel to the field has a lower stimulation threshold than one lying perpendicular to the field. Similarly, cathodal (negative) stimulation has a significantly lower stimulation threshold than anodal (positive) stimulation. Another critical factor determining stimulation threshold is the distance of the closest normal myocyte. The stimulation threshold is inversely proportional to the square of the distance to the closest excitable cell. It can be shown that a displacement of >0.5 mm can significantly change the stimulation threshold. It is probably this factor that results in many of the idiopathic high stimulation threshold problems seen within the first 6-month postimplantation. These cases often present as idiopathic high threshold exit block (voltage stimulation thresholds greater than the output of the pulse generator), and are called micro dislodgment or micro displacement.

An additional factor determining the voltage stimulation threshold is the period of time the stimulus, measured in terms of voltage or current, is applied to the myocardium. This period is referred to as the *pulse duration* or *pulse width*. For obvious reasons, the shorter the pulse duration the higher the stimulation threshold. This nonlinear exponential relationship between the voltage stimulation threshold and the pulse duration can be represented graphically as the *strength–duration* curve. Knowledge that the strength–duration curve is nonlinear is crucial in both design and output programming of pacing systems (Fig. 1.7). For modern atrial or ventricular endocardial leads, the voltage or current stimulation threshold remains relatively constant for pulse durations >0.5 ms. In contrast, a pulse duration <0.2 ms results in a marked elevation of the stimulation threshold with the level approximating to infinity as the pulse duration approaches zero. For most electrodes, the most effective pulse duration range for maximum energy efficiency is from 0.25 to 0.6 ms. Because current or voltage stimulation threshold may rise following lead implantation, the acute and chronic strength–duration curves for the same lead will differ. Therefore, strength–duration curves differ between electrode designs as well as implant times. There are two reference points on a strength–duration curve that are important in determining the quality of a pacing electrode. The first is the lowest point on the curve, called the *rheobase*. The rheobase is by definition the lowest voltage or current that results in myocardial depolarization at infinitely long pulse duration. In practice, the rheobase is almost never determined, because it is rare to measure the stimulation threshold at pulse durations >2.0 ms. Consequently the rheobase usually quoted in the literature is one that is extrapolated from a modified strength–duration curve and can be referred to as an *apparent rheobase*.

The other reference point is the pulse duration time, called the *chronaxie,* which is derived from the rheobase. By definition, the chronaxie is the threshold pulse duration at twice the rheobase voltage or current. The chronaxie can also be referred to as *apparent chronaxie* because the rheobase cannot be accurately determined.

There are a number of lessons to be learnt from the inspection of a strength–duration curve. The ideal pulse duration should be greater than the chronaxie time. When a stimulation threshold is measured or recommended, whether it is voltage or pulse duration, the other determinant of the strength–duration curve must also be quoted. Although this appears obvious, it is not uncommon to try to overcome high threshold exit block by increasing the pulse duration. If the voltage output remains less than the rheobase, then no increase of the pulse duration from normal values will be effective for myocardial stimulation.

Another practical application involves the safety margin discussed earlier. Although 2:1 voltage and 3:1 pulse duration safety margins are usually quoted, this should be used in a practical sense only after inspection of the strength–duration curve. For instance, it may be recommended that for a voltage stimulation threshold of 2.0 V at pulse duration of 0.35 ms, the pulse generator be programmed to 2.0 V and the pulse duration 1.0 ms. However, after inspection of the exponential strength–duration curve, it may be wiser to keep the pulse duration at 0.35 ms and program the voltage to 4.0 V.

As mentioned earlier, there are two controversial derived measurements of lead function that are occasionally used for lead studies (Fig 1.7). The first is the threshold *energy*, which is related to current, voltage, and pulse duration by the formula:

Energy (µJ) = Voltage (V) × Current (mA) × Pulse Duration (PD in ms).

Substituting current as in Ohms Law ($I = V/R$) into the energy formula:

$$E = V^2 \, PD \, / \, R.$$

Like voltage and current, a threshold energy strength–duration curve can be created. Referring to the energy formula, it is not surprising that threshold energy rises with increasing pulse duration. However, with low pulse durations, the exponential rise in voltage threshold results in very marked elevations of energy consumption because the voltage is squared. Knowing this it can be determined that the ideal pacing energy losses occur with a pulse duration of about 0.5 ms.

Because voltage is squared in the energy formula, the voltage safety margin is only 2:1 compared to 3:1 for pulse duration. Similarly, doubling the voltage output of a pulse generator from 1.0 to 2.0 V results in correspondingly smaller energy losses than from 2.5 to 5.0 V. This has important implications when considering pulse generator power source longevity. It is extremely important to measure stimulation thresholds and where possible, lower voltage outputs to 2.5 V or less. However, further energy savings become insignificant with voltage outputs below 1.5 V.

Another derived and equally controversial threshold measurement of electrode function is the charge delivered by the power source of the pulse generator. By definition, this is the current or the number of electrons delivered per unit time and is measured in microcoulombs (μC).

$$\text{Charge (μC)} = \text{Current (mA)} \times \text{Pulse Duration (ms)}.$$

Charge threshold is useful in predicting pulse generator power source longevity. This is because a power source is essentially a limited fuel tank of electrons and the rate at which these are used per unit time, which is essentially charge, identifies the time when the tank will become depleted. On the strength–duration curve, the threshold charge, being the product of current and pulse duration increases in a straight line. The continuing fall in charge threshold with reducing pulse duration is important, although this will plateau as the rising current threshold offsets the effect of the short pulse duration.

Why then, is there a controversy about the use of derived threshold parameters for strength–duration curves? On the surface, the use of energy or charge seems reasonable. The major criticism in using energy or charge is that it is not possible to program these parameters directly with current programmable pulse generators. Being derived parameters, the calculations must take into consideration other parameters such as impedance. As stated earlier, the polarization impedance rises during delivery of current; thus, where the value is measured can be critical. It is essential to measure the voltage before energy can be used in a meaningful way, because the voltage used in any energy calculation must be greater than rheobase for cardiac depolarization to occur. It would be easy to accept what appears to be an appropriate energy value, but because of an inappropriate pulse duration and impedance, the programmed voltage or current could be less than rheobase; thus it would fail to pace the heart. In a practical sense, pacemaker physicians and technologists think and program in terms of voltage and pulse duration. Energy and charge are not used in day-to-day management.

Despite the limitations of the derived parameters, they do help in understanding the concepts of safety margins and energy conservation. It is obvious to see that at very low pulse thresholds, the charge is low, but the energy requirements are high because of elevated current and voltage stimulation thresholds. At pulse durations of 0.4–0.6 ms, all threshold parameters appear ideal. At high pulse durations, the voltage and current requirements may be low, but the energy and charge values are unacceptable. A summary of the optimal pacing outputs is provided in Table 1.1.

Table 1.1 Optimal programming of pacing outputs.

Parameter	Optimal range	Comment
Voltage	1.5–2.5 V	Longevity is markedly reduced when the output is greater than 2.5 V. Voltages less than 1.5 V are not associated with significant increases in longevity.
Pulse duration	0.4–0.6 ms	Pulse durations of 0.4–0.6 ms correspond with the nadir of the threshold energy strength–duration curve (Fig. 1.7).
Safety margin	2:1 voltage 3:1 pulse duration	The strength–duration curve must be taken into account when determining the optimal type of safety margin programming.

Sensing

Besides providing a method for myocardial stimulation, the pacemaker lead is also responsible for retrograde conduction of intrinsic intracardiac signals from the heart back to the pulse generator. The ability of a modern pacing system to adequately sense these signals and respond appropriately depends on both cardiac and pacemaker factors. Cardiac factors determine the quality of these signals, which in turn is dependent on the electrophysiological and anatomical properties of the surrounding myocardium. Once detected, the transfer of an intracardiac signal, without significant attenuation to the pulse generator-sensing circuit is dependent on the shape and materials of the electrode as well as the conductive and insulative properties of the lead. The signal must be amplified and analyzed by the sensing circuitry once it reaches the pulse generator. False or inappropriate signals – caused by extracorporeal interference, skeletal myopotentials and far-field events – must be accurately identified by the sensing circuitry and differentiated from intrinsic cardiac activation.

The foundation of intracardiac sensing involves the ability of the lead system with its cathode and anode to successfully detect spontaneous intracardiac depolarization from within the cardiac chamber it is primarily designed to pace. During Phase 4 or the resting phase of the cardiac action potential, individual myocytes have an electrical gradient of about −90 mV across the cell membrane. As all cardiac cells have a similar gradient; there is, therefore, no potential difference detected between the cathode and anode of a pacing lead during this phase and thus signal is neither conducted to, nor registered in the sensing circuit.

As with a pacing wave of depolarization, the spontaneous cardiac wave of depolarization results from a complex and sophisticated movement of ions across individual cell membranes particularly during Phase 0 of the action potential. The result is an electrical event in both atria and ventricles created by a cascade of depolarizing cells. A potential difference is registered depending on the position of an individual depolarizing myocyte relative to the pacing electrode dipole. Thus, a wave of depolarization throughout the chamber involving millions of cells records a significant difference in electrical potential between the anode and cathode of the pacing system. This results

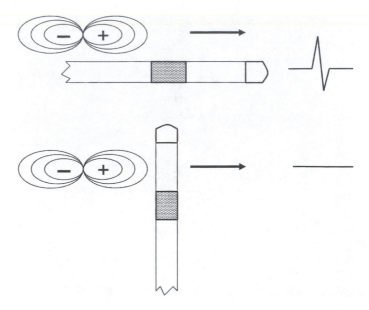

Fig. 1.8 Signal characteristics of the ventricular electrogram are determined in part by the orientation of the electrodes to the signal of cardiac depolarization. *Above*: If the electrodes are oriented parallel to the advancing wavefront of depolarization, a biphasic signal will be recorded, because the electrodes will temporarily be exposed to different electrical fields. *Below*: If the electrodes are oriented perpendicular to the wavefront no signal will be recorded, because the electrical fields that the electrodes "see" will be similar. In actual practice the situation is more complex and the signal recorded by an electrode pair usually has multiple components.

in a biphasic wave, which on the surface electrocardiogram is represented as the P wave for atrial depolarization or the QRS complex for ventricular depolarization.

The shape and voltage of this characteristic wave, which is called the electrogram is dependent on the position of the dipole and the number of cells depolarized. The movement of the wave of depolarization relative to the orientation of the dipole of the electrodes can have a marked effect on the eventual recorded electrogram (Fig. 1.8). For instance, if the inter-electrode dipole is parallel to the wave of depolarization, then the wavefront passes one pole first and then the other, recording the maximum potential with the highest slew rate or voltage change per unit time. The opposite occurs if the electrode dipole is oriented perpendicularly. In this situation, both electrodes record the same potential change simultaneously; thus, there is no relative change in potential between electrodes, despite a normal wave of depolarization in the heart. No electrogram would be recorded in this theoretical situation.

In clinical practice, a generous ventricular electrogram is usually recorded at the time of lead implantation. An atrial or ventricular lead rarely needs to be repositioned, because of failure to sense (Fig. 1.9). The usual cause of a poor voltage ventricular electrogram is loss of ventricular muscle mass such as following infarction. Atrial electrograms are generally smaller than ventricular electrograms, but modern pulse generators can be programmed to high sensitivity to overcome this potential problem.

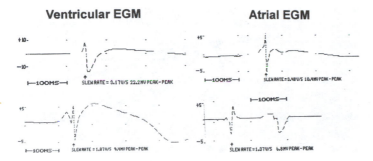

Fig. 1.9 Atrial and ventricular electrograms (EGM) as obtained through a Medtronic Pacing System Analyser Model 5311. *Ventricular*: Above: A typical rS configuration with a minor current of injury pattern. Below: The current of injury pattern is more pronounced. *Atrial*: Above: A typical rS pattern. *Below*: Approximately 150 ms after the atrial electrogram lies a large far-field ventricular electrogram.

The pacing lead not only delivers the electrogram to the sensing circuit of the pulse generator, but is also critical in ensuring that the delivered product is not attenuated below a programmed sub-threshold value. For a lead to deliver an electrogram to the sensing circuit it must pass through two impedance barriers placed in parallel (which should not be confused with the system impedance discussed earlier). The first is the *sensing or source impedance*. This is effectively the sensing impedance of the conductor and electrode–tissue interface that presents itself to a cardiac signal. This was very important in early electrode design, because theoretically the smaller the electrode, the higher the sensing impedance. In turn the higher the sensing impedance, the more markedly the electrogram signal is attenuated. The second impedance barrier is the *input amplifier impedance* within the pulse generator. In this case, the higher the resistance value of the amplifier, the superior the delivered signal to the sensing circuit. Because these impedance barriers lie in parallel, they significantly influence each other. This is demonstrated in Fig. 1.10, where the attenuation of the electrogram signal is plotted against the sensing impedance for different input impedances. Early pulse generators had input amplifier impedances of 1 KΩ. With high sensing impedances, the size of the signal could fall to 20% of that initially seen at the electrodes. However, once the input amplifier impedance was raised to 15 KΩ or greater, the attenuation was only 75% of the initial value. This allowed the introduction of small cathode electrodes.

Ohm's law can also explain this signal attenuation. If a ventricular electrogram signal of 10 mV presents itself to a sensing impedance of 5 KΩ and a very low input amplifier impedance of 1 KΩ, then the total impedance (in parallel) is 6 KΩ.

Current flow (I) = Voltage (V) / Total impedance (R) = 10/6 = 1.67 mA.

The voltage that eventually presents itself to the sensing circuit is thus:

$$V = I \times \text{Input impedance} = 1.67 \times 1 = 1.67 \text{ mV}.$$

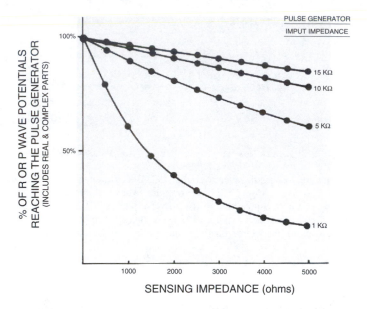

Fig. 1.10 The attenuation of the atrial or ventricular electrogram potential that reaches the pulse generator sensing circuit is graphed against the sensing impedance for a range of input impedances. The higher the sensing impedance, the smaller the amplitude of the received electrogram signals. In turn, the higher the input impedance, the larger the received electrogram signals.

This is 17% of the original signal. However, if the input impedance is increased to 15 KΩ, then the final signal voltage will be:

$$[10\,\text{mV}/(15+5\,\text{k}\Omega)]15\,\text{K}\Omega = 7.5\,\text{mV}.$$

In this case the signal improves to 75% of the original signal. In a practical sense, this was very important, when low input impedance sensing circuits were used with small surface area electrodes. With modern pulse generators, this is not a problem as the attenuation is minimal.

The ventricular electrogram waveform as seen from the apex of the right ventricle is predominantly a negative deflection, although in a majority of cases it is biphasic. The classic pattern is a small initial positive wave followed by a negative deflection and a small positive terminal wave (Fig. 1.9). In about 10% of cases, the electrogram waveform is predominantly positive. Occasionally, a transient current of injury pattern may be seen at the terminal part of the wave. At the time of lead implantation, the amplitude of this deflection and the slew rate are measured by the pacing system analyser. In the ventricle, a bipolar amplitude of >4 mV is recommended for satisfactory sensing. For atrial leads, the amplitude should be >1.5 mV. However, the sensing characteristics of modern pulse generators can usually cater for lower voltages in both chambers. It may be valuable to repeat the measurements in the unipolar configuration as modern pulse generators have programmable sensing polarity.

The *slew rate* is the maximum rate of voltage change (dV/dt) in the electrogram and represents the steepness of the slope over the first derivative or 2-mV voltage excursion. Satisfactory ventricular electrogram slew rates are of the order of 1–4 V/s with the minimum generally accepted being 0.5 V/s. A desirable atrial slew rate is >0.5 V/s.

Lead Polarity

The vast majority of pacing leads implanted today in the atrium and to a lesser extent in the ventricle are bipolar (1). Compared to their unipolar counterparts, early bipolar leads were large, cumbersome and difficult to implant resulting in an early preference for unipolar systems (2). Today, with major technological and engineering advances, bipolar leads are the same as unipolar designs in size and ease of insertion. By definition, all pacemaker electrical circuits are bipolar. To complete the circuit, electrons flow from the cathode to the anode. When applied to transvenous leads, the terms "unipolar" and "bipolar" simply indicate *the number of electrodes in contact with the heart* (Fig. 1.6). A unipolar lead has only one electrode (the cathode), located at the tip. Current flows from the negatively charged cathode to the heart and returns to the anode (the pulse generator) to complete the circuit. In contrast, a bipolar lead has both electrodes, a short distance from each other at the distal end. The tip electrode is the cathode, and a ring electrode proximal to this, serves as the anode. In reality, the differences between unipolar and bipolar pacing are relatively minor. The principal differences between these two electrode configurations are discussed:

Size. The original bipolar lead designs had two parallel conductors individually encased in a stiff, dual-lumen insulated tube and a very bulky bifurcated connector. They were difficult to implant compared to unipolar models. In comparison modern bipolar pacing leads are as thin as their unipolar counterparts and thus size is no longer an issue.

Stimulation Threshold. Because of the larger anode, unipolar pacing has a marginally lower total system resistance compared to bipolar pacing. Unipolar pacing, therefore, should result in a slightly lower stimulation threshold compared with bipolar pacing. In reality, modern, small, low polarization cathodes play a much more important role in determining overall pacing impedance than the larger anode, resulting in essentially the same stimulation thresholds for both configurations.

Sensing of intracardiac electrograms. With its broad inter-electrode distance, the unipolar system "sees" more of the heart in which to detect a spontaneous intracardiac electrical event and thus it was assumed that unipolar was superior to bipolar sensing. In reality, the modern unipolar and bipolar pacing systems show comparable and usually excellent atrial and ventricular electrogram amplitudes and slew rates which usually exceed the standard limits of the sensing circuit by a comfortable margin.

Far-field sensing. The atrial sense amplifier of a dual chamber (or AAI) pacemaker may demonstrate apparent inappropriate sensing related to small amplitude far-field signals arising from the ventricles (Fig. 1.9). In the presence of high atrial sensitivity settings, such signals may be inappropriately interpreted as atrial depolarizations. Generally, this is more likely to occur if the tip of the atrial lead is positioned near the tricuspid valve. Since all leads sense the dipole between the anode and the cathode, a bipolar atrial lead with closely spaced electrodes is less likely to record far-field electrical signals than a bipolar lead with a wider inter-electrode distance or a unipolar lead (3). Sensed, far-field electrical signals may also result in inappropriate mode switching (4). Thus, bipolar leads have a clear advantage with respect to decreasing the size of far-field cardiac signals.

Crosstalk. Crosstalk is an alteration in pacemaker timing induced by the sensing in one chamber of a signal originating in the opposite cardiac chamber. The most commonly described model of crosstalk is the inappropriate sensing of the atrial pacing stimulus by the ventricular channel in dual chamber pacing. The resultant inhibition of ventricular output may in the pacemaker dependent patient, be life threatening. Because of the larger amplitude of the pacing stimulus, crosstalk is far more common with unipolar than with bipolar dual chamber pacing systems.

Skeletal muscle myopotential over-sensing. Unipolar pacing systems are far more susceptible to skeletal myopotential sensing and consequent inhibition than are bipolar systems. Such inhibition represents the most common source of unipolar over-sensing (5) particularly in the atrium, because of the necessity to use high sensitivity settings.

Extra-corporeal over-sensing. Electromagnetic interference (EMI) from a source outside the body may enter a pacemaker sensing circuit either directly into the pulse generator or via the lead. Because the pulse generator is shielded by a metal case, direct penetration by electromagnetic interference is uncommon. The antenna effect of the lead remains a potential problem, although significant cases are limited to a small number of environmental situations. In theory, unipolar sensing should be more sensitive than bipolar sensing to EMI, because of the larger inter-electrode distance, which amplifies the antenna effect. Again, this will be more significant with the higher sensitivity settings that are generally required for atrial sensing.

Right ventricular perforation. Because of their stiffness, certain models of bipolar leads, particularly those insulated with polyurethane, were more prone to right ventricular perforation. The stiff distal end of the lead may damage the endomyocardium and in some cases result in ventricular penetration and perforation (6). Such stiff bipolar leads are no longer available and today there is very little difference in the stiffness between unipolar and bipolar leads.

Skeletal muscle stimulation. The proximity of adjacent skeletal muscle to the anode of a unipolar pulse generator may result in undesirable stimulation of this skeletal muscle. The resultant muscle twitching in coated pulse generators is usually prevented at the time of implantation by positioning the anode toward the subcutaneous tissues, away from the muscle.

Depth of the pulse generator pocket. Because of the potential for local skeletal muscle stimulation from the anode, unipolar pulse generators cannot be buried deep to skeletal muscle, (7) unless very low voltages are programmed. Bipolar pacemakers are not prone to such problems.

Stimulus artifact size. The unipolar stimulus artifact recorded on the surface ECG is significantly larger than a bipolar stimulus of equal voltage (Fig. 1.11). Because of this difference, bipolar pacing may be more difficult to identify on the surface ECG tracing or monitor, from a spontaneous rhythm propagated with a wide QRS complex, such as slow ventricular tachycardia or idioventricular rhythm. In these situations, temporary programming to the unipolar configuration can be very helpful.

Polarity programming flexibility. A bipolar lead connected to a polarity programmable pulse generator allows noninvasive switching between either polarity for pacing and sensing. Polarity programming to unipolar pacing is particularly important in bipolar lead systems with failure of the outer insulation or fracture of the anode conductor. This allows, at least on a

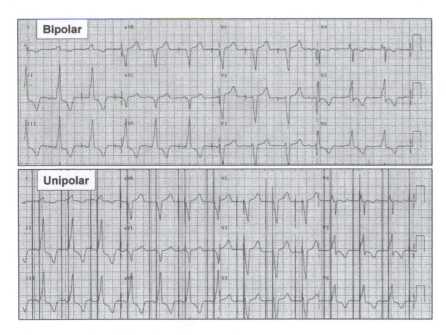

Fig. 1.11 Twelve lead ECGs demonstrating bipolar and unipolar atrial and ventricular pacing. With unipolar pacing, there are prominent atrial and ventricular pacing spikes (stimulus artifact).

temporary basis, intact unipolar pacing. The ability to separately program the polarity configuration for pacing and sensing also allows the advantages of either configuration to be exploited while minimizing its disadvantages.

Vulnerability to ventricular arrhythmias. There is the theoretical risk of ventricular fibrillation whenever a pacemaker stimulus is delivered into the vulnerable period of the ventricle. Experimentally, the ventricular fibrillation threshold is lower with bipolar stimulation than with conventional unipolar cathodal stimulation. Despite these laboratory observations, no clinical differences between permanent unipolar and bipolar systems have been reported with respect to the risk of inducing ventricular arrhythmias.

Special pacing systems/Implantable cardioverter–defibrillator interactions. Because of the specific sensing requirements of automatic anti-tachycardia pacemakers and implantable cardioverter–defibrillators (ICD) with pacing capability, these systems must be bipolar to minimize inappropriate sensing of far-field and extra-cardiac signals. The implantation of a separate dual chamber pacemaker and an ICD is best accomplished with a bipolar pacemaker in order to minimize the chances of over-sensing of pacing stimuli by the ICD, resulting in the delivery of inappropriate shocks. Unipolar pacemakers can inhibit detection of ventricular fibrillation, if the pacing stimuli decrease the automatic sensitivity of the ICD. Indeed some pacemaker physicians are so concerned about the use of unipolar pacing in patients with ICD's as to recommend the banning of unipolar leads in case a patient with a dual chamber pacemaker may later require an ICD (8). A number of sensor-driven pacing systems such as those that utilize impedance measurements (minute ventilation) require a bipolar lead. In others, such as the evoked QT interval sensor, unipolar pacing is preferred, but can be incorporated into a polarity programmable bipolar pacing system.

Reliability. The most quoted reason for choosing a unipolar pacing lead concerns the issue of long-term reliability. Theoretically, the more complex a lead design and the more components that are required for its manufacture, the greater the chances for its failure. Unipolar leads are easier to manufacture than bipolar leads, which have over twice as many components. Transvenous ICD leads are even more complex. Not surprisingly, unipolar leads have a superior track record of fewer mechanical failures than comparable bipolar leads, although this is not as significant today. Over the last decade, there has been a growing incidence of insulation failure, particularly in certain types of polyurethane insulated bipolar leads. Despite this, excellent long-term survival has recently been documented with other types of bipolar leads insulated with polyurethane and silicone rubber. This is discussed in detail later in this chapter. As new lead designs are developed, a clear objective must be to improve reliability, particularly with the more complex bipolar and ICD leads. Ideally, all leads should perform reliably over the lifetime of the patient. If reliability were comparable, bipolar leads appear to be preferable in almost all respects with no clear preferences for unipolar pacing.

The Pacing Electrode

Electrode Size

The earliest transvenous pacing leads had a large stimulating cathode, low pacing impedance; therefore the current drain from these electrodes was excessive (Fig. 1.1) (9). In addition, a large electrode surface area disperses the electron flow over a wide area, resulting in a low current density and a high stimulation threshold. By reducing the cathodal surface area, high current densities and lower stimulation threshold levels were achieved, together with improved longevity of the power source (10). By the late 1970s, most pacing leads had cathodes with surface areas in the range of 8–12 mm^2 and impedance measurements of 400–800 Ω. At that time, further reduction in cathode size was regarded as undesirable, because of the theoretical concerns of micro dislodgment caused by the small electrode surface area coming away from the endocardium. Nevertheless, leads with 4 mm^2 electrodes and later <2 mm^2 electrodes with >1,000 Ω impedance and extremely low stimulation thresholds have been introduced and found to be safe for long-term pacing and sensing (Fig. 1.12) (11).

There are limits to the reduction of the electrode surface area. Small surface area polished electrodes demonstrate significant polarization potentials, which decrease pacing efficiency. In theory, extremely small electrodes may be designed like arrowheads; therefore they may be more likely to penetrate or perforate the myocardial wall. This problem can be overcome by placing a protective soft polymer collar around the base of the electrode to prevent penetration (Fig. 1.12). Such a protective collar, however, may prevent the electrode from making contact with the endocardium. Despite these criticisms, there is no evidence after more than a decade of clinical experience, of any unique problems, associated with very small surface area electrodes.

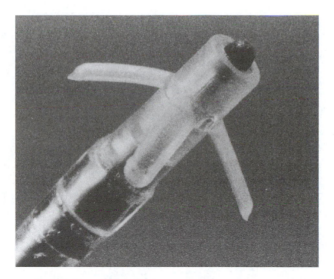

Fig. 1.12 A 1.2 mm^2 porous platinized platinum steroid-eluting electrode. Note the protective ring of silicone rubber immediately behind the electrode to prevent perforation.

Polarization and Electrode Porosity

As already stated, the ideal pacemaker lead should have high electrode-tissue impedance, low ohmic resistance of the conductor and low polarization. The earliest attempt to produce a low polarization electrode was the differential current density (DCD) design. This utilized a small insulating or di-electric, saline filled polymer container with holes drilled at the distal end allowing contact of an enveloped large surface area electrode with the endocardium (12). The current density was high, and having no direct electrode-tissue interface, there was virtually no polarization effect. Subsequently, the trade-off between low stimulation thresholds resulting from small surface area electrodes and the effects of polarization was addressed by designing electrodes with a complex surface structure, which are usually porous. With a porous electrode, the geometric electrode radius can be made small (which maximizes current density); however the electrode surface area is in reality large, because it includes the internal spaces within the electrode pores (which minimizes polarization effects).

The original porous electrode consisted of sintered platinum–iridium fibers, giving the appearance of a fine wire mesh (Fig. 1.13). Because the whole electrode was composed of these fibers, this was referred to as a "totally porous" electrode. The other form of porous electrode involved surface treatment of a solid electrode and was referred to as a "porous surface" electrode. The pores can be created in a number of ways, such as sintering a metal powder or micro-spheres onto a solid metal substrate. The result is an interconnecting network of pores uniformly distributed throughout the coating. Depending on the surface porosity, such electrodes may be macro-porous (constructed with small spheres), or micro-porous (using a fine metal powder). Platinum electroplating using platinum powder is a way of producing a micro-porous surface on an electrode (Fig. 1.12). The electrode appears black because the surface particles are smaller than the wavelength of visible light, which is therefore absorbed. A number of materials can be used to create these

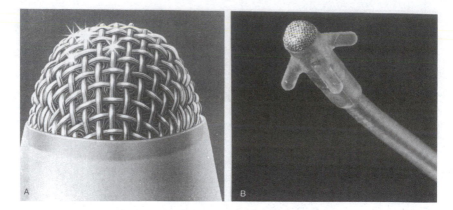

Fig. 1.13 Totally porous electrode. *Left*: Magnified cartoon of the electrode. *Right*: Actual photograph of the distal end of the lead demonstrating the electrode and tines. (Permission for use: Guidant.)

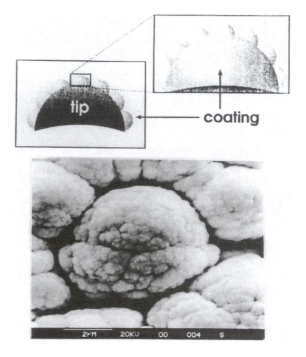

Fig. 1.14 Fractal coated electrode. *Above*: The electrode surface is covered with hemispheres, thus increasing its surface area. These hemispheres are again coated and the process repeated many times. The eventual surface area is thousands times larger than the original surface. *Below*: A scanning electron microscope picture of the fractal microporous surface. (Permission for use: Biotronik.)

micro-surface porous areas including platinum–iridium, titanium nitride, or thermal bonding of iridium oxide onto a titanium substrate. It is also possible to create a micro-porous surface on an endocardial or epi-myocardial screw electrode. Fractal coating is another form of porous electrode (13). The titanium electrode is totally covered with iridium hemispheres. On top of these hemispheres, smaller hemispheres are applied again and again; enlarging the active surface area many thousand fold (Fig. 1.14).

Electrode Composition

The composition of the electrode can be critical to its long-term function. Electrode corrosion or degradation may occur over time. Some metals, such as stainless steel and zinc are clearly unacceptable, as excessive corrosion releases metal ions into the electrode–tissue interface causing an excessive foreign body reaction and a thick peri-electrode fibrous capsule. Platinum is relatively nonreactive and alloying platinum with 10% iridium increases its mechanical strength without altering its electrical performance. For many years, polished platinum or platinum–iridium and later as porous designs, were used in the cathode position. Another cathode material widely used in the past was Elgiloy® an alloy of cobalt, iron, chromium, molybdenum, nickel, and manganese, which was originally developed for noncorrosive watch springs by the Elgin National Watch Company. In European designed leads, carbon was briefly used as a cathode material, because of both its low stimulation threshold and polarization properties (14). Normal carbon or graphite is mechanically weak, brittle, and has poor wear resistance. In contrast, vitreous carbon, a highly purified pyrolytic form of carbon, has excellent mechanical strength, biocompatibility, and complete inertness to body tissues. However, surface contamination resulted in unreliable long-term performance.

In recent years, titanium, titanium oxide, titanium alloys, iridium oxide coated titanium and especially titanium nitride in a variety of shapes and sizes, have become very popular for use as cathode materials, because of low stimulation thresholds and acceptable polarization losses (15–18).

Electrode–Tissue Interface

The rise in stimulation threshold that normally follows lead implantation results from inflammation at the electrode–tissue interface (Fig. 1.15) (19, 20).

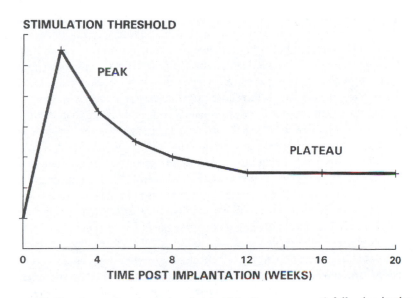

Fig. 1.15 The changes in stimulation threshold (voltage or current) following implantation of a standard nonsteroid-eluting electrode. The acute changes occur within a few days reaching a peak within the first month. The stimulation threshold then falls to a plateau level often considerably higher than the initial stimulation threshold value.

The magnitude of this rise in stimulation threshold is unpredictable and in some cases excessive. In these situations, it is necessary to use relatively high voltage outputs, at least for the first 3- month postimplantation. As the inflammatory process subsides and a fibrous capsule is formed, the stimulation threshold usually falls to a chronic plateau level, often considerably higher than at implantation. Inflammation is the critical factor that must be controlled to achieve a consistently low stimulation threshold postimplantation.

A number of basic bioengineering principles that influence the stimulation threshold are important in the design of pacing electrodes. As discussed, the cathode should be small enough to produce a high current density or electric field strength. However, the electric field strength decreases as a function of the square of the distance between the electrode surface and the tissue to be stimulated. Consequently, the electrode radius should optimally be equal to or less than the thickness of the fibrous capsule that inevitably envelops it. The stimulation thresholds will actually increase if the electrode is smaller than the fibrous capsule. The lead must also provide adequate fixation for the electrode to assure good clinical performance. The development of fixation mechanisms such as tines has greatly reduced the risk of electrode dislodgment. In addition, tissue ingrowth into porous and grooved electrodes may also enhance mechanical stability and ensure intimate electrode contact with the endocardium at the electrode–tissue interface.

The mechanical design of the lead is also important for the control of inflammation. The electrode should be stable and lie gently against the endocardium, causing as little physical irritation as possible. A lead design that allows excessive pressure to be imparted to the distal electrode can traumatize the endomyocardium and provoke an accelerated inflammatory response. In some cases, lead stiffness can result in local myocardial ischemia and ventricular perforation particularly if the design of the distal end acts like an arrowhead. Physical methods aimed at preventing irritation at the electrode–tissue interface should also be considered. For instance an interposing inert biocompatible conductor material such as a hydrogel can be placed between the electrode and endocardium to both reduce mechanical irritation and to present to the endocardium a contaminant-free electrode. It has long been known particularly with vitreous carbon electrodes that a perfectly clean electrode will give a lower stimulation threshold than one contaminated with dust, fiber material, glove powder or other contaminants collected during manufacture or implantation. A variation of the clean electrode concept is the ion-exchange membrane, which allows free flow of current, but the membrane protects the endocardium from the irritating effects of the electrode and contaminants (21). Such membranes can be impregnated with anti-inflammatory drugs such as glucocorticosteroids. Another way of coating the electrode is to use blood soluble materials such as mannitol or polyethylene glycol. Once in the circulation the material dissolves leaving a contaminant free electrode.

The use of local pharmacological agents is a highly effective way to counter the inflammatory reaction at the electrode–tissue interface. Agents investigated include anti-inflammatory drugs, anticoagulants, and drugs that prevent the formation of an extracellular matrix. Apart from glucocorticosteroids, no consistent improvement in stimulation threshold has been found and in some cases significant deterioration in stimulation threshold has occurred. For example, heparin inhibits fibrin formation and prevents the development

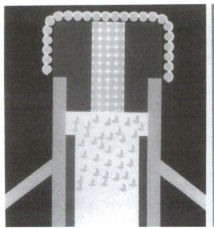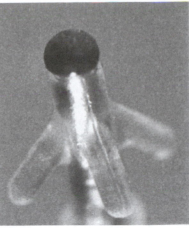

Fig. 1.16 Steroid-eluting electrode. *Left*: Cross sectional diagram demonstrating the silicone rubber plug impregnated with dexamethasone sodium phosphate lying immediately behind the porous electrode and connected to it by a channel. *Right*: Tined lead with a platinized platinum porous, steroid-eluting electrode. (Permission for use: Medtronic.)

of a protective fibrous barrier during acute inflammation, thus allowing more physical damage to occur. Other agents that prevent extracellular matrix formation without altering the inflammatory response, namely tunicamycin and *cis*-hydroxy-proline, cause an elevation in stimulation threshold, indicating that prevention of inflammation is the most important consideration in reducing the chronic stimulation threshold (22, 23). It is not surprising, therefore, that glucocorticosteroid-eluting electrodes, because of their potent anti-inflammatory action, result in a significant reduction in peak and chronic stimulation threshold levels postimplantation (19).

For implantable pacing leads, dexamethasone as the sodium phosphate salt has been found to be much more effective than prednisolone. This is because prednisolone has a high affinity for protein rendering the protein-bound drug pharmacologically inactive. The early edema at the electrode–tissue interface is protein-rich and therefore prednisolone released by a drug-eluting device may be immediately deactivated. Dexamethasone sodium phosphate does not have a high affinity for protein, and is thus suitable for steroid-eluting electrodes. There are a number of ways of presenting steroid to the electrode–tissue interface. The original design, still frequently used for tined leads, is an internal chamber containing a plug of silicone rubber compounded with ≤1 mg dexamethasone sodium phosphate immediately behind a porous electrode. This plug is referred to as a steroid-silicone rubber "monolithic controlled release device" (MCRD). The internal chamber communicates with the outer surface of the electrode and the adjacent electrode–tissue interface through a porous channel (Fig. 1.16) (19). Most of the early clinical studies on steroid-eluting leads utilized this design.

Steroid-eluting electrodes have demonstrated very low acute and chronic stimulation thresholds in both the atrium and ventricle with virtual elimination of the early postoperative peak (19,24–27). In particular, excellent results have been obtained in children, (28) a group known to have a high incidence of elevated stimulation thresholds and in patients with a previous history of high threshold exit block (29). The precise role of the dexamethasone sodium phosphate in this first generation electrode was initially uncertain. It was considered that the unique design and materials of the electrode were responsible for the favorable results. It has been demonstrated conclusively that it is the steroid that prevents the stimulation threshold rise (19). This improvement in stimulation threshold has been shown by the author to persist for more than 20-years clinical follow-up. Steroid-eluting electrodes also demonstrate excellent implantation and long-term P- and R-wave amplitudes and telemetered electrograms.

Today all major pacing companies have incorporated steroid-elution into all tined leads and significant chronic stimulation threshold rises have not been reported, provided mechanical causes such as myocardial penetration, perforation, or lead dislodgment have been excluded. Patients implanted with a steroid-eluting electrode that is coupled with a good passive-fixation lead design and implantation technique can be safely paced from the day of implantation at 2.5 V or less (30). The ability to safely use these low voltages has important ramifications for pulse generator longevity and size, especially with dual chamber and rate responsive systems. With the technical and clinical information that is currently available regarding stimulation threshold and polarization, a number of new leads have been designed with more advanced electrodes. High impedance, steroid-eluting, platinized micro porous-platinum electrodes with surface areas as low as $1.2\,mm^2$ has demonstrated lower stimulation thresholds than the original platinum-coated titanium design (Fig. 1.12) (11, 26). The use of J-shaped tined steroid-eluting leads in the atrial appendage have also shown excellent long-term low stimulation thresholds (27, 31, 32).

Steroid-eluting epicardial leads are also available. Unlike other permanent pacing leads implanted via a transthoracic approach, the electrode is not a helical screw. Therefore, this lead is not myocardial. The electrode is a platinized porous-platinum button shaped configuration, which can be duplicated into a bipolar configuration (Fig. 1.17). As with the original transvenous steroid-eluting electrode, there is a silicone rubber plug impregnated with dexamethasone sodium phosphate behind the electrode (33, 34). The long-term performance is dependent on other characteristics of epicardial leads such as the conductor and the insulator.

A silicone rubber plug within the electrode is not the only method by which steroid can be delivered to the electrode–tissue interface. Another electrode design uses a porous silicone rubber collar impregnated with dexamethasone sodium phosphate or acetate (35, 36). The drug-eluting collar is positioned immediately behind the tip electrode (Fig. 1.18). An obvious advantage would be steroid-eluting active-fixation screw-in leads, which are now widely and very successfully used in both the atrium and ventricle (37). Of interest is that such leads immediately after implantation have higher stimulation thresholds compared to passive-fixation leads. There is, however, a rapid fall in threshold over the first 4- min postimplantation and the next day, the stimulation thresholds are comparable to steroid-eluting tined leads (38). As stated earlier, steroid can be impregnated into an ion-exchange membrane (21).

Although dexamethasone sodium phosphate has been the most widely used glucocorticosteroid in steroid-eluting pacing electrodes, more recently dexamethasone acetate, originally proposed in 1991 (39), has also been

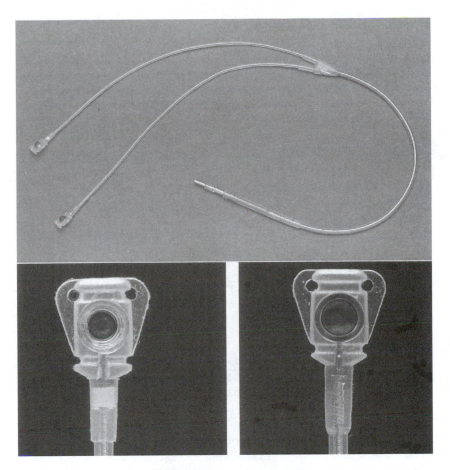

Fig. 1.17 Bipolar, porous platinized platinum, steroid-eluting epicardial electrodes. *Above*: Bipolar configuration demonstrating two separate electrodes. *Below*: Magnified view of the two electrodes. The larger anode is on the right. Above and to the sides of the button electrodes are two sewing holes for attachment of the electrodes to the epicardium. (Permission for use: Medtronic.)

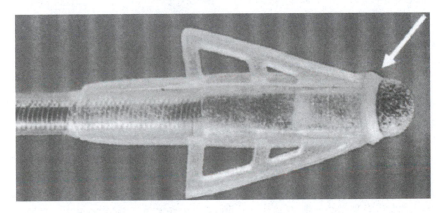

Fig. 1.18 Passive fixation lead demonstrating fins and steroid-eluting collar immediately behind the electrode (white arrow). (Permission for use: St Jude.)

incorporated into both passive- and active-fixation leads. The main differences in the pharmacological properties of the two compounds are due to differences in their water solubility. The acetate salt, being less water soluble should theoretically diffuse slower into the electrode–tissue interface, but there is no evidence that either is superior, particularly with tined leads (40).

Beclomethasone has also been suggested as a glucocorticosteroid for pacemaker electrode use. Being much more potent than the dexamethasone salts, smaller doses could be used. To date, beclomethasone has been applied directly to the screw electrode of very thin leads, where traditional steroid-eluting devices are not practical.

Lead Fixation

Transvenous leads may be attached to the endocardium either actively or passively. Active-fixation leads incorporate devices that invade the endomyo-cardium, whereas passive-fixation leads promote fixation by indirect means. When correctly implanted, both fixation mechanisms result in an extremely low incidence of lead dislodgment.

Passive-Fixation

The first attempt to attach a fixation device to a lead was with the use of a wedge or flange at the tip. Although this probably reduced the incidence of lead dislodgment, this was never proven. Other early passive-fixation electrodes included a helifix electrode (41) and a balloon-tip lead (42), both of which were not commercially successful because of difficulties with implantation and high incidence of operative and postoperative complications. During the late 1970s, small tines positioned immediately behind the electrode were shown to have a very low incidence of lead dislodgment and today these remain the most popular passive-fixation design (Figs. 1.12, 1.13, 1.16) (43). Variations of this concept include wings, cones, and fins (Fig. 1.18). Passive-fixation epicardial leads are also available (Fig. 1.17).

Active-Fixation

Transvenous, active-fixation leads are composed of a screw at the distal end of the lead, which may or may not be electrically active. They can be classified as fixed exposed screws, protected screws, and retractable-extendable screws. The original designs had a fixed, unprotected screw, which could damage venous and intracardiac structures during lead insertion. To overcome this, the lead can be inserted using a steerable catheter (Fig. 1.19) or a protective bullet shaped covering such as mannitol can be used. Following insertion into the venous channels and heart, the mannitol dissolves allowing the bare screw to be secured in the appropriate chamber. Such leads have also been designed with steroid-elution.

The major design available today is the retractable-extendable screw-in lead, which has become popular for both atrial and ventricular use. These designs use a variety of mechanisms to extend and retract the screw (31, 32) This includes an implement to turn the connector pin, which in turn, is mechanically and electrically connected to the electrically active screw via the conductor. A screw driver stylet has also been used to extend and retract the screw. Unlike tined leads, all active-fixation leads traumatize the

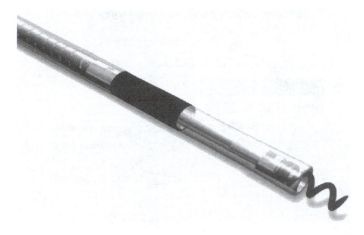

Fig. 1.19 Thin (4.1Fr) bipolar active-fixation lead with a fixed screw and no lumen for a stylet. (Medtronic 3830 SelectSecure™). The screw is coated with beclomethasone. The lead is delivered by a steerable catheter. (Permission for use: Medtronic.)

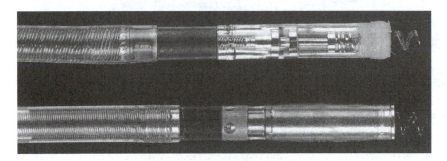

Fig. 1.20 Retractable-extendable active-fixation leads. *Above*: Medtronic 5076 Capsure™ Fix Novus. Note the steroid-eluting collar immediately behind the extended cathode screw. *Below*: St Jude 1488T Tendril™. Both the lead tip and the extended screw are electrically active (cathode). The steroid-eluting plug is housed at the tip of the lead through which the screw passes. (Permission for use: Medtronic and St Jude.)

endomyocardium. This may result in significant elevations of stimulation thresholds postimplantation (31, 32) A steroid-eluting collar surrounding the base of the screw or a monolithic controlled release device through which the screw extends, have demonstrated significantly improved stimulation thresholds in active-fixation leads (Fig. 1.20) (37).

Epi-myocardial leads are all active-fixation. Although, most have a helical screw (Fig. 1.21), stab-on fishhook designs have been available for pediatric use for a long time. All designs have a high incidence of complications and in particular high threshold exit block.

Lead Conductor

The pacing lead conductor is composed of wire that conducts the electrical current from the pulse generator to the stimulating electrode and the sensed cardiac signals (intrinsic or evoked) from the electrode(s) to the sensing amplifier of the pulse generator. Unipolar leads require one conductor, whilst bipolar

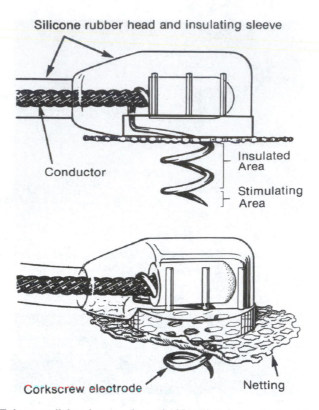

Fig. 1.21 Epimyocardial corkscrew electrode. Note that the conductor is braided.

leads require two. An early and reliable conductor used in the 1960s was composed of four tinsel ribbons of stainless steel wrapped around a central Terylene core (Fig. 1.1). Transvenous implantation of this floppy lead was very difficult, as there was no method for stiffening the lead to guide the tip to the apex of the right ventricle. Consequently a major advance in pacemaker implantation was the introduction of helically coiled conductors (Fig. 1.22). These were composed of a single strand of a tightly coiled wire wound with an empty core, which allowed the passage of a stainless steel stylet to the tip electrode. In this way the lead could be stiffened and shaped during implantation. Helically coiled conductors, however, are prone to fracture at stress points such as sites where anchoring ligatures are applied, where the conductor enters a lead connector or where the lead is encased in an endocardial bridge within the heart (Fig. 1.23). In these situations, the point of fracture is a fulcrum with one side of the conductor moving separate to the other. Thus, one side of the conducting wire is in tension while the other in compression. In order to make the conductor more flexible and to create redundancy, two or more wires were constructed in a multifilar coil arrangement (Fig. 1.22).

The original conductor materials were stainless steel or platinum. These materials were later replaced with more corrosion-resistant alloys with improved fatigue resistance such as MP35N® (SPS Technologies Cleveland OH), an alloy of nickel, chromium, cobalt, and molybdenum. In order to further reduce the resistance to current flow, specialized conductors were designed, including DBS (drawn brazed strand) and DFT (drawn filled tube)

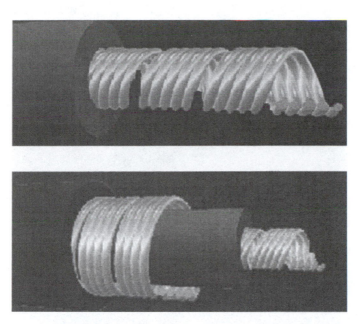

Fig. 1.22 Multifilar helically coil conductors. *Above*: Unipolar. In this example, there are five single uninsulated strands of tightly coiled wire around a central core though which the stylet passes. The coils are covered with insulating tubing. *Middle*: Bipolar coaxial design, which is currently the most common conductor arrangement. There are two multifilar helical coils surrounded by two insulating tubes. The inner is the cathode and the outer surrounding conductor is the anode. This round design is of intermediate size and thicker than a standard unipolar lead. (Permission for use: Medtronic.)

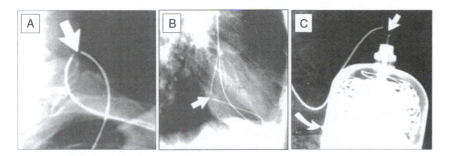

Fig. 1.23 Three examples of fractured unipolar leads occurring at points of stress. A: In the neck where the lead enters the external jugular vein. There is a sharp bend in the lead at the venous entry site and both limbs of the lead move differently with neck movement. B: Within the right atrium. The lead is encased in a short endocardial tunnel, where it makes contact with the wall as it turns to enter the right ventricle. Again both limbs move differently with cardiac contractions. C: At the lead connector site. There is a sharp bend in the lead after it emerges from the connector.

designs. These wires were composed of a central core of highly conductive material such as silver surrounded by a more durable corrosion resistant material such as MP35N®. The resistance of such conductors may be only several ohms and less than 10% of MP35N® alone. Modern conductors undergo intense fatigue and fracture testing by continual bending of the lead to a specific angle or over a specified radius. In recent years, conductor fractures

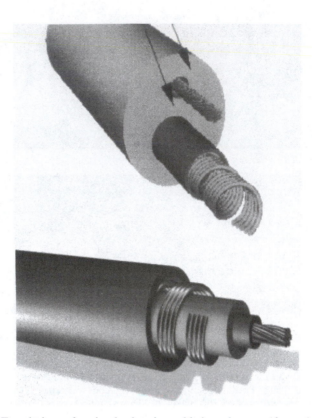

Fig. 1.24 Two designs of pacing leads using cabled conductors. *Above*: A traditional multifilar coiled conductor for stylet delivery lies parallel to a cabled conductor. The lead is slightly oval (Medtronic 5044. Never marketed). *Below*: Coaxial design (Medtronic 3830 SelectSecure™). The cathode cable lies at the center of the lead and is then covered with a protective cover (ETFE) and over that a conventional silicone insulator. It is then surrounded with a polyurethane insulated multifilar coiled anode conductor. There is no lumen for a stylet. (Permission for use: Medtronic.)

have become less common and now represent only a small proportion of chronic pacing lead complications.

Bipolar transvenous leads obviously require two conductors. The original configuration used a parallel arrangement in bi-lumen insulation tubing with a single insulator surrounding both conductors. A major improvement was the coaxial design (Fig. 1.22). This allows the creation of a much smaller circumference lead body with a single inner lumen for stylet control and an even distribution of insulating material around the outer conductor. The inner coil connects to the cathodal tip and is separated from the outer coil by an inner insulating tube. Such leads are only slightly thicker than unipolar designs. More recently a very thin multifilar cable conductor using a nickel alloy to which tantalum can be added has been successfully used with both pacing and ICD leads. The leads are much stronger than conventional leads using helically coiled conductors and in particular; do not require a stylet for forceful lead extraction. The cable can be used in conjunction with a stylet driven helically coiled cathode conductor to allow conventional lead implantation (Fig. 1.24). A cable can also replace the cathode helically coiled conductor of a coaxial lead resulting in a very thin lead without an inner lumen for stylet placement (44). Such a lead (Figs. 1.19 and 1.24) must be inserted using a steerable catheter. Cables are currently widely utilized in ICD lead design and this will be extended to pacemaker leads in the future.

The development of *coated wire technology* has allowed the manufacture of thin bipolar leads whose outside diameter is as small as unipolar leads (46). The technique involves the coating of single strands of conductor wire with a very thin layer of ETFE polymer insulation. Two or more conductors can be grouped together into a multifilar, single coil, which is then placed within another insulative tube to form a lead body with virtually the same flexibility and handling characteristics as a unipolar lead. For example, with a quadrafilar coil, two of the insulated wires can be connected to the cathodal electrode, and the other two, to the anodal electrode of a bipolar lead.

Epimyocardial leads do not require a stylet for implantation and thus there is more flexibility in conductor design conductors. Most epimyocardial leads use a braided wire conductor (Fig. 1.21). Despite this, fractures remain a significant problem because of the stresses imposed by the movement of the heart, diaphragm, and abdominal muscles.

Lead Insulation

The lead insulation extends from the lead connector to the cathode tip and in a bipolar lead is interrupted by the anode ring. The lead collar, used to secure the lead at the venous entry site, is usually manufactured with the same lead insulation material. One of the earliest insulating materials for permanent pacemaker leads was polyethylene (Fig. 1.1). This material had excellent biocompatibility and reasonable biostability. However, as an insulator for pacing leads, polyethylene was stiff, thick, and difficult to bond. It also abraded with nonpolished metals and was found to have poor long-term performance. During the 1960s, silicone rubber (MDX4-4515-50A) became very popular as an insulating material for pacing leads. Although highly biocompatible and biostable, the material has relatively low tear strength and could be easily damaged during surgery using sharp instruments or tight ligatures, thus necessitating a thick layer of insulation. Another disadvantage of silicone rubber is its high coefficient of friction, making it difficult to pass one lead parallel to another during implantation of two leads for dual chamber pacing. This potential disadvantage of silicone rubber has been overcome by the technique of surface polishing or coating the lead with a highly lubricous material called *fast pass coating*.

Polyurethane, a generic name for a very large family of synthetic polymers was first used as an insulator for transvenous pacing leads in 1978. As a group, the polyurethanes exhibit very high tensile and tear strengths, flexibility, and a low coefficient of friction when wetted with blood, making them easier to insert and pass along venous channels compared with silicone rubber insulated leads. Other advantages include biocompatibility, noncarcinogenicity and low thrombogenicity, much like silicone rubber. Unfortunately, many of the polyurethanes rapidly degrade in the body as a result of enzymatic activity. Others cannot be extruded and injection moulded into insulation tubing suitable for pacing leads. One group, Pellethane 2363® (Upjohn Co., CPR Division, Torrance CA.) was found to be biostable and suitable for pacing lead insulation.

The properties of polyurethanes vary according to the *soft* and *hard* segments of the polymer molecular chain. The soft segments are composed of polyether or polyesther chains and the hard segments, urea or urethanes. Structurally, segmented polyurethanes are composed of a core of hard segments surrounded with soft skin comprised of soft segments. The hard and soft segments are thermodynamically immiscible, thus tending to separate. It is this structural feature that determines the mechanical and surface properties of polyurethane. Because it was possible to manufacture very thin polyurethane insulating tubing suitable for pacing leads, polyurethane leads rapidly became very popular. By 1981, however, a number of disturbing reports appeared, questioning the long-term integrity and reliability of this insulating material. These reports described in vivo degradation of implanted polyurethane with surface cracking and subsequent insulation failure (46–48).

Continuing research revealed that some polyurethane insulation failures were at least in part related to specific manufacturing processes in certain leads using the polyurethane insulating material, Pellethane® 80A. The tendency of the hard and soft segments to separate creates inherent stresses in segmented polyurethanes. These, in turn can be intensified during manufacture and in particular during the cooling process following extrusion. This occurs when the molten polymer is forced through a die or into a mould after which it is rapidly cooled. Polyurethane tubing manufactured by the extrusion technique, causes the surface molecules to cool quickly and thus contract, resulting in considerable surface tension. At the same time, the core molecules remain hot and therefore in compression. The result is the creation of a zero stress boundary or neutral axis between the surface and the core, the depth of which will depend on the manufacturing process. This final result of this process is surface cracking or crazing of the polyurethane. The cracking and crazing can be further exacerbated by continuing lead manufacturing such as expansion and shrinking of the insulator during the conductor coil insertion, stretching and bonding as well as surface trauma during and following implantation. In the biologically corrosive environment of the human body, lipid and protein may deposit onto the damaged polyurethane causing swelling, which disrupts the surface organization. This continuing insulation degradation, referred to as *environmental stress cracking* (*ESC*), may lead to insulation failure, when the cracking propagates through the full thickness of the insulator to the conductor.

The most minor and very common change due to ESC is referred to as *surface frosting* and is a whitish haze. This does not result in functional clinical insulation failure. The crack depth is typically 2.5–30 microns and is worst in areas subjected to applied strains either during manufacture or implantation. With time, in the presence of environmental stresses, this may progress to insulation failure. A more significant ESC change occurs in areas where excessive strains are applied during manufacture or at implantation, such as close to the lead connector or where ligatures are placed around the lead. It may also occur where the lead insulation sits between the clavicle and first rib when the lead is introduced by subclavian puncture. Although the subclavian venous access route is frequently blamed for the failure of polyurethane leads, nevertheless, there is still a high failure rate when the cephalic vein is used and care taken with ligatures around the suture collar. Severe frosting may also be seen in intracardiac portions of the lead extracted for other reasons.

Such patches may occur where the lead turns to enter the right ventricle from the right atrium. In these areas, endocardial tunnels may form around the lead, where contact is made with the inner wall of the heart, resulting in excessive stresses on the insulation. It is likely, therefore, those intracardiac sites may also be responsible for insulation failures.

Metal induced oxidation (MIO) is another reported mechanism of insulation failure (49). MIO is a process of oxidative degradation of the polyurethane insulation and involves a reaction of the polymer with oxygen probably released by hydrogen peroxide that comes from inflammatory cells on the outer surface of the lead. For the reaction to occur a catalyst is required. Such catalysts may be metallic corrosion products from the conductor, which accumulate following ingress of body fluids from minor or major insulation breakdown. In order to minimize MIO, conductors can be barrier coated. The objective is to cover the conductor coil with a submicroscopic layer of an inert material such as platinum. As a result of the information gathered on the causes and mechanisms of ESC and MIO, manufacturing changes were instituted to overcome the problems found with the polyurethane Pellethane® 80A. Despite this, questionable long-term implant performance continued to plague subsequent generations of bipolar leads, which used the same Pellethane® 80A polyurethane. Unipolar leads have not shown an increased incidence of insulation problems, apart from those caused by trauma at surgery or at ligature sites.

Almost all currently available polyurethane insulated pacing and ICD leads utilize Pellethane® 55D. This polyurethane is stiffer and harder than Pellethane® 80A due to significantly less polyether segments. New varieties of polyurethane are continually being investigated and combinations of silicone rubber and polyurethane may be clinically acceptable. The major body of the lead may be composed of polyurethane, but at the distal end, where the lead lies inside the ventricle, the insulation may be a softer silicone rubber. The silicone rubber, polyurethane combinations may also be composed of a thin but tough, protective outer coating of polyurethane over a layer of silicone rubber in a coaxial arrangement. Despite improvements in polyurethane, many pacemaker implanters refuse to use leads with this material, because of both the past history of Pellethane® 80A and the stiffness of Pellethane® 55D.

During the late 1970s, a stronger and tougher extra tear resistance silicone rubber (ETR) was introduced that allowed the manufacture of thinner silicone rubber leads. Leads with this material demonstrated elongation or stretching at the time of implantation if the lead was pulled back after entrapment in the trabeculae or chordae. Because of the stretching, the stiffening stylet was unable to reach the tip of the lead if further manipulation was required. A further development during the 1980s was the introduction of high performance silicone rubber insulation (HP). This material had improved tear strength, but still demonstrated a problem found with previous forms of silicone rubber called creep. This results from the movement of molecules over areas of stress such as ligature sites resulting in insulation thinning at the stress points.

Recently a new hybrid form of silicone rubber has been introduced which encompasses the best features of all the previous silicone rubbers allowing very thin leads to be manufactured. This material referred to as Med 4719 (NuSil Technology, Carpinteria, CA, USA) has been introduced either as a pure silicone rubber lead or with a polyurethane outer layer (50). Work continues on the development of new polymers for pacemaker and ICD leads.

One such polymer, Elast-Eon® (AorTech International, Melbourne, Australia) has recently been used as an insulator for ICD leads (Riata® ST Optim, St Jude, Sylmar, CA). This product is part of a large family of polyurethane-silicone rubber hybrids which can be prepared for the specific needs of the pacemaker/ICD industry. An insulator with the strength of Pellethane® 55D can be created with the characteristics of silicone rubber by replacing the polyether soft segment of polyurethane with silicone rubber.

Two other commonly used fluoropolymers can be used as insulating materials within pacing and ICD leads. PTFE (polytetrafluoroethylene) or Teflon® (DuPont) and ETFE (ethylenetetrafluoroethylene) are both strong, nonbiodegradable insulators, which have the disadvantage of being stiff and not easily bondable with other materials such as silicone rubber. PTFE is generally prepared as tubing along which a conducting coil is strung, whereas ETFE is used as a coating with a thickness less than 0.003 in. which for example can be extruded over a cable conductor both as an insulator and to protect the other components of the lead from the abrasive properties of cables. ePTFE (expanded polytetrafluoroethylene) or Gore-Tex® (W. L. Gore and Associates, Newark DE) is a very familiar product in everyday use, which unlike PTFE cannot be used as an insulator. However, being an electrical conductor, ePTFE can be used to cover the shock coils of ICD leads to prevent the inflammatory and fibrotic changes that occur following implantation (Guidant Reliance® Boston Scientific, Boston MA). Such leads can be easily extracted if necessary.

Lead Connector

The lead connector connects the lead to the pulse generator. The original pacing leads had no specialized connector. A small area of conductor at the proximal end was exposed and attached directly to the pulse generator using a small setscrew (Fig. 1.2). Eventually two similar and very reliable unipolar connector designs emerged; one a 5-mm diameter "Medtronic" style and the other a 6-mm "Cordis" style. These connectors were simply a bulbous end to the body of the lead with a terminal area of bare metal, the lead pin, for electrical contact within the pulse generator (Fig. 1.25). For bipolar pacing, two of these unipolar connectors were necessary. A major improvement in lead connectors was the low-profile in-line bipolar design where both electrical terminals lay on a single lead pin with an insulating barrier separating the anode from the cathode. Companies had different designs resulting in connector/pulse generator compatibility problems, particularly during pulse generator replacement. In some cases, large and unreliable adaptors were used, but on other occasions a new lead was required. A plea for standardization was made.

By late 1985, a low-profile 3.2-mm unipolar (Fig. 1.25) and bipolar pacemaker lead connector designated "Voluntary Standard #1 or "VS•1 became available. Pacemaker inter-company rivalry, however, resulted in three variations of lead connector and pulse generator connector block variations; the VS•1, VS•1A and VS•1B (Fig. 1.26). Although similar, these variations were not totally interchangeable. The differences were mainly related to bipolar leads and concerned the length of the lead connector pin and the presence or absence of sealing rings. A VS•1 standard specifies sealing rings on the lead,

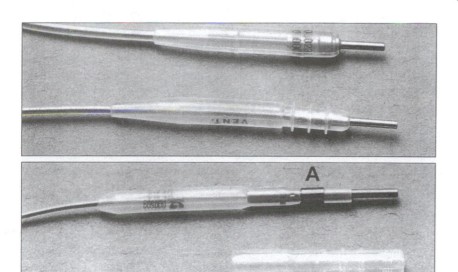

Fig. 1.25 High profile (5-mm) unipolar connectors. *Above*: Two 5-mm connectors with original design above and later version with rings below. *Below*: Unipolar low profile (3.2-mm) lead with anodized (A) ring being converted to high profile unipolar using an adaptor. The same adaptor can be used to convert a low profile bipolar connector to a 5-mm unipolar one. (Permission for use: Medtronic and St Jude.)

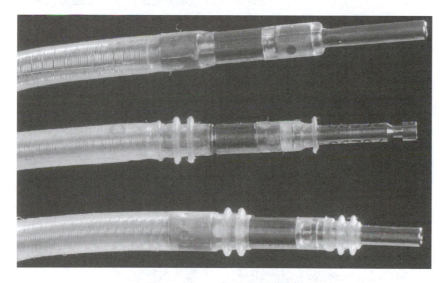

Fig. 1.26 VS•1 style connectors. *Above*: VS•1B. The lead connector has no sealing rings and a long lead pin. Suitable for a 3.2-mm style (long pin receiving port and sealing rings) pulse generator connector block. *Middle*: VS•1A. The lead connector has sealing rings and a long pin. Suitable for a 3.2-mm style pulse generator connector block. *Below*: VS•1. The lead connector has sealing rings and a short lead pin. Suitable for both 3.2-mm or IS•1 style pulse generator header blocks. (Permission for use: Medtronic and St Jude.)

whereas, VS•1A is similar but the lead pin is longer as is the receiving port in the pulse generator connector block. The receiving port of the VS•1B pulse generator has both sealing rings and a long receiving port. Although a long connector pin (VS•1A or VS•1B) will fit into the short receiving port of the VS•1 pulse generator, the proximal anodal ring contact of the connector may not mate correctly with the anodal terminal of the pulse generator. As a consequence, bipolar pacing and sensing may not be possible. To many pacemaker implanters, these subtle differences are not obvious until confronted with lead and pulse generator incompatibility either at surgery or postoperatively during pacemaker testing. Such errors are expensive and potentially hazardous to the patient. Sealing rings are an integral part of the insulating mechanism of low-profile in-line connectors. They do not need to be on the lead connector itself, since they can also reside within the receiving port of the pulse generator. Engineering principles usually demand that any sealing rings, which could be damaged, should reside on the component to be replaced, in most cases the pulse generator. However, a pulse generator connector block with sealing rings is significantly larger than one without them.

With these controversies in mind, a formal international connector standard was created, which called for a low-profile connector with sealing rings on the lead. This final standard, designated "IS-1 UNI" for unipolar leads and "IS-1 BI" for bipolar leads is now the official international lead connector standard. To help with the problem of VS•1, IS-1 incompatibility, it is imperative that prior to pulse generator replacement, the implanter check the compatibility of the implanted lead and the proposed pulse generator. In addition, the IS-1 standard calls for unipolar and bipolar lead connectors to be interchangeable. To prevent damage to a unipolar IS-1 lead connector from the anode setscrew of a bipolar connector, a protective ring may be present over the unipolar lead connector at the appropriate position (Fig. 1.25). This ring, however, may be mistaken for a true anode terminal and the lead regarded as bipolar. Although the manufacturer's intentions are good, the results at surgery may be potentially disastrous unless the pulse generator can automatically revert to unipolar pacing on contact with body tissues. In terms of backward compatibility of the IS-1 leads to older pulse generators, unipolar and bipolar low-profile connectors can be easily converted to the standard 5-mm unipolar design by the use of a sleeve (Fig. 1.25).

Future lead designs demand even lower profile connectors with more than two poles. This is to satisfy the need for new physiological sensors to be added to pacing leads as well as to create multipole left ventricular leads to allow different combinations of pacing to overcome high stimulation thresholds and phrenic nerve stimulation. Such a low voltage standard using four poles is currently being prepared and has been designated IS-4. A similar standard for ICD leads has been designated DF-4.

Specific Purpose Pacing Leads

Right Atrial Leads

The physiologic advantages of pacing the atrium were appreciated soon after the establishment of cardiac pacing. Although, atrial leads were available in the 1970s, the problems of where to pace in the atria, specific programmable atrial pacing algorithms and the slow development of appropriate low stimulation threshold leads, limited this approach. For the same reasons, atrial epicardial or epimyocardial leads, either specifically designed or modified from ventricular designs never became established. The development of a transvenous passive fixation atrial lead presented specific challenges. Unlike the ventricle, the atrium is predominantly smooth walled, apart from ridges, such as the *crista terminalis* or fine shallow muscle bands which traverse the anterior wall from the crista terminalis, referred to as the *pectinate muscles*. The right atrial appendage is a heavily trabeculated extension of the pectinate muscles and is suitable for endocardial lead placement. In order to enter this cul-de-sac, tined atrial endocardial leads are J-shaped to allow cathode positioning well within the atrial appendage close to its apex. The fixed J is usually achieved by a permanent bend in the conductor or occasionally by creating a thickened bend in the insulator. It was not surprising, therefore, that tines similar to those used with ventricular leads became popular for atrial J leads (Figs. 1.12, 1.13, 1.16). Interestingly, positions outside the atrial appendage but close to it, such as on the anterior wall also show good fixation and low dislodgement for tined leads. This is particularly so if the patient has had open-heart surgery, where the right atrial appendage may have been cannulated or excised.

The next evolutionary step in atrial lead development was the endocardial active-fixation, screw-in lead. Such leads, even without steroid-elution became popular for right atrial use, with the anticipated high stimulation thresholds and exit block accepted as an inevitable consequence of endocardial trauma (31). It was believed that the incidence of lead dislodgement was lower than with the use of tined passive-fixation leads. As experience was obtained with both systems, the actual incidence of lead dislodgement was found to be very low, with high volume implanters reporting an incidence of 1–4% with no clear preference for either design (31).

With the clinical success of dual chamber pacing systems during the 1980s, the search for low atrial stimulation threshold leads intensified. Once the value of steroid-elution was confirmed, the technology was incorporated into atrial tined J leads which provided very low stimulation thresholds and excellent sensing, comparable to results in the ventricle (27, 31, 32). Steroid-elution technology has also been successfully extended to active-fixation leads placed in the atrium (Figs. 1.18, 1.20) (37) In general, the straight leads are preferred and are inserted using a J shaped stylet. Shorter lead lengths than those used in the ventricle are preferred (52–53 cm). Because of active-fixation, they can be placed anywhere in the atrium using a curved stylet. However, an area close to or within the right atrial appendage is desirable to prevent far-field sensing. More recently, other areas in the right atrium such as Bachmann's bundle and high and low atrial septum have been suggested to prevent delay in left atrial depolarization. Specialized techniques such as a steerable catheter will be necessary to position leads in these areas.

Not all active-fixation leads have an extendable-retractable screw. Some models have a fixed screw coated in mannitol which dissolves in blood prior to fixation (Guidant, Sweet Tip®). As discussed previously, a thin diameter cabled lead inserted through a steerable catheter has a fixed screw which is essentially covered by the catheter until it is attached to the endocardium (Medtronic SelectSecure® Medtronic Inc., Minneapolis MN) (Fig. 1.19). Active-fixation leads can also be attached to the endocardium using a steerable stylet (St Jude

Medical, Locator®) (Fig. 1.27). Such a stylet has been found to be useful in patients with enlarged atria, difficult anatomy, congenital abnormalities or the need for positioning in unusual locations.

Single Pass Leads

With the popularity of dual chamber pacing, it was not surprising that a dual chamber pacing system using a single lead would be developed to overcome the need for two separate leads. By definition, a single pass lead incorporates both the atrial and ventricular leads within a single lead body (Fig. 1.28). The main limiting factor of a single pass lead is the necessity for the atrial electrode

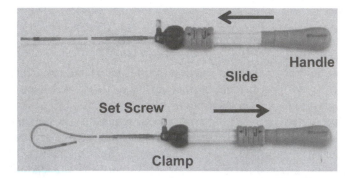

Fig. 1.27 A steer able stylet (Locator®, St Jude), operated with one hand, for positioning an active fixation lead in the heart. The stylet can be used to continually and temporarily alter the curvature of the distal part of the lead without the necessity to remove or replace the stylet. *Above*: The lead pin is attached to the guiding stylet by a setscrew attached to the bulbous clamp of the stylet handle. For a straight stylet, the arrow indicates the position of the slide next to this clamp. *Below*: Moving the slide along the handle away from the lead gradually curves the stylet and hence the lead. The amount of movement each way determines the curvature of lead. Turning the whole handle also turns the distal curved lead within the heart. The clamp can be released from the handle and rotating the detached clamp turns the lead pin, which extends or retracts the screw mechanism. (Permission for use: St Jude.)

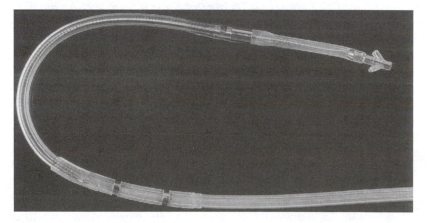

Fig. 1.28 Bipolar single pass lead for atrial sensing and ventricular pacing. (Permission for use: Medtronic.)

to make contact with the atrial wall to allow atrial pacing. Because of this, single pass leads are only suitable for atrial synchronous, ventricular pacing (VDD). Despite the long and extensive evolution of the modern bipolar single pass lead, its use today is limited to small numbers in relatively few centers. Because of their inability to achieve low threshold atrial pacing, such leads are only implanted in patients with high degree atrioventricular block with normal sino-atrial function. A normal size right atrium is preferable. For best atrial sensing, the bipolar atrial dipole, which is from five to ten mm, should lie close to the mid-to-high atrial wall. A number of designs, some quite exotic, have been proposed in an attempt to achieve DDD(R) pacing (51–55).

Coronary Sinus Leads

Atrial pacing from the coronary sinus using specialized pacing leads was reported as early as the 1960s. With the development of specialized automatic tachycardia reversion pacing systems to interrupt a re-entry circuit in the left atrium, coronary sinus leads were once again used to pace near the mouth of the coronary sinus (56). To achieve this, the cathode was positioned about 4 cm behind the tip of an angled lead which was introduced well into the coronary sinus. The lead between tip and cathode was stiffened usually with conductor coil. Leads with a distal cathode were also designed to pace the atrium deeper in the coronary sinus. As electrophysiologic techniques evolved to cure these tachyarrhythmias, the pacing techniques became redundant and so did the use of coronary sinus leads. More recently with interest in dual-site atrial pacing, there was a resurrection of coronary sinus pacing. However, this interest was only transient as pulse generators designed to cater for two atrial leads were never developed and the adaptors used to create a single connector were cumbersome and unreliable.

Left Ventricular Pacing Leads

The coronary venous system has also been used for cardiac resynchronization therapy. Using either a standard lead or a coronary sinus lead with a distal tip cathode, pushed as far as possible into the coronary sinus, left ventricular pacing could be achieved. This principle has been used to establish bi-ventricular pacing with the other lead in the right ventricle (57). The technique requires tools or work stations to cannulate the coronary sinus and then allow positioning of specialized leads well into the coronary venous system generally on the lateral left ventricular wall. Such placement is technically difficult, very time consuming and the leads, implantation techniques and pacing algorithms are rapidly evolving. Unlike conventional leads, specialized left ventricular leads positioned on the epicardial surface using the coronary venous system use a floppy wire to guide the lead into the distal vein, where it is then wedged (Fig. 1.29). The guide wire usually passes through the center of the cathode. Generally the leads are much thinner than standard leads and may use the same lumen to pass a larger gauge stiffening wire which is useful when removing the coronary sinus catheter work station.

On occasion, a larger diameter lead may be useful if the coronary venous system is large. Lead dislodgement remains a problem. Tines have been used (Fig. 1.29) as well as bends in the distal lead to hopefully ensure entrapment (Fig. 1.30). Steroid-eluting collars have also been introduced. The original

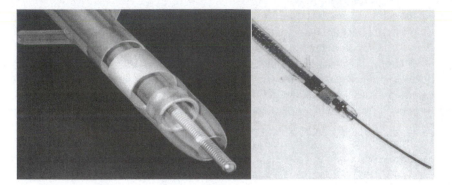

Fig. 1.29 A left ventricular lead demonstrating the "over the wire" concept. *Left*: Cartoon showing the guide wire passing through the lead. The guide wire is positioned in a cardiac vein tributary on the epicardial left ventricular wall and the lead is gradually passed over this wire until it becomes wedged. *Right*: The lead and guide wire. (Permission for use: Guidant.)

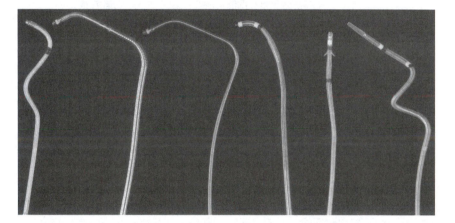

Fig. 1.30 Range of "over the wire" left ventricular leads for positioning in cardiac veins. (Permission for use: Guidant, Medtronic, St Jude.)

leads were unipolar using the anode of the right ventricular lead to achieve pacing. Bipolar leads are now available and can be coupled to a range of programmable polarity options to overcome high thresholds and phrenic nerve stimulation. It can be envisioned that multipolar leads will be available in the future to increase the number of polarity options. Despite the marked advances in left ventricular lead design, high stimulation thresholds, phrenic nerve stimulation and lead dislodgement remain significant problems. Coupled with a failure to cannulate the coronary sinus or position the lead in a satisfactory position or failure of therapy to improve symptoms (nonresponder) makes cardiac resynchronization, a therapy with a potentially high complication and failure rate. Despite this rapid progress is currently being made.

Concluding Remarks

In recent years, there have been remarkable advances in cardiac pacing leads. The most important changes have been the establishment of safe bipolar leads with small, porous, steroid-eluting electrodes that provide extremely low chronic stimulation threshold and low polarization characteristics. It is important not to forget the less heralded advances in conductor and insulator technology. These advances not only have contributed to the safety of these leads but also allowed much thinner leads to be manufactured. There has also been a remarkable international and inter-company co operation in the development of lead connector standards, which has allowed all modern leads to be compatible with competitor products.

References

1. Mond H, Irwin M, Morillo C et al.: The World survey of cardiac pacing and cardioverter defibrillators: Calendar year 2001. PACE 2004; 27:955–964.
2. Mond HG: Unipolar versus bipolar pacing - Poles apart. PACE 1991; 14:1411–1424.
3. Griffin JC: Sensing characteristics of the right atrial appendage electrode. PACE 1983; 6:22–25.
4. Mond H. and Barold SS: Dual chamber, rate-adaptive pacing in patients with paroxysmal supraventricular tachyarrhythmias: Protective measures for rate control. PACE 1993; 16:2168–2185.
5. Mymin D, Cuddy TE, Sinha SN, et al.: Inhibition of demand pacemakers by skeletal muscle potentials. JAMA 1973; 223:527–532.
6. Cameron J, Ciddor G, Mond H, et al.: Stiffness of the distal tip of bipolar pacemaker leads. PACE 1990: 13;1915–1920.
7. Kistler PM, Eizenberg N, Fynn SP et al.: The subpectoral pacemaker implant: It isn't what it seems! PACE 2004; 27:361–364.
8. Weiss DN, Zilo P, Luceri RM et al.: Should unipolar pacemaker leads be banned? Lessons from pacemaker/implantable cardioverter defibrillator interactions. PACE 1997; 20:237–239.
9. Mond H: The Cardiac Pacemaker. Function and Malfunction. New York: Grune and Stratton, 1973, pp. 60–66.
10. Schuchert A and Kuck KH: Influence of internal current and pacing current on pacemaker longevity. PACE 1994; 17:13–16.
11. Ellenbogen KA, Wood MA, Gilligan DM, et al.: Steroid eluting high impedance pacing leads decrease short and long term current drain: Results from a multicenter clinical trial. PACE 1999; 22:39–48.
12. Parsonnet V, Gilbert L, Lewin G et al.: A non polarizing electrode for endocardial stimulation of the heart. J Thorac Cardiovasc Serg. 1968; 56:710–715.
13. Schaldach M, Hubman M, Weikl A, et al.: Sputter-deposited TiN electrode coatings for superior sensing and pacing performance. PACE 1990; 13:1891–1895.
14. Elmqvist H, Schueller H, Richter G: The carbon tip electrode. PACE 1983; 6:436–439.
15. Moracchini PV, Cappelletti F, Melandri PF, et al.: Titanium oxide tip electrode, A solution to minimize polarization and threshold increase (Abstract). PACE 1985; 8:A–85.
16. Schaldach M, Hubman M, Weikl A, et al.: Sputter-deposited TiN electrode coatings for superior sensing and pacing performance. PACE 1990; 13:1891–1895.
17. Tang C, Yeung-Lai-Wah JA, Qi A, et al.: Initial experience with a co-radial bipolar pacing lead. PACE 1997; 20:1800–1807.
18. DelBufalo AGA, Schlaepfer J, Fromer M et al.: Acute and long-term ventricular stimulation thresholds with a new, Iridium oxide-coated electrode. PACE 1993; 16:1240–1244.
19. Mond H and Stokes KB: The electrode–tissue interface: the revolutionary role of steroid elution. PACE 1992; 15:95–107.
20. Sibille Y and Reynolds H: Macrophages and polymorphonuclear neutrophils in lung defence and injury. Am Rev Respir Dis 1990; 41:471–501.

21. Guerola M and Lindegren U: Clinical evaluation of membrane-coated 3,5 mm2 porous titanium nitride electrodes. In Aubert AE, Ector H and Stroobandt R (eds). Euro-pace'93 Monduzzi Editore, 1993, pp. 447–450.

22. Stokes K, Bornzin G: The electrode - biointerface: Stimulation. In Barold SS (ed). Modern Cardiac Pacing. New York: Futura Publishing, 1985, pp. 33–77.

23. Brewer G, McAuslan BR, Skalsky M, et al.: Initial screening of bio-active agents with potential to reduce stimulation threshold (Abstract). PACE 1988; 11:509.

24. Kruse IM: Long-term performance of endocardial leads with steroid-eluting electrodes. PACE 1986; 9:1217–1219.

25. Mond HG: Development of low stimulation-threshold, low-polarization electrodes. In: New Perspectives in Cardiac Pacing. 2. Barold SS and Mugica J (eds). Mount Kisco, NY: Futura Publishing Company, Inc., 1991, P133–162.

26. Pioger G: Low surface area electrodes: comparison between Synox 60 BP (1.3 mm2), Capsure Z 5034 (1.2 mm2) and Stela BT26 (2 mm2):158 cases (Abstract). PACE 1997; 20:1443.

27. Hua W, Mond HG, and Strathmore N: Chronic steroid eluting lead performance: A comparison of atrial and ventricular pacing. PACE 1997; 20:17–24.

28. Till JA, Jones S, Rowland E, et al.: Clinical experience with a steroid eluting lead in children. Circulation 1989; 80:II–389.

29. Stokes K, Church T: The elimination of exit block as a pacing complication using a transvenous steroid eluting lead (Abstract). PACE 1987; 10:748.

30. Hiller K, Rothschild JM, Fudge W et al.: A randomized comparison of a bipolar steroid-eluting lead and a bipolar porous platinum coated titanium lead (Abstract). PACE 1991; 14:695.

31. Mond HG, Hua W and Wang CC: Atrial pacing leads: the clinical contribution of steroid elution. PACE 1995; 18:1601–1608.

32. Hua W, Mond H and Sparks P: The clinical performance of three designs of atrial pacing leads from a single manufacturer: the value of steroid elution. Eur J.C.P.E 1996; 6:99–103.

33. Stokes KB: Preliminary studies on a new steroid eluting epicardial electrode. PACE 1988; 11:1797–1803.

34. Karpawich PP, Hakimi M, Arciniegas E: Improved chronic epicardial pacing in children: Steroid contribution to porous platinised electrodes. PACE 1992; 15:1151–1157.

35. Mathivanar R, Anderson N, Harman D et al.: In vivo elution of drug eluting ceramic leads with a reduced dose of dexamethasone sodium phosphate. PACE 1990; 13:1883–1886.

36. Schuchert A, Kuck KH: Benefits of smaller electrode surface area (4 mm²) on steroid eluting leads. PACE 1991; 14:2098–2104.

37. Kistler PM, Liew G and Mond HG: Long-term performance of active-fixation pacing leads: a prospective study. PACE 2006; 29:226–230.

38. Kistler PM, Kalman JM, Fynn SP et al.: Rapid decline in acute stimulation thresholds with steroid-eluting active fixation pacing leads. PACE 2005; 28:903–909.

39. Anderson N, Mathivanar R, Skalsky M et al.: Active fixation leads – long term threshold reduction using a drug-infused ceramic collar. PACE 2004; 14:1767–1771.

40. Singarayar S, Kistler PM, DeWinter C et al.: A comparative study of the action of dexamethasone sodium phosphate and dexamethasone acetate in steroid-eluting pacemaker leads. PACE 2005; 28:311–315.

41. Bergdahl L: Helifix, an electrode suitable for transvenous and ventricular implantation. J Thorac Cardiovasc Surg 1980; 80:794–799.

42. Sloman JG, Mond HG, Bailey B et al.: The use of balloon-tipped electrodes for permanent cardiac pacing. PACE 1979; 2:579–585.

43. Mond H and Sloman G: The small-tined pacemaker lead – Absence of dislodgement. PACE 1980; 3:171–177.

44. Gammage MD, Swoyer J, Moes R et al.: Initial experience with a new design parallel conductor, high impedance, steroid-eluting bipolar pacing lead (Abstract). PACE 1997; 20:1229.

45. Tang C, Yeung-Lai-Wah JA, Qi A, et al.: Initial experience with a co-radial bipolar pacing lead. PACE 1997; 20:1800–1807.

46. Byrd CL, McArthur W, Stokes K et al.: Implant experience with unipolar pacing leads. PACE 1983; 6:868–882.

47. Scheuer-Leeser M, Irnich W, Kreuzer J: Polyurethane leads: facts and controversy. PACE 1983; 6:454–458.

48. Timmis GC, Westveer DC, Martin R et al.: The significance of surface changes on explanted polyurethane pacemaker leads. PACE 1983; 6:845–857.

49. Stokes K, Urbanski P, Upton J: The in vivo auto-oxidation of polyether polyurethanes by metal ions. J Biomatr Sc, Polym 1990; 1:207.

50. Medtronic family of Novus® Leads. Medtronic, Minneapolis, MN.

51. Morgan K, Bornzin GA, Florio J et al.: A new single pass DDD lead (Abstract). PACE 1997; 20:1211.

52. Hirschberg J, Ekwall C and Bowald S: DDD pacemaker system with single lead (SLDDD) reduces intravascular hardware. Long-term experimental study (Abstract). PACE 1996; 19:601.

53. DiGregorio F, Morra A, Bongiorni M et al.: A multicenter experience in DDD pacing with single-pass lead (Abstract). PACE 1997; 20:1210.

54. Hartung WM, Strobel JP, Taskiran M, et al.: "Overlapping bipolar impulse" – Stimulation using a single lead implantable pacemaker system first results (Abstract). PACE 1996; 19:601.

55. Lucchese F, Halperin C, Strobel J et al.: Single lead DDD pacing with overlapping biphasic atrial stimulation – First clinical results (Abstract). PACE 1996; 19:601.

56. Vohra J, Hamer A, Mond H, Sloman G, Hunt D: Patient initiated implantable pacemakers for paroxysmal supraventricular tachycardia. Aust N Z J Med 1981; 11:27–34.

57. Leclercq C, Cazeau S, Le Breton H et al.: Acute hemodynamic effects of biventricular DDD pacing in patients with end-stage heart failure. JACC 1998; 32:1825–1831.

The Pulse Generator

Richard S. Sanders

Basic Pacing Concepts and Terminology

A cardiac pulse generator is a device having a power source and electronic circuitry that produce output stimuli. Functionally, at its simplest, current sourced by the device's battery travels through a connecting pathway to stimulate the heart and then flows back into the pacemaker to complete the circuit.

Although numerous and varied designs of cardiac pacemakers are available, all have the same basic components:

- A power source in the form of a battery
- Circuitry (output, sensing, telemetry, microprocessor or microsequencer, memory)
- A metal casing (can) welded shut to keep out fluids
- A feedthrough (a piece of wire surrounded by glass or sapphire) that maintains a hermetic seal to provide an electrical connection through the can
- A means of connecting a pacing lead (wire to the heart) to the header of the pacemaker
- Sensors (e.g., acceleration, vibration, impedance)

Modern pacemakers are extremely sophisticated and highly programmable, capable of storing a rather impressive array of diagonstic data. Weighing about 25 g, they can pace and sense in one, two, or three chambers and adjust their rate by tracking intrinsic atrial activity or by responding to input from a sensor.

Because the pacemaker is an electronic device, the clinician may be unfamiliar with the engineering nomenclature associated with this technology. The more common terms are listed in Table 2.1. How the pacemaker works and factors to take into consideration when programming a pacemaker are discussed in the following sections.

Table 2.1 Engineering nomenclature.

Ampere	A unit of electric current equaling one coulomb per second
Amplifier	Device or circuit that amplifies, enlarges, or extends an electrical signal
Anode	Positive pole electrode
Capacitor	Device that can store an electrical charge
Cathode	Negative pole electrode
Circuit	A closed path followed by an electric current
Coulomb	A measure of charge equal to the amount of electricity transported by 1 A of current for 1 s
Current (I)	Flow of electrons through a conductor
Current drain	Current drawn from a battery
Impedance	The total opposition to the flow of current (including that through the conductor and across the interface to the stimulation site). Often used interchangeably with the term "resistance"
Insulation	Material that offers high resistance to the flow of electric current
Joule	Unit of measurement for energy or work (one joule = one coulomb flowing across a potential of 1 V for 1 s)
Ohm (Ω)	Basic unit of electrical resistance and/or impedance (one ohm = resistance produced when one ampere of current produces a voltage of 1 V across a conductor)
Ohm's Law	Voltage = current times resistance ($V = IR$)
Resistance	The electrical property of a material that resists the flow of electric current
Resistor (R)	Electronic circuit component that produces a known resistance
Volt (V)	Basic unit of measurement of electrical potential difference
Watt	Unit measure for power

Power Source (Battery)

Pacemakers directly benefited from advances in battery technology; thus, a variety of power sources have been employed in cardiac pacemakers over the last four decades. The first chemical cell to achieve wide-scale use was composed of mercury–zinc (HgZn) also known as the Rueben or Mallory cell (1,2). Unfortunately, mercury–zinc had some undesirable characteristics. The cell voltage was 1.35 V, so most pacemakers incorporated four to five cells in series to provide the 5.0–6.0 V deemed necessary to produce consistent capture or depolarization of the heart. In addition, as the cell is depleted, the voltage decreases to almost zero precipitously with little or no warning. As a consequence, pacemaker patients had to be followed frequently to assure that the battery voltage did not decrease to a point where capture was lost. Several manufacturers flirted with nuclear-powered cells but this much-touted battery failed to achieve much popularity because of the government restrictions and bulky radiation shielding, which made them rather large (3). One manufacturer produced a rechargeable cell (nickel–cadmium); however, these devices required constant recharging and the memory effect of these rechargeable batteries had an adverse effect on the overall longevity.

Prior to 1975, pacemaker longevity in excess of 3–4 years was the exception (4,5). This changed in the mid-1970s as the industry migrated almost exclusively to a lithium iodide-based cell. This cell had many of the characteristics that were considered ideal for a pacemaker power source. It was highly reliable and had a very long shelf-life. Its energy density was better than previous cells, enabling manufacturers to provide many ampere-hours in a small volume. This allowed for significant size–volume reductions in the pacemaker. In contrast to the mercury–zinc cell, which exhibited a sudden decrease in voltage just before depletion, the lithium iodide cell had a more predictable and gradual decrease of voltage as it approached depletion. The chemical reaction between lithium and iodine produces lithium iodide, a resistive barrier.

$$2L_i \rightarrow 2L_i^+ + 2e^- \quad \text{(anode reaction)}$$

$$2L_i^+ + 2e^- + I_2 \rightarrow 2L_iI \quad \text{(cathode reaction)}$$

$$2L_i + I_2 \rightarrow 2L_iI$$

At the interface where the anode (positively charged electrode) and the cathode (negatively charged electrode) interact, a lithium iodide barrier grows, building up internal resistance in the cell. This has two distinct advantages: first, it allows the manufacturer to select a predefined depletion level known as the *elective replacement point*, after which the device can be expected to function another 3–6 months; second, it creates a system that effectively prevents any internal shorts because the lithium iodide layer forms wherever the anode and cathode come in contact (6). Yet another advantage of lithium iodide was the absence of outgasing (any gaseous result of the chemical reaction). Mercury–zinc batteries produced hydrogen gas as a byproduct and therefore had to be encapsulated in gas-permeable epoxy or a chemical "getter" was necessary for sealed devices. In the case of the epoxy-encapsulated device, the epoxy allowed the hydrogen to diffuse into body tissues. Unfortunately this allowed water to enter and contact the pacemaker circuit. With some models, the water dissolved ionic contaminants left on the circuit, which produced shorts or dendrites (essentially mineral deposits) and resulted in premature battery depletion and several pacemaker recalls (7). Lithium iodide batteries produced no gases and allowed engineers to hermetically seal the battery and circuit inside a metal can, eliminating a significant mode of failure while better protecting the electronic circuit from spurious electrical interference.

Lithium iodide chemistry, which has a favorable energy density, has a low power density and can only supply currents in the very low milliampere range. This limited power density makes lithium iodine batteries less suitable for some of today's high current requirements, such as long-range telemetry. Additional chemistries are being introduced into today's pacemakers, including carbon monofluoroide (CFx) and manganese dioxide (MnO2) chemistry. These new cell formulations achieve many of the benefits of the lithium iodide chemistry and provide significantly better power delivery. These new chemistries may well totally supplant lithium iodide as the power source of choice for pacemakers.

Gradual Decay of Battery Voltage (Elective Replacement Indicator)

All cells experience self-discharge; the decrease in capacity occurs as a result of the reaction of cathodal and anodal materials, even when the cell is not connected to a circuit. Lithium iodide cells have a relatively low self-discharge. Once a cell is connected to the circuit, power is supplied to keep the pacemaker awake in what is called a quiescent state, still executing logic commands and looking for sensed inputs. Thus, even when a pulse generator is sitting in its packaging, not connected to a lead, its battery capacity is being slowly depleted as a result of the quiescent current requirements of the circuitry and the self-discharge of the cell. This factor, along with considerations regarding the ability to maintain sterility of the device in its packaging, has led manufacturers to provide device-specific "use-before" or "shelf-life" dates. By specifying the maximum time between device cell connection and implantation, manufacturers assure that clinicians can expect the device to meet its published postimplant longevity specifications despite the effects of preimplant depletion of the power source.

At beginning-of-life (BOL) a lithium iodide cell will have a voltage output of around 2.8 V and an internal impedance <1,000 Ω (Fig. 2.1). As it ages, cell impedance rises because of the progressive buildup of lithium iodide. This generally continues until the elective replacement point is reached, and the cell impedance rises above 8,000 Ω. The cell should not be allowed to deplete to lower levels because the pacemaker's circuitry requires a minimum voltage level to operate. Manufacturers designate a specific point that triggers the elective replacement indicator (ERI) significantly in advance of the point where circuit operation is threatened. It is at this point that replacement is advisable (or at least follow-up monitoring of the patient should be intensified).

One should always consult the physicians' manual to determine the specific behavior that indicates the need for elective replacement. A mode conversion from dual-chamber to single-chamber (e.g., DDD to VVI), rate response to nonrate response or a change in magnet rate behavior may be observed when the ERI is triggered. Some pulse generators also provide an additional pre-ERI alert known as an intensified follow-up indicator (IFI), a safety feature that

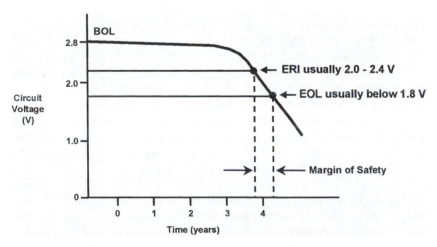

Fig. 2.1 At beginning-of-life (BOL), the lithium iodide battery exhibits an output voltage of 2.8 V, which slowly decays until it nearly depletes, whereupon the voltage decays more rapidly. At around 2.0–2.4 V, the elective replacement indicator is triggered, which usually leaves 6 months before the pulse generator will begin to behave abnormally as it reaches its end of useful life (EOL).

signifies that the frequency of follow-up visits should be increased because the unit is approaching ERI. This is particularly useful if the pacemaker is programmed to settings that require higher battery current drains (e.g., high voltage outputs or pacing rates) (8).

Longevity

At the simplest level, pacemaker longevity is determined by the battery capacity and the current drain. In reviewing longevity specifications for a device as published in physicians' manuals and promotional materials, one should pay particular attention to the associated conditions and assumptions. Pacemaker manuals usually describe longevity using an assumption of nominal outputs and pacing rate (Table 2.2). Nominal values adequately pace the heart in the majority of patients, and are preset in the device before it is shipped by the manufacturer. The longevity of the device is affected by the output settings, as is the margin between the triggering of the ERI and the onset of compromised behavior (9).

Physicians' manuals sometimes provide two different battery ratings: the stoichiometric capacity, or total amount of energy stored in the battery and the usable battery capacity. The latter is significantly lower than the stoichiometric capacity and is the value most relevant to the clinician, because the battery effectively becomes useless once the voltage drops below the circuit-operating threshold. Battery capacity is expressed in ampere-hours or A h. A common rating for a pacemaker's battery capacity is in the range of 1.0–1.5 A h (10).

The total current drain on the battery is primarily composed of: (a) quiescent current (i.e., that required to keep the circuitry running (sensing circuitry, amplifiers, and central processing unit), and (b) pacing current that is required to produce the output pulse used to stimulate the heart. Total current drain of a dual-chamber pacemaker set to nominal outputs (quiescent current + pacing current) is typically 10–15 μA per pacing cycle. Fifty to sixty percent of the total current drain is quiescent, and is relatively constant. This type of current drain is wholly determined by the circuit design – there is little that a clinician can do to change it. In addition, as the pacing output is reduced the proportion attributed to the quiescent current increases. Thus, a pacemaker that is

Table 2.2 Effect of current drain on longevity for Intermedics Marathon DDDR Pulse Generator.

	Rate	Years of service life			
		100% Pacing	100% Pacing	50% Pacing	50% Pacing
Nominal output		500 Ω load	750 Ω load	500 Ω load	750 Ω load
DDDR mode, 3.5 V pulse amplitude	60	6.3	7.4	7.1	8.0
0.45 ms pulse width	70	5.8	6.9	6.8	7.7
Low output					
DDDR mode, 2.5 V pulse amplitude	60	7.4	8.4	8.0	8.7
0.45 ms pulse width	70	6.8	7.8	7.7	8.4

From Baker RGJ, Falkenberg EN. Bipolar versus unipolar issues in DDD pacing (Part II). *PACE* 1987;10:125–132, with permission.

Table 2.3 Effect on longevity of output voltage, output pulse width, pacing rate, and lead impedance.

Parameter	Effect on longevity	Factor
Increasing output voltage	Decrease in longevity	Exponential
Increasing output pulse width	Decrease in longevity	Linear
Increasing pacing rate	Decrease in longevity	Linear
Increasing lead impedance	Increase in longevity	Linear

not pacing or has its output near zero still drains some amount of energy from its battery. For this reason, reducing output does not always have a profound longevity benefit.

The pacing current drain during each paced cycle is a function of output voltage, pulse width, and lead impedance. The interrelationship between these factors can be expressed by the following equations:

$$E_P = V_P \cdot I_P \cdot T$$

Using Ohm's law we can substitute

$$I_P = V_P / R_L$$

Thus

$$E_P = V_P^2 T / R_L$$

where E_P, energy of each pacing pulse (μJ); V_P, output pulse voltage (V); I_P, output pulse current (mA); T, output pulse width (ms); and R_L, lead impedance (Ω).

The mathematical relationship indicates that the energy extracted from the battery per pulse is linearly related to the pulse width and lead impedance but varies by the square of the output voltage. It follows that, when programming output, the voltage will have a more pronounced effect on energy consumption than a proportional change in pulse width (Table 2.3).

Battery Impedance and Output Programming

Despite the fact that the battery generates 2.8 V, it is possible to program the device to higher outputs through the use of specialized circuits that step up the voltage to higher levels. The selection of output voltages varies by manufacturer but generally covers the range of 0.5–8.0 V.

If a pacemaker is close to its elective replacement point, programming from a low- to a high-output setting immediately increases current drain on the battery, causing the terminal voltage of the battery to fall. This is an effect of Ohm's law and is the result of high battery impedance in a partially depleted cell. This has been shown to cause premature activation of the ERI (11).

In rate-responsive devices, current drain will increase as the exercise rate increases, which will decrease the battery voltage. In rate-responsive devices with a mature battery and a high battery impedance, exercise could trigger the ERI. In the same device, a reasonably normal battery voltage may be observed during follow-up with the patient at rest. Generally, standard reprogramming disengages an ERI that has occurred in response to a transient increase in current drain.

Effects of Cold and Heat on the Battery

Lithium iodide batteries are also affected by extremes of cold or heat. Although these effects are not seen when a device is implanted, be aware that:

1. A pacemaker can be exposed to cold before implant such as during shipping. Low temperatures slow down the reaction between lithium and iodine, which causes the internal resistance to rise and voltage to drop. This condition is temporary and exists only during the exposure to low temperatures. The battery recovers immediately at room temperature, but the ERI could already be triggered. Occasionally, if a device is not interrogated after implant, the clinician might see the ERI at the first follow-up and falsely assume there is something wrong. If this occurs, it is possible that the unit has been exposed to cold prior to implant, activating the ERI, which at this point could usually be reset during normal programming (12).
2. Exposure to extreme heat can cause a pacemaker to explode. If a deceased patient is to be cremated, it is recommended that the unit be removed. Most funeral directors are now aware of this, particularly if they have experienced this unfortunate phenomenon.

Circuitry

Cardiac pacemakers incorporate some of the most advanced, high-reliability electronic circuitry available. The basic building block is the integrated circuit (IC), which starts as a silicon wafer and has a number of miniaturized circuit elements etched into its surface during the manufacturing process. Modern pulse generators incorporate custom-designed, very large-scale integrated (VLSI) circuits (13). ICs are built up layer by layer and can incorporate millions of electronic elements. The elements are so fine that they can barely be seen with an optical microscope.

Some components are not integrated into the IC, such as larger-value capacitors, diodes, inductors, transmission coil, and so on. These components that cannot be incorporated on the IC must be added as discrete components. It is the goal of the pacemaker designer to minimize the number of discrete components to save cost and space. The ICs and discrete components are mounted onto a layered substrate, which, like a matrix of major highway interchanges, provides pathways on its surface, and within and between its layers, by which the components are interconnected. Historically, this substrate was composed of a ceramic material. Today, these substrates are almost exclusively constructed of a flexible polymer. This combination of discrete components and ICs, mounted on a substrate, are known as hybrid circuits (Fig. 2.2). The hybrid circuit and the battery together comprise 80–90% of the space in the pacemaker's can (13).

It is often useful to think of a pacemaker's circuit not in terms of specific components, but rather according to their various functions. These functional sections include: logic and control, memory, timing, sensing, output, data transmission, and programming. Figure 2.3 illustrates the functional block diagram of a typical pulse generator, the Sulzer Intermedics Marathon. The circuitry associated with each of these functions is described in the following sections (14).

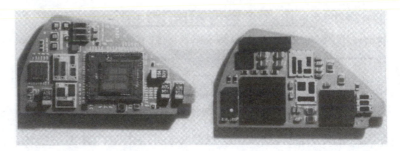

Fig. 2.2 Hybrid circuit (front and back), consisting of one or more integrated circuits and a number of discrete components mounted on a ceramic substrate.

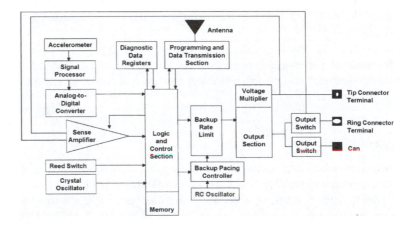

Fig. 2.3 Block diagram showing functional organization of Intermedics Marathon SR pulse generator.

The Microprocessor

In most modern pacemakers the logic functions are controlled by microprocessors. A pacemaker microprocessor is very similar to the central processing unit (CPU) in a desktop computer. A pacemaker microprocessor operate with currents millions of times less than low-power microprocessors in today's laptop computers. This low-power operation is necessary in order to achieve overall size and longevity and can limit its processing power. The pacemaker CPU is generally customized and integrated with other components such as memory on one IC.

The microprocessor is constantly accessing its memory for instructions on what to do next. Processor speed is somewhat dependent on a crystal oscillator or clock. The higher the speed, the more instructions that can be executed per second, but more current is required. Fortunately, because of the nature of pacing, the processor does not need to be on all the time. It can be in a sleep mode, a good deal of the pacing cycle, and only needs to be awakened when it receives an input or needs to execute a particular function. The percentage of time the processor is awake and performing tasks is called the duty cycle. The higher the duty cycle, the higher the current drain and the shorter the device longevity. Thus, even in the absence of pacing, frequent sense events can increase current drain. Actually, the microprocessor receives inputs from

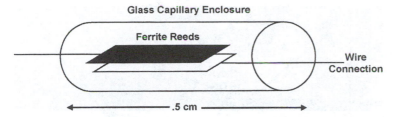

Fig. 2.4 Schematic representation of magnet-activated pacemaker reed switch.

several circuits other than sensing and crystal oscillator circuitry. It checks to see if the reed switch (a magnet-activated switch composed of two very small ferrite reeds placed close together inside a tiny glass tube) is open or closed (Fig. 2.4). It is used as a way for an ordinary magnet to activate or deactivate certain features or functions, such as temporarily suspending sensing.

The processor also receives inputs from the sensor(s) for rate-response and telemetry/programming commands. All these inputs are used by the microprocessor to determine whether when and to which chamber to deliver an output pulse. Some inputs, such as from the crystal oscillator, occur as fast as millions of times per second. Other inputs, such as from the reed switch, might not occur for months or years. In the case of a totally pacemaker-dependent patient, there may be no sensed inputs for the life of the patient.

Sensing Circuitry

Pacemaker leads connect the sensing and output circuitry to the outside world via feedthroughs. The feedthroughs function like a single-lane highway that handles two-way traffic, like a serial bus in computer lingo. The pacemaker spends much more of the pacing cycle looking for sense events than it does actually providing pacing output, which generally has a duration of half a millisecond or less. How a pacemaker senses depends on the particular device, but there are some similarities.

The sensing circuitry of a pulse generator is used for both the amplification and filtering of intracardiac signals. To prevent the sensing of noncardiac signals by the pacemaker, the intracardiac signal is processed by the circuitry to determine whether it has sufficient amplitude and the appropriate frequency content. This relationship between amplitude and frequency may be characterized by plotting a frequency–response curve. This curve is derived in the laboratory by inputting sine-squared ($\sin^2$) or some other test waveforms of varying amplitudes and frequencies into the circuit. Although intracardiac signals are far more complex than the $\sin^2$ signals, the latter are easy to generate and can be reproduced with precision (15).

The frequency–response curve shown in Fig. 2.5 illustrates several key points. First, everything above the curve is sensed by the pacemaker, while everything below is not. Second, the sensing circuit is designed and tuned to be most sensitive to signals within a specific frequency range. This point may differ somewhat between various manufacturers' sensing circuits, but is usually in the range of 20–30 Hz. Signals with frequencies at or near the center point are passed through the filters with little or no loss of amplitude, whereas signals far from the center frequency will be significantly attenuated. Once

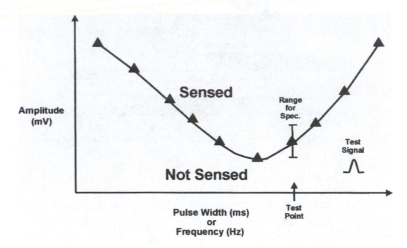

Fig. 2.5 Frequency–response curve of pacemaker sense amplifier exposed to $\sin^2$ input signals. Signals above the curve are sensed, whereas those below are not. Another characteristic of pacemaker sensing circuits is the preference given to frequencies within the range of 20–60 Hz, a significant frequency component of cardiac IEGMs.

the signal passes through the filters, if it has sufficient amplitude, it will be detected by the pacemaker.

These characteristics of the sensing circuit have many clinical implications. The programmable sensitivity settings of a pacemaker, usually expressed in millivolts, correspond to the device's response to a $\sin^2$ signal at or near the 0 dB frequency. Often, manufacturers will use different test signals for their atrial and ventricular sense amplifiers to better approximate the frequency content of the signals originating in each chamber called the intracardiac electrogram (IEGM). When a complex signal like an IEGM, made up of various frequencies, is encountered, those portions of the signal at or near the zero dB frequency are preferentially passed through, whereas other portions are attenuated (run-on). Thus, a large intracardiac signal with frequency components outside the central range will appear significantly smaller to the pacemaker. Moreover, owing to differences in this so-called bandpass filtering from one pacemaker model to another, a particular sensitivity setting (e.g., 2 mV) may not be equivalent in different devices. One further note: the body itself acts like a filter, and the morphology of the IEGM may differ significantly from the surface EKG. Unlike the surface EKG, the IEGM reflects more of a local electrical event near the electrode within the heart (Fig. 2.6).

It is impractical to analyze the frequency content of an intracardiac signal in the implant setting; therefore, clinicians often calculate a surrogate value, known as the slew rate, which is related to frequency (Fig. 2.7). The slew rate is the slope of a straight segment (the intrinsic deflection) of the electrogram; this corresponds to the change in voltage with respect to time ($\Delta V/\Delta T$), and is expressed in mV/ms. A signal with a slew rate of approximately 0.5 mV/ms is considered the minimum requirement to ensure an appropriate signal frequency for sensing.

Some portions of the signal may not have adequate amplitude and slew rate to be sensed because of the complex nature of the IEGM. Typically, the portion

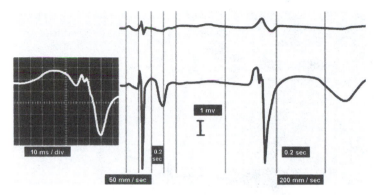

Fig. 2.6 Surface EKG (*Top*) and ventricular electrogram (*Bottom*) demonstrate the difference in amplitude and frequency content. Sweep speed has been increased from 50 to 200 mm/s.

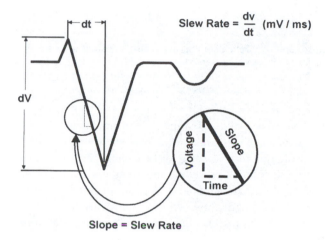

Fig. 2.7 Slew rate, or the change in voltage divided by the change in time of an intracardiac signal.

of the signal with the highest slew rate and amplitude is in the middle of the electrogram, representing the moment when the wave of depolarization passes directly under the sensing electrode. Thus, the earliest parts of the signal, which may be visible on the surface ECG, may not be sensed by the device. In this case, the pacemaker output is delivered into already depolarized tissue, rendering the pulse ineffective. This should not be considered a sensing malfunction, but is simply a delay in the timing of sensing the event by the generator. It is most commonly observed in dual-chamber devices in patients with right bundle branch block. Arrival of localized depolarization in the area of the right ventricular lead is significantly delayed, allowing the output pulse to be delivered during left ventricular depolarization and well into the surface QRS (Fig. 2.8). Clinically, this may manifest itself in the apparent undersensing of a P-wave or QRS, a surface ECG phenomenon known as pseudofusion. Either shortening or extending the A-V delay might alleviate the pseudofusion.

Clinicians should follow certain precautions to ensure appropriate sensing of a patient's intrinsic electrograms. The amplitude and slew rate of the

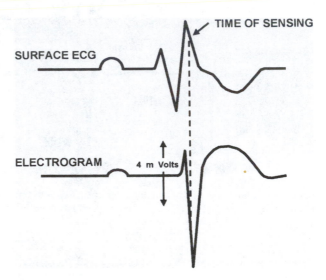

Fig. 2.8 Illustration of mechanism that may cause apparent undersensing. Pulse generator with a lead in the RV apex senses electrogram during the large second deflection. Thus, an output at any time prior to the corresponding point on the surface EKG is normal but may result in fusion or pseudofusion phenomenon.

electrogram should be evaluated at the time of implantation, and, if either or both appear inadequate or marginal, the lead should be repositioned. A specialized piece of equipment (pacing systems analyzer or PSA) which should be used during the implant procedure measures both of these characteristics and provides the required quantitative measure of the electrogram. Assuring a robust sensing signal at the time of implant provides the most programming flexibility to deal with problems that may arise later. Because the characteristics of the signal may change over time, owing to fibrotic encapsulation and/or inflammatory reactions following implantation, or owing to the activity of certain cardioactive drugs, a sensing threshold test should be performed prior to hospital discharge, during the acute-to-chronic phase (typically, the first 6–8 weeks postimplant), and periodically thereafter (16,17). During this test, the pacemaker's sensitivity is progressively programmed to less sensitive settings (i.e., higher mV values) to determine the setting at which reliable sensing is lost (18). The device is then programmed to a value that provides an adequate margin to ensure continued sensing, while minimizing the possibility of inappropriate sensing of extracardiac signals.

Many modern pacemakers incorporate a means to automatically adjust the sensing circuit to be more or less sensitive (autogain function). The auto gain function constantly monitors the intracardiac signal and maintains a preset safety margin to should any changes in the amplitude or slew rate occur over time. This minimizes the need to evaluate and adjust the sensing setting during follow-ups.

Sensing Circuitry and Electromagnetic Interference

Unwanted signals from external and endogenous sources can be sensed by the pacemaker. Endogenous sources include myopotentials generated by skeletal muscles and far field signals originating in the chamber opposite to which sensing was intended (e.g., R-waves would be considered far field when sensed in the atrium) (19,20). External sources are numerous and include cellular phones, electronic article surveillance systems, diathermy equipment, electrocautery, some large electronic motors and, in fact, any equipment generating a large electromagnetic field. Their effects are usually temporary and may include inhibition, asynchronous pacing, and high-rate ventricular pacing in dual-chamber modes. In rare cases (e.g., electrocautery, external defibrillation) EMI can trigger the backup mode or ERI. Proximity is an important factor, because energy generally falls off by a factor related to the square of the distance. Lower sensitivities and bipolar sensing make devices less susceptible to electromagnetic interference (EMI); medical professionals are encouraged to follow warnings in physicians' manuals to avoid serious interaction with these sources of interference (21). In most cases, simple precautions are extremely effective, like not putting a cell phone in a breast pocket over the pacemaker (22).

Pacemaker circuitry also contains feed through filters and noise discriminating capabilities that provide an additional level of protection against sources of EMI. Feed-through filters help protect the circuit from damage owing to high-voltage EMI by shunting the energy away from the circuit. Lower energy EMI signals that pass through the protective circuitry are evaluated by a noise discrimination function. If the number of sense events in a given cardiac cycle is greater than what would normally be expected from anything cardiac in origin, the pacemaker may revert to a noise mode. Noise reversion tends to occur if the sensed rate is greater than 7 events/s. A pacemaker's noise response is usually fixed-rate pacing at a rate set by the manufacturer and lasts as long as the interference is present, although the specific behavior should be verified by referencing the physicians' manual included with the pacemaker.

Output Circuitry and Pacing Thresholds

Output circuitry is usually composed of capacitors and electrical switches controlled by the microprocessor or logic circuitry. Output circuitry can deliver voltage in excess of the battery voltage, generally through the use of a charge pump. A charge pump provides the flexibility to program many discrete voltages and also allows for voltage regulation. The charge pump uses a number of small capacitors to dump charge into a larger capacitor. The larger capacitor is then discharged through the lead and heart tissue for a controlled period corresponding to the pulse width.

As mentioned previously, the voltage the battery can supply decreases as it depletes. Older pulse generators used voltage doublers to provide programmable output voltage that would decrease output as the battery depleted. For example, when battery voltage was at BOL, output settings provided by the manufacturer were roughly multiples of the BOL battery voltage (e.g., 2.8, 5.4, or 8.1 V). At or near ERI the device might actually be delivering the same multiples of the now diminished capacity (e.g., 2.2, 4.4, or 6.6 V). Even if a patient's pacing threshold remained constant, the output of the device might thus require readjustment because of declining battery voltage (23,24).

In the preceding example, the voltage is considered unregulated (i.e., there is no guarantee that the delivered voltage will match the programmed value). Use of unregulated outputs can affect the value reported for the

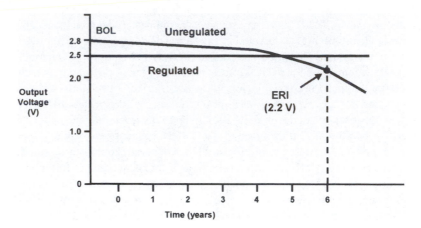

Fig. 2.9 Unregulated voltages decline as battery voltage declines, whereas regulated voltages are maintained at the programmed value.

pacing threshold, because the actual output does not necessarily match the programmed value (or, put another way, the programmed value may overstate the actual voltage being delivered). Toward ERI, it may appear as though the pacing threshold is increasing, requiring even more energy to stimulate the heart, whereas this may merely be the result of diminishing battery voltage. Therefore, it should not be mistaken as an impending lead or physiologic problem, especially when the lead impedances are relatively constant (25). Modern manufactured pacemakers with charge pumps have regulated output voltage so that even near the elective replacement point the device will deliver the programmed output (Fig. 2.9).

The output capacitor delivers its voltage, which decays exponentially throughout the pulse. The beginning voltage, called leading edge voltage (V_1), is nearest the programmed value, and the voltage at the end of the pulse, called the trailing edge (V_2), is dependent on the impedance of the lead system or load and the capacitance of the output capacitor. The amount of current delivered to the heart is related to the programmed voltage and the lead impedance, and is governed by Ohm's law ($V = IR$). An illustration of a typical pacemaker output is shown in Fig. 2.10.

Both the amplitude and width of the output pulse should be defined when expressing pacing threshold. As discussed in greater detail in Chapter 1, successful stimulation (or capture) of cardiac tissue follows a strength–duration relationship. At narrower pulse widths, it requires higher voltages to stimulate tissue, whereas at longer pulse widths the curve becomes asymptotic and flattens out (23,26).

Programming the output near the flat end of the strength–duration curve tends to be inefficient, as a point of diminishing returns is reached (prolonging pulse width does not enable further reductions in voltage). This minimum voltage at which the heart can be stimulated regardless of the pulse width is called the *rheobase* (Fig. 2.11). The pulse width that corresponds to two times the voltage at rheobase is known as the *chronaxie*; it closely approximates the point of minimum threshold stimulation energy (27,28).

The following formula describes the relationship of stimulus voltage, current, and pulse duration to stimulus energy:

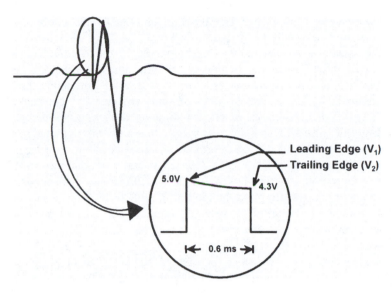

Fig. 2.10 Typical pacemaker output pulse showing leading and trailing edge voltage.

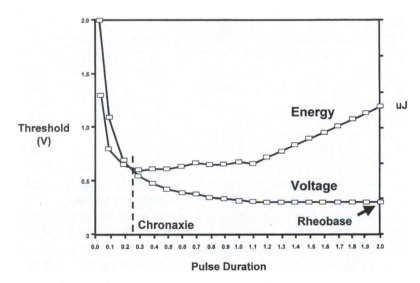

Fig. 2.11 Strength–duration curve shows relationship between stimulation voltage and pulse width. Points on and above the curve capture, whereas those below do not. At short pulse widths, a small change in pulse width is associated with significant change in threshold amplitude; however, this is not the case at longer pulse durations, where only a small change is seen. (Reprinted from Ellenbogen KA, ed. *Cardiac Pacing*, 2nd ed. Oxford: Blackwell Science, 1992, with permission.)

$$E = V^2 / R \times t$$

where E is the stimulus energy in microjoules; V, the stimulus voltage in volts; R, the total pacing impedance in KΩ; and t, the pulse width in ms. The chronaxie represents the point of minimum threshold energy on the strength–duration curve; at greater pulse widths only a slight reduction in threshold voltage is seen, whereas at lesser pulse widths threshold voltage and stimulation energy steeply increase. Thus, chronaxie pulse width and the point of minimal stimulation energy are usually fairly close.

It is essential to understand the threshold strength–duration relationship in order to be able to appropriately program stimulus amplitude and pulse width. For the most part, pulse generators allow evaluation of stimulation threshold by automatically decrementing either stimulus voltage (at a constant pulse width), or of pulse width (at a constant stimulus voltage). Considered independently of pulse width, stimulation voltage is usually programmed to about twice the threshold value so as to provide an adequate safety margin; if only pulse width is considered, the pulse width is generally programmed to at least three or more times the threshold value. Such methods provide similar safety margins with a threshold pulse duration of 0.20 ms or less; however, because of the flattened right tail of the strength–duration curve, an adequate stimulation safety margin may not result from tripling a threshold pulse duration greater than 0.3 ms (24).

Most modern pulse generators can reliably detect if an output pulse has resulted in appropriate cardiac depolarization by sensing the evoked potential of repolarizing tissue. This allows the pulse generator to automatically vary the output "on the fly" while maintaining an adequate safety margin. The result is some increase in longevity and reduction in the burden of checking thresholds and output adjustments during follow-up.

Factors such as method of measurement, type of electrode, drugs, and duration of lead implantation affect the threshold and strength–duration curve (29–31). In addition, a factor known as the *Wedensky effect* should sometimes be taken into consideration (32). The Wedensky effect posits that, when stimulation thresholds are measured by decrementing the stimulus voltage until loss of capture, the threshold is usually lower by 0.1–0.2 V than when gradually increased from subthreshold until capture is achieved.

Residual voltage may reside on a capacitor following discharge. This is because the pulse width may terminate discharge before all stored energy has had a chance to dissipate. This is an advantage because, when it is time for the next pacing pulse, it does not need to be charged from ground zero. When doing manual thresholds, however, this can create some distortions in threshold measurement. When a device is programmed from very high to very low voltage, it may take several cycles for the output capacitor to discharge enough energy to reach a lower voltage. Some manufacturers design in a means to accelerate the draining of energy following pulses. If taking threshold measurements and jumping from 8 to 1 V, wait a few cycles (8–10) to make sure the lower voltage has been reached.

Telemetry and Communications Circuit

Telemetry is a term used to describe measurement at a distance. Pacing devices are capable of wireless bidirectional telemetry; that is, the pulse generator and the programmer are able to transmit from one to the other. Telemetry is essential for modern pacemakers, which have so many programmable parameters and unique functions that may need to be adjusted or turned on or off (18,33). Some of the programmable parameters in modern pacemakers can be found in Table 2.4.

Table 2.4 Programmable parameters in modern pacemakers.

Pacing mode	A-V delay after pace/sense
Polarity	Magnet response
Lower rate	ERI mode reversion
Maximum pacing rate	Mode switching adjustments
Atrial/ventricular pulse widths	Setup of diagnostic functions (e.g., storage of IEGMs)
Atrial/ventricular pulse amplitudes	
Atrial/ventricular sensitivity	Antitachycardia features
Atrial/ventricular refractory period	Noninvasive programmed stimulation
Atrial/ventricular blanking period	Sleeping rate
Postventricular atrial refractory period	Hysteresis rate
Atrial refractory extension	Telemetry ON/OFF
Adaptive A-V delay	Rate responsive or sensor settings

When devices were nonprogrammable or had one or two programmable parameters, the ability to interrogate was not that important. One of the first units capable of transmitting information was a rechargeable pacemaker sold in the 1970s; telemetry was used to confirm proper alignment of the recharging head (18).

The next evolution was confirmation of programming. This was important, especially for parameters that were not obvious or visible on the surface ECG, such as pulse width and sensitivity. When multiprogrammable devices were introduced, telemetry was broadened to include stored programmable settings so that the physician could interrogate and get the programmable rate, output, and sensitivity. In the late 1970s pacemakers still were not able to assess information about the battery or lead system through the pacemaker programmer. The decay of the output pulse is dependent on the lead impedance. The slope of the wave-form between the pulse leading and trailing edge has been used as a relative indicator of lead impedance, so it was possible to tell if lead impedance was increasing or decreasing by looking at the slope from one visit to the next. Similarly, amplitude was examined as a reflection of battery voltage, because pacemakers in those days did not have regulated outputs (Fig. 2.12).

By the early to mid-1980s most pacemakers could directly measure lead impedance and battery voltage via telemetry. Some could even transmit this over the telephone along with programming data. As devices became more sophisticated – with a dozen or more programmable parameters – faster communication schemes were required to keep total communication time down to acceptable levels. One way to minimize communication time involved single-parameter programming. For example, initially if you wanted to program rate and output, you would have to do so sequentially. Faster communication schemes allowed programming of multiple parameters at the same time known as batch programming. All modern pacemakers allow batch programming (34).

A diagnostic tool that has achieved popularity is the ability to transmit an intracardiac electrogram, or IEGM, which enables the clinician to assess what the pacemaker is seeing. Much of this information is analyzed and transmitted in digital format. IEGMs can be transmitted in real time or stored and

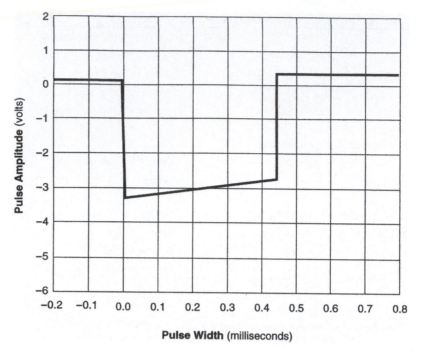

Fig. 2.12 Diagrammatic representation of an output pulse as it would appear on an oscilloscope.

retrieved for later use. Stored waveforms capability arrived later because it required considerable memory.

Pacemaker Interrogator

Programming Methods and Schemes

One of the simplest programming schemes involved the use of a magnet. Some early pacemakers could be programmed merely by holding a magnet directly over the pulse generator. When the reed switch closed, the pacemaker would step through a series of programmable rates; once the desired rate was achieved, the magnet was removed. In order to program a lower rate, the magnet would be held in place until the highest rate was achieved, after which the rate would jump to the lowest rate option, and the cycle would start again.

A more sophisticated magnetic programming scheme involves a pulsed electromagnetic field, usually generated by an electromagnet and picked up by a coil. Inductive coupling is used, whereby the magnetic field permeates the wire coil, inducing current flow in the coil. These currents are then picked up and decoded to form a programming command.

Better communication circuits involve the use of radiofrequency transmission, and incorporate a coil that acts as an antenna to receive incoming signals and encoded instructions. The same radiofrequency coil is used to transmit information back to the programmer. One relatively simple scheme is called *pulse position modulation*. This is a form of digital communication using what amounts to a Morse code, involving electromagnetic signals that are usually of a

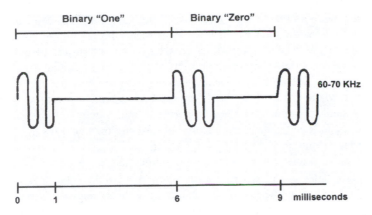

Fig. 2.13 Pulse position modulation scheme for radiofrequency communication between pacemaker and programmer.

specific frequency. The receiving coil is tuned to that frequency (called the *carrier frequency*). The carrier frequency is modulated to encode the information transmitted. There are two methods: amplitude modulation (AM) and frequency modulation (FM). In pacemakers, the common method is to turn the radiofrequency carrier on and off very rapidly to represent a binary code so that a "1" or a "0" would be represented by pulses (short versus long) (Fig. 2.13).

The higher the frequency of the radiofrequency transmission, the narrower the time interval between energy pulses and the more "1s" and "0s" that can fit into a unit of time. There are constraints with low-power radiofrequency transmission having to pass through the skin, air, body tissues, and metal shielding of the can; these become more pronounced at higher frequencies. All this serves to limit the transfer rate of information. In addition, because of the critical nature of the information, it needs to be encoded to provide security against error misprogramming. Therefore, for example, if a single parameter is programmed, signals will often echo back to the programmer to ensure that it was interpreted correctly. This takes additional time. Sometimes redundant information is sent just to ensure accuracy (or for security). Data encoding schemes for modern pacemakers are very sophisticated, so misprogramming owing to external sources of interference should be extremely rare. Encoded pulses generally occur with very precise timing. In addition, the transmission has to satisfy several conditions, one of which is that the electromagnetic energy detected by the pacemaker must be high enough to overcome the insensitivity of its receiving coil. This eliminates interference from other noise sources that have relatively low field strengths, and may also eliminate signals with frequencies outside the tuned range.

Sources of interference can prevent programming or communication, although misprogramming is unlikely as a result of these conditions. For example, a cathode-ray TV screen or similar medical equipment, if in close proximity to the programmer, might prevent programming from occurring. In addition, the programmer has to receive signals back from the pacemaker, very limited power source. Thus means that signals from the pacemaker are much weaker than those able to be sent by the AC line-powered programmer. Further, if the pacemaker is buried deep in a pocket, it usually requires that the wand of the programmer increase its receiving sensitivity, making it more susceptible to environmental noise.

Some programming schemes require dual interlock, where a reed switch must be closed before the device will be able to accept programming commands. Reed switch closure can also instruct the pacemaker to transmit a signal. This can be used as a locator beacon to properly align the programming wand.

Programmer software is constantly being updated by manufacturers to correct errors or malfunctions, add features, and expand or limit the range of programmable parameters. If there is a problem interrogating or programming a device, check with the manufacturer to ensure that the software level is appropriate for the model being programmed.

The latest improvement allows communication to occur over greater distances (20 ft.) and increased speeds without the aid of the programming wand or head. Specific frequency bands have been dedicated to medical devices so as to avoid interference with other types of equipment which rely on radio frequencies for their operation. This also enables pulse generators to be interrogated at home without active participation by the patient and has opened the door to remote patient follow-up.

Pacemaker Interrogation

Interrogation is important for modern pacemakers to ascertain the pacemaker's programmed parameters, and the state of the battery and lead; it also allows downloading of stored diagnostic data to evaluate the pacemaker–patient interaction. Interrogation often includes identification of the pacemaker model and serial number as well as determination of whether some special condition exists (e.g., replacement indicator, noise reversion, backup mode, etc). It is recommended that, prior to programming, the clinician routinely interrogate the system and, in fact, many programming protocols require interrogation to be the first operation (34,35).

There are a variety of interrogation data, generally falling into two categories: real-time measured data and stored event or programmed data. The former are immediate and instantaneous events as they occur, whereas the latter are previously recorded or programmed. Interrogation should include real-time measured data, which enable checking of lead integrity and battery status. A number of parameters can be measured for each pacing cycle and displayed as real-time data, including pulse amplitude, pulse width, sensitivity (if auto-gain is present in the device), current consumption, battery voltage, battery impedance, and lead impedance. Because these are measured values, they are only accurate within a specified tolerance. Repeated interrogation of measured parameters may seem very consistent and not vary by the tolerance specified, but the absolute value of that parameter may vary by the tolerance. For example, taking three readings of battery voltage might result in readings of, perhaps, 2.75, 2.74, and 2.75. Yet the actual values might be off by 10% from the real value of the voltage. This is why the battery voltage measured by telemetry is rarely the sole indicator of battery replacement. Instead, it is used for looking at trends in battery voltage. For example, an abnormal drop in battery voltage from one visit to the next might signify a problem that needs closer scrutiny. Knowing the total current drain from the battery allows for a rough calculation of longevity. Some of the newer devices have a gas gauge to estimate longevity. These are rough approximations because the exact battery capacity also varies from battery to battery and is dependent on many other variables.

Lead Impedance

The noninvasive measurement of lead impedance was one of the earliest uses of measured pacemaker telemetry. Following the deployment of lithium iodide it soon became clear that the pacing lead was more likely to fail than the pulse generator. In fact, lead failure has been responsible for most of the serious recalls and advisories in the pacing industry in the past 30 years (7,36,37). Therefore, it should come as no surprise that lead impedance telemetry became a valuable diagnostic tool to help with the assessment of lead integrity (38,39).

There are various techniques for measuring lead impedance. Voltage at the beginning and end of the output pulse is measured on the output capacitor in some pacemakers. This voltage decay is a function of the lead impedance. The higher the lead impedance, the slower the decay on the output capacitor. Because impedance changes throughout a pacing pulse, this method provides an average impedance and may differ slightly when compared to values obtained at implant by a pacing analyzer that generally measures impedance at the beginning of the pulse. Lead impedances generally do not change dramatically (>200 Ω) from one follow-up to the next unless there is a pending or immediate problem (40).

A drop in impedance is generally the result of failing insulation. In the case of a unipolar lead, this failure exposes the pacing coil to blood and allows current to leak directly back to the can from the site of the insulation breach. This results in less energy reaching the heart, which may cause loss of capture. In bipolar pacing systems an insulation breach sometimes occurs between the two conductor coils, which can result in a direct short, attenuating the energy being delivered to the heart and also causing sensing failure. When this occurs in a coaxial bipolar lead, a couple of things can happen. Inhibition or triggering can occur when the two conductors make and break contact (which will appear to be oversensing on the surface ECG); and/or loss of capture or inappropriate sensing may occur owing to the attenuation of pacing current and IEGM amplitude. Programming to a unipolar configuration may temporarily alleviate the loss of capture but does not prevent oversensing when the conductors make and break contact, so prompt lead replacement is recommended.

Both conductor fractures and connection problems can cause lead impedance to rise, often to high levels. This sets off a chain of events: the flow of current lessens so there is an attenuated output and capture is lost, and battery current drain decreases. Sensing can also be affected, with oversensing due to make-or-break connections or undersensing. Because the measurement of lead impedance occurs only during the pacing pulse, which is a fraction of the pacing cycle, intermittent fracture may not be reflected in the measured values; therefore, repeated measurements should be made if trouble is suspected. When troubleshooting, it may also be necessary to try other techniques for placing stress on the lead to induce the coils to separate (e.g., applying pressure or asking the patient to raise or move the arm on the side where the device is implanted). Some devices have the capability of taking beat-by-beat lead impedance measurements over a prolonged period and displaying them graphically, increasing the sensitivity/specificity of lead impedance as a diagnostic tool (Fig. 2.14) (41).

Once again, the cautious approach is to take repeated measurements if an unanticipated value is encountered. Repeat the measurement and correlate

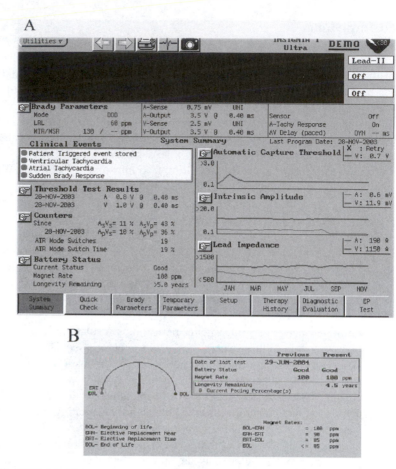

Fig. 2.14 (**a**). Status screen and modern pulse generator capable of storing sequential measurements of lead impedance and displaying the trend graphically. (**b**). Interrogator screen shows battery status in an easily understandable pattern.

with clinical symptoms (such as lack of sensing) if readings are high. It is an unusual case when a physician would take remedial action based on telemetry alone, with the possible exception of a device under an advisory that has a failure mechanism with a known footprint related to a dramatic change in lead impedance or other measured value.

Stored Data

Implantable devices are now capable of accumulating information on patient–device interaction. This is stored digitally and accessible via the programmer. Most devices report on the percentage of paced versus sensed events by chamber. This can be further subdivided by rate range. An example of one such display is shown in Fig. 2.15.

These data are useful for assessing device utilization as well as for providing information on tuning the lower rate and rate–response settings. For example, making a 5 ppm adjustment in the lower rate can dramatically lower the percentage of pacing during sleeping hours.

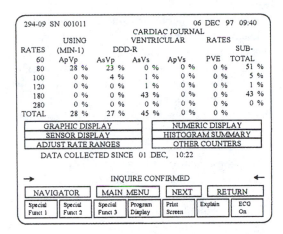

Fig. 2.15 Interrogation screen from Intermedics Marathon DR pacemaker showing percentages of cycles in five categories by rate range (ApVp, atrial pace followed by ventricular pace; AsVp, atrial sense followed by ventricular pace, etc.; PVE, premature ventricular event).

Stored data are particularly useful in helping to assess the frequency and duration of tachyarrhythmias. Digital stored data include mode switching episodes, tachycardia counters, and segments of stored IEGMs from either or both chambers. Most of the aforementioned are time stamped. The amount of stored data is constantly increasing because of the availability of low-power memory and may, in the very near future, have many of the capabilities of external cardiac event recorders (42). The physician is also given the option of clearing the diagnostic data registers, and should be aware that certain programming operations may clear them unintentionally. It is always prudent to print out any diagnostic data that you would like to access at the time of the initial interrogation, before any reprogramming takes place.

Clinical Issues

Although the historical evolution of cardiac pacing technology is interesting from an engineering perspective and bears directly on the operating characteristics of today's devices, it is the clinical observations that are of overriding interest. Knowing how the pacemaker works can help the clinician distinguish a true malfunction that requires intervention from seemingly "quirky" behavior that can arise in the presence of external interference or unusual cardiac rhythms. An understanding of the design considerations and operating characteristics can prevent an inappropriate intervention (e.g., explant) in response to a behavior that may appear wrong to the clinician, yet may in fact represent normal operation. Just like a computer, pacemakers generally "do what they are told."

All the major pacing companies have 24h technical assistance help lines staffed with individuals trained to assist with troubleshooting their company's devices. The physicians' manual is an excellent reference for learning how the device works, although it rarely covers all the idiosyncrasies one might encounter in the clinic.

Without getting into the complexity of design, it should be noted that each manufacturer has its own way of implementing even basic functions. This chapter focuses on some of the more common behaviors, and the reader should recognize that a specific device may be at variance with what has been presented here.

New circuit designs and battery chemistries in future devices will, in all likelihood, change the way devices work. The trends are already apparent, with increasing automatic functions and greater degrees of data storage and retrieval. Many of these efforts are focused on improving ease of use rather than changing the therapeutic benefits of pacing. For example, devices now have the ability to continuously adjust the pacing output, sensitivity, and AV delay. When combined with the capability of longer-distance telemetry the need for an in-office assessment may be reduced or eliminated. Design engineers are constantly trying to balance the need for clinical flexibility and ease of use. Future generations of microprocessors and improvements in packaging technology will enable pacemakers to take on tasks that normally require the intervention of the clinician. Although increasing automation and ease of use appear likely to decrease the amount of time and effort needed to administer pacemaker therapy, a basic understanding of the engineering considerations always benefits both physician and pacemaker recipient.

References

1. Euler KJ. Electrochemical and radioactive power sources for cardiac pacemakers. In: Shaldach M, Furman S, eds. *Advances in pacemaker technology*. New York: Springer-Verlag, 1975:329–343.
2. Sanders RS, Lee MT. Implantable pacemakers. *Proc IEEE* 1996;84(3):480–486.
3. Parsonnet V, Berstein AD, Perry GY. The nuclear pacemaker: is renewed interest warranted? *Am J Cardiol* 1990;66:837–842.
4. Furman S, Garvey J, Hurzeler P. Pulse duration variation and electrode size as factors in pacemaker longevity. *J Thorac Cardiovasc Surg* 1975;69(3):382–389.
5. Tyers GFO, Brownlee RR. Power pulse generators, electrodes, and longevity. *Prog Cardiovasc Dis* 1981;23:421–434.
6. Levine PA. Magnet rate and recommended replacement time and indicators of lithium pacemakers. *Clin Prog Pacing Electrophysiol* 1986;4:608–618.
7. Tyers GF. FDA recalls: how do pacemaker manufacturers compare? *Ann Thorac Surg* 1989;43(3):390–396.
8. Sanders RS, Barold SS. Understanding elective replacement indicators and automatic parameter conversion mechanisms in DDD pacemakers. In: Barold SS, Mugica J, eds. *New perspectives in cardiac pacing*. Mount Kisco, NY: Futura Publishing, 1988.
9. Schuchert A, Kuck K-H. Influence of internal current and pacing current on pacemaker longevity. *PACE* 1994;17(1):13–16.
10. Intermedics Technical Manual. *Relay DDDR pacing system*. Angleton, TX: Intermedics, 1992.
11. *Medtronic News*. Winter 1986–1987:15.
12. Barold SS, Falkoff MD, Ong LS, et al. Resetting of DDD pulse generators due to cold exposure. *PACE* 1988;11:736–743.
13. Schroeppel EA. Current trends in cardiac pacing technology. *Biomed Sci Technol* 1992;1:90–102.
14. Marathon DDDR pacing system technical manual. Angleton, TX: Intermedics, 1996.
15. Furman S, Hurzeler P, DeCaprio V. Cardiac pacing and pacemakers: III. Sensing the cardiac electrogram. *Am Heart J* 1977;93:794–801.
16. Barold SS, Ong LS, Heinle RA. Stimulation and sensing thresholds for cardiac pacing: electrophysiologic and technical aspects. *Prog Cardiovasc Dis* 1981;24:1–29.
17. Platia EV, Brinker JA. Time course of transvenous pacemaker stimulation impedance, capture threshold, and electrogram amplitude. *PACE* 1986;9:620–625.

18. Levine PA. *Why programmability? Indications for and clinical utility of multiparameter programmability*. Sylmar, CA: Pacesetter Systems, 1981.

19. Halperin JL, Camunas JL, Stern EH, et al. Myopotential interference with DDD pacemakers: endocardial electrographic telemetry in the diagnosis of pacemaker-related arrhythmias. *Am J Cardiol* 1984;54:97–102.

20. Irnich W. Muscle noise and interference behavior in pacemakers: a comparative study. *PACE* 1987;10:125–132.

21. Baker RG Jr, Falkenberg EN. Bipolar versus unipolar issues in DDD pacing (Part II). *PACE* 1984;7:1178–1182.

22. Belott PH, Sands S, Warren J. Resetting of DDD pacemakers due to EMI. *PACE* 1984;7:169–172.

23. Furman S, Hurzeler P, Parker B. Clinical thresholds of endocardial cardiac stimulation: a long-term study. *J Surg Res* 1975;19:149–155.

24. Furman S, Hurzeler P, Mehra R. Cardiac pacing and pacemakers: IV. Threshold of cardiac stimulation. *Am Heart J* 1977;94:115–124.

25. Tanaka S, Nanba T, Harada A, et al. Clinical experience with telemetry pacing systems and long-term follow-up: clinical aspects of lead impedance and battery life. *PACE* 1983;6:A30–A110.

26. Hill WE, Murray A, Bourke JP, et al. Minimum energy for cardiac pacing. *Clin Phys Physiol Meas* 1988;9(1):41–46.

27. Irnich W. The chronaxie time and its practical importance. *PACE* 1980;3:292–301.

28. Kay GN. Basic concepts of pacing. In: Ellenbogen KA, ed. *Cardiac pacing*, 2nd ed. Boston, MA: Blackwell Science, 1996:37–123.

29. Furman S, Parker B, Escher DJW, et al. Endocardial threshold of cardiac response as a function of electrode surface area. *J Surg Res* 1968;8(4):161–166.

30. Stokes K, Bornzin G. The electrode-biointerface: stimulation. In: Barold SS, ed. *Modern cardiac pacing*. Mount Kisco, NY: Futura Publishing, 1985:37–77.

31. Mugica J. Progress and development of cardiac pacing electrodes (Part I). *PACE* 1990;13:1558.

32. Timmis GC, Westveer DC, Holland J, et al. Precision of pacemaker thresholds: the Wedensky effect. *PACE* 1983;6:A60–A220.

33. Sholder J, Levine PA, Mann BM, et al. Bidirectional telemetry and interrogation in cardiac pacing. In Barold SS, Mugica J, eds. *The third decade of cardiac pacing: Advances in technology and Clinical Applications*. Mt. Kisco, NY: Futura Publishing, 1982:145–166.

34. Sanders RS, Levine PA, Markowitz HT. Pacemaker diagnostics: measured data, event marker, electrogram, and event counter telemetry. In: Ellenbogen KS, Kay N, Wikoff B, eds. *Clinical cardiac pacing*. Philadelphia: WB Saunders, 1995:639–655.

35. Castellanet MJ, Garza J, Shaner SP, et al. Telemetry of programmed and measured data in pacing system evaluation and follow-up. *J Electrophysiol* 1987;1:360–375.

36. Phillips R, Frey M, Martin RO. Long-term performance of polyurethane pacing leads: mechanisms of design-related failures (Part II). *PACE* 1986;9:1166–1172.

37. Furman S, Benedek ZM. The implantable lead registry. Survival of implantable pacemaker leads (Part II). *PACE* 1990;13:1910–1914.

38. Clarke M, Allen A. Early detection of lead insulation breakdown. *PACE* 1985;8:775.

39. Schmidinger H, Mayer H, Kaliman J, et al. Early detection of lead complications by telemetric measurement of lead impedance. *PACE* 1985;8:A23–A90.

40. Winokur P, Falkenberg E, Gerard G. Lead resistance telemetry: insulation failure prognosticator. *PACE* 1985;8:A85–A339.

41. *Pulsar technical manual*. St. Paul, MN: Guidant Corp, 1999.

42. Sanders R, Martin R, Frumin H, et al. Data storage and retrieval by implantable pacemakers for diagnostic purposes. *PACE* 1984;7:1228–1233.

Modes of Pacemaker Function

Paul J. Wang, Amin Al-Ahmad, Henry H. Hsia, and Paul C. Zei

NASPE/BPEG Generic Pacemaker Code

The method of classifying pacemaker function originated in 1987 as the NASPE/BPEG (North American Society of Pacing and Electrophysiology/ British Pacing and Electrophysiology Group). The classification has subsequently been modified to incorporate rate modulated pacing and multisite pacing (Table 3.1). The first position of the code indicates the cardiac chamber paced, which may include the atrium (A), ventricle (V), both the atrium and ventricle (dual or D), or none (O). The second position represents the cardiac chamber sensed, which may include the atrium (A), ventricle (V), both the atrium and ventricle (dual or D), or none (O). Manufacturers may also designate S for a single chamber that is sensed, or paced, either the atrium or the ventricle. The third position represents the function that the pacemaker performs: triggered (T), inhibited (I), triggered and inhibited (dual or D), or none (O). *Triggered* refers to pacing in the chamber paced after the sensing of intrinsic activity in the chamber sensed. The sensing and pacing may occur in different chambers. For example, in the VAT mode, the atrium is sensed and the ventricle is paced. If the response is *inhibited*, sensing of intrinsic electrical activity results in no pacing in the designated chamber. In dual sensing, the sensing of intrinsic ventricular events inhibits pacing (inhibited) in the ventricle or atrium for a programmed time interval. Sensing of intrinsic atrial events results in inhibition of an atrial pacing and triggers pacing in the ventricle after a specified AV delay or interval.

The fourth position represents rate modulation. Rate modulation is the ability of the pacemaker to adjust the timing events according to signals from a sensor. Sensors such as motion, acceleration, temperature, or impedance may be used to adjust the pacing rate to the physical activity or metabolic demands of the patient.

The fifth position in the code is the site of multisite pacing. There may be only a single site in each chamber that is paced (O). There may be two sites within the atria that are paced (A) or there may be two sites within the ventricles that are paced (V). There may be two pacing sites within both the atria or ventricles (D).

Table 3.1 NASPE/BPEG code.

I Chamber paced	II Chamber sensed	III Response to sensing	IV Rate modulation	V Multisite pacing
O = None	O = None	O = None	O = None	O = None
A = Atrium	A = Atrium	I = Inhibited	P = Rate modulation	A = Atrium
V = Ventricle	V = Ventricle	T = Triggered		V = Ventricle
D = Dual (A + V)	D = Dual (A + V)	D = Dual (both inhibited and triggered)		D = Dual (A + V)

Table 3.2 Commonly encountered pacing modes.

Mode	Advantages	Disadvantages	Clinical uses
AAI (R)	Requires only a single lead Simple	Slow ventricular rates may develop if AV block occurs.	Sinus node dysfunction without AV node dysfunction
VVI (R)	Requires only a single lead Simple	During pacing, atrioventricular synchrony is not preserved.	AV block in a patient with atrial fibrillation
DDD (R)	AV synchrony is maintained for patients with sinus node and AV node disease.	Requires two leads More complex	Bradycardia caused by sinus node disease or AV node disease
VDD (R)	AV synchrony is maintained for patients with AV node disease. One specially designed lead can be used.	AV synchrony is lost if the patient develops sinus bradycardia.	Bradycardia caused by AV node disease
DDI (R)	AV synchrony is maintained during atrial pacing.	AV synchrony is not maintained during atrial sensing.	For patients with sinus bradycardia and intermittent sensing of atrial arrhythmias. Occasionally used as a stand-alone pacing mode but more frequently as a mode switching pacing mode.

Pacing Modes

Pacing modes are programmed according to the needs of the patient. Pacing modes that are commonly used are shown in Table 3.2.

Single Chamber

AAI Mode

In the AAI mode, atrial pacing will occur when the atrial rate falls below the programmed atrial rate (Fig. 3.1). When no intrinsic atrial activity has occurred within a specified interval (lower rate limit, LRL), atrial pacing occurs. The letter "P" is commonly used to indicate an atrial sensed event and the letter "A" is commonly used to indicate an atrial paced event. The intervals used in the AAI timing intervals are PP, AA, AP, and PA. Ventricular events such as a conducted QRS complex or a premature ventricular beat are not sensed in the AAI mode. The AAI mode is only appropriate in patients with intact

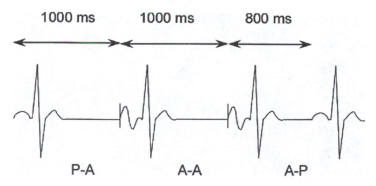

Fig. 3.1 Normal function in the AAI mode. P refers to a sensed atrial event. A refers to a paced atrial event. Two successive events may be described as one of the following intervals: AA, PP, PA, and AP. The LRL (also called the low rate timer) in the example shown is 60 bpm. Thus, the PA and AA intervals are 1,000 ms. The P wave is sensed and after 1000 ms the low rate timer expires. An atrial paced event occurs (A). A second atrial paced event occur after 1000 ms. Sensing atrial activity inhibits the pacemaker output and resets the low rate timer. In the AAI mode, timing is based on the time between atrial events.

atrioventricular (AV) conduction. The selection of AAI as a permanent pacing mode compared to VVI and DDD modes is dependent on many factors and is highly influenced by individual physician and regional practice patterns. The patient suspected to have AV conduction disturbances should receive a DDD pacemaker. Some clinicians assess the AV conduction system by pacing the atrium at rest; if AV Wenckebach occurs at atrial pacing rates of 120 bpm or greater, some clinicians implant an AAI pacemaker without a ventricular lead. In contrast, many physicians implant a dual chamber pacemaker in patients with sinus rhythm and intact AV conduction; the device can be programmed to the AAI mode of function until ventricular pacing is required because of the development of AV block.

In summary, the patient receiving an AAI pacemaker should be in sinus rhythm without evidence of AV conduction abnormalities.

VVI Mode

In the VVI mode, the ventricular rate is not allowed to fall below the programmed rate (Fig. 3.2). This is achieved through sensing and pacing in the ventricle so that pacing will occur when no intrinsic ventricular activity has occurred within a specified interval (LRL). Inhibition of ventricular pacing occurs after a sensed ventricular event to prevent ventricular pacing at rates above the programmed rate. Atrial events are not sensed in the VVI mode.

In general, patients with AV conduction abnormalities and organized atrial activity should be programmed to the DDD mode. Patients with chronic atrial fibrillation are the best candidates for VVI or VVIR pacing modes.

Dual Chamber

DDD Mode

In the DDD mode, atrial and ventricular sensing and pacing are present (Fig. 3.3). Atrial and ventricular stimulus delivery are inhibited by ventricular-sensed events. In addition, intrinsic atrial events are "tracked" (or followed) by ventricular-paced events if AV conduction does not occur within a specified interval (the AV

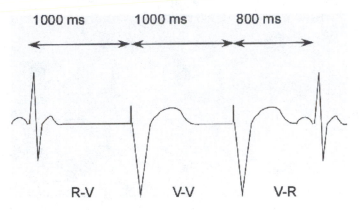

Fig. 3.2 Normal function in the VVI mode. R refers to a sensed ventricular event. V refers to a paced ventricular event. The two successive events may be expressed as the following intervals: VV, RR, RV, and VR. The LRL (also called the low rate timer) in the example shown is 60 bpm. Thus, the VV and RV intervals are 1,000 ms. A sensed ventricular event (first QRS complex) resets the low rate timer. The low rate timer expires without a sensed ventricular event and a ventricular stimulus is provided. After two successive ventricular-paced events (second and third QRS complexes), sinus rhythm at a rate of 75 bpm (800 ms) with normal AV conduction inhibits pacing. In the VVI mode, AV synchrony is not maintained during pacing.

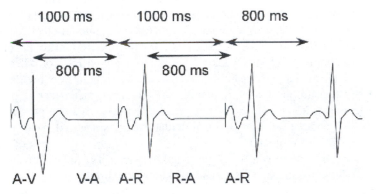

Fig. 3.3 Normal function in the DDD mode. R refers to a sensed ventricular event. V refers to a paced ventricular event. P refers to a sensed atrial event. A refers to a paced atrial event. The atrioventricular relationship is described by the intervals PR, AR, AV, PV. P waves (sensed atrial events) may be tracked and followed by ventricular-paced events (PV) or P waves may be conducted to the ventricle (PR). Atrial-paced events may be followed by a ventricular-paced event (AV) or may be conducted to the ventricle (AR).

interval, AVI). Thus, in the patient with sinus rhythm and AV block, the paced ventricular rate will follow the sinus rate as it responds to metabolic changes. Atrial pacing occurs when intrinsic atrial activity is not present (e.g., sinus arrest or sinus bradycardia). DDD pacing in patients with impaired AV conduction and sinus rhythm permits the most physiologic pacing, particularly when sinus bradycardia is also present.

VDD Mode
In the VDD mode, there is sensing in both the atrium and the ventricle and pacing only in the ventricle (Fig. 3.4). Sensed ventricular events result in inhibition of ventricular pacing, as in the DDD mode. Sensed atrial events

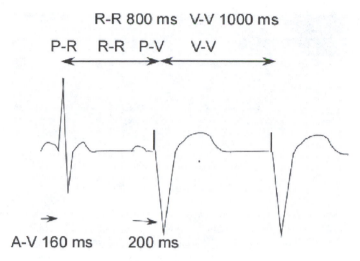

Fig. 3.4 VDD mode. Sensing occurs in both the atrium and the ventricle but pacing only occurs in the ventricle. Atrial events may be tracked and followed by ventricular-paced events (PV). When there is a sinus pause or a PVC not followed by a P wave, the next event will be a ventricular-paced event rather than an atrial-paced event in DDD mode. The AV and PV intervals can be programmed separately in some pulse generators.

are tracked as in DDD mode. The VDD mode has been used in patients with AV block and sinus rhythm. However, because the atrium is not paced, VDD mode generally is not used in patients with impaired sinus node function. Atrioventricular synchrony is not maintained in the VDD mode if sinus bradycardia develops. The VDD mode is most commonly used with a special pacing system that employs a single lead with a specially designed "floating" atrial electrode for sensing and a conventional ventricular electrode for pacing and sensing.

DDI Mode
In the DDI mode, ventricular events result in inhibition of pacing stimulus delivery in the atrium and ventricle, although the atrium and ventricle are sensed and paced; therefore, it is very similar to the DDD mode (Fig. 3.5). However, atrial tracking does not occur because sensing atrial activity only inhibits an atrial stimulus and does not trigger the AVI. Therefore, the atrial and ventricular rates are fixed and cannot adjust to metabolic needs.

The absence of tracking prevents rapid ventricular pacing during transient atrial tachyarrhythmias. Prior to the development of mode switching (described later), the DDI and DDIR modes were frequently used to prevent tracking of atrial tachyarrhythmias. When sinus bradycardia is present, AV pacing at the programmed rate occurs. However, when the sinus rate exceeds the programmed rate, there is no coordination between the atrial event and the ventricular-paced event.

Other Modes
The less commonly used modes fall into several groups. Asynchronous modes (AOO, VOO, DOO) are not frequently used as permanent modes. They may be used as temporary modes to assess capture and prevent sensing of electromagnetic interference (Fig. 3.6). Triggered modes (e.g., VVT and AAT) also

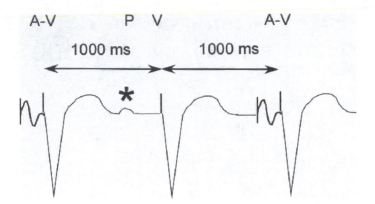

Fig. 3.5 In DDI mode, sensing and pacing occur in both the atrium and ventricle. A sensed atrial event results in inhibition of pacing in the atrium. A sensed ventricular event results in inhibition of pacing in the atrium and the ventricle. Atrial tracking is not present. In the example, after delivering an atrial stimulus, a ventricular stimulus is delivered, because no intrinsic ventricular activity was detected. After the first AV paced QRS complex, a P wave is sensed (*), which inhibits atrial pacing. A ventricular stimulus is delivered because no ventricular activity is sensed. After the second paced QRS complex, no atrial activity is sensed so an atrial stimulus is provided. In the DDI pacing mode, if the patient has intact AV conduction the pacemaker functions essentially as an AAI pacing system. However, if AV conduction block occurs, AV synchrony is maintained during atrial pacing but not during atrial sensing.

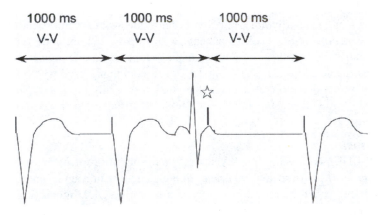

Fig. 3.6 In the VOO mode, ventricular output occurs at a constant rate and no ventricular sensing occurs. In the example, the low rate is 60 bpm (1,000-ms intervals). Stimulus output occurs despite the presence of an intrinsic QRS complex. The third stimulus do not result in ventricular capture because it was delivered during a period when the ventricular tissue was still refractory.

are not frequently used as permanent modes. They were used diagnostically prior to the introduction of marker channels and intracardiac electrograms. A pacing stimulus is delivered at the precise time of sensing a ventricular or atrial event in VVT and AAT, respectively (Fig. 3.7). In this way, the pacing stimulus is used to mark each sensed event and may be used for evaluating undersensing or oversensing. Lower rate pacing is also present in the VVT- and AAT-triggered modes.

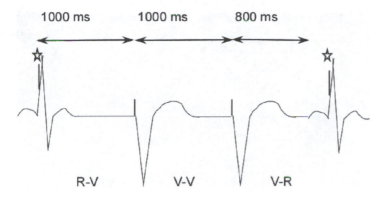

Fig. 3.7 In the VVT mode, a pacing stimulus is given immediately on sensing of ventricular events.

VDI is used infrequently as a permanent mode; however, some devices mode switch to VDI or VDIR. It has the same function as the VVI mode but with atrial sensing capability for diagnostic purposes (e.g., counting episodes of atrial tachyarrhythmias). Pacing only occurs in the ventricle while sensing occurs in both the atrium and ventricle.

The DVI mode provides pacing in the atrium and the ventricle, but sensing occurs only in the ventricle (Fig. 3.8). Therefore, like the DDI mode, atrial tracking does not occur. However, unlike DDI, atrial events do not inhibit atrial output. Because atrial output occurs without regard to intrinsic atrial activity, in the DVI mode atrial pacing after an intrinsic atrial event may precipitate an atrial tachyarrhythmia. This pacing mode is essentially obsolete.

Timing Cycles

There is a series of programmable parameters that determine the intervals between intrinsic and paced events for each mode. These intervals are often called "timing cycles." Pacing intervals can be described in milliseconds (ms) or beats per minute (bpm). There are 60,000 ms in each minute because there are 1,000 ms in each second and 60 s in each minute. The value of 60,000 is derived by using the number of milliseconds in one second (1,000) and multiplying by the number of seconds in 1 min (60). It is useful to keep several equivalent values in mind because clinicians are more familiar with bpm: 200-bpm and 300 ms intervals, 150-bpm and 400-ms intervals, 120-bpm and 500-ms intervals, 100-bpm and 600-ms intervals, and 60-bpm and 1,000-ms intervals.

Single Chamber Timing Cycles

VVI

The VVI mode is characterized by sensing and pacing in the ventricle so that pacing will occur when no intrinsic ventricular activity has occurred within a specified interval defined by the LRL. There are four intervals in the VVI pacing mode: VV, VR, RV, and RR where R is an intrinsically sensed R wave and V is a ventricular-paced event. VVI pacemakers have three basic timing cycles that must be considered: LRL, hysteresis rate, and the ventricular refractory period.

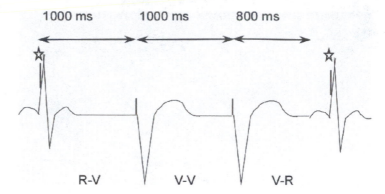

Fig. 3.8 In the DVI mode, the atrium and ventricle are paced with sensing only in the ventricle. The LRL is 1,000 ms. The AVI is set at 200 ms. An intrinsic P wave (star) is not sensed. AV pacing occurs because no R wave is sensed.

Lower Rate Limit: The most basic interval in the VVI mode is the LRL (Fig. 3.2). The LRL determines the maximum length of time the pacemaker circuitry will wait for intrinsic ventricular activity (R wave) to occur before initiating a ventricular output stimulus. When there is no hysteresis (see the following), this interval applies both to the period from the last intrinsic event to the first-paced event or the period from the last-paced event to the next-paced event (Fig. 3.2). Therefore, the LRL determines the longest interval permitted between any two ventricular events. The LRL may also be called the minimum rate, lower rate timer, and basic (or base) pacing rate. The LRL is usually expressed in pulses per minute.

Hysteresis Rate: When the parameter called hysteresis is programmed ON, the maximum interval from the last intrinsic event to the first paced event may exceed the interval from the last paced event to the next paced event (Fig. 3.9). Therefore, the pause following any intrinsic R wave is greater than the interval from one paced beat (V) to the next paced beat (V). This results in the pacemaker being inhibited from delivering an output pulse if the intrinsic rate exceeds or is equal to the hysteresis rate. The word *hysteresis* is derived from Latin, meaning "to lag behind."

When hysteresis is programmed ON, the maximum V-to-V interval is defined as the lower rate interval and the maximum R-to-V interval is defined as the hysteresis interval. The hysteresis rate is expressed either in the absolute rate in beats per minute or the hysteresis interval is expressed in milliseconds. Alternatively, the hysteresis rate may be expressed as the number of beats per minute subtracted by the lower rate or the number of milliseconds added to the lower rate interval. In some cases the hysteresis rate is recorded as a percentage subtracted by the lower rate.

Hysteresis permits initiation of pacing only when the intrinsic rate has slowed significantly. However, the pacing occurs at a more rapid rate once pacing is initiated. Hysteresis is used most commonly to decrease the frequency of pacing. For example, the patient's intrinsic rate may range from 45 to 60 bpm. If hysteresis were programmed OFF, setting the LRL to 55 bpm would result in pacing a large proportion of the time. If the hysteresis rate was 40 bpm and the LRL was 55 bpm, pacing would only occur occasionally when

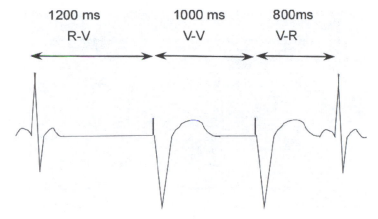

Fig. 3.9 VVI mode with hysteresis. The ventricular-paced rate is 60 bpm, so the LRL is 1,000 ms. However, pacing will not occur after an intrinsic R wave until the hysteresis interval of 1,200 ms is reached. When pacing begins, the pacing rate will be the lower rate interval of 1,000 ms.

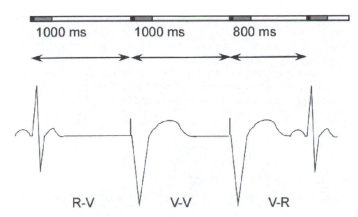

Fig. 3.10 Example of VVI pacing from Fig. 3.2 with refractory periods added. The ventricular refractory period (VRP) has an initial absolute blanking period (solid black). During the absolute blanking period, no sensed events are noted in the marker channel. During the remaining portion of the VRP, the relative refractory period (gray), sensed events may be noted, but the LRL will not be reset.

the intrinsic rate dropped to 40 bpm. When pacing occurred, it would continue at 55 bpm until the intrinsic rate exceeded this rate. The LRL is thought to be the slowest rate that is hemodynamically desirable. The hysteresis interval is selected as an interval longer than the lower rate interval that does not result in symptoms. Therefore, it would be unusual to program a hysteresis interval longer than 1,500 ms (<40 bpm).

Ventricular Refractory Period: The ventricular refractory period (VRP) (expressed in milliseconds) is the interval following a paced or sensed ventricular event during which the pacemaker is not responsive to detectable ventricular signals (Fig. 3.10). It contains two parts: the absolute refractory period and the relative refractory period. All signals are ignored during the absolute refractory period. Noise sampling occurs within the relative refractory period. The purpose of the VRP is to prevent oversensing of the T wave or the output pulse stimulus afterpotential.

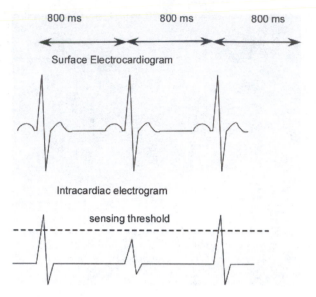

Fig. 3.11 Intrinsic cardiac depolarization can be recorded at the pacing lead electrode and measured by the pacemaker. This signal is called an electrogram. In this example, the electrogram is measured from the ventricular lead and is caused by ventricular depolarization. The signal has an amplitude of 8 mV. This signal would not be "seen" by the pacemaker if the sensitivity is set to 10 mV. However, by lowering the sensitivity value to 5 mV (making the pacemaker more sensitive), the intrinsic depolarization would be "seen" and pacemaker timing cycles would be reset when appropriate.

Problems with Sensing in VVI Mode

Intrinsic cardiac activity results in a wave of depolarization that is detected by the pacing electrodes and generates a signal called an electrogram. The pacemaker uses a programmable setting called the sensitivity to identify cardiac signals (Fig. 3.11). Any electrical signal that is larger than the programmed sensitivity setting is defined as intrinsic cardiac activation. The signal is defined as ventricular if it is sensed in the ventricular channel (which presumably receives input from a pacing lead placed in the ventricle), and atrial if the signal is detected in the atrial sensing channel. Setting the sensitivity value to a higher value makes the pacemaker less sensitive (a larger signal is required to be defined as intrinsic activity). Problems with undersensing and oversensing can be observed.

Oversensing: Oversensing is the sensing by the pacemaker circuitry of cardiac or extracardiac signals other than the ventricular depolarization, resulting in inappropriate inhibition or triggering. In the VVI mode, oversensing does not result in triggering; therefore, it is manifested only by inhibition (Fig. 3.12).

Oversensing can be caused by myopotentials, T-wave sensing, lead fracture, a loose set screw, electromagnetic interference, environmental noise, or a malfunction of the pacemaker circuitry. The diagnosis of oversensing in the VVI mode is made because of longer than expected intervals. For example, an RR interval greater than 1,000 ms is most consistent with ventricular oversensing if the lower rate interval is 1,000 ms and hysteresis is not programmed ON.

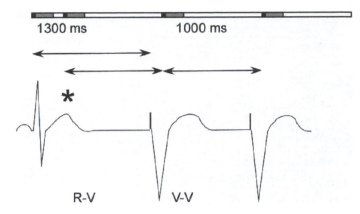

1300 ms   1000 ms

R-V   V-V

Fig. 3.12 Oversensing of the T wave in the VVI mode. In this example, the lower rate interval is 1,000 ms. The T waves following the intrinsic QRS complex and the paced complex are sensed, resulting in a longer than programmed escape interval. The problem would be solved by programming a longer VERP.

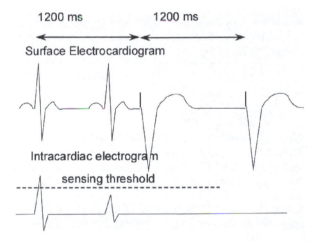

1200 ms   1200 ms

Surface Electrocardiogram

Intracardiac electrogram

sensing threshold

Fig. 3.13 Undersensing of an intrinsic R wave in the VVI mode. In this example, the lower rate interval is 1,200 ms. The first intrinsic R wave is sensed, initiating the lower rate interval timing. However, because the second intrinsic R wave is not sensed, a paced ventricular event occurs shortly after it. The interval between the ventricular-paced events (VV) is 1,200 ms.

Undersensing: Undersensing is the failure of the pacemaker circuitry to recognize and respond to appropriate cardiac signals (Fig. 3.13). Undersensing can occur if the pacemaker is programmed to a low sensitivity setting, a lead insulation break is present (which can lead to attenuation of the intracardiac signal), the amplitude of the signal is too low, an event falls within a refractory period (functional undersensing), the rate of change in voltage per change in time (slew rate) is too slow, or there is a malfunction of the pacemaker circuitry. In the VVI mode, undersensing results in paced events occurring earlier than expected as defined by the LRL. Premature ventricular beats may generate an electrogram with a lower amplitude than normal ventricular activation and result in undersensing (Fig. 3.14).

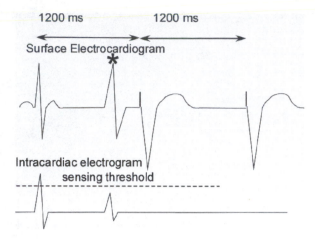

Fig. 3.14 Undersensing of a premature ventricular contraction. In the example, surface ECG, refractory periods and intracardiac electrograms (EGM) are shown. The electrograms generated by native QRS complexes are 7 to 8 mV and are appropriately sensed (because the sensitivity is set to 5 mV). The electrogram from the premature ventricular contraction is only 4 mV and is not sensed by the pacemaker. The problem can be corrected by reducing the sensitivity value to 3 mV (making the pacemaker "more" sensitive).

AAI

The AAI mode is characterized by sensing and pacing in the atrium so that pacing will occur when no intrinsic atrial activity has occurred within a specified interval defined by the LRL. The timing cycles in the AAI pacing mode are very similar conceptually to the timing cycles of the VVI pacing mode.

Lower Rate Limit: The most basic interval in the AAI mode is the LRL. The LRL determines the maximum length of time the pacemaker circuitry will wait for intrinsic atrial activity (P wave) to occur before initiating an atrial output stimulus (Fig. 3.1). When there is no hysteresis (see the following), this interval applies both to the period from the last intrinsic event to the first paced event or the period from the last paced event to the next paced event.

Hysteresis Rate: When the parameter called hysteresis is programmed ON, the maximum interval from the last intrinsic event to the first paced event exceeds the interval between consecutive paced events (Fig. 3.15). Therefore, the pause following an intrinsic P wave is greater than the interval from one paced beat (A) to the next paced beat (A). This results in the pacemaker being inhibited from delivering an output pulse if the intrinsic rate exceeds or is equal to the hysteresis rate.

When hysteresis is programmed ON, the maximum A-to-A interval is defined as the lower rate interval and the maximum P-to-A interval is defined as the hysteresis interval.

Atrial Refractory Period: The atrial refractory period (ARP) (expressed in milliseconds) is the interval following a paced or sensed atrial event during which the pacemaker ceases to be responsive to detectable atrial signals. It contains two parts: the absolute refractory and relative refractory periods (Fig. 3.16).

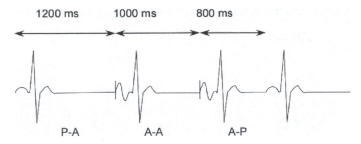

Fig. 3.15 AAI mode with hysteresis. In this example, the LRL is 1,000 ms with a hysteresis interval of 1,200 ms. Pacing occurs after the hysteresis interval of 1,200 ms. The next atrial paced event (third P wave) occurs after 1000 ms.

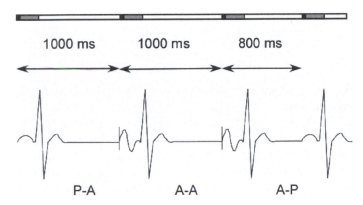

Fig. 3.16 Example of AAI pacing from Figure 3.1 with refractory periods added. The ARP has an initial absolute refractory period (abs). No sensed events are noted in the marker channel during the absolute refractory period. During the remaining portion of the ARP, the relative refractory period (rel), sensed events may be noted, but the LRL will not be reset.

All signals are ignored during the absolute refractory period, and noise sampling occurs within the relative refractory period. The purpose of the ARP is to prevent oversensing of the output pulse stimulus afterpotential, the atrial electrogram produced by the atrial stimulus, or ventricular depolarization.

Sensing Problems in AAI Mode

Oversensing: Oversensing is the sensing by the pacemaker circuitry of cardiac or extracardiac signals other than the native atrial depolarization, resulting in inappropriate inhibition (Fig. 3.17).

Oversensing can be caused by sensing of the farfield R wave, myopotentials, lead failure, a loose set screw, electromagnetic interference, environmental noise, or a malfunction of the pacemaker circuitry. The diagnosis of oversensing in the AAI mode is made because of longer than expected intervals. For example, if the lower rate interval is 1,000 ms and hysteresis is not programmed ON, an AA interval greater than 1,000 ms is most consistent with atrial oversensing.

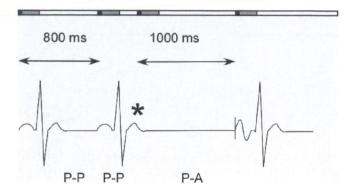

Fig. 3.17 Oversensing in AAI. In this example, the lower rate interval is 1,000 ms. After the second appropriately sensed atrial event, atrial oversensing occurs (asterisk), resetting the timing cycles.

Undersensing: Undersensing is the failure of the pacemaker circuitry to recognize and respond to appropriate cardiac signals (Fig. 3.18). Undersensing can occur if the pacemaker is programmed to a low sensitivity setting; for example, undersensing will occur if the intrinsic P wave amplitude is 3 mV and the sensitivity is set to a value of 5 mV. Other potential causes of undersensing include lead insulation breaks (which cause attenuation of the signal amplitude), an event falling within a refractory period ("functional undersensing"), or malfunction of the pacemaker circuitry. In the AAI mode, undersensing results in paced events earlier than expected as defined by the LRL.

Dual Chamber Timing Cycles

The DDD mode combines dual chamber pacing, inhibition of pacing by atrial and ventricular-sensed events, and atrial tracking (Fig. 3.19). Atrial-sensed events result in the inhibition of atrial pacing output; ventricular -sensed events result in the inhibition of ventricular pacing output. Tracking is a function in which atrial-sensed events are followed by a ventricular-paced event within a specified range of rates. There are four forms of the atrioventricular interval in the DDD mode: AV, PV, AR, PR, where P and R are sensed intrinsic P waves and R waves and A and V are paced atrial and ventricular events. There are several fundamental intervals in the DDD mode, including the AVI, the postventricular atrial refractory period (PVARP), the total atrial refractory period (TARP), the ventricular refractory period (VRP), low rate interval, and upper rate interval.

AV Interval

Fundamentals of the AVI
The AVI is an important programmable parameter in dual chamber pacing modes. It represents the interval between the atrial event and the ventricular event (Fig. 3.19). Hemodynamically, the pacemaker AVI simulates the human PR interval, allowing time for atrial contraction and ventricular filling. Therefore, the AVI must be adjusted to optimize hemodynamic function. There are

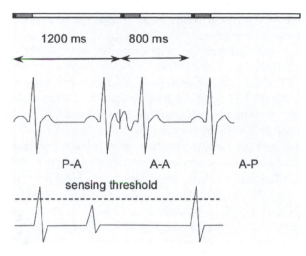

Fig. 3.18 Undersensing in AAI. In this example, the lower rate interval is 1,200 ms. The first P wave is sensed but the second P wave is not sensed. An atrial-paced event occurs 1,200 ms after the first P wave.

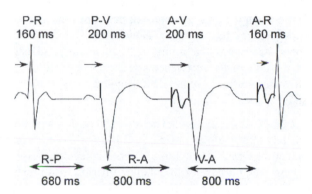

Fig. 3.19 DDD mode. P and A refer to intrinsic and paced atrial events, respectively. R and V refer to intrinsic and paced ventricular events, respectively. Four successive events result in the intervals PR, PV, AV, and AR. In ventricular-based timing, the interval from an intrinsic or paced ventricular event (R or V) to the subsequent atrial-paced event is defined by the atrial escape interval (AEI).

several factors that play roles in determining the optimal programming for the AVI at rest: (a) optimizing the timing of atrial contraction and ventricular contraction, (b) attempting to maintain intrinsic AV conduction, and (c) desiring to conserve battery energy. The maintenance of intrinsic AV conduction has some hemodynamic benefit because normal activation of the ventricles is associated with improved ventricular contraction and cardiac output. However, the optimal range for the AVI at rest is approximately 100–200 ms, centering at approximately 150 ms. Patients with markedly prolonged PR intervals may exhibit impaired left ventricular filling because atrial contraction occurs so far in advance of ventricular contraction. In addition, in patients without AV block, often one tries to minimize pacing in the ventricle in order to conserve battery energy and optimize the hemodynamics of ventricular contraction. Therefore, there are a number of factors that determine the optimal programmed AVI at rest. In patients with AV block or markedly prolonged PR interval, the AVI is typically programmed at 150 ms to optimize ventricular filling. In patients with a normal PR of about 150 ms, the AVI may be programmed at 200 ms or greater in order to prevent fusion of the paced depolarization and the intrinsic ventricular depolarization, permitting normal ventricular activation and conserving battery energy. In PR intervals of approximately 240 ms or greater, one balances the potential improvement in hemodynamics with intrinsic depolarization with the optimal AV delay for filling and battery energy consumption. Although these are general guidelines, currently, the optimal method is to use Doppler echocardiographic measurements of cardiac output and mitral flow.

There may be special circumstances in which the AVI is programmed to be short. Pacing at the right ventricular apex with a short AV delay decreases the left ventricular outflow tract gradient in obstructive hypertrophic cardiomyopathy. Depolarization initiated from the right ventricular apex results in motion of the right ventricular septum away from the outflow tract, which diminishes the gradient. When AV conduction is intact, the AVI interval must be short enough to achieve capture of the right ventricle before intrinsic conduction depolarizes the ventricle. However, a short AVI can be associated with poor atrioventricular timing and worsening of diastolic function. Although some individuals experience significant improvement with pacing, several multicenter studies have not demonstrated a large functional improvement measured by exercise testing.

AVI and Ventricular Safety Pacing: The AVI may be divided into several periods. Immediately after the onset of the AVI is a period of absolute blanking, during which atrial signals are not used for timing cycles, noise reversion, or mode switching. The purpose of the blanking period is to prevent sensing of the afterpotential after a pacing stimulus, double counting of an intrinsic atrial depolarization, and inappropriate inhibition of ventricular output by oversensing of the atrial stimuli on the ventricular channel, a phenomenon called ventricular crosstalk. During AV pacing, the atrial stimulus may be sensed on the ventricular channel (crosstalk), resulting in inhibition of pacing, and possibly ventricular asystole. Therefore, a mechanism to prevent crosstalk is particularly important. Ventricular safety pacing was designed specifically to prevent ventricular crosstalk inhibition or inhibition caused by noise in the ventricular channel (Fig. 3.20). After an atrial-paced event, any sensed event after the absolute blanking period within the safety pacing (or crosstalk sensing) window results in a ventricular-paced event at a shorter AVI, usually between 80 and 120 ms. As a result, if the atrial stimulus is detected on the ventricular channel, a ventricular-paced event will occur rather than be inhibited, as it otherwise would be. The short AVI is easy to identify and also makes the possibility of a ventricular-paced event falling on the T wave less likely. Factors that increase the likelihood of crosstalk include high atrial output settings (e.g., 5 V at 1 ms) coupled with high ventricular sensitivity (e.g., 1 mV).

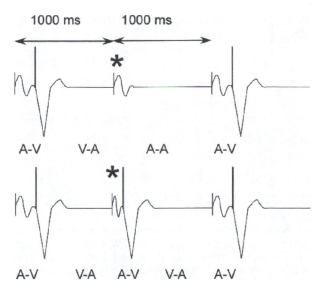

Fig. 3.20 Safety pacing. In the upper and lower panels, the first complex is an AV paced beat. In the upper panel, the second complex is only an atrial paced complex not followed by a ventricular paced complex (asterisk). The electrical stimulus of ths atrial complex is sensed on the ventricular channel, resulting in ventricular inhibition, a phenomenon called crosstalk. In the lower panel, the second complex is an AV paced beat but the AV interval is marked shorter, approximately 110 ms (asterisk). This shortened AV represents safety pacing, a feature in which a ventricular paced complex occurs when sensing occurs during the second phase of the AV interval. The first phase of the AV interval is the absolute blanking period. The third phase of the AV interval is the alert period, during which a ventricular sensed event results in ventricular inhibition.

Differential AVI: Differential AVI is present when there is a difference in the AVI following an atrial-sensed event (PV) compared to the AVI following an atrial-paced event (AV). In most cases, there is a modest delay from the time of onset of the P wave to the time that the atrial depolarization is sensed by the atrial lead. This time varies based on intracardiac conduction properties, the site of spontaneous depolarization, and the location of the atrial lead. By programming the AVI after a sensed atrial event shorter than the AVI after a paced atrial event, the time from onset of depolarization (whether spontaneous or owing to an atrial stimulus) to the end of the AVI will be approximately the same.

AVI Hysteresis: With positive AV/PV hysteresis, one interval of a PV will result in lengthening of the PV to permit conduction (Fig. 3.21). There may be a search function in which the AVI is extended so that intrinsic conduction may resume, resulting in maintenance of the extended AVI. The purpose of positive hysteresis is to provide a shorter AVI when there is AV block, necessitating pacing, and a longer AVI when there is AV conduction, permitting normal ventricular activation. Positive hysteresis is most suited for the patient with variable AV conduction times. Negative AV/PV hysteresis, in contrast, is designed to maintain ventricular capture without fusion. If an R wave is sensed within the AVI, the AVI is shortened (Fig. 3.22). A search function may be used to look for intrinsic AV conduction, resulting in a shorter AVI on the subsequent beats.

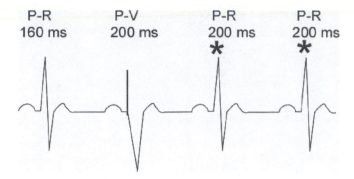

Fig. 3.21 Positive AV hysteresis. In the first complex, there is intrinsic conduction more rapid than the programmed AV interval of 200 ms. In the second complex, AV conduction has slowed, resulting in a P-synchronous ventricular complex. In positive AV hysteresis there is prolongation of the AV interval to promote AV conduction. This extension of the AV interval is seen in the second and third complexes (asterisks). Only if the AV conduction further slows would ventricular pacing resume.

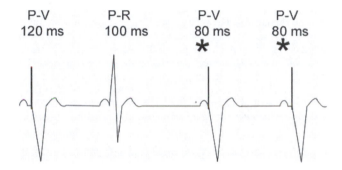

Fig. 3.22 Negative AV hysteresis. Negative AV hysteresis has been employed in order to maintain ventricular pacing in conditions such as hypertrophic cardiomyopathy. The PV interval is 120 ms in the first cycle. Intrinsic conduction has spontaneously become faster, resulting in a shortened PR interval of 100 ms in the second cycle. The AV interval is automatically shortened by 20 to 80 ms in order to maintain ventricular pacing (asterisks).

Postventricular Atrial Refractory Period

The PVARP is an interval during which the atrial channel is refractory to intrinsic atrial signals and is initiated by a paced or sensed R wave. The PVARP is used to prevent retrograde P waves from being tracked, resulting in pacemaker-mediated tachycardia (PMT). As discussed later, the PVARP also limits the maximum rate that tracking can occur, the maximum tracking rate (MTR).

PMT is the consequence of a repetitive sequence of retrograde conduction to the atrium and tracking of this atrial activity, resulting in a paced ventricular event (Fig. 3.23). When this sequence continues, the PMT may continue without cessation and require termination. PMT often occurs at the MTR but may be below it if the retrograde conduction time is long. The PVARP is generally programmed longer than the retrograde conduction time in order to prevent PMT.

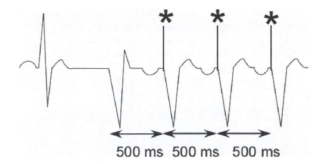

Fig. 3.23 Pacemaker mediated tachycardia (PMT). In this case, a premature ventricular contraction (second QRS complex) leads to retrograde ventriculo-atrial (VA) conduction. The atrial activity occurs after the PVARP has expired, is sensed, and leads to ventricular pacing, which again is associated with VA conduction. An incessant tachycardia can be initiated and sustained in this way.

There are several important consequences of programming a PVARP that is unnecessarily long. As indicated in the following, the PVARP has important effects on the behavior of the pacing system at high atrial rates. In addition, the occurrence of atrial pacing after an intrinsic P wave may result in the induction of paroxysmal atrial arrhythmias such as atrial fibrillation.

Total Atrial Refractory Period

The TARP is the total period of time that sensed activity on the atrial channel does not result in tracking. The TARP is the sum of the PVARP and the AV interval, because during both these periods atrial activity does not result in a paced ventricular event (Fig. 3.24). Atrial activity may be tracked during the remaining part of the timing cycle. As discussed in the following, the TARP defines the atrial rate at which 2:1 atrial tracking occurs.

Ventricular Refractory Period

The ventricular refractory period (VRP) is the period following a paced or sensed ventricular event during which a sensed ventricular event during which a sensed ventricular event will not reset the timing cycle. The ventricular refractory period for dual chamber pacing systems and single chamber ventricular pacing systems have a similar range of values and functions. The purpose of the interval is to prevent oversensing of the T wave or the output pulse stimulus afterpotential. The VRP is usually programmed at approximately 180 to 280 ms.

Lower Rate Behavior

Atrial pacing occurs when intrinsic atrial activity is not present at the programmed lower interval or shorter. This is referred to as lower rate behavior. The most basic interval in the DDD mode is the LRL. The LRL determines the maximum length of time the pacemaker circuitry will wait for intrinsic atrial or ventricular activity (P wave or R wave) to occur before initiating an atrial output stimulus. Because both atrial and ventricular events may be used in determining the timing cycles, one must consider two basic methods of establishing the LRL rules: ventricular based timing and atrial-based timing (Figs. 3.25 and 3.26).

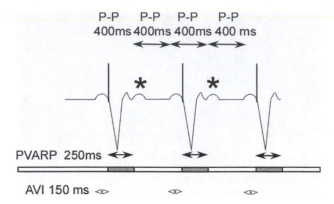

Fig. 3.24 The TARP is the sum of the AVI and postventricular refractory period (PVARP). The TARP defines the interval in which the shortest interval at which atrial activity is tracked because atrial events do not lead to atrial tracking during the TARP. In this case, the TARP is 400 ms, the sum of the AV interval of 150 ms and the PVARP of 250 ms.

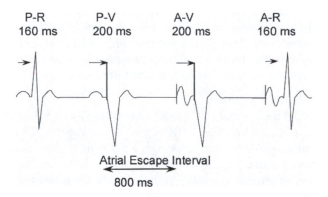

Fig. 3.25 Ventricular-based timing DDD lower rate behavior. The atrial escape interval (AEI) is initiated after a ventricular-paced or sensed event. Ventricular based timing leads to slightly faster heart rates if native conduction is present. In this example, the LRL is set to 60 bpm, so the AEI is 800 ms for an AVI of 200 ms.

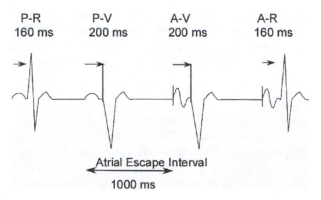

Fig. 3.26 Atrial-based timing DDD lower rate behavior. The timing of atrial-paced events is determined by the previous atrial-sensed or paced events. A short PR or AR interval owing to intrinsic conduction will not affect the timing of the next atrial-paced event, in contrast to ventricular based timing.

In ventricular-based timing, the occurrence of a ventricular-sensed event results in creation of an atrial escape interval (AEI). If another ventricular-sensed event occurs within the AEI, another atrial escape interval will begin after the second ventricular-sensed event, and so on. If an atrial-sensed event follows a ventricular event after the PVARP expires, the atrial-sensed event will trigger the AVI. If neither an atrial-sensed event nor a ventricular-sensed event occurs within the AEI, then an atrial-paced event will occur. All atrial-paced events are followed by a ventricular-paced event unless an intrinsic ventricular event has occurred within the AVI. In ventricular-based timing, the atrial escape interval (AEI) is determined by subtracting the AVI from the lower rate interval. In the presence of intact AV conduction, ventricular-based timing may result in the effective ventricular rate faster than the programmed LRL. This phenomenon occurs because the interval from the atrial-paced event to the ventricular-sensed event is shorter than the programmed AVI and the atrial escape interval (AEI) is calculated by subtracting the AVI from the LRL (Fig. 3.25).

In atrial-based timing, the interval between atrial-sensed or atrial-paced events and subsequent atrial-paced event is the lower rate interval (Fig. 3.26). If a ventricular-sensed event not preceded by an atrial event occurs, the time to the next atrial-paced event will be the atrial lower rate interval. In some pacemakers, the time to the next atrial-paced event is the lower rate interval minus the programmed AVI. Sensed atrial events are tracked and followed by a ventricular-paced event at the AVI unless the ventricular-paced events following atrial-sensed events raises the ventricular rate above the upper rate limit. In that case the ventricular-paced event is delayed so that the VV interval is at the upper rate limit (see the following).

Upper Rate Behavior

When the intrinsic atrial activity exceeds the LRL, the atrial events will be followed by a ventricular-paced event if an intrinsic R wave does not occur by the end of the programmed AVI. For most patients, during sinus rhythm, "tracking" atrial activity is desirable at all physiologic rates. However, it is possible for pathologic atrial arrhythmias to result in an intrinsic atrial rate far in excess of the appropriate sinus rate. In such cases, it is particularly important to have an algorithm that limits the tracking rate. Otherwise, a rapid atrial tachyarrhythmia could result in rapid ventricular-paced rates that might result in hypotension, hemodynamic collapse, or dangerous ventricular arrhythmias. Therefore, for the DDD and VDD pacing modes a separate upper rate interval is required. The upper rate interval defines the shortest interval at which tracking of atrial activity can occur. The maximum rate at which atrial activity is tracked 1:1 is called the upper rate limit or maximum tracking rate (MTR).

The DDD upper rate behavior defines the function of the pacemaker at atrial rates above the upper rate limit. When the intrinsic atrial rate exceeds the upper rate limit, the ventricular-paced events are delayed until the upper rate interval is reached (Fig. 3.27). This results in extension of the AVI. After one or more cycles of extension of the AVI, the P wave may occur within the PVARP. When the atrial event falls within the PVARP, it is not sensed and therefore does not result in a ventricular-paced event. The subsequent atrial-sensed event is tracked or followed by a ventricular-paced event. This results in a pattern of progressively prolonging atrial-sensed (P) to ventricular-paced events (V) intervals followed by an atrial event that is not tracked. This pattern

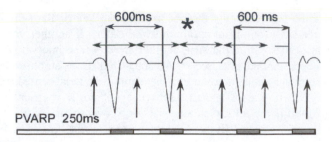

Fig. 3.27 DDD upper rate behavior. The arrows indicate the P waves that occur at 500 ms cycle length or 120 bpm. In this case the upper tracking rate cycle length is 600 ms or 100 bpm. In the first complex the P wave is followed by a ventricular paced event with a normal AV interval. However, the second P wave is followed by a ventricular paced event at a longer than normal AV interval because the VV interval cannot exceed the upper rate limit cycle length. The third P wave occurs with the PVARP and therefore is not tracked (asterisk). The fourth P wave is again tracked and followed by a ventricular paced event.

resembles AV Wenckebach behavior during AV conduction and therefore is termed "pseudo-" or "electronic"-AV Wenckebach.

When the intrinsic atrial rates are sufficiently rapid, they reach the 2:1 interval. At these rates, there are exactly two intrinsic atrial events for every ventricular-paced event. The 2:1 tracking occurs when one P wave falls within PVARP and one P wave falls outside PVARP. This occurs exactly when the intrinsic atrial interval is equal to the sum of the PVARP and the AVI, called the TARP.

For patients with complete AV block, attention should be paid to the appropriate upper rate interval and 2:1 interval. The upper rate interval should be sufficiently high to permit 1:1 tracking through most activities. In addition, the TARP should be programmed to a value that is lower than the interval equal to the upper rate limit. This maneuver provides a period of "electronic" Wenckebach before the development of 2:1 block (Fig. 3.27). However, as described in the following, programming the TARP to allow a maximal tracking rate greater than the maximal sinus rate provides the most physiologic method for pacing. There are several factors that may be important in programming the upper rate interval appropriately.

For patients with intrinsic AV conduction, programming the upper rate limit is mainly focused on avoiding tracking atrial arrhythmias at rapid rates. Therefore, the upper rate limit can be programmed at a relatively low rate, particularly when a specific response to atrial arrhythmias, such as mode switching (discussed later), is not available. In contrast, for patients with AV block, there is a need to program the upper rate so that ventricular tracking occurs during exertion. However, for patients with AV block it is particularly important to avoid 2:1 AV block at rapid sinus rates. It is important to calculate the 2:1 rate using the total atrial refractory period (TARP = AVI + PVARP). It is most desirable to have the 2:1 rate exceed the expected maximal sinus rates. This is particularly challenging when two conditions are present: the retrograde conduction time is long and the maximum sinus rate is extremely fast. For example, if the patient achieves sinus rates of 200 bpm, using a PVARP of 200 ms and an AV delay of 140 ms, 2:1 block will occur at 340 ms, or about 170 bpm. Thus, as the patient exercises, the ventricular rate will precipitously fall to about 85 bpm when the sinus rate reaches 171 bpm. In such situations there are a number of possible solutions. One solution is to program the pacemaker to a DDDR mode, allowing sensor-driven pacing to occur during exertion. Another solution is to program the AVI to a "rate adaptive" AVI so that at rapid ventricular rates the AVI shortens. Another solution is to program the PVARP to an extremely short interval, relying on the PMT termination algorithms if retrograde conduction is present. Both of these maneuvers reduce the TARP, which increases the rate at which 2:1 block occurs. In the example, if the TARP at peak exercise was <300 ms, 2:1 block would not occur. Finally, β-blockers can be used to reduce the maximal sinus rate.

Rate Adaptive Pacing

Hemodynamics of Exercise and Rate
Both heart rate and stroke volume increase significantly during exercise, resulting in a marked increase in cardiac output. Both heart rate and stroke volume are determined by sympathetic stimulation. Normal individuals are able to increase their heart rate severalfold during exercise. There are a number of algorithms that have been used to estimate the heart rate during exercise. The following simple equation has been used to estimate the maximum predicted heart rate for age:

$$\text{maximum heart rate} = 220 - \text{age}$$

Exercise protocols that incorporate graded levels of work have also been used to observe the increase in heart rate at multiple levels of exercise.

Chronotropic Incompetence
Some individuals exhibit an impaired heart rate response to increased metabolic demand. Patients in sinus rhythm may have sinus node dysfunction, leading to decreased maximal sinus rates with exertion. Patients in chronic atrial fibrillation may have a slow ventricular response that does not increase adequately with exertion. In both these cases, the heart rate response to exertion may be blunted, a condition termed chronotropic incompetence. The definitions of chronic incompetence are varied: It is sometimes defined as failure to achieve 75% of the maximal predicted heart rate. "Relative" chronic incompetence refers to a blunted heart rate response at lower levels of exertion and is more difficult to define.

Rate-Adaptive Pacing
Rate-adaptive pacing was developed to provide a heart rate response to meet the metabolic needs of the patient with chronotropic incompetence. For the patient in sinus rhythm, DDDR pacing provides an adequate heart rate with atrial pacing at rates that may exceed the maximal sinus rates. For the patient in chronic atrial fibrillation, VVIR pacing provides an adequate heart rate response with ventricular pacing.

Rate-adaptive pacing relies on the performance of sensors to provide input to the pacemaker regarding the appropriate heart rate for the activity. An algorithm then converts the sensor data to a specific heart rate response. Currently available sensor systems are so-called "open loop" because an external algorithm must be applied to the sensor data to determine an appropriate heart rate. A "closed-loop" system would internally regulate the heart rate response based on the sensor data without requiring adjustment of an external algorithm.

Sensors

Motion Sensors

Activity or motion sensors are the simplest and most widely used sensors in pacemakers today. The basic motion sensor is a piezoelectric crystal that creates a small amount of electrical energy when subjected to force. The electrical energy is measured and used as an indicator of activity. The piezoelectric crystal is mounted on the generator case so that it detects vertical motion. Basic activities such as walking and running activate this vertical motion sensor.

The activity sensor generates signals that vary in amplitude and frequency. These signals from the activity sensor are counted and used with the algorithm to determine the sensor-driven rate. The activity sensing pacemakers generally respond rapidly to motion, resulting in an almost immediate increase in heart rate with activity. The heart rate response continues to rise with increasing workloads. Most pacemakers utilizing sensor driven pacing have a programmable threshold and slope of response to modulate the heart rate response to each individual patient. The threshold determines the amount of activity that is required to initiate sensor-driven pacing and may be programmed from low to high. The slope determines the change in heart rate for a given increase in sensor-indicated activity and also may be programmed from low to high. Most pacemakers have a deceleration mode that permits the rate to decrease gradually rather than fall precipitously after termination of exercise because cessation of activity rapidly results in an absence of sensor activity. A rapid deceleration results in a rapid fall in heart rate.

A piezoelectric crystal mounted within the pacemaker generator case may be used to sense forward and backward motion rather than vertical motion. Such a sensor is considered an accelerometer. The accelerometer may be more sensitive to many activities such as bicycling because the accelerometer is able to detect anterior and posterior motion, whereas the vertical motion is minimal. Activities such as riding on a subway or horseback are less likely to cause an excessive increase in the heart rate response using an accelerometer-based pacemaker compared to an activity motion sensor. Clinical studies in normal volunteers have suggested that the accelerometer-based sensors may simulate sinus rate behavior more closely than vibration-based piezoelectric sensors (1). In a study of 63 patients, an accelerometer-based sensor DDDR pacemaker demonstrated longer exercise time, 9.15 ± 0.65 min versus 8.23 ± 0.71 min for the DDDR and DDD modes, respectively, during metabolic exercise testing (2).

Minute Ventilation

The transthoracic impedance varies with each respiration because the volume of air in the lungs changes. The transthoracic impedance may estimate the lung tidal volume. An estimate of minute ventilation is obtained by multiplying the estimated tidal volume by the respiratory rate. Minute ventilation correlates well with oxygen consumption and measurements of metabolic need.

A pacemaker system has been developed to measure the transthoracic impedance through the delivery of a series of minute electrical impulses from the pacemaker lead. These impulses are of such low amplitude that they do not result in myocardial capture and do not result in significant battery depletion. A minute ventilation sensor is commercially available, including in the United States, and has been shown to correlate well with oxygen consumption during exercise. In addition, minute ventilation sensors have been combined with activity sensors in the same pulse generators, providing the option of using either sensor or a "blended" sensor (3). Clinical studies have demonstrated that a variety of lead configurations may be used for minute ventilation devices (4).

Evoked QT Interval

Ventricular repolarization is highly dependent on sympathetic stimulation. The QT interval of the paced complex also varies with sympathetic tone. Therefore, it has been proposed that the QT interval from an evoked or paced complex might be used as a sensor. The T wave after a paced complex is measured. Various algorithms may be used to result in pacing slightly faster than the intrinsic rate if the intrinsic rate is faster than the programmed lower rate. Measurements of the evoked QT must also take under consideration the pacing rate because the pacing rate also affects the QT. Patients may vary according to the effect of sympathetic tone on the change in evoked QT and adjustments may need to be made for individual patients. In a clinical study of nine patients with activity sensor pacemakers and five patients with QT sensor pacemakers, the activity sensor provided a more prompt response, whereas the QT sensor resulted in rates more proportional to the level of exertion (5). Combinations of the evoked QT sensor and the activity sensor are currently being explored.

Other Sensors

There are a variety of other sensors that have been developed and studied experimentally or clinically. The paced depolarization integral, similar to the evoked QT, also utilizes an evoked potential but instead examines the ventricular depolarization. The sensor measures the area of the poststimulus ventricular depolarization, which increases with activity (6).

A temperature sensor has also been used clinically for adaptive rate pacing. As exercise continues, the body temperature rises in a nonlinear manner. Cooler blood returns from the extremities with the onset of activity, resulting in a fall in core temperature. Algorithms using temperature as a sensor must consider these phenomena and respond appropriately.

The intracardiac impedance has been used to estimate right ventricular volume. Similar to the minute ventilation sensor, a minute electrical current is emitted. The impedance across the right ventricular lead may reflect the volume of the right ventricle, potentially providing an estimate of cardiac output and stroke volume. The pre-ejection interval also may be used to reflect sympathetic tone. This interval is the time from the onset of electrical ventricular depolarization to the onset of ventricular ejection. The onset of ventricular ejection is determined using the right ventricular impedance signal to indicate a change in ventricular volume. In a clinical study of 10 patients, the pre-ejection interval decreased significantly with exercise from 137.7 ± 17.8 to 103.0 ± 21.6 ($p < 0.05$) (7).

Sensors that measure pH, mixed venous O_2, and oxygen saturation have been investigated. In a study of 14 patients with an implanted pacemaker with central venous oxygen saturation sensor, the oxygen saturation measured by the pacemaker correlated well with samples from the right ventricle ($n = 105$; $r = 0.73$; $p < 0.001$) (8). These sensors have been shown to correlate with activity; however, it has been difficult to develop a durable, robust sensor for an implantable device.

A recent sensor has been the incorporation of a microaccelerometer into the pacemaker lead tip itself. This sensor may detect changes in peak endocardial acceleration (PEA), which may correlate with the dP/dt maximum of the heart. Clinical results have suggested this sensor may be effective in determining the sensor driven rate in exertion and pharmacologic stimulation. In a clinical study of 15 patients, dobutamine resulted in PEA from $1.1\,g \pm 0.5$ to $1.4\,g \pm 0.5$ ($p < 0.001$) (9). Early studies have also suggested that hemodynamic changes in neurocardiogenic syncope may be detected using this system.

Sensor Combinations

Each sensor has its own limitations that prevent it from accurately simulating metabolic needs during all conditions of exertion and sympathetic stimulation. Activity sensors do not respond to mental stress, anxiety, or fever, which are all potent causes of sinus tachycardia in normal individuals. In addition, some forms of exertion, such as cycling, may not be adequately sensed by activity sensors. In addition, sensors such as minute ventilation may not react as rapidly as some activity sensors to changes in activity.

Sensors may also result in inappropriate sensor-driven pacing. Mechanical vibration or tapping of an activity pacemaker generator, for example, result in rates that are inappropriate for metabolic demands.

Combination sensors have been introduced in order to provide a means of achieving the optimal responsiveness and appropriateness of sensor-driven pacing. In such devices, one may select the individual sensor or a combination or integrated sensor. For example, a minute ventilation sensor may be combined with an activity sensor. Using a blended sensor, an algorithm is used to describe the contribution of each sensor. The simplest algorithm is the use of the sensor that results in the most rapid rate. This permits the most responsiveness but will not prevent inappropriate response to stimulation of various kinds. More complex algorithms provide a check of one sensor against the other, modulating the response of one sensor if it is outside a range specified by the other sensor (10). The combination sensor resulted in a higher heart for ascending stairs compared with descending stairs in a clinical study comparing an activity sensor to a combination activity and minute ventilation sensor. In contrast, the activity sensor alone resulted in a higher heart rate with descending stairs (11).

Currently, minute ventilation and activity, QT interval and activity, and accelerometer and microaccelerometer (PEA) are clinically be used as dual sensor combinations.

Rate Adaption Algorithms

There are several algorithms that involve rate-modulation of a programmable parameter. The rate adaptive AV delay is one such example. By programming a rate adaptive AV delay, the physiologic shortening of the AVI with exercise may be mimicked. As the atrial rate increases, the AVI automatically decreases. The rate adaptive AVI permits a higher maximum tracking rate and 2:1 tracking rate, because the latter is equal to the sum of the PVARP and the AVI. Programming a rate adaptive interval may be quite important in the patient with impaired AV conduction but persistent retrograde conduction in whom a shorter PVARP cannot be programmed.

A sensor-adaptive PVARP is available in some generators. The PVARP decreases as the sensor-determined rate increases. This permits maintaining a longer PVARP at rest while permitting a higher maximum tracking rate and 2:1 atrial tracking rate. However, the use of this parameter is based on a physiologic decrease in the retrograde conduction time with exertion. Although this is expected with normal conduction, some individuals who have retrograde conduction may not shorten the retrograde conduction time to the extent that is assumed by the algorithm.

Noise Response

In addition to safety pacing, manufacturers have developed noise response algorithms that reduce the effects of "noise" owing to lead problems and from internal and external sources of interference. Most commonly, a noise sampling period within or just after the ventricular refractory period is used. The noise sampling period can have a duration of 60 to 200 ms and sensed event during this period is interpreted as noise. The sensed noise will reset the ventricular refractory period or noise sampling period without resetting the lower rate timer. A ventricular stimulus is delivered when the lower rate timer expires. The effects of noise on pacing system function depend on the effects on the size of the sensed signals in the ventricular channel. If the signals are relatively small (e.g., an environmental source with a low field strength), no effects on pacing system function are observed. Inhibition of pacemaker outputs is observed in the presence of intermittent noise. Asynchronous pacing at the programmed low rate occurs as the noise becomes more continuous.

Special Pacing Algorithms

Pacemaker-Mediated Tachycardia Termination Algorithms

Pacemaker-mediated tachycardia arises from retrograde conduction via the normal conduction system of the heart of a paced or intrinsic ventricular event to the atrium. The tracking of the retrogradely conducted atrial complex must occur for PMT to occur. The successive ventricular-paced event that tracks this atrial complex also results in retrograde conduction to the atrium.

Algorithms have been developed to automatically terminate PMT. The first step in a PMT algorithm is detection. Some algorithms are triggered when atrial tracking occurs at a specific rate. Other algorithms may be started when repetitive atrial-sensed events occur after ventricular-paced events with a VA duration of less than 400 ms. After detection, the intervention may be extension of PVARP, the nontracking of an atrial event for one beat cycle, or an atrial paced beat before the ventricular paced event. The PMT algorithms may be repeated within a specified period of time. However, often this period is relatively long to prevent repetitive nontracking of atrial rhythms.

Another form of a PMT algorithm is the PVC PVARP extension. PMT most commonly is initiated by a PVC because atrial activity has not had the chance to enter the AV conduction system, making retrograde conduction much more likely. Therefore, a pacemaker may define a PVC as a ventricular-sensed event not preceded by an atrial event. When such a PVC occurs, the pacemaker automatically extends the PVARP in order to decrease the likelihood of sensing of a retrograde P wave.

Mode Switching

Mode switching algorithms have been developed in order to decrease symptoms owing to tracking of atrial tachyarrhythmias. In the DDD or DDDR mode, pacemakers may sense the rapid rate of the atrial arrhythmias and produce rapid ventricular pacing, often at the upper rate limit of the pacemaker. These arrhythmias therefore may become symptomatic and require reprogramming of the device to a nontracking mode such as VVI or DDI.

Mode switching was developed as a method of automatically changing from a tracking mode such as DDD(R) or VDD(R) to a nontracking mode such as DDI(R) or VVI(R). These algorithms may be triggered by a specific atrial rate, frequently the upper rate limit or a rate above the programmed upper rate interval. A specified number of beats may activate the detection algorithm.

The mode switching algorithms available in the current generation of pacing systems are overall effective and well-tolerated. The main difficulty associated with the mode switching algorithms is detection of atrial arrhythmias. Frequently, the atrial electrograms in atrial arrhythmias are attenuated when compared to electrograms during sinus rhythm. Bipolar sensing reduces the likelihood that far field signals generated by myopotentials and other sources of interference will be inappropriately sensed as an atrial tachycardia and lead to inappropriate mode switching.

Rate Smoothing

Manufacturers have developed rate smoothing algorithms that can be turned "on" in a number of pulse generators in order to reduce marked changes in heart rate (e.g., when the pacing system develops 2:1 AV block at high atrial rates). The rate smoothing algorithm limits the maximal change in pacing rate from cycle to cycle. The rate smoothing algorithm also may be useful for stabilizing the ventricular rate in patients with atrial fibrillation.

Rate Drop Response

Pacing therapy may ameliorate symptoms in patients with vasovagal syncope. Some manufacturers have developed a ratedrop response algorithm that employs a programmable heart rate-time duration "window" that can detect a rapid decrease in heart rate, which then triggers pacing at a relatively high rate. In a small study this programming feature reduced the symptoms associated with vasovagal syncope; a large randomized trial (Vasovagal Pacemaker Study II or VPS II) did not demonstrate any significant reduction in the incidenced of syncope.

Regularization of Ventricular Rate During Atrial Fibrillation

There are several algorithms that are used to initiate ventricular pacing during atrial fibrillation in order to regularize the ventricular rate. Ventricular pacing typically results in concealed conduction into the AV node, decreasing the conduction of the subsequent beats. There may be a marked reduction in the variability of the RR intervals during this algorithm.

Atrial Overdrive Pacing for Atrial Fibrillation Prevention

There are a number of studies that have examined the incidence of atrial fibrillation while atrial overdrive pacing has been programmed ON to decrease the initiation of atrial fibrillation. In the Atrial Dynamic Overdrive Pacing

Trial (ADOPT) study, there was a significant decrease in the incidence of atrial arrhythmias in patients programmed with the atrial overdrive pacing. Additional studies are underway to determine the effectiveness of atrial over-drive pacing in different patient populations.

Minimizing Ventricular Pacing

There is evidence that ventricular pacing may result in decreased hemodynamic performance compared to intrinsic depolarization. In the Dual Chamber and VVI Implantable Defibrillator (DAVID) trial, patients undergoing implantable defibrillator implantation demonstrated an excess incidence of cardiovascular events in patients programmed to DDD. Additional retrospective analyses of the Mode Selection Trial (MOST) and the Multicenter Automatic Defibrillator Implantation Trial -II(MADIT II) trial have demonstrated that an increased percentage of ventricular pacing is associated with an increased incidence of heart failure in patients with sinus node dysfunction and cardiomyopathy respectively. Since it is often difficult to avoid ventricular pacing in many patients with DDD pacing, there are algorithms that have been developed to avoid ventricular pacing. One algorithm (Fig. 3.28) switches between AAIR mode while avoiding ventricular pacing in the presence of intact AV conduction and DDDR mode when ventricular pacing is needed.

Pacing for Cardiac Resynchronization

General Principles of Cardiac Resynchronization

Patients with significant interventricular and intraventricular conduction abnormalities have been shown to benefit hemodynamically from pacing the right and left ventricles in a coordinated manner, so-called cardiac resynchronization. Such pacing began with simultaneous pacing of the right and left ventricles. More recently, the ability to pacing in one ventricle to precede pacing in the other ventricle has recently been added. In addition, pacing one chamber after sensing an intrinsic event in the other chamber (usually right ventricle) may be possible.

Cardiac resynchronization pacing is based on the principle that hemodynamic benefits result from pacing even the absence of bradycardia. There the programmed settings of cardiac resynchronization should be made in order to ensure pacing at all times.

Timing Cycles for Cardiac Resynchronization

As discussed above, both ventricles are usually pacing at all times. In current cardiac resynchronization devices, the timing cycles are essentially the same as for conventional pacing. However, it is particularly important that the parameters be programmed to promote pacing and avoid intrinsic activity.

First, it is important to consider circumstances that promote intrinsic activity. In sinus rhythm, it is necessary for the AV interval to be sufficiently short to permit capture of both ventricles. In left bundle branch block for example, if the AV interval is not sufficiently short, the right ventricle may still be activated first and it may not be possible to activate the left ventricle in time to avoid mechanical dyssynchrony. Since in sinus rhythm AV conduction is usually relatively constant from beat-to-beat it may be possible to pacing the left ventricle

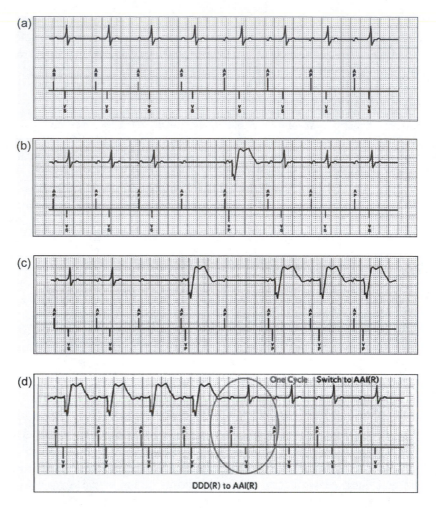

Fig. 3.28 Algorithm to avoid ventricular pacing. One algorithm to minimize ventricular pacing varies between the AAIR and DDDR function. In (a), AAIR is present. As shown in (b), when there is AV block for one transient beat, dual chamber pacing will occur. In (c), there is back-up dual chamber pacing. In (d), AV block has subsided and atrial pacing again occurs.

at a time earlier than the onset of right ventricular conduction. The right ventricle may be paced or be activated via the AV conduction system.

There are number of strategies to promote ventricular pacing in sinus rhythm. Rate-adaptive AV delay is generally employed in order to promote ventricular pacing. Negative AV hysteresis is used to promote ventricular pacing by shortening the AV interval when intrinsic conduction is detected in the AV interval.

Loss of ventricular pacing occurs at or above the upper rate limit in patients with intact AV conduction and in sinus rhythm. In patients with intact AV conduction, this phenomenon has not been recognized in conventional pacing since it was of no hemodynamic consequence. In cardiac resynchronization therapy, it results in a failure to deliver pacing. In fact

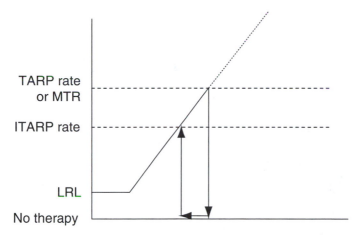

Fig. 3.29 Loss of Biventricular Pacing. On the Y axis the atrial rate is shown. As the atrial rate exceeds the LRL, biventricular pacing is maintained. However, when the atrial rate reaches the TARP, which equals the sum of the PVARP and the AV interval, biventricular pacing will stop. However, biventricular pacing will not resume even after the atrial rate falls until the atrial rate reaches the intrinsic total atrial refractory period (ITARP), which is the sum of the PVARP and the PR interval. From Wang PJ, Kramer A, Estes NAM III, Hayes DL. Timing cycles for biventricular pacing. PACE 2002; 25:52–75. (12).

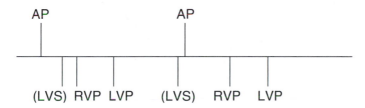

Fig. 3.30 Biventricular Pacing timing cycles. The basic biventricular system utilizes right ventricular sensing and biventricular pacing. In the first complex, atrial pacing is followed by right ventricular and left ventricular pacing. The right ventricular and left ventricular pacing may be simultaneously performed or at a programmed off-set. The left ventricle is not sensed. From Wang PJ, Kramer A, Estes NAM III, Hayes DL. Timing cycles for biventricular pacing. PACE 2002; 25:52–75. (12).

under certain circumstances the failure of pacing will continue despite a decrease in the atrial rate. The point of resumption of ventricular pacing is in fact lower than the rate at which ventricular pacing is first lost. As soon as the PP interval is less than the AV interval plus PVARP, a P wave will fall within PVARP and not be tracked. Since the PR interval is greater than the AV delay, the next P wave will also fall within the PVARP. As long as the PR interval plus PVARP is greater than the PP interval, atrial tracking will not occur (Fig. 3.29).

Biventricular pacing timing cycles are similar to DDD timing cycles. In the simplest form, right ventricular sensing only is present and right ventricular and left ventricular pacing are simultaneous. However, there also may be a timing difference between right and left ventricular pacing (Fig. 3.30).

References

1. Candinas R, Jakob M, Buckingham TA, et al. Vibration, acceleration, gravitation, and movement: activity controlled rate adaptive pacing during treadmill exercise testing and daily life activities. *PACE* 1997;20:1777–1786.
2. Lazarus A, Mitchell K. A prospective multicenter study demonstrating clinical benefit with a new accelerometer-based DDDR pacemaker. *PACE* 1996;19: 1694–1697.
3. Leung S-K, Lau C-P, Tang M-O, et al. An integrated dual sensor system automatically optimized by target rate histogram. *PACE* 1998;21:1559–1566.
4. Bonnet J-L, Geroux L, Cazeau S. Evaluation of a dual sensor rate responsive pacing system based on a new concept. *PACE* 1998;21:2198–2203.
5. Mehta D, Lau C-P, ward DE, et al. Comparative evaluation of chronotropic responses of QT sensing and activity sensing rate responsive pacemakers. *PACE* 1988;11:1405–1412.
6. Callaghan F, Vollman W, Livingston A, et al. The ventricular depolarization gradient: effects of exercise, pacing rate, epinephrine, and intrinsic heart rate control on the right ventricular evoked response. *PACE* 1989;12:1115–1130.
7. Ruiter J, Heemels JP, Kee K, et al. Adaptive rate pacing controlled by the right ventricular preejection interval: clinical experience with a physiological pacing system. *PACE* 1992;15:886–894.
8. Faerestrand S, Ohm O-J, Stangeland L, et al. Long-term clinical performance of a central venous oxygen saturation sensor for rate adaptive cardiac pacing. *PACE* 1994;17:1355–1372.
9. Rickards AF, Bombardini T, Corbucci G, et al. An implantable intracardiac accelerometer for monitoring myocardial contractility. *PACE* 1996;19:2066–2071.
10. Clementy J, Barold S, Garrigue S, et al. Clinical significance of multiple sensor options: rate response optimization, sensor blending, and trending. *Am J Cardiol* 1999;83:166D–171D.
11. Alt E, Combs W, Willhaus R, et al. A comparative study of activity and dual sensor: activity and minute ventilation pacing responses to ascending and descending stairs. *PACE* 1998;21:1862–1868.
12. Wang PJ, Kramer A, Estes NAM III, Hayes DL. Timing cycles for biventricular pacing. PACE 2002;25:52–75.

Section II

Device Implantation

4

Implant Techniques

Peter H. Belott

The implantation of devices for the management of both bradyarrhythmias and tachyarrhythmias has come together from divergent clinical pathways. There has, however, been an interesting parallel in the development of their methods of implantation (1). This has largely been driven by the dramatic advances in technology. In 1958, Seymour Furman and J.B. Schwedel passed the first transvenous endocardial electrode for prolonged cardiac pacing (2). Almost simultaneously, Rune Elmqvist and A.K.E. Senning developed a totally implantable pacemaker system with an epigastric pocket and the electrodes connected subcutaneously to the heart (3). These two events simultaneously introduced both the transvenous and epicardial approaches to cardiac pacing. Similarly, Mirowski and associates in 1980 implanted the initial cardioverter-defibrillator (ICD) (4). Its evolution has been identical to that of the cardiac pacemaker. The ICD, initially placed epicardially with an abdominal pocket, has given way to a transvenous approach and a pectoral pocket. To this day, these two fundamentally different approaches have stood the test of time as safe and reliable methods for device implantation (5,6). Initially, the cardiothoracic surgeon using the epicardial approach under general anesthesia performed the majority of implantations of pacemakers and ICDs. This was largely due to the fact that many device implantations were associated with open cardiac procedures such as value replacements and repair of congenital defects. The early pacemakers and ICDs were large and more easily placed in a subcutaneous abdominal pocket. This approach was further reinforced by the lack of a truly reliable endocardial lead system for pacing as well as for defibrillation. With the development of reliable endocardial lead systems, the transvenous endocardial approach by cutdown soon replaced an open chest procedure. This approach generally precluded the use of anesthesia but required some form of imaging for appropriate electrode placement. As technology advanced, electrode systems became extremely reliable. The development of fixation mechanisms has all but eradicated the complication of lead dislodgement. In addition, the pulse generator, either pacemaker or ICD, over time has become greatly reduced in size. Dramatic reduction in pacemaker as well as ICD size has radically reduced the required surgery. What once required a major open chest procedure under general anesthesia can now be carried out by a simple cutdown and relatively minor surgery. In the late 1970s, Littleford and Spector introduced the percutaneous sheath set technique for venous access via the subclavian vein (7). This technique and variations on this theme have revolutionized device implantation. The percutaneous technique has also generated controversy with respect to its safety. Subsequently, the implantation procedure, previously exclusively the domain of the cardiothoracic surgeon, has become the review of the invasive cardiologist and electrophysiologist. Similarly, the procedure has undergone a transition from the operating room to the cardiac catheterization laboratory or special procedures room. The luxury of having an anesthesiologist, except in special circumstances, has disappeared. The implanting physician has assumed additional responsibilities. In addition, the procedure that once required a rather protracted hospital stay can now be performed on an ambulatory basis. The "subclavian crush" phenomenon has resulted in a rethinking of the percutaneous approach to the subclavian vein. There has been a shift back to the cephalic vein cutdown and the development of alternate percutaneous techniques for access to the axillary vein. The transmyocardial or epicardial approach has long been abandoned for permanent pacing, but has continued to be used for ICD implantations. Transthoracic endocardial lead placement techniques by atriotomy and limited thoracotomy for unusual patho-physiologic and congenital anomalies have been developed. More recently, thoracoscopy has been used for the placement of epicardial electrodes, particularly with respect to the implantable cardioverter defibrillator. Thus, there have been radical changes in anatomic approach, preoperative planning, implantation personnel, and implant facility over the past 40 years for the modern pacemaker, and as little as 20 years for the ICD. The disciplines that were once exclusively those of the cardiac surgeon have been passed on to the invasive cardiologist and electrophysiologist. The procedure, initially reserved for the operating room, is now performed in a special study room or cardiac catheterization laboratory. General anesthesia has been replaced by simple conscious sedation, and the procedures that once required a lengthy hospital stay are now carried out on an ambulatory basis. Similarly, the ICD devices, once simple, are now complex, offering total arrhythmia control as well as backup dual-chambered, rate-adaptive pacemakers. These changes have not been without a price.

Now, the advent of resynchronization therapy has added a new level of complexity to pacemaker and defibrillator implantation. Not only is a third lead required but reliable left ventricular stimulation is essential for positive clinical results. Resynchronization therapy has brought new challenges to device implantation with respect of venous access, coronary sinus cannulation, lead positioning, effective stimulation and as well as new complications. And finally the new popularity of selective or alternative site pacing for optimal hemodynamics and arrhythmia management has challenged the traditional sites of lead placement. As one can see the advances in device implantation have brought new challenges, problems, and concerns. This chapter attempts to explore all the aspects of modern pacemaker and ICD implantation from a practical point of view. It addresses the new challenges, problems, and concerns.

Personnel

Qualifications of the Implanting Physician

An often hotly debated topic is who should be allowed to implant a permanent pacemaker or ICD (8). Traditionally, the cardiac surgeon has been responsible for device implantation procedures. Historically, this stems from the original implantation experience. Early systems were large and were implanted on an epicardial basis, requiring extensive surgery under general anesthesia. This clearly was the responsibility of the cardiac surgeon. Over the years, the surgical requirements, as previously stated, have gradually diminished. This is largely owing to the ever-diminishing size of the device and the introduction of the percutaneous and nonthoracotomy approach for venous access.

At the same time, catheterization skill requirements have increased greatly. The complexities of a modern arrhythmia management system call for precise placement of multiple electrodes, sophisticated endocardial mapping, and a complete understanding of electrophysiology. Clearly, device implantation, which was once a purely surgical responsibility, now appears to be a cardiac catheterization and electrophysiological procedure. As a result, many more procedures are performed by the cardiologist and fewer by the cardiac surgeon. In certain instances, the cardiologist, electrophysiologist, and cardiac surgeon perform as a team. The surgeon achieves venous access and creates the pocket, and the cardiologist positions the required electrodes. As the cardiologist performs many more procedures, the cardiothoracic surgeon's experience has become more limited. It has now reached the point where numerous cardiothoracic surgical training programs offer the trainee little or no exposure to device implantation. At the same time, a cardiac fellow trained in internal medicine has little or no exposure to surgical techniques and procedures and is expected to perform surgery. There is a clear need to develop training of all parties interested in implanting devices for arrhythmia management, whether they are cardiac surgeons or interventional cardiologists (9–12). Regardless of how one has become trained to implant pacemakers, careful review (by those responsible for credentialing in a given institution) of the training and experience of individuals in pacing will assist in preventing inadequately trained individuals from performing independent, unsupervised pacemaker implantation. Criteria for adequate training and experience should include a minimum number of pacemaker procedures, including single-chamber and dual-chamber implantations, lead replacements, pulse generator replacements, and upgrades to dual-chamber from single-chamber systems. Also, some documentable experience in an active pacemaker service clinic should be required.

The personnel required for the insertion of the ICD are very similar to those for pacemaker implantation. There is a primary surgeon, who may either be an electrophysiologist or cardiac surgeon. Of course, if an epicardial approach is instituted, the cardiothoracic surgeon is mandatory. In addition, an electrophysiologist and electrophysiology nurse should also be available.

Support Personnel

Historically, pacemaker procedures were carried out in the operating room, and pacemaker procedures were generally add-on cases at the end of the surgical day. The surgical team was never the same as a rule, with continuous change in nursing staff and anesthesiologist. Basic support personnel included a scrub nurse, a circulating nurse, and an anesthesiologist. Either the manufacturer's representative or a cardiovascular technician carried out threshold testing. More often than not, this was delegated to the manufacturer's representative.

The support personnel are critical to the safe and expeditious outcome of both a permanent pacemaker and ICD implanting procedure. Therefore, it would appear somewhat suboptimal to have continuous change in nursing staff or support personnel. The transition of the pacemaker procedure from the operating room to the special studies laboratory or the cardiac catheterization laboratory has consequently enhanced the safety and outcome of the procedure. The support personnel for a permanent pacemaker procedure, no matter where it is performed, should essentially include a registered nurse who can administer drugs and deliver surgical supplies to the surgical field, a scrub nurse who is familiar with the particular needs of any implanting physician, and a cardiovascular technician who is familiar with operating the sophisticated radiologic equipment. The same individual can assist with the electrophysiologic recordings and measurements required for the pacemaker implantation. Standard operating room procedure requires either a nurse anesthetist or a physician anesthesiologist for any surgical procedure. This is not the case in the cardiac catheterization laboratory, where the implanting physician is responsible for conscious sedation. However, the anesthesiology team should always be readily available for any unexpected cardiovascular or respiratory emergency. The role of the pacemaker manufacturer's representative in a pacemaker implantation varies from institution to institution (13). A highly trained manufacturer's representative can be invaluable in the pacemaker procedure. This is particularly true in small remote institutions that perform cardiac pacemaker implantations. There are, however, institutions that view the presence of the manufacturer's representative in a permanent pacemaker procedure as inappropriate. They limit his or her role to that of merely a courier of the hardware to the institution. In our experience, a well-trained and highly experienced manufacturer's representative is an invaluable member of the support team. In many institutions, he or she not only functions as a courier of leads and devices, but also substitutes as the cardiovascular technician for threshold testing and measurements. The manufacturer's representative also offers a level of consistency with respect to record keeping. The manufacturer's representative is usually responsible for registering the pacemaker patient and precisely recording the threshold information.

The personnel required for insertion of an ICD are very similar to those of the pacemaker implantation. The ICD manufacturer's representative, however, as stated, is controversial. He or she can be an important member of the implantation team and can prove invaluable for providing leads, defibrillators, and support equipment. The earlier ICD implantations that were limited to epicardial placement required a minimum of two trained physicians (an electrophysiologist and a cardiac surgeon). With the transition to the nonthoracotomy approach, a well-trained electrophysiologist working with an ICD manufacturer's representative is frequently all that is required. The ideal constitution of an ICD implantation team is listed in Table 4.1. Each member of the ICD implant team should be completely familiar with the unique requirements of an ICD implantation. This includes a protocol for patient rescue, should it be required. The circulating nurse is responsible for running

Table 4.1 Personnel required for ICD implantation and testing.

Implanting physician (cardiothoracic surgeon, electro-physiologist)

Anesthesiologist

Electrophysiologist

Technical support personnel

Engineer

Technician

EP nurse

Manufacturer's representative

the external defibrillator for rescue as directed by the electrophysiologist and implanting physician. Similarly, the manufacturer's representative should not only be responsible for equipment and supplies, but also for threshold testing, programming, arrhythmia induction, and even rescue. This is, of course, all under the guidance and supervision of the implanting physician or electrophysiologist. It should be noted that as the ICD implantation procedure becomes more simplified, there is a growing desire on the part of non-electro-physiology-trained physicians to implant ICDs. The ICD implant technique has become very similar to that of a permanent pacemaker. Unfortunately, today there are no formal published guidelines with respect to obtaining privileges for the insertion of an implantable cardioverter defibrillator. One must remember that there are two parts to the ICD implantation; first, the implantation of a lead and device, and second, and more important, the intraoperative electro-physiologic protocol that includes not only pace-and-sense threshold determinations, but arrhythmia induction, defibrillation threshold (DFT) determination, patient rescue and, finally, defibrillator programming. Only a trained electrophysiologist can perform the second part of an implantation. It is hoped in the future that the American College of Cardiology and the North American Society of Pacing and Electrophysiology will establish formal guidelines for ICD implantation and credentialing.

Implant Facility and Required Equipment

The operating room has been the traditional location for both permanent pacemaker and ICD procedures. The operating room offers optimal sterile technique and conditions ideal for insertion of a foreign body such as a pacemaker. Another benefit of the operating room is its endless supply of surgical instruments for difficult situations. If a more extensive surgical procedure becomes necessary, the operating room is ideally suited for such situations. However, the radiographic equipment in the operating room is considerably limited when compared to that of the cardiac catheterization laboratory. In addition, radiographic supplies, such as contrast and catheterization materials, are also lacking in the operating room. Frequent time delays may be encountered because there is a tendency to be technically unprepared. Disruptions in the flow of the procedure and unnecessary time delays are frequent consequences. The cardiac catheterization laboratory can be an ideal place for performing permanent pacemaker and ICD procedures, and it offers unlimited radiologic capabilities (14,15). High-quality images for precise electrode placement are usually obtained. In addition, the cardiac catheterization laboratory is the resource for all types of catheters, guidewires, sheaths, and angiographic material that may be required in a given situation. It is also the location of sophisticated physiologic recording and monitoring equipment for the required electrophysiologic measurements in such procedures. The early concerns over safety and sterility have now proven to be unfounded. This is mainly the result of the institution of rigid protocols for sterile technique.

Physiologic Monitoring

The monitoring requirements for a permanent pacemaker are actually quite simple. From a practical point of view, all that is required is continuous electrocardiographic monitoring on a reasonable quality oscilloscope (16). Threshold information can be obtained easily from the combined use of a pacemaker system analyzer and an oscilloscope. The availability of complex multichannel recording systems is truly a luxury. Such systems, which offer both surface and intracardiac recordings, are not necessary from a practical point of view. In addition, patient-monitoring equipment should include an automatic blood pressure cuff. The presence of continuous oxygen saturation monitoring is also extremely important with conscious sedation. A pacemaker implantation procedure should not be performed without the presence of a DC defibrillator and a thoroughly equipped crash cart. In some institutions, external pacing and defibrillation pads are applied throughout the case. Basic monitoring equipment for ICD implantation is similar to that of a permanent pacemaker procedure. Placement of an intraarterial line for blood pressure monitoring during arrhythmia induction and termination is recommended.

Surgical Instruments

Both the permanent pacemaker and ICD procedure merely require a minor surgical tray with a limited number of instruments (17). The recommended instruments are shown in Fig. 4.1 and listed in Table 4.2. There are several instruments that the nonsurgically trained implanting physician should become familiar with and that deserve special mention. It should be remembered that the surgical instruments are designed to help, not hinder, the implanting physician. The three instruments that are extremely helpful in implantation of an arrhythmia device are the Weitlaner self-retaining retractor, the Senn retractor, and the Goulet retractor. The Weitlaner retractor is extremely useful for maintaining good exposure and anatomic planes of dissection. The Senn retractor is used for more delicate tissue retraction and is very helpful when elevating tissue planes and edges. The Goulet, a flat strip of metal that has smooth scalloped ends, is especially useful when creating the pacemaker or ICD pocket. It is capable of gentle tissue retraction, exposing large tissue areas.

The operating room offers optimal lighting through the use of an array of high-intensity lamps. This is not the case in the cardiac catheterization laboratory, where the lighting is marginal at best. The use of a high-intensity headlamp in situations of marginal lighting, particularly for wound inspection, can be extremely helpful. For the nonsurgically trained implanting physician, the use of a headlamp takes practice to coordinate head, eye, and lamp movement.

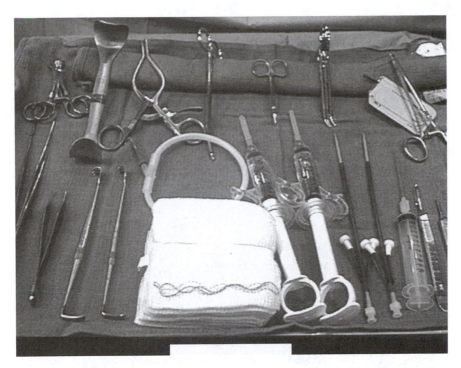

Fig. 4.1 Minor surgical tray that includes a limited number of instruments and supplies. From the upper left and clockwise: towel clips, Goulet retractor, Weitlaner self-retaining retractor, Metzenbaum scissors, iris scissors, hemostats, needle holder, scalpel, 10-cc syringe with #18 gauge thin-walled needle, sheath sets, local anesthetic, guidewire, Senn retractor, Adson (toothed) forceps, and non-toothed forceps.

Traditionally electrocautery has been considered contraindicated in permanent pacemaker procedures (18–20). Yet, electrocautery has been found to be invaluable for cutting as well as coagulation and plays an essential role in device-related procedures.

A reliable pacemaker system analyzer is indispensable in any pacemaker or ICD procedure (21). The Pacemaker System Analyses (PSA) should be able to perform all the measurements required for any pacemaker or ICD procedure. It should also offer heart rate support during such measurements. Modern PSAs offer every programmable feature that is available in any modern pulse generator. In many instances, the PSA has been incorporated into the pacemaker or ICD programmer. There should also be an emergency capability such as high output or, if needed, high-rate pacing for arrhythmia management. The ability to supply hard copy for analysis and record keeping, although not essential, is desirable.

Miscellaneous Supplies and Spare Parts

One should never undertake a device procedure without a complete assortment of spare parts that are readily available. An example of the required spare parts is shown in Table 4.3. In any given procedure, one should have readily available splice kits, an assortment of stylets, lead adapters, wrenches, lubricants, lead caps, and wire cutters for unique situations. It is recommended

Table 4.2 Pacemaker surgical instrument tray.

One Army-Navy retractor

One smooth forceps

One small Weitlaner

One medium blunt Weitlaner

One small Metzenbaum scissor

One mouse-tooth forceps

Four baby towel clips

Two curved Kelly clamps

One Bozeman uterine dressing forcep

One Peers clamp

Two Senn retractors

One Goulet retractor

Two Adson forceps with teeth

One curved Mayo scissor; one #3 knife handle

Two small needle holders

Five curved mosquitos

One package of 2–0 Polyglactin nonabsorbable suture

One package of 4–0 Polyglactin nonabsorbable suture

One package of 0 silk 18′ suture

#10 scalpel blade

#3 or #4 French eye needle

Table 4.3 Pacemaker supplies and spare parts.

Lead stylets

Variable stiffness

Straight and variable J curve

Varying lengths

Screwdriver kit and torque wrenches

Sterile medical adhesive

Wire crimper/cutter

One set of connecting cable introducer sets, 11 and 12 French

Silicone oil

Adapter sleeves

Helical coil adapter with 5 mm pin

Lead connector caps, 3.2-, VS1-, and 5-mm sizes

Step up and step down adapters

that the institution establish a cart, similar to the crash cart, which contains every imaginable component that may be necessary for a given pacemaker or ICD situation. A checklist of supplies and parts should be established and a periodic and timely inventory carried out. One or more staff members should

Table 4.4 Recommended ICD supplies.

AC fibrillator box

Lead adapter sleeves and caps

External defibrillator

Large Parsonnet Dacron pouches ($1.5' \times 6'$)

Guidewires

Imaging contrast material

Introducers (long and short lengths, 9, 10, 11, 12, and 14 French)

Jackson-Pratt drainage system

Multiple stylets

Multiple torque wrenches

Tunneling tool with multiple lead adapters

Transvenous rate sensing lead

Subcutaneous patches

Y-adapters

Subcutaneous array

Extra transvenous rate sensing leads

Lead extensions

Lead repair kit

be placed in charge of the servicing and performing of timely inventory of the cart. In addition to the spare parts, the cart should also be stocked with a complete array of sheath sets, dilators, and guidewires, as well as the components and equipment for electrode extraction. Some additional components might include a complete assortment of Parsonnet pouches, equipment and components for tunneling as well as drainage procedures. The basic required equipment for ICD insertion is identical to that for a pacemaker procedure. Additional requirements include the equipment and supplies unique to the ICD. These would include high-voltage cables, programmable stimulator, external defibrillator with sterile external and internal paddles, AC defibrillator, sterile programming wand for ICD communication, external programmer, and tunneling tools unique to the ICD implantation (Table 4.4). Similar to the pacemaker implantation procedure, one cannot have enough supplies and spare parts.

Preoperative Planning

If the procedure is to proceed in a smooth and expeditious fashion, careful preoperative planning is essential. The first such decision is whether the patient requires a single-chamber or dual-chamber pacemaker. As a rule, if the patient has intact atrial function, every effort is made to preserve atrial and ventricular relationships. Single-chamber ventricular pacing is usually reserved for the patient with chronic atrial fibrillation or atrial paralysis. A device is selected with acceptable size, longevity, and programmability. If the heart is chronotropically incompetent, a device that offers some form of rate adaptation is considered. Just as important is the lead selection. One necessary decision is whether to use passive-fixation or active-fixation leads. Generally, an active-fixation electrode is selected when problems of dislodgment are expected, such as in the patient with a dilated right ventricle or amputated atrial appendage. Active-fixation leads are one of several factors that enhance removability of the lead, if it is necessary in the future. Also important is the pacing configuration (unipolar versus bipolar). This decision relates to both electrodes and the pulse generator. Although the use of bipolar pacing and sensing has definite advantages, bipolar leads have historically been more complicated and prone to problems. Bipolar leads are also larger in diameter. The compatibility of electrodes and the pulse generator is extremely important, particularly when using an older existing electrode with a modern new pulse generator. If incompatibility exists, an appropriate adapter must be obtained.

Directly related to the device selection process is whether an AICD or Biventricular system should be placed. These decisions also effect type of device, and lead systems employed.

An important component of this process is careful documentation of the indications (22). This should be reflected in the history to document symptoms, medications, and conditions that are essential. In addition, the physical examination is also supported by demonstrating arrhythmias and its side effects on the vital signs for evidence of cardiac decompensation and neurologic deficits. Of course, any other documentation of bradyarrhythmias or tachyarrhythmias can be extremely helpful. Comments on the results of Holter monitoring, event recording, and 12-lead electrocardiography are essential. Documenting rhythm strips and electrophysiologic studies for the chart are mandatory for peer review.

The laboratory data that exclude any transient causes of arrhythmia—digitalis level, thyroid panel, and other chemistries—should be obtained. It is obvious that all of the documentation does not have to be present on the chart or medical record but should be readily available if requested.

Historically, most pacemaker and ICD procedures have been performed on an inpatient basis. As a rule, under the circumstance, the preoperative evaluation, the actual procedure, as well as postoperative care are rendered in the hospital. In the case of both permanent pacing and ICD implantation, individuals are generally admitted with major symptoms such as syncope. The patient is formally admitted, and the procedure is scheduled after a complete workup. After the procedure, the patient is observed briefly in the hospital and subsequently discharged and referred for outpatient device follow-up. In today's cost-containment environment, such an approach is inefficient and not cost effective. Thus, there has been an attempt to abbreviate the patient's hospital stay and render care on an ambulatory basis.

Hospitalizations were frequently prolonged in the early days, when devices were large, surgery was more involved, and catastrophic complications, such as lead dislodgement, perforation, and wound infections were frequent. The prospect of a brief hospital stay would appear heretical and unthinkable. Today, where experience is high and surgery is limited, complications are rare. Most important, the major concern over lead dislodgement, potential asystole is virtually nonexistent with the newer modern, positive electrode systems. With respect to pacemakers, if one reflects on the current pacemaker

Table 4.5 Ambulatory pacemaker procedure analysis, 1983–1995.

Year	83	84	85	86	87	88	89	90	91	92	93	94	95	Total
TP	99	102	112	110	112	123	100	107	135	119	145	113	97	1474
TA	34	34	56	60	78	87	70	87	124	94	128	104	87	1043
TRUE	8	16	44	56	78	86	68	83	124	90	125	102	87	967
<24	26	18	12	4	0	1	2	4	0	4	3	2	0	76
%AMB	34	34	50	60	69	70	70	77	91	78	88	92	88	69

TP, total patients; TA, total ambulatory; TRUE, cases discharged the same day of procedure; < 24, cases discharged within 24 h (overnight hospitalization); %AMB, percent ambulatory procedures.

population, truly pacemaker-dependent patients are few and far between. The patients are generally worked up on an ambulatory basis with symptoms of presyncope and syncope that are detected by outpatient ambulatory monitoring. They are subsequently admitted to the hospital for a permanent pacemaker. If this procedure were performed on an ambulatory basis and one experienced total failure, the worst that would occur is a patient who is no better off than prior to the procedure. Today, when issues of cost containment are at their highest, the prospect of an ambulatory pacemaker procedure is very appealing.

The safety and efficacy of this approach has been demonstrated both in Europe and the United States (23,24). Concerns with respect to potential complications continue to be expressed (25–27). Questions about lead selection, timing of discharge, and the intensity of follow-up are raised frequently. In addition, economic input has yet to be fully appreciated—although it is believed that more pacemaker procedures are being performed on an ambulatory basis, it has not been reflected in the literature. Since the original reports of Zegeleman and colleagues and Belott, Haywood and associates have reported a randomized control study of the feasibility and safety of ambulatory pacemaker procedures (23,24,28). Our own experience now stands over 13 years with over 1,474 pacemaker procedures, of which 1,043 have been performed on an ambulatory basis (Table 4.5) (29). Of these procedures, 967 were performed on a true ambulatory basis with the patient admitted and discharged on the same day. It appears that over the last 15 years 69% of all pacemaker procedures were ambulatory. From 1990 to 1995, 85% of the procedures were ambulatory. There were no pacemaker deaths or emergencies. Two axioms have been borne out from this experience. First, if there are any doubts or concerns, any patient's hospitalization can be extended; and second, any operator is always truly aware of the problem patient and for such as patient, who has potentially sustained a complication, hospitalization can always be extended. Given the gratifying results of this 13-year experience, all elective permanent pacemaker procedures at our pacemaker center are performed on an ambulatory basis (30). This includes new implants, electrode repositions, upgrade procedures, electrode extractions, and pulse generator changes. Today, because of the dramatically reduced ICD size and required surgery, as well as protocols for more expeditious device testing, even these procedures are performed on an ambulatory basis.

The management of surgery in the anticoagulated patient is controversial. There is a paucity of information throughout the literature with respect to the handling of a patient requiring anticoagulation. One thing is clear: The patient receiving anticoagulants, including heparin and platelet antagonists, is at risk for hematoma formation. It is commonly held that patients who require oral anticoagulants should have the prothrombin time brought to normal prior to the implantation. Anticoagulants can be resumed between 24 and 48 h after the pacemaker procedure. Reducing the prothrombin time to normal in patients requiring anticoagulants, such as those with artificial heart valves, places the patient at grave risk for thromboembolic complications. Addressing this issue, many operators choose to admit the patient to the hospital and start intravenous heparin while the warfarin is withheld and the prothrombin time is brought to normal values. This often takes days. The patient is scheduled for surgery once the prothrombin time has reached control. On the day of surgery, the heparin is stopped and reversed, and the surgery is carried out. Several hours after surgery, heparin is resumed. Then, after 24 to 48 h, if there is no evidence of significant hematoma, the warfarin is resumed; and, once therapeutic, the heparin is stopped and the patient is discharged on oral warfarin therapy. In this day and age of cost control and managed care, this maneuver can prove to be quite costly. In addition, despite vigorous attempts at hemostasis, large hematomas have resulted from the use of heparin. Although anecdotal, it is the general impression of this author that the greatest risk of bleeding complications, hemorrhage, and hematoma occur with the use of heparin as well as platelet antagonists such as aspirin. Having experienced a devastating thromboembolic complication from the withdrawal of warfarin as well as multiple large hematomas from the use of heparin, this author has chosen to perform pacemaker and ICD procedures with the patient fully anticoagulated on the oral agent warfarin. This policy has been in effect for a minimum of 10 years. As a rule, the patient on oral anticoagulants has the INR dropped to approximately 2. There have been no devastating hematomas or thromboembolic events. It is this author's opinion that pacemaker and ICD procedures can be performed safely with the patient fully anticoagulated. Recently, this approach has been supported by a 4-year experience reported by Goldstein et al. (31). There was no difference in the incidental bleeding complications between anticoagulated and nonanticoagulated patients. There were no wound hematomas, blood transfusions, or clinically significant bleeding in any patient receiving warfarin. Recently Guidici in a large series of patients further substantiated the safety and efficacy of implanting devices without reversing warfarin therapy (32). The interruption of anticoagulant therapy in pacemaker and ICD procedures to prevent hemorrhage is unfounded. The medicolegal risks from interrupted continuous anticoagulant therapy and the resultant thromboembolic event are real. Although there is a theoretical risk of hemorrhage after pacemaker procedures in patients with therapeutic levels of anticoagulation, the risk appears to be minimal. The bleeding can generally be treated by local measures, such as placement of drains or reoperation. The risk of bleeding is greatly outweighed by the risk of thromboembolism after withdrawal of anticoagulant therapy. In addition, if a major hemorrhage should occur, resulting in tamponade caused by a perforation, such bleeding will not cease on the basis of thrombus formation, because it is mechanical and requires emergency surgical intervention. The issue of pacemaker and

ICD surgery on anticoagulated patients will become more prevalent as more patients receive anticoagulation therapy for the arrhythmia of atrial fibrillation as well as coronary artery interventions.

Pacemaker and ICD Implantation: General Considerations

Anesthesia

Most pacemaker procedures are performed under local anesthesia with some form of sedation (33). In the centers where the procedure is routinely performed in the operating room, there is generally an anesthesiologist or nurse anesthetist as part of the implant team. With the recent transition from the operating room to the cardiac catheterization laboratory, the implant physician is responsible for most conscious sedation.

The challenge at hand is to achieve optimal patient comfort while avoiding the risks of oversedation and respiratory depression. The type of local anesthetic and the dose delivered are important in addition to appropriate conscious sedation. As a general rule, it is desirable to select an anesthetic agent that is rapid in onset in combination with one that offers sustained action. A list of pharmacologic properties of commonly used local anesthetic agents is found in Table 4.6.

As with many variables in the procedure, patient sedation is largely a personal preference. Despite the agents to be utilized, it is important that the operator become completely familiar and comfortable with one or more agents. A popular practice is combining a sedative agent with a narcotic, thus achieving optimal sedation, anesthesia, and analgesic effect. A popular combination is the use of a diazepam derivative with a semisynthetic narcotic.

Occasionally, total sedation is required. In this setting, an anesthesiologist or nurse anesthetist is required for the administration of Pentothal or nitrous oxide.

Table 4.6 Pharmacologic properties of commonly used local anesthetic agents.

	Duration (h)	Onset (min)	Maximum adult dose	Protein binding
Esthers				
Chloroprocaine	Short	Slow	800 mg	5%
(Nesacaine)	(0.5–1.5)	(5–10)	(11 mcg/kg)	
Chloroprocaine	Short	Fast	800 mg	
(Novocaine)	(0.5–1.5)	(5–15)	(11 mcg/kg)	
Tetracaine	Long	Slow	200 mg	85%
	(3.3–5)	(20–30)		
Amides				
Bupivacaine	Long	Mod	100 mg	82–96%
(Marcaine)	(3–5)	(10–20)		
Lidocaine	Mod	Fast	300 mg	55–65%
(Xylocaine)	(1–3)	(5–15)	(4 mcg/kg)	

From Belott PH, Reynolds DW. Permanent pacemaker implantation. In: Ellenbogen KA, Kay N, Wilkoff BL, eds. Clinical cardiac pacing. Philadelphia: WB Saunders, 1995, with permission.

Table 4.7 Conscious sedation drug protocols.

Drug name	Route of administration	Dosage range	Maximum dose	Comments
Droperidol	IV	8–17 mcg/kg	17 mcg/kg	
Fentanyl	IM/IV	50–100 mcg	100 mg	Short-acing, very potent
Ketamine	IV	0.5 mg/kg	0.5 mg/kg	Temporary loss of consciousness
Meperidine	M/IV	25–100 mg	100 mg	Long-acting
Midazolam	IV	1.0–2.5 mg	5 mg	
Morphine	IM/IV	1.5–15 mg	20 mg	Long-acting
Nitrous oxide	Inhalation	30–50%	50%	
Thiopental	IV	1–4 mg/kg		Temporary loss of consciousness
Valium	IV	2–10 mg	10 mg	

From Belott PH, Reynolds DW. Permanent pacemaker implantation. In: Ellenbogen KA, Kay N, Wilkoff BL, eds. Clinical cardiac pacing. Philadelphia: WB Saunders, 1995, with permission.

A new agent requiring the assistance of an anesthetist is propofol. With this agent, the patient's sedation can be very effectively titrated and the analgesic and sedative effect rapidly reversed. With the growing use of the ambulatory approach and conscious sedation, the Joint Commission of Hospital Accreditation has mandated the establishment of protocols for safe and effective utilization. In addition, physicians administering conscious sedation must be credentialed. Conscious sedation protocols generally require thorough patient assessment prior to the institution of therapy. Appropriate resuscitation equipment should be readily available. Any patient undergoing conscious sedation requires continuous monitoring of pulse oximetry, cardiac rhythm, and blood pressure. The period of postprocedure monitoring directly relates to the pharmacologic agent that is administered. Table 4.7 outlines popular conscious sedation drug protocols. With respect to the ICD, the choice of anesthesia is related to operator preference or hospital protocol. As previously mentioned, the procedure may be performed under general anesthesia or with conscious sedation. In a patient who requires multiple DFT determinations as well as a subpectoral dissection, general anesthesia would probably be a better selection. General anesthesia offers optimal patient comfort as well as airway control. Many centers that advocate a simple subcutaneous ICD implantation utilize conscious sedation with local anesthesia. For periods of ventricular fibrillation induction, the patient receives brief deep sedation with a short acting barbiturate such as barbital or propofol.

On May 3, 1995, a North American Society Pacing Electrophysiology Policy Conference on IV sedation was held in Boston. A NASPE expert consensus document on the use of IV conscious sedation/analgesia by nonanesthesia personnel in patients undergoing arrhythmia-specific diagnostic, therapeutic, and surgical procedures was generated (34). The policy conference (a) reviewed the current state of the art with respect to conscious sedation, (b) reviewed current position statements developed by other relevant health professional groups, (c) reviewed the legal and licensing applications of IV conscious sedation, (d) developed recommendations for the use of IV sedation, (e) specified the minimum training requirements for professional administration of IV sedation for arrhythmia-specific procedures, and (f) reviewed the cost effectiveness and economic impact of IV-conscious sedation.

Antibiotics and Antiseptic Solutions

Although there is no substitute for good infection control practices in a rigid surgical environment, the controversy over prophylactic antibiotics continues (35). As a general rule, antibiotics have been used in pacemaker and ICD procedures because the risk of infection carries an extreme monetary penalty (36–38). It is well known that surgical procedures that are prolonged are associated with increased risk of infection. Unfortunately, the literature does not reflect any specific requirements with respect to antibiotic prophylaxis in pacemaker and ICD procedures (39).

When considering antibiotic prophylaxis, the primary offending agents are usually *Staphylococcus epidermidis* or *Staphylococcus aureus*. In this situation, a broadspectrum antibiotic, such as a cephalosporin, appears to be ideal. If one is concerned over Staphylococcus resistance, then vancomycin should be considered. It has been our practice to administer IV cephalosporins during the intraoperative period followed by oral cephalosporins for 2 to 4 days. It is a common practice to administer topical antibiotics for wound irrigation as an additional strategy for prevention of wound infection. Once again, there are no data to support such an approach (40). It should be pointed out that there is a major concern over potential systemic toxicity from such antibiotic irrigations. Despite the lack of supporting scientific data, Table 4.8 outlines several antibiotic irrigation protocols. It has been our practice to administer 1 g of cefazolin intraoperatively followed by cefuroxime monohydrate 500 mg twice daily for 4 days. A povidone iodine-soaked sponge is generally placed in the device pocket just after its formation. Following this protocol in a series of more than 1,500 pacemaker procedures, the results have been quite gratifying, with only two wound infections. Despite the fact that antibiotics and antibiotic irrigation are controversial, wound infections in a setting of device procedures are so catastrophic that they should be avoided at all cost.

Table 4.8 Common antimicrobial irrigation protocols.

Agent	Concentration
Bacitracin	50,000 U in 200 mL of saline
Cephalothin	1 g/L of saline
Cefazolin	1 g/L of saline
Cefuroxime	750 mg/L of saline
Vancomycin	200–500 mg/L of saline
Povidone iodine	Concentrated or diluted in aloquats of saline

From Belott PH, Reynolds DW. Permanent pacemaker implantation. In: Ellenbogen KA, Kay N, Wilkoff BL, eds. Clinical cardiac pacing. Philadelphia: WB Saunders, 1995, with permission.

Anatomic Approach

There are two basic anatomic approaches to permanent cardiac pacing and ICD therapy (5,6).

The first is the epicardial, which requires general anesthesia and surgical access to the epicardial surface of the heart. The second is the transvenous approach, which involves passage of the electrodes through a vein into the endocardial surface of the heart. This approach is performed under local anesthesia with conscious sedation.

Initially, almost all pacemaker and ICD procedures were approached exclusively from the epicardial point of view. But with the development of a transvenous approach, either by cutdown or percutaneous techniques, now almost all pacemaker and ICD procedures are approached on a transvenous or nonthoracotomy basis. Today, the epicardial approach is reserved for certain unique circumstances. Electrodes can be placed on the epicardium by a variety of techniques. This involves a subxiphoid incision, and limited thoracotomy, or direct application of electrodes on an exposed heart. Recently, mediastinoscopy and thoracoscopy have been used to apply permanent pacing and rate-sensing electrodes as well as patch electrodes. The transvenous approach can be performed by venous cutdown, percutaneous venous access, or a combination of the two.

A thorough understanding of the venous anatomic structures of the head, neck, and upper extremities are imperative for safe venous access (Fig. 4.2) (41). The precise location and orientation of the internal jugular, innominate, subclavian, and cephalic veins are important for safe venous access (42). Their anatomic relation to other structures is crucial in avoiding complications. The venous anatomy of interest from a cardiac pacing and ICD point of view starts peripherally with the axillary vein (43).

The axillary vein is a large venous structure that represents the continuation of the basilic vein. It starts at the lower border of the teres major tendon and

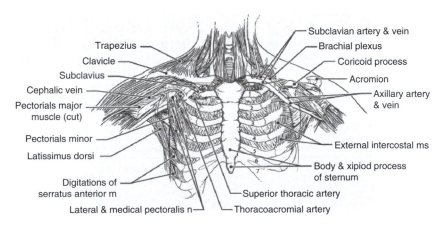

Fig. 4.2 Detailed anatomy of the anterolateral chest, demonstrating the axillary vein with the pectoralis major and minor muscles removed. (From Belott PH, Reynolds DW. Permanent pacemaker and cardioverter defibrillation implantation. In: Ellenbogen KA, Kay N, Wilkoff BL, eds. Clinical cardiac pacing and defibrillation, 2nd ed. Philadelphia: WB Saunders, 2000, with permission.)

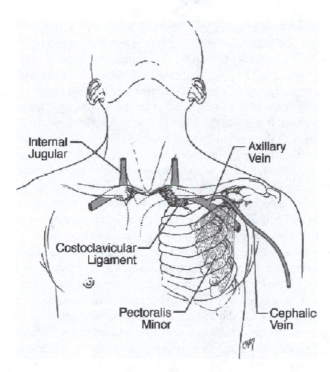

Fig. 4.3 Anatomic relationship of the axillary vein to the pectoralis minor muscle. The pectoralis major has been removed. Note the cephalic vein draining directly into the axillary vein at approximately the first intercostal space. (From Belott PH. Unusual access sites for permanent cardiac pacing. In: Barold SS, Mugica J, eds. Recent advances in cardiac pacing: Goals for the 21st century. Armonk, NY: Futura Publishing, 1997, with permission.)

latissimus dorsi. The axillary vein terminates immediately beneath the clavicle at the outer border of the first rib, where it becomes a subclavian vein. The pectoralis minor and pectoralis major muscles and costocoracoid membrane cover the axillary vein anteriorly. It is anterior and medial to the axillary artery, which it partially overlaps. The axillary vein is covered by the clavicular head of the pectoralis major at the level of the coracoid process (Fig. 4.3). At this juncture, the axillary vein receives the more superficial cephalic vein. It is important to note that the cephalic vein terminates in the deeper axillary vein at the level of the coracoid process beneath the pectoralis major muscle. The cephalic vein commonly used for pacemaker venous access is classified as a superficial vein in the upper extremity. This vein, which actually commences near the antecubital fossa, travels along the outer border of the biceps muscle and enters the deltopectoral groove. The deltopectoral groove is an anatomic structure formed by the deltoid muscle and clavicular head of the pectoralis major. The cephalic vein traverses the deltopectoral groove and superiorly pierces the costocoracoid membrane, crossing the axillary artery, and terminates in the axillary vein just below the clavicle at the level of the coracoid process. The subclavian vein is a continuation of the axillary vein. The subclavian vein extends from the outer border of the first rib to the inner end of the clavicle, where it joins with the internal jugular vein to form the innominate vein. The subclavian vein is just inferior to the clavicle and subclavius muscle. The subclavian artery is located posterior and superior to the vein. The two structures are separated internally by the scalenus anticus muscle and phrenic nerve. Inferiorly, this vein leaves a depression in the first rib and on the pleura. The junction of the internal jugular and subclavian veins form the brachiocephalic trunk or innominate veins. These are two large venous trunks located on each side of the base of the neck. The right innominate vein is relatively short. It starts at the inner end of the clavicle and passes vertically down to join with the left innominate vein just below the cartilage of the first rib. This junction forms the superior vena cava. The left innominate vein is larger and longer than the right, passing from left to right for approximately 2½ in. where it joins with the right innominate vein to form the superior vena cava. The left innominate vein is in the anterior and superior mediastinum. The internal and external jugular veins have also been used for device venous access. The external jugular vein is a superficial vein of the neck receiving blood from the exterior cranium and face. This vein starts in the substance of the parotid gland at the angle of the jaw and runs perpendicular down the neck to the middle of the clavicle. In this course, it crosses the sternocleidomastoid muscle and runs parallel with its posterior border. At the sternocleidomastoid muscle's attachment to the clavicle, this vein perforates the deep fascia and terminates in the subclavian vein just anterior to the scalenus anticus muscle. The external jugular vein is separated from the sternocleidomastoid by a layer of deep cervical fascia. Superficially, it is covered by the platysma muscle, superficial fascia, and skin. The external jugular vein can be variable in size and even duplicated. Because of its superficial orientation, the external jugular vein is less frequently used for cardiac venous access.

The internal jugular vein, although an unusual site for pacemaker venous access, is utilized more frequently than the external jugular vein (Fig. 4.4). This is because of its larger size and deeper and more protected orientation. The internal jugular vein starts just internal to the jugular foramen at the base of the skull. It drains blood from the interior of the cranium as well as superficial parts of the head and neck. This vein is oriented vertically as it runs down the side of the neck. Superiorly, it is lateral to the internal carotid and inferolateral to the common carotid. At the base of the neck, the internal jugular vein joins the subclavian vein to form the innominate vein. The internal jugular vein is large and lies in the cervical triangle defined by the lateral borders of the omohyoid muscle, the inferior border of the digastric muscle, and the medial border of the sternocleidomastoid. The superficial cervical fascia and platysma muscle cover the vein. It is usually identified just lateral to the easily palpable external carotid artery.

Byrd underscores the concept of thoroughly understanding anatomy with his description of the anteriorly and posteriorly displaced clavicle (44). The posteriorly displaced clavicle commonly seen in chronic obstructive pulmonary disease patients can make venous access from the percutaneous point of view extremely hazardous. Similarly, the anteriorly displaced clavicle, as found in the elderly kyphoscoliotic patient with interiorly bowed clavicles, renders percutaneous venous access next to impossible. An appreciation of these anatomic variations is essential to avoid the complications of pneumothorax, hemopneumothorax, and unsuccessful venipuncture. It should also be appreciated that the right ventricle is an anterior structure, the apex of which is usually located anteriorly and to the left (Fig. 4.5). Although the normal location is distinctly to the left of the midline, occasionally it can be rotated anteriorly

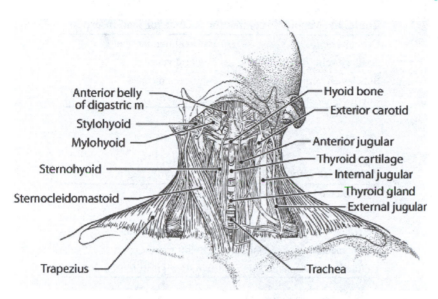

Fig. 4.4 Detailed anatomy of the neck demonstrating the relationship of the venous structures, and superficial and deep anatomy. (From Belott PH, Reynolds DW. Permanent pacemaker and cardioverter defibrillation implantation. In: Ellenbogen KA, Kay N, Wilkoff BL, eds. Clinical cardiac pacing and defibrillation, 2nd ed. Philadelphia: WB Saunders, 2000, with permission.)

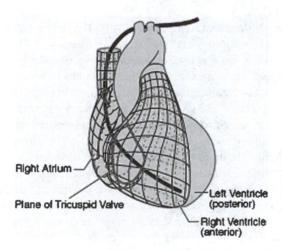

Fig. 4.5 Anterior orientation of the right ventricle. (From Belott PH. A practical approach to permanent pacemaker implantation. Armonk, NY: Futura Publishing, 1995, with permission.)

and to the right. In extreme circumstances, this displacement will rotate the right ventricular apex to the right of the midline. If this is not appreciated, lead placement can be extremely difficult if not impossible.

Transvenous Pacemaker Lead Placement

Historically, the venous cutdown technique has been the primary means of venous access for pacemaker electrode insertion (45). The cephalic vein has been commonly used in this approach, either from the right or left side.

Table 4.9 Venous structures for pacemaker lead insertion.

Cephalic vein	External jugular vein
Axillary vein	Femoral vein
Subclavian vein	Inferior vena cava
Internal jugular vein	

Table 4.10 Venous access for dual-chambered pacing.

Venous cutdown: Isolate one or two veins
Percutaneous: Two separate sticks and sheath applications
Percutaneous: Two electrodes down one large sheath
Percutaneous: Retained guidewire (Belott technique)
Cutdown with cephalic vein guidewire (Ong-Barold technique)

Occasionally, the more experienced surgeon has cannulated the internal jugular and the deeper axillary vein via this approach. Little departure from this pacemaker implantation technique had occurred until the late 1970s, when Littleford and Spector introduced the percutaneous sheath-set technique for venous access via the subclavian vein (46–49). This technique and variations on its theme have revolutionized pacemaker implantation. The percutaneous technique, however, has generated considerable controversy with respect to its safety. The percutaneous sheath-set technique has proven to be especially efficacious for dual-chambered pacing. With the development of the peel-away sheath, the problem of sheath removal from the permanent electrode was resolved. All that remained was in puncturing the desired venous structure. Once again, a thorough knowledge of the normal and abnormal anatomy was obviously essential. In more recent times, a combination of cutdown and percutaneous technique has been used to successfully access the venous structure. This involves the cutdown on a vein for vascular control and subsequent direct percutaneous access to a vessel by means of the Salinger technique. Common venous structures for pacemaker lead insertion are listed in Table 4.9.

Dual-chambered pacing calls for the introduction of an atrial and ventricular electrode. The cutdown technique is less suited for this approach because all too often the cephalic vein can hardly accommodate one electrode, and even less two. The percutaneous approach appears ideally suited for dual-chambered pacing as there is potential for unlimited access to the venous circulation. Various options for dual-chambered pacing venous access are listed in Table 4.10. There are four percutaneous approaches for dual-chambered pacing.

1. The first approach uses two separate percutaneous sticks and the application of two sheaths (50). This approach increases the risk of complications related to the venipuncture process in addition to possibly not finding the vessel a second time. There is also increased risk of pneumothorax, air embolism, bleeding, and vascular trauma.

2. The second technique utilizes one percutaneous stick and the use of a large sheath set that will accommodate the passage of both atrial and ventricular electrodes (51,52). The passage of two electrodes down one sheath is less desirable because the large sheath may increase the risk of air embolization and blood loss. In addition, there is increased frustration from electrode dislodgement and entanglement.

3. The retained-guidewire technique appears to be the most desirable approach. It also provides unlimited access to the central circulation (53–55). One is never committed or compromised. There is less risk of bleeding, pneumothorax, and air embolization. This author prefers the retained-guidewire technique. The ventricular electrode should be positioned first. This is both safe and practical. It is safe because, once positioned, there is always electrical support of the ventricle should asystole occur. It is also preferred, because the initially placed ventricular electrode is less susceptible to dislodgement during the positioning of the second (atrial) electrode. Once the ventricular electrode is in position, leaving the stylet in the vicinity of the lower right atrium stabilizes it. The electrode is also secured by use of a suture sleeve at the puncture site. After the ventricular electrode is stabilized, a second sheath set is applied to the retained guidewire (Fig. 4.6). The atrial electrode is introduced, positioned, and secured. The retained guidewire is only removed after one is completely satisfied with both electrode positions and there is no need to exchange. Hemostasis is achieved by a figure-of-eight suture stitch.

4. A fourth approach uses a combination of the sheath-set technique and a venous cutdown approach. Ong and associates have described the cephalic-guidewire technique (56). This technique involves the cutdown and isolation of the cephalic vein (Fig. 4.7). Instead of performing a venotomy, the vein is punctured percutaneously and a guidewire and sheath set applied. Unlike the cutdown technique, the cephalic vein is completely sacrificed. If the guidewire is retained, multiple sheath set exchanges and lead placements can be carried out. Once again, hemostasis is achieved by compression and/or the application of a figure-of-eight suture stitch. Despite sacrificing the cephalic vein, there have been no reports of venous complications.

Venous Cutdown of the Cephalic Vein: Cephalic Venous Access

The cephalic vein is found, as previously noted, in the deltopectoral groove. The lateral border of the pectoralis major muscle and the medial border of the deltoid muscle at the level of the coracoid process define the deltopectoral groove. An incision is made along the deltopectoral groove extending approximately 1½ to 2 in.. The incision is carried down directly through the dermis to the surface of the pectoralis muscle. The skin incision should be carried out in a single stroke. Once the initial incision has been made, a Weitlaner self-retaining retractor can be applied for exposure. The deltopectoral groove is then clearly identified. The deltopectoral groove is opened using Metzenbaum scissors. Further reapplication of the Weitlaner self-retaining retractor to the medial head of the deltoid and lateral head of the pectoralis major muscle affords excellent exposure. Careful dissection of the deltopectoral groove eventually exposes the cephalic vein. At times, this vessel is extremely diminutive and atretic.

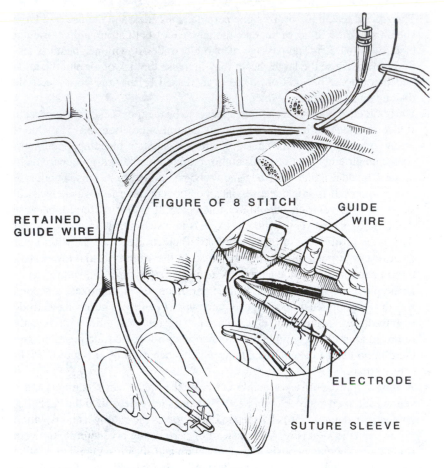

Fig. 4.6 The retained guidewire technique. The insert shows the secured ventricular electrode and suture sleeve, figure-of-eight stitch held by a clamp, and a second sheath set applied to the retained guidewire. (From Belott PH. New developments. In: Belott PH, et al. Implant techniques. Armonk, NY: Futura Publishing, 1988, with permission.)

If the cephalic vein is too small, further dissection may be carried proximally. In rare instances, dissection will actually be carried to the deeper axillary vein. Once exposed, the cephalic vein is freed from its fibrous attachments and O silk ligatures are applied proximally and distally (Fig. 4.8). Once adequate venous control has been obtained, a horizontal venotomy is made with an iris scissor or a #11 scalpel blade (Fig. 4.9). The vein should be supported at all times with a smooth forceps. Using mosquito clamps, forceps, or vein pick, the venotomy is opened and the electrode(s) introduced (Fig. 4.10). Once venous access has been achieved, the electrodes are positioned in the appropriate chambers using standard techniques.

Percutaneous Access to the Subclavian Vein

Cardiologists have used the Seldinger technique for percutaneous access for years. In this technique, a large-bore needle (#18 gauge) is used to percutaneously puncture the vascular structure. A guidewire is introduced through the needle into

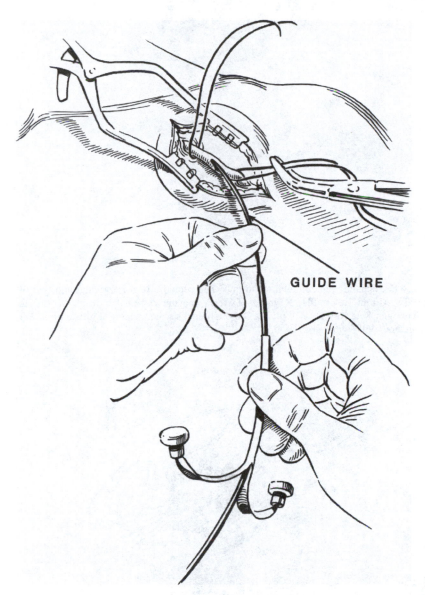

GUIDE WIRE

Fig. 4.7 The Ong-Barold technique. (From Belott PH. New developments. In: Belott PH, et al. New perspectives in cardiac pacing implantation techniques. Armonk, NY: Futura Publishing, 1988, with permission.)

the vessel and the needle is removed over the wire and exchanged for a catheter or sheath. Today, prepackaged introducer sets are used for this purpose.

Once again, it is important for the operator to be completely familiar with normal anatomy and superficial anatomic landmarks. The traditional subclavian puncture is carried out in the middle third of the clavicle. This location is frequently associated with an increased risk of vascular trauma, pneumothorax, and a lack of success. An alternate approach calls for the puncture at the apex of an angle formed by the clavicle and first rib (Fig. 4.11) (57). This location is remote from the apex of the lung, and the venous structure is generally much larger.

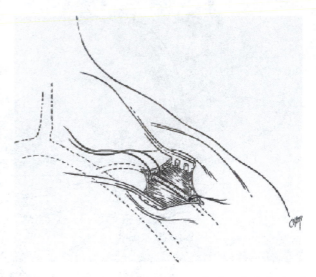

Fig. 4.8 Cephalic vein cutdown technique. The cephalic vein is isolated and tied off distally. (From Belott PH, Reynolds DW. Permanent pacemaker implantation. In: Ellenbogen KA, Kay N, Wilkoff BL, eds. Clinical cardiac pacing. Philadelphia: WB Saunders, 1995, with permission.)

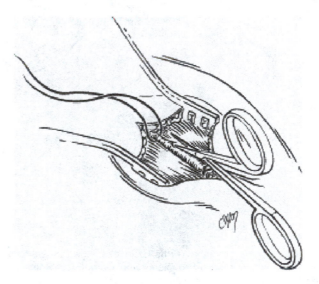

Fig. 4.9 Venotomy is performed with an iris scissors. (From Belott PH, Reynolds DW. Permanent pacemaker implantation. In: Ellenbogen KA, Kay N, Wilkoff BL, eds. Clinical cardiac pacing. Philadelphia: WB Saunders, 1995, with permission.)

It is important to maintain the patient in the anatomic position. Maneuvers that artificially open the costoclavicular and infraclavicular spaces should be avoided. The common practices of placing towels between the scapulae or extending the arm may result in undesirable puncture of the costoclavicular ligament or subclavius muscle. The medial venous puncture clearly increases the success rate as well as dramatically reduces the risk of pneumothorax and vascular injury.

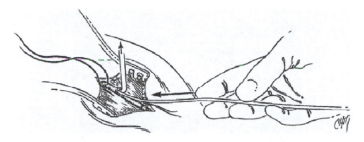

Fig. 4.10 The lead is inserted while the venotomy is held open with a vein pick. (From Belott PH, Reynolds DW. Permanent pacemaker implantation. In: Ellenbogen KA, Kay N, Wilkoff BL, eds. Clinical cardiac pacing. Philadelphia: WB Saunders, 1995, with permission.)

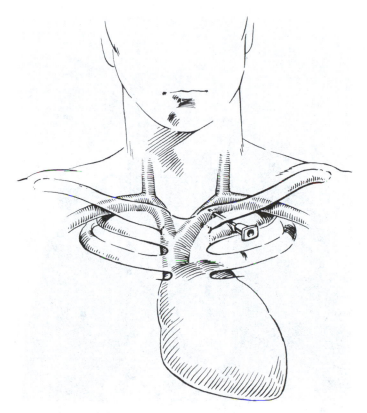

Fig. 4.11 Extreme medial subclavian puncture. (From Belott PH. New developments. In: Belott PH, et al. New perspectives in cardiac pacing implantation techniques. Armonk, NY: Futura Publishing, 1988, with permission.)

An #18 gauge thin-walled needle is used for venipuncture. Once the vessel has been entered, the guidewire is inserted with its tip position in the mid-right atrium (Fig. 4.12). Fluoroscopy should always be used to check the position of the wire. The wire should never be forced; if any resistance is encountered, readvancement is advised. The guidewire tracks superiorly into

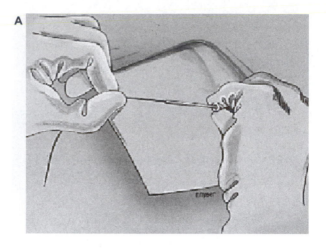

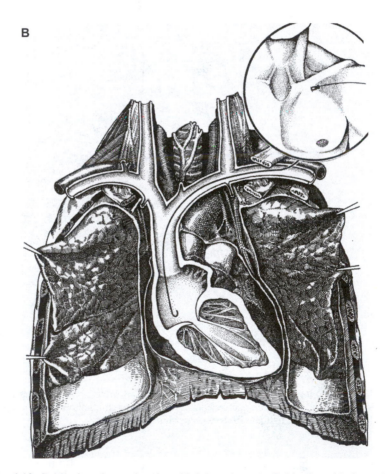

Fig. 4.12 Guidewire advanced to the mid right atrium. A: Guidewire with tip occluder is passed down the needle. B: Guidewire is advanced to the mid-right atrium.

the internal jugular vein. Once venous access has been achieved, every effort should be made to retain it. As the guidewire tracks into the internal jugular vein, a subtle change in the needle angle should be effected and the guidewire retracted into the needle while the needle is still in the vascular structure. The wire is readvanced, usually resulting in passage through the innominate vein to the superior vena cava. If this maneuver fails, a small-gauge rubber dilator may be passed over the guidewire and used as a catheter to steer the guidewire into its proper trajectory. The dilator may also be used for injection of contrast material to define the venous anatomy.

Once successful venous access has been achieved, the skin incision is created. The incision should be directed along anatomic lines. The skin incision is carried medially and inferiorly for approximately 2 in.. Once the incision has been carried out, the Weitlaner self-retaining retractor is applied similar to that described for the venous cutdown. The Weitlaner retractor holds tissue under tension as broad-based scalpel strokes are carried around to the surface of the pectoralis muscle.

After the incision has been carried to the surface of the pectoralis muscle and there is good exposure of the puncture site, a figure-of-eight suture stitch is applied about the needle (Fig. 4.13). This stitch serves for hemostasis throughout the procedure. With the initial preparations of the wound completed, the needle may be removed from the guidewire and a sheath set applied. The dilator and sheath are advanced over the guidewire with a continuous forward motion. It is important to avoid twisting and rotating the dilator sheath because this motion may result in tearing of the sheath's leading edge at the sheath dilator transition. The sheath should always be advanced under fluoroscopic observation. This avoids the inadvertent puncture or tearing of the right innominate vein and superior vena cava. After successful passage of the sheath set, the dilator is removed and the electrode passed down the sheath. It is recommended that when the dilator is removed, the guidewire be retained and the electrode passed alongside the guidewire. The sheath is then retracted and peeled away. Positioning of the electrode with the sheath in situ is unwise because it may result in air embolism or unnecessary blood loss. With the sheath removed, hemostasis is achieved by applying tension to the figure-of-eight stitch (Fig. 4.14) (58). The retention of the guidewire is a variation of the standard introducer technique. The retained guidewire may provide unlimited venous access and the ability to exchange and introduce additional electrodes by simply applying another sheath to the guidewire. The retained guidewire should be held to the drape with a clamp to avoid inadvertent dislodgement. The retained guidewire can also serve as a ground for unipolar threshold analysis. It can also be used as an intracardiac lead for the recording of electrograms or for emergency pacing. The guidewire should be retained in both single- and dual-chambered procedures until satisfactory lead position is attained.

Axillary Venous Access

Frequently, the solution to one problem creates another problem. A case in point is this author's proposed extreme medial subclavian percutaneous technique. Although this approach is safe, avoids the complication of pneumothorax, and expedites venous access, it has been implicated in the case of

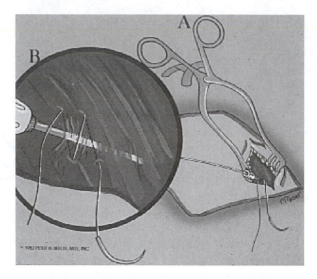

Fig. 4.13 Initial dissection complete, the figure-of-eight stitch is placed about the needle.

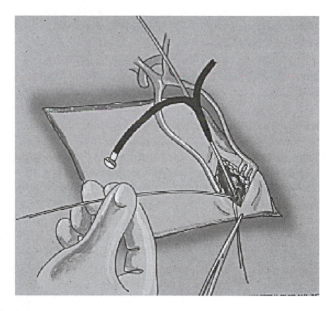

Fig. 4.14 The sheath is retracted and tension is applied to the figure-of-eight stitch. The guidewire is retained and clamped to the drape.

premature pacemaker lead failure by conductor fracture and insulation damage (59). Electrode failure as a result of an extreme medial approach has been called "the subclavian crush phenomenon." Fyke was first to report insulation failure of two leads placed side by side in the percutaneous approach to the subclavian vein where there was a tight costoclavicular space (60,61). This phenomenon has now been extensively reported in the literature.

There are a number of proposed mechanisms and potential solutions (62–65). Electrodes of a more complex design, such as bipolar coaxial construction, are most susceptible to this phenomenon. A more lateral percutaneous approach

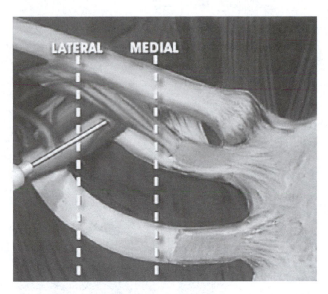

Fig. 4.15 Safe access of the extrathoracic portion of the subclavian vein as described by Byrd. (From Byrd CL. Clinical experience with the extrathoracic introducer insertion technique. PACE 1993;16(9):1781–1784, with permission.)

has been suggested to avoid the crush phenomenon. More recently, the axillary vein has been suggested as an alternate site of venous access to avoid the crush phenomenon. This was first suggested by Byrd in his proposed "safe introducer technique" (66).

Byrd defines a safety zone for percutaneous venous access that is very similar to the subclavian window. In addition, several conditions must be fulfilled. An essential condition of puncture is adequate ease of needle insertion that avoids friction and puncture of bone, cartilage, or tendon (Fig. 4.15). If a puncture cannot be safely conducted within the safety zone, the axillary vein is then percutaneously cannulated. As mentioned in the descriptive anatomy, the axillary vein is actually a continuation of the subclavian vein after it exits the superior mediastinum and crosses the first rib. It is frequently called the extrathoracic portion of the subclavian vein. This vein is usually quite large. The axillary vein traverses the anterolateral chest wall into the axilla (Fig. 4.16). It crosses the deltopectoral groove at approximately the level of the coracoid process. At the level of the teres major and latissimus dorsi muscle, it becomes the basilic vein. Both pectoralis major and minor muscles cover the axillary vein. It runs medial and parallel to the deltopectoral groove for approximately 1–2 cm.

The cephalic vein, a common venous access site for pacemaker implantation, drains directly into the axillary vein just superior to the pectoralis minor. The axillary vein is an excellent site for venous access, but is usually not considered because it is a rather deep structure. The surface landmarks of note are the infraclavicular space, deltopectoral groove, and the coracoid process.

The axillary venous approach was initially reported in 1987 by Nichalls as an alternate site of venous access for large central lines (67). Nichalls developed a technique from cadaver dissection by which he established reliable landmarks. He defined the axillary vein as an infraclavicular structure. In his technique, the needle is always anterior to the thoracic cavity, generally

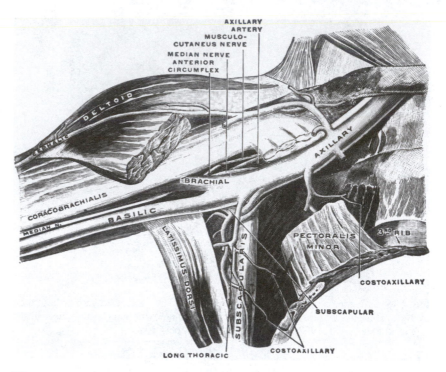

Fig. 4.16 Detailed anatomy of the anterolateral chest demonstrating the axillary vein with the pectoralis major and minor muscles removed. (From Belott PH. Unusual access sites for permanent cardiac pacing. In: Barold SS, Mugica J, eds. Recent advances in cardiac pacing: goals for the 21st century. Armonk, NY: Futura Publishing, 1997, with permission.)

tangential to the chest wall to avoid pneumothorax and hemopneumothorax. The landmarks used by Nichalls are as follows (Fig. 4.17). The vein starts medial at a point below the medial aspect of the clavicle where the space between the clavicle and the first rib becomes palpable. The vein extends laterally to a point three fingerbreadths below the inferior aspect of the coracoid process. The skin is punctured along the medial border of the pectoralis minor muscle at a point above the vein as surface landmarks define it. The axillary vein is punctured by passing the needle anterior to the first rib, maneuvering posteriorly and medially. It is corresponding to the lateral-to-medial course of the axillary vein. The needle passes between the first rib and clavicle. In this technique, the arm is usually adducted 45 degrees. The Nichalls experience was further reinforced by Taylor and Yellowlees, who reported an experience with the technique in 102 consecutive patients (68). There were only four failures and one pneumothorax. In the technique described by Byrd, an #18 gauge thin-walled needle is guided by fluoroscopy and directed to the medial portion of the first rib. The needle is held perpendicular to the first rib, as it is walked laterally until the axillary vein is punctured. This is indicated by the aspiration of venous blood (Fig. 4.18). The guidewire is inserted and the introducer is subsequently applied per standard technique. It is important to note that the needle path is always directed anterior to the thoracic cavity to avoid the risk of pneumothorax. Byrd reported a series of 213 consecutive cases where the

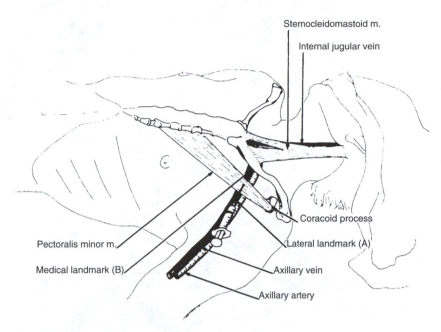

Fig. 4.17 Nichalls' sketch of the landmarks for axillary vein puncture. (From Belott PH, Byrd CL. Recent developments in pacemaker and load retrieval. In: Belott PH. New perspectives in cardiac pacing implantation techniques, 2nd ed. Armonk, NY: Futura Publishing, 1991, with permission.)

extrathoracic portion of the subclavian vein (axillary vein) was successfully cannulated as a primary approach (69).

Magney (70) and associates have reported a new approach to percutaneous subclavian venipuncture to avoid lead fracture (69). This technique, very similar to Byrd's, only uses extensive surface landmarks for veni-puncture (Fig. 4.19). The technique involves puncture of the extrathoracic portion of the subclavian vein or axillary vein. The location of the axillary vein is defined as the intersection with a line drawn between the middle of the sternal angle and the tip of the coracoid process. This is generally near the lateral border of the first rib. Recently, this author has described blind axillary venous access using a modification of the Byrd and Magney recommendations (71,72). In this technique, the deltopectoral groove and coracoid process are primary landmarks. The deltopectoral groove and coracoid process are palpated and the curvature of the chest wall noted. An incision is made at the level of the coracoid process. It is carried medially for approximately 2½ in. and is perpendicular to the deltopectoral groove (Fig. 4.20). The incision is carried to the surface of the pectoralis major muscle. The deltopectoral groove is directly visualized.

The needle is inserted at an angle of 45 degrees parallel to the deltopectoral groove, 1–2 cm medial (Figs. 4.21 and 4.22).If the vein is not entered, fluoroscopy is then used to define the first rib. The needle is advanced and touches the first rib. Sequential needle punctures are walked laterally and posteriorly until the vein is entered. It should be noted that one cannot palpate the axillary artery pulse and, thus, it is not a reliable landmark. The axillary artery and brachial plexus are usually much deeper and more posterior structures. This simple technique using basic anatomic landmarks of the

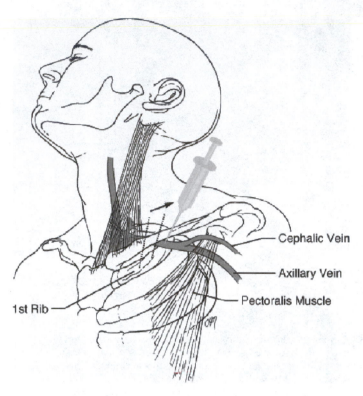

Fig. 4.18 Byrd's technique for access of the extrathoracic portion of the subclavian vein. Sequential needle punctures are walked posterolaterally along the first rib until the vein is entered. (From Belott PH, Reynolds DW. Permanent pacemaker implantation. In: Ellenbogen KA, Kay N, Wilkoff BL, eds. Clinical cardiac pacing. Philadelphia: WB Saunders, 1995, with permission.)

deltopectoral groove and a blind venous stick has been used successfully in 168 consecutive pacemaker and ICD procedures. There have only been three failures. These required an alternate approach. With a thorough knowledge of regional anatomy, the axillary vein can be safely used as a primary site for venous access.) If the vein is not entered, fluoroscopy is used to define the first rib (Fig. 4.23). The first rib is an extremely reliable land mark for axillary venous access.Using fluoroscopy guidance, the needle is advanced and touches the first rib.Caution should be used so as to avoid passing the needle into the interspace between the first and second rib causing a pneumothorax. This can be avoided by placing the needle tip over the rib using fluoroscopy and gradually increasing the needle angle while advancing until the rib is touched. Then one can walk along the rib medially and laterally until the vein is entered. At present the blind venous access has been abandoned for this first rib approach as it reduces the risk of pneumothorax to zero. Critical is the ability to identify the first or second rib radiographically. In addition if the first rib is poorly visualized or set to far under the clavicle one can always use the second rib in a similar fashion. Sequential needle punctures are walked laterally and posteriorly until the vein is entered. Occasionally, in a thin patient the axillary artery can be easily palpated. This makes the axillary vein stict easy as the percutaneous stick can be make just medial and inferior

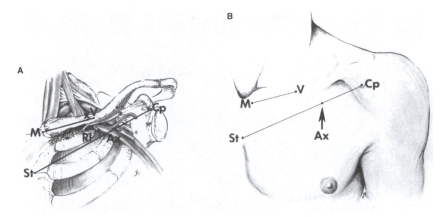

Fig. 4.19 Deep (A) and superficial (B) anatomic relationships of the Magney approach to subclavian vena puncture. Point M indicates the medial end of the clavicle. X defines a point on the clavicle directly above the lateral edges of the clavicular/subclavius muscle (tendon complex). R1. Point D overlies the center of the subclavian vein as it crosses the first rib. St, the center of the sternal angle; Cp, coracoid process; Ax, axillary vein; star, costoclavicular ligament; open circle with closed circle, costo-clavicular ligament; open circle with closed circle inside, costoclavicular ligament; sm, subclavius muscle. The arrow points to Magney's ideal point for venous entry. (Magney JE, Staplin DH, Flynn DM, et al. A new approach to percutaneous subclavian venipuncture to avoid lead fracture or central venous catheter occlusion. Pacing Clin Electrophysiol 1993;16(11):2133–2142, with permission.)

to the palpable axillary pulse. Because one cannot always palpate the axillary pulse, it is not a reliable landmark. The axillary artery and brachial plexus are usually much deeper and more posterior structures. The needle is advanced and touches the first rib and sequential needle punctures are walked laterally and posteriorly until the venous structure is entered. The axillary vein may also be isolated by direct cutdown. Using Metzenbaum scissors, the fibers of the pectoralis major muscle are separated adjacent to the deltopectoral groove at the level of the coracoid process. This is just above the level of the superior border of the pectoralis minor. The pectoralis major is split in this area and the fibers are gently teased apart. This is carried out in an access parallel to the muscle bundles; the axillary vein is found directly underneath the pectoralis major. A pursestring stitch is applied to the vein and it can be cannulated by either percutaneous or the cutdown approach. A pursestring stitch serves for hemostasis and ultimately assists in anchoring the electrode(s) after positioning. A number of techniques have been developed to assist access of the axillary vein. Varnagy and associates have described a technique for isolating the cephalic and/or axillary vein (73). This technique consists of introducing a J-ended Teflon guidewire through the vein in the antecubital fossa under fluoroscopic control. The metal guidewire is then palpated in the deltopectoral groove or identified by fluoroscopy. The palpated guidewire guides the subsequent cutdown for puncture of the vessel by fluoroscopy. The cutdown can be performed on the vein or the intravascular guidewire pulled out of the venotomy to allow application of an introducer. It is felt that this technique offers the benefits of rapid venous access while avoiding the hazard of pneu-mothorax associated with the percutaneous approach. If the percutaneous

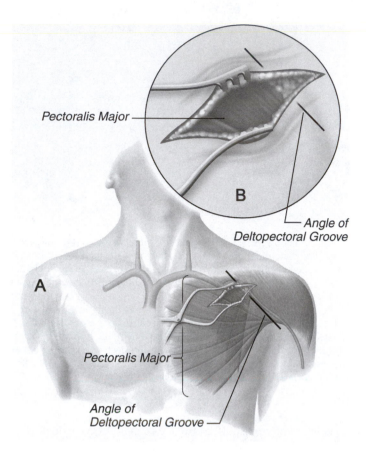

Fig. 4.20 A: Incision carried down to the surface of the pectoralis major muscle and its orientation with respect to the deltopectoral groove noted. B: Insert demonstrating the deltopectoral groove and orientation of the lateral border of the clavicular head of the pectoralis major. (From Belott PH. Blind axillar venous access. Pacing Clin Electrophysiol 1999;22(7):1085–1089, with permission.)

approach is used, the puncture can always be extrathoracic using fluoroscopy to guide the needle to the guidewire. Axillary venipuncture can also be facilitated by the use of contrast venography. The venous anatomy can be observed by fluoroscopy in the pectoral area and, if possible, recorded for repeat viewing. The needle trajectory and venipuncture are guided by contrast material in the axillary vein (74). Laboratories fortunate enough to have sophisticated imaging capabilities can create a mask. Spencer and associates reported the use of contrast venography for localizing the axillary vein in 22 consecutive patients (75,76). Similarly, Ramza and associates demonstrated the safety and efficacy of the axillary vein for placement of pacemaker and defibrillator leads when guided by contrast venography (77). Lead placement was successfully accomplished in 49 of 50 patients using this technique. Venous access of the axillary vein can also be guided by Doppler and ultrasound techniques. Fyke has described a Doppler-guided extrathoracic introducer insertion technique in 59 consecutive patients (total of 100 leads) with a simple Doppler flow detector (78). A sterile Doppler flow detector is moved along

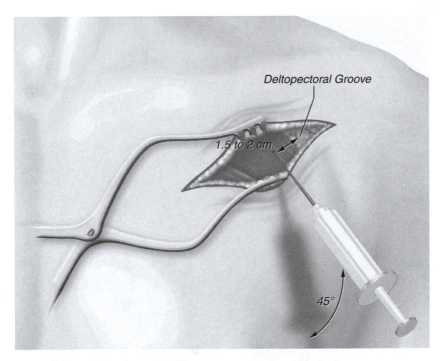

Fig. 4.21 Needle trajectory and angle with respect to the deltopectoral groove, pectoralis major, lateral border of the cephalic head of the pectoralis major muscle, and the chest wall. (From Belott PH. Blind axillar venous access. Pacing Clin Electrophysiol 1999;22(7):1085–1089, with permission.)

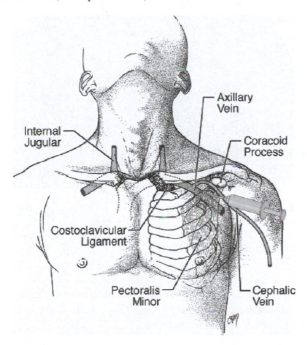

Fig. 4.22 Axillary vein puncture and its relationship to surface landmarks as well as the first rib. (From Belott PH. Unusual access sites for permanent cardiac pacing. In: Barold SS, Mugica J, eds. Recent advances in cardiac pacing: goals for the 21st century. Armonk, NY: Futura Publishing, 1997, with permission.)

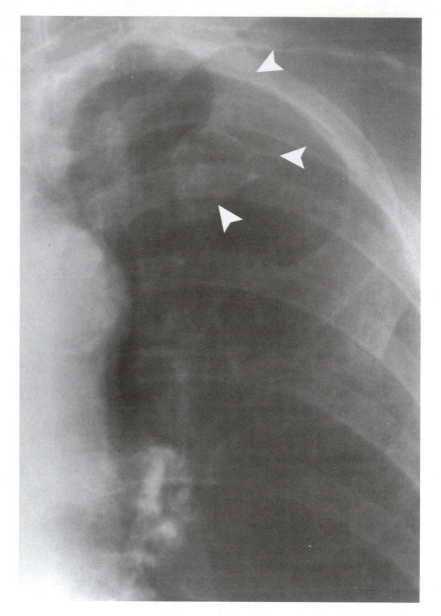

Fig. 4.23 Radiograph demonstrating the location of the first rib. (From Belott PH. Unusual access sites for permanent cardiac pacing. In: Barold SS, Mugica J, eds. Recent Advances in Cardiac Pacing: Goals for the 21st Century. Armonk, NY: Futura Publishing, 1997, with permission.)

the clavicle and, once the vein is defined, the location and angle of the probe are noted and the venipuncture carried out (Fig. 4.24). Care is taken to avoid directing the Doppler beam beneath the clavicle. Gayle and associates have developed an ultrasound technique that directly visualizes the needle puncture of the axillary vein (79,80). A portable ultrasound device with sterile sleeve and needle holder is used. The ultrasound head is placed over the skin surface in the vicinity of the axillary vein. Once identified, the puncture and

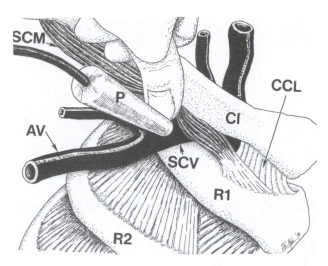

Fig. 4.24 Doppler location of the axillary vein crossing the first rib. AV, axillary vein; CCL, costo-clavicular ligament; CL, clavicle; P, Doppler probe; R1, first rib; R2, second rib; SCM, subclavius muscle; SCV, subclavian vein. (From Fyke FE. Doppler guided extrathoracic introducer insertion. Pacing Clin Electrophysiol 1995; 18 (5 Pt 1):1017–1021, with permission.)

Seldinger technique are used. Because this technique directly visualizes the axillary vein, it has been used with considerable success for both pacing and defibrillator electrodes. There have been no pneumothoraces. The technique can be carried out transcutaneously or through the incision on the surface of the pectoralis muscle.

The axillary vein is becoming a common venous access site for pacemaker and defibrillator implantations, given the concerns of the subclavian crush and the requirement for insertion of multiple electrodes for dual-chambered pacing and a large complex electrode for transvenous nonthoracotomy defibrillation. There are now a number of reliable techniques for axillary venous access (Table 4.11).

Given the recent interest in the axillary vein, it is recommended once again that the implanting physician become thoroughly familiar with the anatomy of the anterior thoracic wall, shoulder, and axilla. It is imperative that the physician visit the anatomic laboratory to refresh and review the regional anatomy and surface landmarks.

Contrast Venography

As previously mentioned, contrast venography may be used to facilitate percutaneous venous access of both the subclavian and axillary vein. Hayes and colleagues first described this technique (74). In this technique, a venous line is established on the side of planned venous access. It is advisable to use a large-gauge needle. Contrast material (10–20 mL) is injected rapidly into the intravenous line followed by a saline flush. Occasionally, a nonsterile assistant massaging the contrast material through the peripheral venous system underneath the sterile drape facilitates this. Fluoroscopy is then used to direct the

Table 4.11 Techniques for axillary venous access.

Blind percutaneous puncture using surface landmarks

Blind puncture through pectoralis major muscle using deep landmarks

Direct cutdown on the axillary vein

Fluoroscopy: needle the first rib for reference

Contrast venography

Doppler-guided

Ultrasound-guided

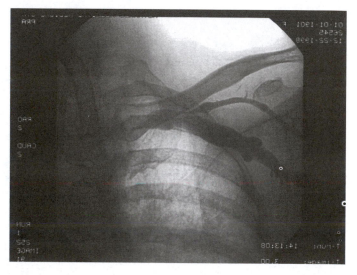

Fig. 4.25 Contrast venography of the larger axillary vein with a smaller cephalic vein draining into it at a right angle. (From Belott PH, Reynolds DW. Permanent pacemaker and cardioverter defibrillation implantation. In: Ellenbogen KA, Kay N, Wilkoff BL, eds. Clinical cardiac pacing and defibrillation, 2nd ed. Philadelphia: WB Saunders, 2000, with permission.)

needle to the site of venous access as defined by the contrast material (Fig. 4.25). In the cardiac catheterization laboratory or special studies room, a mask or map may be obtained for guidance after the contrast material has dissipated. This technique has been extremely helpful in locating both the subclavian and axillary veins and has been applied to other venous structures. When this technique is used regularly, one becomes aware of the extreme medial-to-lateral variability of the location of the axillary vein's course and location. Occasionally, this approach is used after multiple attempts at blind venipuncture where contrast venography demonstrates a proximal complete obstruction of the venous structure with collaterals to the internal jugular (Fig. 4.26).

Jugular Venous Access

The jugular vein has been used for permanent pacemaker implantation as an alternate cutdown site (81). As a rule, the jugular vein has not been utilized for nonthoracotomy lead systems. This is a large venous structure that lies in the cervical triangle defined by the lateral border of the omohyoid muscle, inferior

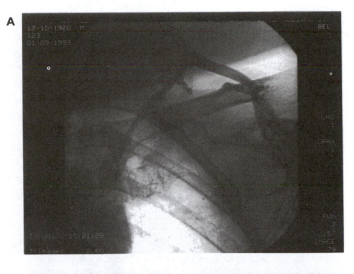

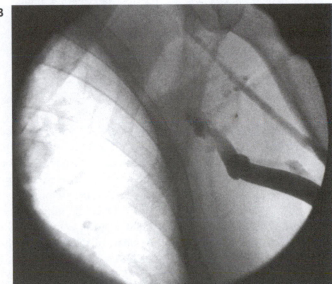

Fig 4.26 A: Complete absence of the axillary vein. (Note plexus of veins draining over the clavicle into the external jugular vein and subsequently the innominate vein.) B: Totally obstructed axillary vein.

border of the digastric muscle, and the medial border of the sternocleidomastoid. The superficial cervical fascia and platysma muscle covers it. It can be identified by palpation because it is just lateral to the external carotid. Many authors have described exotic and sophisticated landmarks to define its location when, in reality, simple palpation of the carotid pulse defines the jugular vein. Punctures immediately lateral to the carotid pulse are frequently rewarded with success. Historically, jugular venous access has been considered when traditional venous cutdown of the cephalic vein has been unsuccessful. This approach is somewhat less desirable than the subclavian, axillary, and cephalic vein placement because of increased risk of lead fracture and the potential for lead erosion. The acute angle that is created on the lead after it exits the venous structure as it is brought down over the clavicle to the pocket creates circumstances for this problem. Also, this procedure is somewhat more involved because tunneling is required to bring the lead to the pocket. If tunneling is performed under the clavicle, there is increased risk of pneumothorax and vascular injury. If the lead is tunneled over the clavicle, tissue is typically thin and there is a greater risk of erosion. As a rule, the right internal jugular approach is preferred. In early reports jugular venous access was performed by the cutdown technique. An alternate percutaneous approach has been proposed that requires little attention to anatomic landmarks and dissection. Additionally, an initial supraclavicular incision is not required. This approach involves percutaneous access of the right internal jugular vein. Access to the internal jugular vein is best obtained with the patient in the normal anatomic position with the head facing anterior. Rotating the head to the left only distorts the anatomy. The carotid artery is palpated in the lower third of the neck. The internal jugular vein is lateral to the common carotid artery. The two structures are parallel. Addressing the patient on the right side for the right internal jugular approach, the implanting position places the middle finger over the course of the common carotid artery. The course of the internal jugular will be under the index finger. In fact, the index and middle fingers side by side are generally analogous to the size and orientation on the surface of the skin to the deeper internal jugular vein and common carotid artery because they run side by side underneath the skin. The venipuncture anywhere along the course should enter the internal jugular vein. If the puncture is made above the clavicle, pneumothoraces are avoided. The needle is generally held perpendicular to the plane of the neck rather than angled. This helps avoid infraclavicular puncture and potential pneumothorax. Once the needle has entered the vein, it is gently angled inferiorly for the passage of the guidewire. If the internal carotid artery is inadvertently punctured, the needle is simply removed and pressure held. A repeat attempt at venipuncture is made slightly lateral to the initial stick. Once the internal jugular vein is entered, the technique is essentially identical to a standard procedure. A small incision is carried laterally down the shaft of the needle to the surface of the sternocleidomastoid muscle. If more tissue depth is required, the muscle can be split and the incision carried directly down over the vein. A small Weitlaner retractor is used for more adequate exposure. It is important to place a figure-of-eight suture for vascular control, hemostasis, and anchoring (Fig. 4.27). The retained-guidewire technique may be used for placement of both the atrial and ventricular electrodes. After adequate lead position, the figure-of-eight stitch is secured for hemostasis and the lead anchored to the muscle body using the suture sleeve. A second incision for the pocket formation is made infraclavicularly. The leads are then tunneled to the pocket by standard tunneling techniques (Fig. 4.28). When the electrodes are tunneled under the clavicle, care must be taken to avoid vascular trauma. Conversely, when tunneling over the clavicle, every effort should be made to ensure optimal tissue depth to avoid potential erosion. The tunneling technique described by Roelke and associates for submammary pacemaker implantation may also be used for infraclavicular tunneling (82). A long #18 gauge spinal needle can be passed from the infraclavicular incision to the supraclavicular incision. The guidewire is passed, and the sheath set is applied and tunneled to the supraclavicular inci-

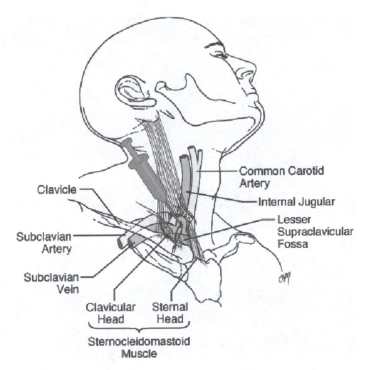

Fig. 4.27 Percutaneous venous access of the right internal jugular vein. Weitlaner retractor placed demonstrating the figure-of-eight stitch. (From Belott PH, Reynolds DW. Permanent pacemaker implantation. In: Ellenbogen KA, Kay N, Wilkoff BL, eds. Clinical cardiac pacing. Philadelphia: WB Saunders, 1995, with permission.)

sion. The rubber dilator is removed. The lead to be used is inserted in the distal end of the sheath and tied. Once secured, the lead and sheath are pulled through to the infraclavicular incision.

The external jugular vein is less frequently used for venous access because it is more inferiorly located and there is a higher risk of pneumothorax as well as vascular complications; it is less precise, and successful cannulation may be more frustrating.

Femoral Venous Access

The femoral vein has been reported as an alternate site for pacemaker implantation. If one punctures the venous structure above Poupart's ligament, it is anatomically the iliac vein; below Poupart's ligament, it is designated as the femoral vein. Iliac venipuncture has been reported as an alternate source for single and dual-chambered pacemaker implantation (83,84). It has not been utilized for defibrillator electrode placement. Ellestad and French have reported a 90-patient experience utilizing the iliac vein. This vein can be used for transvenous lead placement when an abdominal pocket is desired. It is usually reserved for patients with little pectoral tissue, such as in the case of bilateral mastectomy, extensive pectoral radiation damage, or for a variety of other cosmetic reasons. A small incision is made above the inguinal ligament above the vein, just medial to the palpable femoral artery (Fig. 4.29). The incision is carried down to the surface above the vein. The vein is then punctured via the

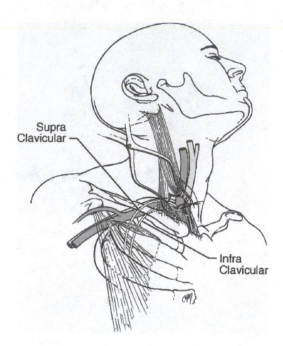

Fig. 4.28 Pacemaker leads (S) tunneled over and under the clavicle to the infraclavicular pocket. (From Belott PH. Unusual access sites for permanent cardiac pacing. In: Barold SS, Mugica J, eds. Recent advances in cardiac pacing: goals for the 21st century. Armonk, NY: Futura Publishing, 1997, with permission.)

Seldinger sheath-set technique with the guidewire retained for dual-chambered implants. A figure-of-eight stitch or a pursestring suture is placed for hemostasis. The suture is placed through the fascia, around the lead as it enters the vein. Special long (85 cm) leads are positioned in a conventional manner and secured to the fascia by use of a tie around the suture sleeve and lead. A horizontal incision is made at the second site, just lateral to the umbilicus. This is carried down to the surface of the rectus sheath. A pacemaker pocket is created in the conventional manner. Preparations are then made for tunneling of the leads from the initial incision to the newly created pocket by use of one of the standard tunneling techniques. Active fixation electrodes are recommended for both atrial and ventricular lead placement. In the Ellestad experience, lead dislodgments have been reported as a major weakness in this approach. Venous thrombosis and lead fracture do not appear to be a problem, although the published experience with this approach is relatively small and the latter is difficult to discern. Obviously, the complication of pneumothorax associated with the percutaneous approach does not exist. Similarly, the complication of air embolism is not a problem.

Upgrading Techniques for Dual-Chambered Pacing and Defibrillator Systems

It is now appreciated that when approaching a patient for a permanent transvenous pacemaker or modern AICD system, every effort should be made to preserve atrial and ventricular relationships.(In addition there are patients

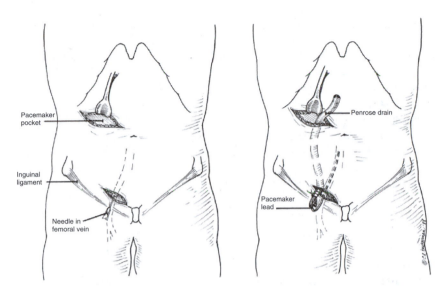

Fig. 4.29 Use of the right iliac vein for placement of pacemaker leads. The leads are ultimately tunneled using a Penrose drain to a pocket created in the right upper quadrant. (From Ellestad MH, French J. Iliac vein approach to permanent pacemaker implantation. Pacing Clin Electrophysiol 1989;12(7 Pt 1):1030–1033, with permission.)

with an existing pacemaker system who require an upgrade to an automatic implantable cardioverter defibrillator or a biventricular system for resynchronization. These patients require the addition of a pacing and shocking electrode and/or a left ventricular lead.) Sensitive to this concept, the majority of patients today receive dual-chambered pacing and ICD systems. There is, however, a large group of patients who have previously received single-chambered, ventricular-demand pacing systems. There is also a smaller group of patients who have previously received single-chambered atrial pacing systems. In addition, more recently, there are individuals who require an upgrade of their pacing system, which requires the abandonment of a pacing system and the addition of an implantable defibrillator. Many of the patients with VVI pacing and single-chamber defibrillator systems are symptomatic with the "pacemaker syndrome." In addition, a small group of atrially paced patients who have previously received single-chamber atrial systems are symptomatic with the development of AV block. Many of the symptomatic patients with such systems require pacemaker system upgrades with the addition of an atrial electrode. These patients, who are atrially paced and symptomatic with AV block, require ventricular support with the addition of a ventricular electrode. A patient previously paced either atrially or ventricularly who requires a defibrillator system will require the addition of a nonthoracotomy shocking lead. These groups of patients require system upgrades with the addition of one or more electrodes. The conventional pacing system upgrade techniques and pacing and defibrillator upgrading techniques involve the placement of a second electrode. In addition, this procedure is also combined with a pulse generator change. The dilemma with pacemaker and ICD system upgrades is the required supplemental venous access for placement of a second lead.

Venous access can be carried out by either cutdown or the percutaneous approach. If the initial electrode has been placed via cutdown, the isolation of a second vein for venous access will prove extremely difficult. In this case, percutaneous approach should be attempted. Conversely, if the initial electrode has been placed percutaneously, then a second percutaneous approach or a cutdown is always possible. The second percutaneous puncture is usually carried out just lateral to the initial venous entry site. The initial lead can be used as a marker of the venous anatomy. If any difficulty is encountered, fluoroscopy is used to guide the lead using the chronic ventricular lead for reference (85,86). There is potential risk of damaging the initial electrode and care should be taken to avoid its direct puncture. The use of radiographic materials can also help define the venous structure as well as its patency.

Occasionally, the vessel to be recanalized is thrombosed or obstructed, precluding venous access on the same side. In this case, contralateral venous access should be considered (87). In this instance, the desired electrode is passed via the contralateral subclavian vein, positioned, and subsequently tunneled back to the original pocket (Fig. 4.30). The contralateral puncture site requires a limited skin incision of about 1–2 cm. It is carried down to the surface of the pectoralis muscle. The pectoralis muscle is used for anchoring the electrode with its suture sleeve. The electrode is anchored and secured once it has been positioned. The proximal end of the electrode is then tunneled back to the original pocket.

Ventricular Lead Placement

Each implanting physician develops her or his own technique for ventricular lead placement (88). Common fundamental principles are used in the positioning of every electrode. Virtually every ventricular lead placement involves the passage through the right heart utilizing simultaneous manipulation of the electrode and stylet to achieve appropriate placement. Lead placement is virtually impossible without the lead stylet. The stylet is usually performed into a gentle curve that allows the electrode to negotiate a course through the right heart. The size and tightness of the curve directly relate to one's personal preference. As a general rule, curves that are too tight do not negotiate venous structures in the superior mediastinum, whereas curves that are too gentle fail to cross the tricuspid valve. Pacemaker and ICD lead movement is entirely different from the diagnostic catheters used in the cardiac catheterization laboratory. These leads cannot be torqued or rotated into position. Lead placement depends solely on manipulation of the lead body and stylet. Slight adjustments in the stylet by retraction and advancement result in subtle changes in the lead tip orientation. It is this combination of slight retraction and advancement of the curved stylet that ultimately points the electrode in the proper direction and effects precise lead placement. The ventricular lead placement can be expedited by placing the fluoroscopy in the right anterior oblique projection (Fig. 4.31). This maneuver helps define the apex of the right ventricle. Once again, it is important to point out that the right ventricular apex is an anterior structure. By placing the fluoroscopy in the right anterior oblique projection, one creates the illusion that the apex of the right ventricle is oriented toward the left lateral chest wall. An inexperienced operator will spend hours trying to position the ventricular electrode to the left of the spine when, in reality, the right ventricle

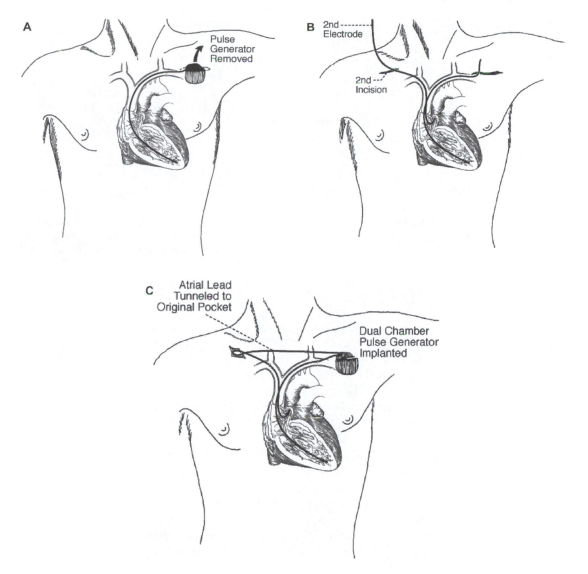

Fig. 4.30 A: Pacemaker system upgrade using contralateral subclavian vein. The pacemaker pocket is opened and the old pulse generator and lead and dissected free, externalized and disconnected. B: A second lead is inserted via the contralateral vein using the percutaneous technique. C: The second lead is tunneled back to the initial pocket. The chronic ventricular and new atrial electrodes are connected to the pulse generator. (From Belott PH. Unusual access sites for Permanent Cardiac Pacing. In: Barold SS, Mugica J, eds. Recent advances in cardiac pacing: Goals for the 21st century. Armonk, NY: Futura Publishing, 1997, with permission.)

is directly anterior. By simple rotation of the fluoroscopy into the right anterior oblique projection, the apex of the right ventricle is now oriented in the left chest. This is the same maneuver that angiographers use when performing left ventriculography. With the curved stylet in place, it is recommended that the ventricular lead be passed across the tricuspid valve and out to the pulmonary artery (Fig. 4.32). This maneuver documents right heart passage. If there are

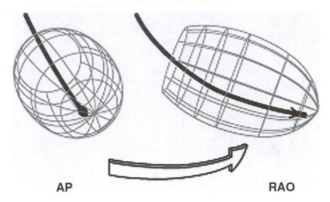

Fig. 4.31 Computer-generated wire form demonstrating the spatial orientation of the lead in the apex of the right ventricle in both the anterior-posterior and right antero-oblique projections. (From Belott PH, Reynolds DW. Permanent pacemaker implantation. In: Ellenbogen KA, Kay N, Wilkoff BL, eds. Clinical cardiac pacing. Philadelphia: WB Saunders, 1995, with permission.)

any doubts of the electrode position, one can manipulate fluoroscopy into the lateral projection. The lead tip should be observed to point anterior to be just beneath the sternum. This documents the right ventricular apex placement as opposed to the coronary sinus, which is posterior.

Passage of the electrode to the pulmonary artery is facilitated by retraction of the curved stylet approximately 1–2 cm, rendering the electrode tip floppy. Passive blood flow usually carries the lead to the right or left pulmonary artery. The curved stylet is then readvanced to the lead tip. With the lead stylet in the ventricular lead tip, the electrode body is gently retracted along the interventricular septum (Fig. 4.33). In the midpoint of the interventricular septum, the lead stylet is retracted 1–2 cm, rendering the lead tip floppy. The floppy lead tip then drops into the right ventricular apex. With the stylet retracted, the lead body is advanced, firmly seating the electrode tip in place. Because the lead is retracted, the lead tip is supple, precluding perforation of the right ventricular apex. It is not uncommon when retracting the lead down the interventricular septum for fixation mechanisms to hang up on right ventricular trabeculations. In this case, the stylet is removed and a straight stylet is advanced toward the lead tip. This maneuver usually frees the tip and directs it toward the apex of the right ventricle. Once the lead tip is appropriately oriented, the stylet should be retracted to render the tip floppy. Gentle electrode body advancement will seat the lead in the apex of the right ventricle.

Subtle adjustment in the lead tip orientation and position may be achieved by gentle lead retraction and readvancement with the stylet slightly retracted. With the lead in its desired position, the lead body can be advanced until slight resistance is encountered. This usually guarantees good ventricular lead tip seating. All stylet maneuvers should be observed under fluoroscopy. Occasionally, when exchanging the curved stylet for the straight stylet, the straight stylet, when advanced, dislodges the ventricular lead from the right ventricular apex. In extreme circumstances the stylet actually dislodges the tip back into the right atrium. When this problem is encountered, the lead placement is repeated as in the preceding, but a more flexible stylet is recommended.

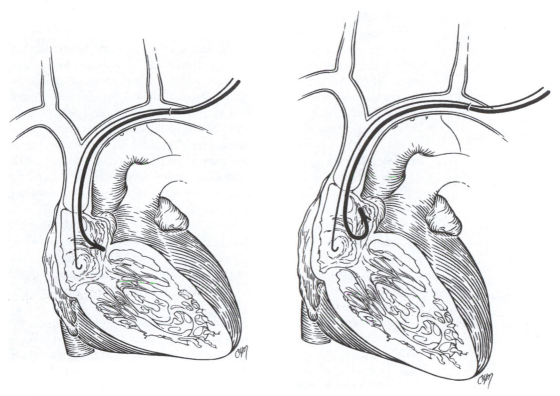

Fig. 4.32 Electrode with curved stylet is advanced to the tricuspid valve. The electrode is pressed against the tricuspid valve and flipped across into the right ventricular outflow tract. (From Belott PH. A practical approach to permanent pacemaker implantation. Armonk, NY: Futura Publishing, 1995, with permission.)

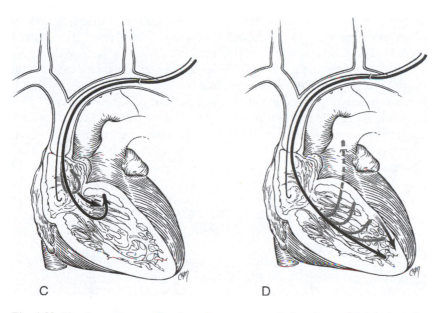

C   D

Fig. 4.33 The electrode passed to the pulmonary artery is then dragged down along the intraventricular septum and allowed to fall into the right ventricular apex. (From Belott PH. A practical approach to permanent pacemaker implantation. Armonk, NY: Futura Publishing, 1995, with permission.)

Ventricular lead dislodgement during stylet exchange can be avoided by straightening the lead body prior to advancement of the stylet across the tricuspid valve. This maneuver is carried out by gentle retraction of the ventricular lead under fluoroscopic observation. The straightened and retracted ventricular lead avoids the buildup of a loop in the lower right atrium that can result in lead dislodgement with subsequent stylet manipulations. Right ventricular lead fixation is validated by gently pulling on the electrode until resistance is encountered. This is an extremely reliable sign that fixation of the lead has been achieved by the tines or other passive fixation mechanisms. The same maneuver should never be performed with a positive fixation screw-in electrode. In this case, good fixation is documented by acceptable threshold measurements. This is because the active fixation or screw-in lead tissue bond is extremely delicate and retraction usually results in dislodgement, weakened fixation, and further tissue damage. Occasionally, right ventricular placement by retracting the electrode from the pulmonary artery is unsuccessful. In this case, the lead may be readvanced to the pulmonary artery and the curved stylet removed. A stiff stylet is then inserted. It usually points toward the apex of the right ventricle. By simply dragging the electrode over the stiff stylet as it is pointing away to the right ventricular apex, the electrode can be positioned.

Right ventricular perforation is avoided by simultaneously advancing the electrode body while retracting the stylet. In this maneuver, the lead stylet is merely pointing the way to the right ventricular apex. Ventricular lead placement is much more expeditious after left venous access. It is as if the heart were designed for permanent pacemaker and ICD lead placement from the left. Once left venous entry access is achieved, the ventricular lead tracks in a gentle curve from the superior vena cava, right atrium, right ventricle, and pulmonary artery with the curved stylet. On fluoroscopy, the track of the electrode forms a giant letter C. Because there are no acute angles or bends, the lead advances with little or no difficulty. Occasionally, the advancing lead tip hangs up on the tricuspid valve. With the curved stylet in place, the tricuspid valve is usually negotiated by backing the lead across the valve with a loop. An alternate method calls for retraction of the curved stylet, rendering the tip floppy. The floppy tip is observed to point in the appropriate direction. Brisk movement across the tricuspid anulus will achieve right heart passage. This is known as the "floppy-tip technique." Occasionally, in the extreme elderly patient, venous structures in the superior mediastinum are extremely tortuous, with many acute angles and bends. This situation can render even a left-sided approach extremely difficult. Such tortuosity usually causes passage of the curved stylet to be particularly difficult. The curved stylet can even drag the electrode tip back into these tortuous venous structures. Generally, a more gentle stylet curve is indicated. In this situation, multiple stylet exchanges may be required. On a rare occasion, such tortuosity may even preclude actual passage from the left side.

Lead passage and placement via right venous access is intrinsically difficult because of the multiple natural acute angles and bends that are encountered from this approach. Just as a left venous approach forms a gentle C-shaped curve that is counterclockwise, the right venous access results in a clockwise curve that directs the electrode to the right lateral atrial wall when the curved stylet is in place (Fig. 4.34). It then takes considerable skill, ingenuity, and even luck to cross the tricuspid valve. Because the lead tip consistently points to the right lateral atrium, right heart passage is usually achieved by backing a large loop across the tricuspid valve (Fig. 4.35). Occasionally, tined leads hang up on the tricuspid valve, adding further frustration. The floppy-tip technique is not as helpful in this situation. A variety of lead stylet configurations may ultimately be required to achieve right heart passage. As a rule, less exaggerated stylet curves are more helpful, whereas exaggerated curves tend to increase the electrode tip orientation toward the right lateral atrial wall.

The commonest lead-related complication is dislodgment. Pacemaker and defibrillator lead fixation mechanisms have resolved this problem. Fixation mechanisms may be passive, such as tines, or active, such as some forms of screw-in mechanisms. Although the implanting physician usually develops a preference, in any given circumstance, one fixation mechanism may be preferred to another. The experienced implanting physician should be completely familiar with the complete armamentarium of electrodes to effectively deal with any given circumstance. The exclusive use of positive or passive fixation leads should be avoided. There is an argument for exclusive use of the screw-in positive fixation lead as it can easily be removed should this become necessary. By the same token, this electrode causes tissue damage and is subject to potential sensing and threshold problems. The passive fixation tined lead is more easily placed and, because little or no tissue damage is

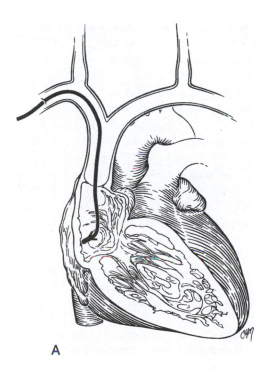

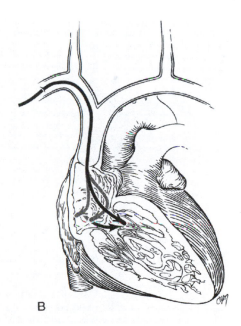

A   **B**

Fig. 4.34 Lead passage from the right side, causing the lead tip to track laterally to the right atrial wall. (From Belott PH. A practical approach to permanent pacemaker implantation. Armonk, NY: Futura Publishing, 1995, with permission.)

Fig. 4.35 The lead is backed into the right ventricle across the tricuspid valve. (From Belott PH. A practical approach to permanent pacemaker implantation. Armonk, NY: Futura Publishing, 1995, with permission.)

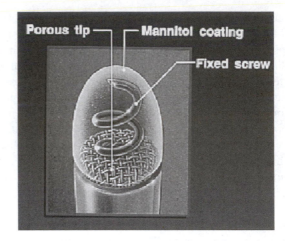

Fig. 4.36 The Guidant fixed exposed screw. Sweet tip covered with mannitol.

involved, thresholds and sensing tend to be superior. With the advent of steroid elution, these arguments no longer hold true. It should be pointed out that tines render removal much more challenging and increase the risk of life-threatening complications with their removal. With the development of modern lead extraction techniques, these arguments also no longer hold true.

It has been this author's practice to reserve the positive screw-in fixation lead in the ventricle for unique circumstances. Such circumstances include a dilated cardiomyopathy where the right ventricle is extremely thin with little or no trabeculations for tined fixation. The positive fixation screw-in lead is also ideal if atypical electrode position is desired. Such a circumstance includes electrode placement high on the interventricular septum.

No matter what type of lead is used, there is always a definite learning curve. Tines can engage endocardial structures resulting in resistance to passage. If this situation is encountered, the lead should be retracted completely into the right atrium. Tines frequently hang up on endocardial structures, preventing placement in the right ventricular apex. Subtle adjustments in the lead body as well as the stylet, ultimately overcome this problem.

There are essentially two types of active fixation leads; both involve a helix or screw as a fixation mechanism. The first and simplest design incorporates a continuously exposed screw. Because the screw is exposed, problems may be encountered as the exposed screw seemingly catches on every endocardial structure. Usually, the lead tip is freed by counterclockwise rotation of the lead body. In an attempt to avoid this problem, some manufacturers have coated the exposed screw with some form of sugar that dissolves, ultimately exposing the screw (Fig. 4.36). The problem with this remedy is that, once the coating dissolves, the exposed screw once again can hook on any endocardial structure.

The second type of common active fixation lead design employs a retractable/extendable screw that is mechanically activated (Fig. 4.37). This lead avoids the problem of hang-up and is much easier to work with. One merely maps a point of fixation and activates the fixation mechanism.

Fig. 4.37 Positive fixation electrode

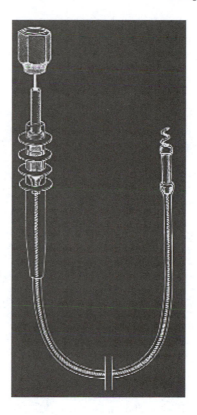

Once successful ventricular lead placement has been achieved, the lead must be secured. The first step in this process is withdrawal of the lead stylet to the vicinity of the lower right atrium (89) (Fig. 4.38). The stylet is not totally removed, but retained to add support if a second lead is to be placed. With a straight ventricular lead stylet in the vicinity of the lower right atrium, the lead is anchored at the venous entry site. The lead suture sleeve should be used for anchoring to avoid lead injury. Care is also taken not to cut through the suture sleeve and also injure the lead. Once the ventricular lead is anchored and after no further leads are to be added, the lead stylet is removed.

Atrial Lead Positioning

Atrial lead placement directly relates to the type of atrial electrode selected, regardless of fixation mechanism. Similar to the ventricular lead, proper placement is a symphony of the lead and stylet.

There are essentially two techniques. The first involves placement of an atrial lead with a preformed curve or atrial "J" (90). In this case, the straight stylet is used to straighten the preformed J. After venous access, the lead is advanced to the mid-right atrium. The atrial J electrode placement does not require special positioning of the fluoroscopy as discussed in ventricular lead placement. With the lead tip in the mid-right atrium, the straight stylet is withdrawn several centimeters. The atrial lead tip will begin to assume its J configuration, with the tip now pointing cephalad. The lead body is then slowly advanced at the venous

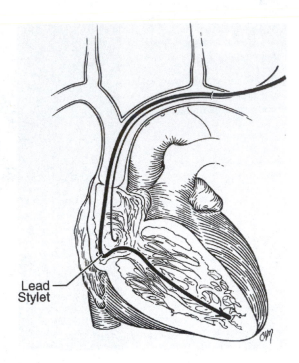

Fig. 4.38 With the ventricular electrode in place, the lead stylet is positioned in the lower right atrium for stability, the guidewire is retained. (From Belott PH. A practical approach to permanent pacemaker implantation. Armonk, NY: Futura Publishing, 1995, with permission.)

entry site. This maneuver rolls the atrial lead tip into the atrial appendage (Fig. 4.39). Occasionally, if the initial right atrial position is too low, the lead tip will hook the tricuspid valve. Conversely, too high a position will prevent the preformed J from assuming its curve. Once the lead has been positioned in the atrial appendage, rolling or twisting the electrode body clockwise and counter-clockwise should establish neutral torque on the lead. Good atrial lead positioning is confirmed by fluoroscopy. In the anterior–posterior projection, the electrode is observed to move to and fro, medial to lateral (Fig. 4.40) (91,92). In the lateral projection, the tip should be observed to be anterior just under the sternum; it will bob up and down with each atrial contraction. Selecting proper-sized J or proper size of the J loop is only gained with experience. A loop either too large or too small will result in dislodgment. Occasionally, even the best of efforts from the most experienced physician will be frustrated by dislodgement. As a rule, it is better to create a more generous loop. If one chooses a preformed atrial J lead with an active fixation mechanism, the same technique is employed as described in the preceding. Once the lead is in position, the active fixation mechanism is activated. It is important to note that the fixed or exposed active fixation electrode is unavailable in a preformed J configuration.

The second technique involves atrial placement of an active fixation lead that is straight. In this case, desired lead position is achieved by preforming the stylet into a shape that will achieve the desired position. Such leads

Fig. 4.39 The preformed atrial J electrode is positioned by partially withdrawing the lead stylet and allowing the lead to partially assume its J shape and subsequently advancing the lead body to allow the lead tip to move into the right atrial appendage. (From Belott PH. A practical approach to permanent pacemaker implantation. Armonk, NY: Futura Publishing, 1995, with permission.)

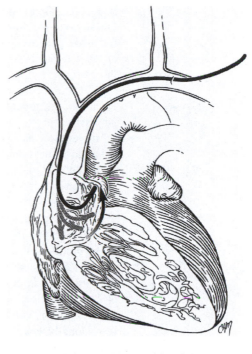

Fig. 4.40 A well-placed atrial lead in the atrial appendage moves to and fro, medial to lateral radiographically in PA projection. (From Belott PH. A practical approach to permanent pacemaker implantation. Armonk, NY: Futura Publishing, 1995, with permission.)

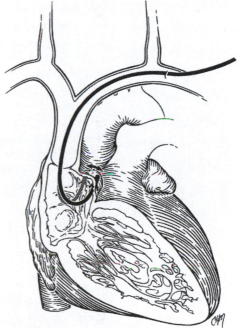

are usually prepackaged with an assortment of stylets. With practice, stylet manipulation can gain access to unusual atrial locations. The nonpreformed atrial J technique allows the physician to map the atrium for ideal threshold lead physiology (93). When using this approach, it is recommended that a positive fixation lead be used. Straight nonpreformed tined leads have been placed in this manner in the atrial appendage without dislodgment. Their use, however, is not recommended because of the risk of dislodgement. It has been this author's practice to reserve the use of an active fixation lead in the atrium for those patients who have undergone open-heart surgery where the atrial appendage has been amputated. There are also occasions when placement of the preformed atrial J tined lead in the atrial appendage will result in unacceptable thresholds. In this case, this electrode is removed and exchanged for a nonpreformed active fixation lead. The atrium is then mapped for ideal pace/sense thresholds.

Unlike the ventricular lead, good fixation is not documented by retraction. Good position is documented by fluoroscopy and acceptable threshold measurements. This is particularly true with active fixation leads where pulling should be avoided, because it may result in easy dislodgment.

The floppy-tip technique may be used for achieving unusual atrial lead placement with a straight active fixation lead. This is particularly useful for placement along the right lateral atrial wall. With the curved stylet retracted 1 to 2 in., the lead tip assumes a more lateral position. By simply advancing the lead to a point of contact, the fixation mechanism can be activated and threshold measurements carried out.

Active fixation extendable retractable leads that require the lead stylet to be fully advanced for placement preclude the use of this floppy-tip technique. Occasionally, in a setting of a giant right atrium, atrial endocardial lead contact is difficult to achieve. In this circumstance, a stiffer stylet is recommended. This stylet is preformed into a more exaggerated curve. Subsequently, frustration is encountered because the stiffer stylet with a more exaggerated curve will not negotiate the venous system in the superior mediastinum.

Unlike ventricular lead placement, venous access has little effect on atrial lead positioning. Whether from the right or left venous access, the preformed J or straight electrode with preformed J stylet is easily maneuvered into the atrial appendage or desired position. It should be noted that a right lateral atrial position is more easily achieved by a right venous access. Atrial septal positions are more easily achieved from the left.

Once an acceptable atrial lead position has been achieved, the lead is secured. The suture sleeve should always be used. Care should be taken to avoid cutting the lead. Ties should be snug to avoid slippage.

Epicardial Lead Placement

Initially, epicardial pacemaker lead placement was the implant technique of choice. This was because of the large size of the pacemaker pulse generator as well as unreliable leads for transvenous placement. Today, epicardial pacemaker lead placement is reserved for those patients undergoing cardiac surgery. Even in this circumstance, the transvenous approach is frequently employed. This is largely owing to the safety and efficacy of the transvenous approach. Today, only rare and unusual circumstances result in an epicardial pacemaker implant. These include patients undergoing cardiac surgery, patients with recurrent transvenous dislodgment, and patients with a prosthetic tricuspid valve or a congenital anomaly such as tricuspid atresia. More recently, the epicardial approach regained popularity with the development of the automatic implantable cardioverter defibrillator. This system initially required the placement of epicardial patch electrodes as well as ratesensing

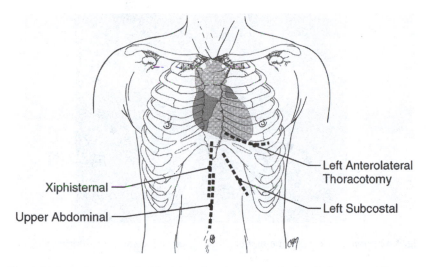

Fig. 4.41 Location of surgical incisions for placement of epicardial systems. The common median sternotomy is not shown. (From Belott PH, Reynolds DW. Permanent pacemaker implantation. In: Ellenbogen KA, Kay N, Wilkoff BL, eds. Clinical cardiac pacing. Philadelphia: WB Saunders, 1995, with permission.)

leads. With the development of the nonthoracotomy defibrillator lead, once again, the epicardial approach has fallen by the wayside. There has been some resurgence of this approach with the development of four-chambered pacing for dilated cardiomyopathy.

The epicardial approach offers the advantage of mapping for ideal pacing thresholds and other electrophysiologic parameters. The leads or patches are directly attached to the epicardium and pulled to a subcutaneous pocket. This pocket is usually in the upper abdomen. Historically, multiple epicardial approaches have been developed (Fig. 4.41). These include the median sternotomy, left anterolateral thoracotomy, subxiphoid, left subcostal, and thoracoscopic approaches. The subxiphoid and the left subcostal preclude a thoracotomy. General anesthesia is almost always required for all epicardial pacemaker and ICD implantation techniques. In addition, these procedures are generally performed in the operating room by the cardiothoracic surgeon.

The identical epicardial approaches have been used for both pacing and ICD implantation. The more recent use of the epicardial approach for ICD implantation was necessitated to configure defibrillation patch electrodes around the heart for optimal DFTs. Historically, the first clinical implants used an epicardial cup electrode for the ventricular apex in conjunction with a helical spring electrode in the superior vena cava (4). The high DFTs from this system ultimately led to the preference for two epicardially placed patch electrodes. It should be pointed out that epicardial patch electrodes might even be placed extrapericardially. This approach reduces epicardial adhesions. In addition to the patches, ratesensing leads must also be applied. This is usually achieved by placement of two sutureless screw-in electrodes side by side (Fig. 4.42). These electrodes can serve for both pacing and sensing. Both the patches and rate sensing leads must be tunneled to the device pocket using standard tunneling techniques. Because of the early ICD pulse generator size, epicardial leads and patch electrodes required an abdominal pocket. As there is little call for epi-

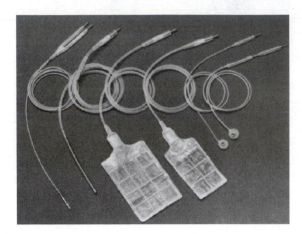

Fig. 4.42 From left to right: the first electrode is an endocardial rate sensing and pacing electrode. Endocardial high-energy spring electrode in the middle pair. Epicardial patches and pair on the extreme left epicardial rate sensing electrodes. (Courtesy of Guidant, Inc., St. Paul, MN.)

cardial pacemaker placement, the following discussion reviews the epicardial approach as it applies to the automatic implantable cardioverter defibrillator.

The median sternotomy is the most popular approach because it provides optimal exposure and access to the entire heart (94–96). It is used in patients undergoing an open-heart procedure who also require ICD implantation. The incision is well tolerated and associated with much less patient discomfort. Two large patches may easily be placed extrapericardially (Fig. 4.43). Excellent exposure is achieved as the procedure is generally performed under cardiopulmonary bypass with the lungs deflated. The rate sensing leads are directly screwed to the epicardial surface. The patch electrodes are sutured to the pericardium.

The left anterolateral thoracotomy also offers excellent exposure of the heart and left ventricle. An incision is created in the fifth intercostal space (Fig. 4.44). This approach is ideal for extrapericardial placement of a large patch electrode over the posterior surface of the left ventricle as well as a smaller patch anteriorly between the sternum and pericardium. This approach is associated with considerable postoperative pain and is its major drawback. This pain frequently results in atelectasis and transient pleural effusions. Today, a more lateral approach has been adopted that eliminates pain associated with division of the latissimus dorsi. Once again, the leads are tunneled to an abdominal pocket by use of a small chest tube or hemostat.

The subxiphoid approach was developed for patients undergoing simple ICD implantation (Fig. 4.45). There is decreased morbidity and discomfort with this approach. There is, however, a slight increase in resultant DFTs. Wound discomfort postoperatively is much less. The major disadvantage of this approach is limited surgical exposure and the requirement for intrapericardially placed patches. Frequently, because of unacceptable DFTs, an additional transvenous coil must be placed. This approach is generally not used in patients who have undergone a prior cardiac surgical procedure.

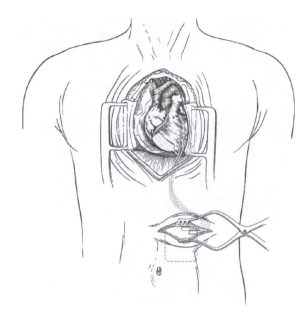

Fig. 4.43 Median sternotomy. (From Belott PH, Reynolds DW. Permanent pacemaker and cardioverter defibrillation implantation. In: Ellenbogen KA, Kay N, Wilkoff BL, eds. Clinical cardiac pacing and defibrillation, 2nd ed. Philadelphia: WB Saunders, 2000, with permission.)

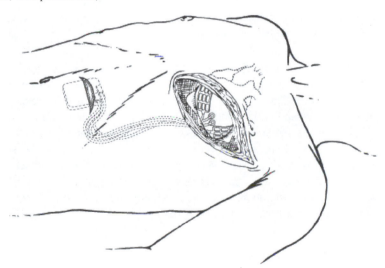

Fig. 4.44 Left lateral thoracotomy with epicardial rate-sensing and patch electrodes tunneled to the subcutaneous pocket in the left upper quadrant. (From Belott PH, Reynolds DW. Permanent pacemaker and cardioverter defibrillation implantation. In: Ellenbogen KA, Kay N, Wilkoff BL, eds. Clinical cardiac pacing and defibrillation, 2nd ed. Philadelphia: WB Saunders, 2000, with permission.)

The left subcostal approach was originally developed for placement of rate pacing and sensing leads. It is now also used for placement of ICD patches. This approach is associated with minimal morbidity (97–98). The left subcostal approach is carried out with an incision in the left subcostal area. This approach can also be used in patients who have had prior cardiac

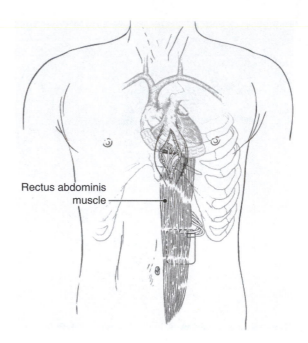

Rectus abdominis muscle

Fig. 4.45 Subxiphoid epicardial approach with rate-sensing and patch electrodes tunneled to the subrectus pocket in the left upper quadrant. (From Belott PH, Reynolds DW. Permanent pacemaker and cardioverter defibrillation implantation. In: Ellenbogen KA, Kay N, Wilkoff BL, eds. Clinical cardiac pacing and defibrillation, 2nd ed. Philadelphia: WB Saunders, 2000, with permission.)

surgery (99,100). The left subcostal approach is extrathoracic and avoids the complications of a thoracotomy. There is, however, greater postoperative wound discomfort when compared to the subxiphoid approach. Occasionally, both pacing leads and ICD patches have been placed using thoracoscopy. A small incision is made on the anterior chest and the pacing leads and/or defibrillator patches introduced into the left pleural space. The thoracoscope is used to guide the leads and patches to the pericardial surface for attachment (101,102). Thoracoscopy, a relatively new approach, appears to be safe and efficacious. Because thoracotomy and sternotomy are avoided, it carries the lowest morbidity of all the epicardial approaches.

Pacemaker and ICD Pocket Creation

The timing of pocket creation is a personal preference. Usually, the pocket is created at the end of the procedure. Some implanters prefer to create the pocket at the time of initial incision. It is argued that bleeding is more easily controlled and the risk of electrode damage less if the pocket is created early in the procedure. Proponents of late pocket creation feel that the highest priority in any pacemaker or ICD procedure is establishment of early backup pacing to protect the patient. Thus, pacemaker and ICD pocket creation is of low priority and deferred to the end of the case. The proposed pocket location, whether pectoral for pacing and ICD or abdominal for the ICD, the pocket should be generously infiltrated with local anesthesia. The plane of dissection should always be created at the junction of the subcutaneous tissue and the underlying muscle fascia. This is best achieved by placing the

Table 4.12 Subcutaneous versus submuscular ICD pocket.

Site	Advantages	Disadvantages
Subcutaneous	Limited surgery	Less cosmetic
	Better control of bleeding	Increased risk of erosion
	Better analgesia	Increased risk of dislodgment from Twiddler syndrome
	Easier pulse generator change	
Submuscular	Optimal cosmetics	Increased pr oblems with hemostasis
	Less risk of dislodgment from twiddling	Greater postoperative pain
	Greater patient acceptance	Potential migration laterally to the axilla

subcutaneous tissue under tension with a retractor. A plane of dissection is established with Metzenbaum scissors or the cutting function of electrocautery. Once the plane of dissection has been established, it is continued until the pocket is complete. The plane is maintained at the subcutaneous tissue and muscle fascia junction to effect optimal tissue thickness. The pocket should always be created under direct visualization and blunt dissection avoided. With blunt dissection, there is no visualization and a lack of control with respect to tissue depth. Blunt dissection can result in inconsistencies in pocket thickness and increased risk of erosion. This is a particular concern with the larger ICD devices. A well-formed pocket should be as deep as possible, right on top of the muscle. This can only be carried out by direct visualization. As today's devices become smaller, the required dissection has been gradually limited. If the subcutaneous tissue is held under gentle tension, the desired plane of dissection is easily defined and maintained. Pocket creation by precise dissection is less traumatic and offers optimal pocket thickness. In addition, bleeding is more easily controlled and optimal hemostasis achieved. Visualization can be enhanced by use of the headlamp. The risk of hematoma is reduced as all bleeding is directly visualized and managed with electrocautery. An abdominal pocket may be required for some ICD implantations. Subpectoralis muscle pocket implantation has been used for both pacemaker and ICD implantations in patients with little or no subcutaneous tissue. Initially, ICD pockets were created almost exclusively in the left upper quadrant of the abdomen. This was because of the predominant use of the epicardial approach and the generous size of the device. With the advent of the nonthoracotomy approach, the ICD pocket is now almost exclusively placed in the left pectoral area. The abdominal pocket may be either subcutaneous or submuscular. In the pectoral area, initially because of device size, a submuscular approach was used. With the radical reduction in device size of both the pacemaker and ICD, the subcutaneous pocket is becoming more common. The concern with a subcutaneous pocket, whether abdominal or pectoral, is the increased risk of erosion (Table 4.12).

If an abdominal pocket is to be created, one must be completely familiar with the anatomy of the anterior abdominal wall. This includes the multiple muscular and fascia layers (Fig. 4.46). One must be completely familiar with the anterior rectus sheath, rectus muscle and posterior rectus sheath, linea alba, and peritoneum. Failure to appreciate the anatomic relationships of the abdominal wall may result in inadvertent access of peritoneal cavity. An abdominal pocket

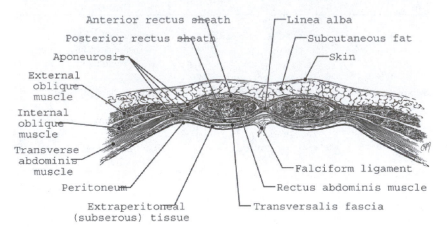

Posterior rectus sheath

Anterior rectus sheath   ⌐Linea alba
Posterior rectus sheath   ⌐Subcutaneous fat
Aponeurosis   ⌐Skin
External
oblique
muscle
Internal
oblique
muscle
Transverse
abdominis
muscle   ⌐Falciform ligament
Peritoneum   ⌐Rectus abdominis muscle
Extraperitoneal   ⌐Transversalis fascia
(subserous) tissue

Fig. 4.46 Crosssectional anatomy of the rectus sheath above the arcuate line. (From Belott PH, Reynolds DW. Permanent pacemaker and cardioverter defibrillation implantation. In: Ellenbogen KA, Kay N, Wilkoff BL, eds. Clinical cardiac pacing and defibrillation, 2nd ed. Philadelphia: WB Saunders, 2000, with permission.)

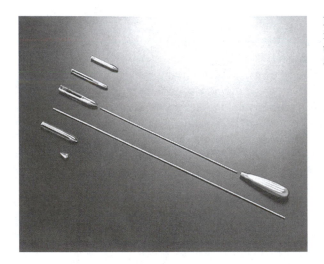

Fig. 4.47 Subcutaneous tunneling tool with interchangeable handle, tunneling rod, and tunneling bullet. (Courtesy of Guidant, Inc., St. Paul, MN.)

is created by carrying an incision through the subcutaneous tissue and fat to the surface of the anterior rectus sheath. A plane is created directly on top of the anterior rectus sheath and an attempt is made not to violate this structure. The subcutaneous tissue is separated from the anterior rectus sheath by direct visualization, creating a pocket large enough to accommodate the particular device. The pocket is carefully inspected for hemostasis and lavaged with antibacterial solution. The pocket will receive the leads using standard tunneling techniques. In the case of an ICD where an epicardial approach is used, most leads are tunneled using a small chest tube and Kelly clamp for guidance. In the case of the nonthoracotomy transvenous system, tunneling may be achieved to the abdominal pocket by using a tunneling tool (Fig. 4.47).

No matter which technique is used, care should be taken to achieve optimal depth of the tunneling track to avoid future lead erosion. The submuscular

Fig. 4.48 Crosssectional anatomy of the rectus sheath above the arcuate line with the ICD in place. A: Device placed posterior to the anterior rectus sheath. B: Device placed anterior to the anterior rectus sheath. C: ICD placed on top of the posterior rectus sheath beneath the rectus muscle. (From Belott PH, Reynolds DW. Permanent pacemaker and cardioverter defibrillation implantation. In: Ellenbogen KA, Kay N, Wilkoff BL, eds. Clinical cardiac pacing and defibrillation, 2nd ed. Philadelphia: WB Saunders, 2000, with permission.)

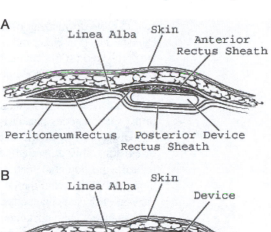

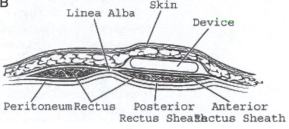

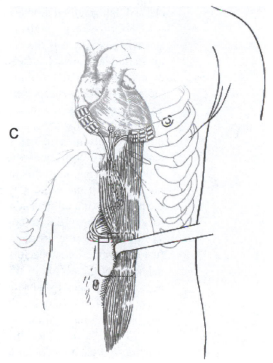

abdominal pocket is a modification of the subcutaneous approach. This has been used for abdominal ICD placement. A space is created between the posterior rectus sheath and rectus muscle. The deeper submuscular approach is associated with potential violation of the peritoneal cavity as well as postoperative erosion into the peritoneal cavity (Fig. 4.48). As a general rule, abdominal pockets should not be located over previous surgery or in the vicinity of abdominal hernias.

The pectoral pocket, once exclusively used for permanent pacemakers, is now employed for nonthoracotomy ICD placement. This is because of the considerable downsizing of the ICD pulse generator. The ICD pectoral pocket can be created in either the right or left pectoral area but with the left pectoral area preferred (103). This is because of lower achievable DFTs with an active can device. As stated previously, the pacemaker pocket is generally subcutaneous. The ICD pocket may be created either subcutaneously or submuscularly. Physicians less skilled in surgery prefer the subcutaneous approach. The benefit of the subcutaneous pocket is its simplicity and avoidance of deep dissection. The disadvantage of the subcutaneous approach is obviously the concerns of erosion. This is particularly true of the larger ICD where pressure points increase the potential for erosion. The subcutaneous pocket should be made large enough to avoid the buildup of tension or pressure points. A final disadvantage of the subcutaneous pocket for ICD placement at its current size is one of cosmetics. The subcutaneous approach results in a large visible bulge that does not occur with a deeper submuscular approach. The submuscular pectoral pocket remains the most popular approach for nonthoracotomy ICD placement. This offers optimal cosmetics and is virtually free from erosion. The submuscular approach requires a complete understanding of the regional anatomy. The important superficial landmarks are the clavicle, deltoid muscle, pectoralis muscle, and deltopectoral groove. The pectoralis major muscle, as previously noted, is superior to the pectoralis minor. The pectoralis major muscle has two major subdivisions. There is the clavicular head, which attaches to the clavicle, and the sternal head, which attaches to the lateral border of the sternum. Both heads ultimately fuse and attach to the humerus. It is the fascial plane that separates these two heads that represents an ideal fascial plane of dissection for creating a subpectoral pocket. The deeper pectoralis minor muscle has two connections. Its superior head is attached to the coracoid process. The muscle then fans out inferiorly, attaching to the anterior ribs. The thoracoacromial neurovascular bundle can be easily identified on the surface of the pectoralis minor muscle (Fig. 4.49). Trauma to this neurovascular bundle can result in hematoma, and interruption of the nerve may result in pectoral atrophy. The lateral border of the pectoralis major clavicular head defines the deltopectoral groove. The inferolateral border of the sternopectoralis major muscle head defines the anterior axillary fold. There are three distinct submuscular pectoral approaches. The first is the anterior subpectoral approach created between the clavicle and sternal heads of the pectoralis major (Fig. 4.50). The second submuscular pectoral approach is created by a lateral reflection of the clavicular head of the pectoralis major (Fig. 4.51). And, finally, a lateral submuscular approach or anterior axillary approach through the inferolateral border of the pectoralis major muscle (Fig. 4.52). Each approach has its benefits and potential complications. The anterior approach is similar to that of a subcutaneous pacemaker pocket creation. It requires the creation of a plane of dissection between the sternal and clavicular portions of the pectoralis major muscle. The resultant pocket is anterior and does not interfere with the axilla. The lateral approach requires dissection of the pectoralis major along the deltopectoral groove. There is a tendency for the ICD or pacemaker to drift into the axilla because this approach is more lateral. Similarly, the axillary approach requires dissection and establishment of a plane at the anterior axillary fold. This approach also can result in device drift into the axilla and cause discomfort. The lateral and axillary approaches can also potentially interrupt the long thoracic nerve, which will result in "winged scapula." The incision for the anterior approach is initiated just medial to the

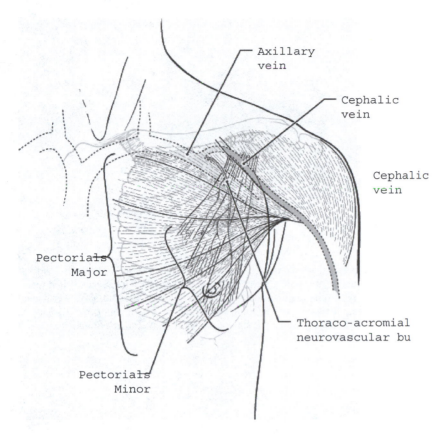

Axillary
vein

Cephalic
vein

Cephalic
vein

Pectoralis
Major

Thoraco-acromial
neurovascular bu

Pectoralis
Minor

Fig. 4.49 Superficial and deep anatomy of the deltopectoral area demonstrating the relationship of the superficial pectoralis major, the pectoralis minor axillary and cephalic veins, and the thoracoacromial neurovascular bundle. (From Belott PH, Reynolds DW. Permanent pacemaker and cardioverter defibrillation implantation. In: Ellenbogen KA, Kay N, Wilkoff BL, eds. Clinical cardiac pacing and defibrillation, 2nd ed. Philadelphia: WB Saunders, 2000, with permission.)

B

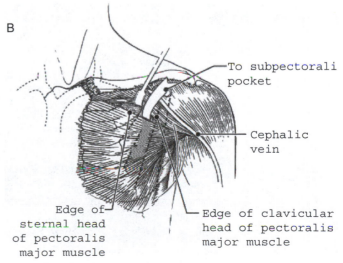

To subpectorali
pocket

Cephalic
vein

Edge of
sternal head
of pectoralis
major muscle

Edge of clavicular
head of pectoralis
major muscle

Fig. 4.50 Anterior subpectoralis muscle approach. The clavicular and sternal heads of the pectoralis major are gently retracted and a plane of dissection established subpectorally. (From Belott PH, Reynolds DW. Permanent pacemaker and cardioverter defibrillation implantation. In: Ellenbogen KA, Kay N, Wilkoff BL, eds. Clinical cardiac pacing and defibrillation, 2nd ed. Philadelphia: WB Saunders, 2000, with permission.)

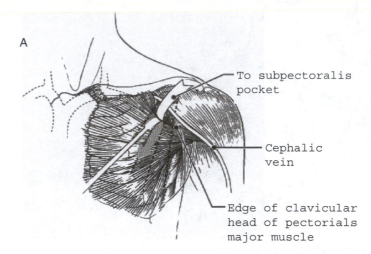

To subpectoralis pocket

Cephalic vein

Edge of clavicular head of pectorials major muscle

Fig. 4.51 Deltopectoral groove subpectoral approach. The lateral border of the pectoralis major clavicular head is gently retracted and a plane of dissection established medially behind the pectoralis major muscle. (From Belott PH, Reynolds DW. Permanent pacemaker and cardioverter defibrillation implantation. In: Ellenbogen KA, Kay N, Wilkoff BL, eds. Clinical cardiac pacing and defibrillation, 2nd ed. Philadelphia: WB Saunders, 2000, with permission.)

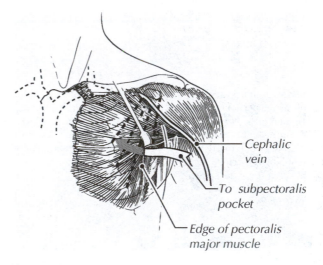

Cephalic vein

To subpectoralis pocket

Edge of pectoralis major muscle

Fig. 4.52 Anterior axillary fold subpectoralis major muscle approach. The lateral border of the pectoralis major muscle sternal head at the anterior axillary fold is gently retracted and a plane of dissection established retropectorally. (From Belott PH, Reynolds DW. Permanent pacemaker and cardioverter defibrillation implantation. In: Ellenbogen KA, Kay N, Wilkoff BL, eds. Clinical cardiac pacing and defibrillation, 2nd ed. Philadelphia: WB Saunders, 2000, with permission.)

coracoid process and carried inferomedially perpendicular to the deltopectoral groove (Fig. 4.53). In the anterior approach, the clavicular and sternal heads of the pectoralis major muscle are identified and retracted, establishing a plane to the anterior chest wall (Fig. 4.54). Once in the chest wall, the pocket may be enlarged as needed using blunt dissection.

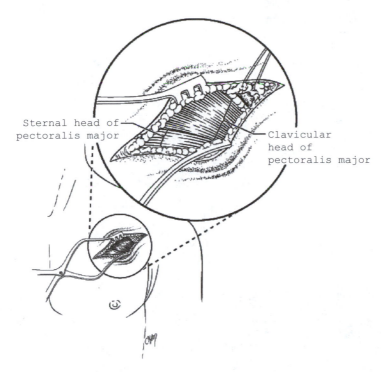

Fig. 4.53 Initial incision for subpectoralis ICD placement. Insertion demonstrates the deltopectoral groove, and the clavicular and sternal heads of the pectoralis major muscle. (From Belott PH, Reynolds DW. Permanent pacemaker and cardioverter defibrillation implantation. In: Ellenbogen KA, Kay N, Wilkoff BL, eds. Clinical cardiac pacing and defibrillation, 2nd ed. Philadelphia: WB Saunders, 2000, with permission.)

Reflecting the lateral clavicular head of the pectoralis major muscle creates the lateral submuscular approach. In this case, an initial vertical incision is made along the deltopectoral groove. The dissection is carried down to the surface of the pectoralis fascia. The lateral border of the pectoralis major clavicular head is retracted medially and a subpectoralis major muscle plane of dissection established.

The lateral anterior axillary submuscular pectoral approach calls for creation of a dissection plane in the anterior axillary fold (104). A dissection plane is easily established as the pectoralis major is separated at the planes created between the pectoralis major and minor muscles. A skin incision is created inferiorly along the anterolateral axillary fold. It is carried down to the surface of the pectoralis major muscle. Both the pectoralis major and minor muscles are identified and separated and a plane of dissection is created between them. This approach usually requires a separate incision for venous access and tunneling to the axillary fold incision. The inferolateral margin of the pectoralis major muscle is easily separated from the adjacent subcutaneous tissue for establishing a large plane of dissection. The ICD should be placed as medial as possible with the leads lateral to avoid the risk of CAN abrasion. With the ICD or pacemaker in the pocket, a careful multilayered closure is used.

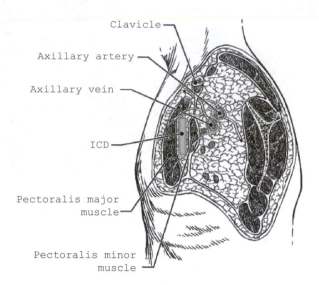

Clavicle

Axillary artery

Axillary vein

ICD

Pectoralis major
muscle

Pectoralis minor
muscle

Fig. 4.54 Sagittal section of the shoulder girdle demonstrating superficial and deep anatomy with automatic implantable cardioverter defibrillator placement under the pectoralis major muscle. (From Belott PH, Reynolds DW. Permanent pacemaker and cardioverter defibrillation implantation. In: Ellenbogen KA, Kay N, Wilkoff BL, eds. Clinical cardiac pacing and defibrillation, 2nd ed. Philadelphia: WB Saunders, 2000, with permission.)

Tunneling

Tunneling generally refers to the passage of a lead through tissue from one location to another. Although rarely used in cardiac pacing, it has become extremely popular with the recent development of the nonthoracotomy implantable defibrillation lead systems. Such systems require the passage of a lead from one wound in the pectoral region subcutaneously through the tissue to a second wound in the abdomen. In addition, any epicardial pacemaker or ICD system requires tunneling techniques of leads and patch electrodes from the epicardial site to the abdominal or pectoral pocket. Multiple techniques have been developed for tunneling. The simplest technique is the use of a Penrose drain. The proximal end of the lead or leads is placed in the Penrose drain. Then, a nonconstricting tie applied about the Penrose drain just distal to the lead connectors. The proposed tract is infiltrated. A long clamp is pushed bluntly through the subcutaneous tissue from the receiving wound directly to the wound containing the lead to be tunneled (Fig. 4.55). The free end of the Penrose drain is grasped and pulled back to the receiving wound, dragging the new lead with it. When passing the clamp from one wound to another, care should be taken to establish as deep a track as possible. Once the Penrose drain with leads has been pulled to the receiving wound, the drain is released and removed. A variation of this technique calls for the delivery of the Penrose drain to the receiving wound by using a passer. The passer may be a thin, blunt rod, knitting needle, or even a sheath-set dilator. The Penrose drain is attached to the free end of the passer; the passer is advanced from the wound of the new lead origin to the receiving wound. Once again, the Penrose drain and leads are pulled through to the receiving wound. Roelke and associates have described in a unique tunneling technique (Fig. 4.56). A 20-cm, #18 gauge

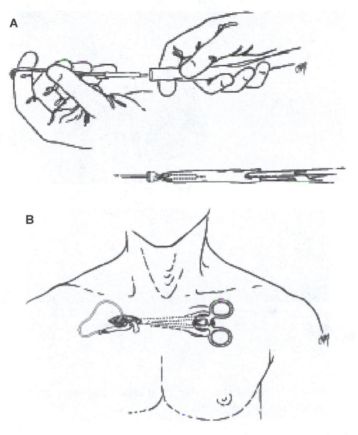

Fig. 4.55 A: The lead is placed and secured in a Penrose drain. B: The lead and Penrose drain are grasped by a clamp and pulled from a donor site to the recipient wound. (From Belott PH, Reynolds DW. Permanent pacemaker implantation. In: Ellenbogen KA, Kay N, Wilkoff BL, eds. Clinical cardiac pacing. Philadelphia: WB Saunders, 1995, with permission.)

pericardiocentesis needle is directed from the receiving pocket to the origin of the leads. A J guidewire is then passed from the receiving pocket through the needle to the donor incision. The needle is removed and a 10 French introducer passed over the guidewire. The free end of the lead to be tunneled is placed in the sheath and secured with a tie. The sheath is then withdrawn to the receiving wound.

The initial epicardial ICD systems required epicardial pacing, and ICD systems required tunneling of leads from the epicardium to an abdominal pocket. This was usually carried out using a large chest tube. The proximal ends of the leads were stuffed into the back end of the chest tube for protection and the chest tube was guided by a clamp percutaneously to the abdominal pocket. The tip of the chest tube was grasped with a large, curved Kelly clamp and, using an index finger for palpation, the clamp guided the chest tube through the tissue to the abdominal pocket. Distance from the epicardium to the abdominal pocket was relatively short; this tunneling technique has proven to be simple and expeditious. This is not the case when tunneling is required from a transvenous insertion site in the upper chest to a distal abdominal

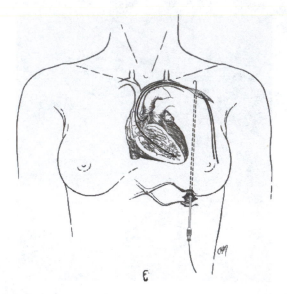

Fig. 4.56 Subcutaneous tunneling with guidewire and sheath. (From Belott PH. Unusual access sites for permanent cardiac pacing. In: Barold SS, Mugica J, eds. Recent advances in cardiac pacing: goals for the 21st century. Armonk, NY: Futura Publishing, 1997, with permission.)

pocket. Such is the case of the earlier nonthoracotomy pacing systems connected to the larger ICD pulse generator.

To assist in long stretches of tunneling, one manufacturer developed a tunneling tool to resolve this problem. The tunneling tool basically consists of a rod with a handle at one end and a distal bullet that could be replaced with a lead adapter (Fig. 4.47). Tunneling over large areas can prove to be extremely challenging. It is important to maintain optimal depth of the track. Care should be taken to avoid intrathoracic entry as well as superficial cutaneous exit. Once the tunneling track was established, the bullet was exchanged for the lead adapter. With the leads placed in the adapter, a tie is required to secure them. After the leads are secured, the tunneling tool is retracted back to the abdominal pocket.

Occasionally ICD systems require the placement of additional leads and/or patches to achieve adequate DFTs. An additional patch electrode may be added through a small, left anterior chest incision (Fig. 4.57). This incision is generally placed along the left inframammary skin fold. A subcutaneous pocket is developed and a supplemental patch placed. The patch is sutured to the chest wall. The proximal lead is then tunneled to the ICD. A variation on this system is the subcutaneous array developed by CPI (Fig. 4.58). The array consists of three flexible defibrillator leads that are joined at a common connector. The leads are designed to be placed subcutaneously along the contour of the chest wall. The leads fuse as a common electrode that connects to the ICD. Creating a small incision in the left lateral inframammary skin fold places the array. Three separate subcutaneous tracts are created using a blunt-tipped malleable stylet. The stylet is loaded with a sheath that is advanced down each tract. The stylet is removed and the limbs of the array are passed down each sheath.

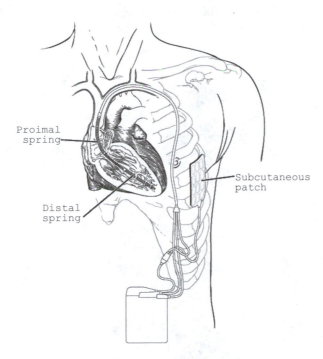

Fig. 4.57 Endocardial pacing and shocking electrode position in the apex of the right ventricle. The electrode has been tunneled to the ICD in the right upper quadrant; a subcutaneous patch has been placed and similarly tunneled to the ICD. (From Belott PH, Reynolds DW. Permanent pacemaker and cardioverter defibrillation implantation. In: Ellenbogen KA, Kay N, Wilkoff BL, eds. Clinical cardiac pacing and defibrillation, 2nd ed. Philadelphia: WB Saunders, 2000, with permission.)

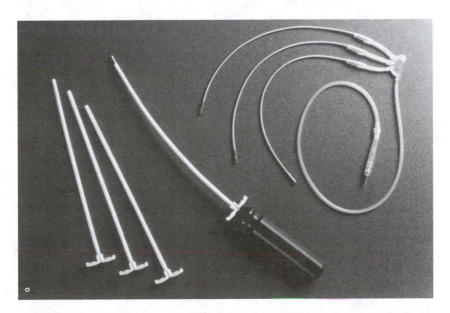

Fig. 4.58 Subcutaneous array system. Left-sheaths; middle tunneling tool loaded with sheath; and right subcutaneous array. (Courtesy of Guidant, Inc., St. Paul, MN.)

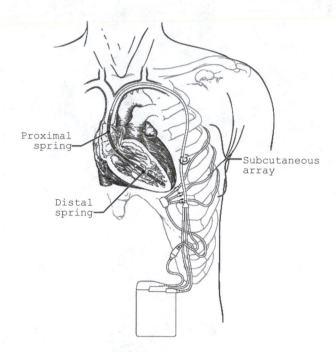

Fig. 4.59 Endocardial pacing and shocking electrode tunnel to the pocket in the left upper quadrant. Subcutaneous array similarly positioned and fixed to the left anterior chest wall and tunneled to the ICD. (From Belott PH, Reynolds DW. Permanent pacemaker and cardioverter defibrillation implantation. In: Ellenbogen KA, Kay N, Wilkoff BL, eds. Clinical cardiac pacing and defibrillation, 2nd ed. Philadelphia: WB Saunders, 2000, with permission.)

The sheaths are split and peeled away, leaving the array limb in position (Fig. 4.59). The proximal end of the array lead is then tunneled to the ICD pocket.

Immediate Postoperative Care

Postoperative monitoring has changed dramatically over the past several years. Intensive monitoring and prolonged hospital stays are no longer required for pacemaker and ICD patients. Patients admitted electively usually return to a cardiac monitoring area and are subsequently discharged. A brief period of rhythm monitoring is all that is required. In the case of the ICD, predischarge evaluation of DFTs may be carried out.

The activity level of the patient in the immediate postoperative period is limited merely by the amount of sedation. Prolonged periods of bed rest are to be avoided. The modern lead systems with active and passive fixation mechanisms offer a new dimension of security. It is important to have the patient active immediately or shortly after arrival in the monitored area. The intention is to detect early those patients with potential pacemaker or ICD system malfunctions. Prolonged periods of inactivity merely result in a false sense of security. The reliability of the pacing or ICD system is demonstrated by early activity. The patient's approach from the ambulatory point of view is made active as soon as sedation has worn off. Postoperative pacemaker and ICD system evaluation with noninvasive studies, monitoring, and reprogramming are carried out at the time of initial postoperative visit to the pacemaker and ICD clinic. This is usually within 24–48 h.

ICD and pacemaker procedures require documentation from both a clinical and medicolegal point of view. The operative report should clearly identify the following: indications, device and lead manufacturer, make and model, and details of the implant procedure. Final device program settings are equally important. There should be a clear description of the entire procedure, as well as any problems encountered. Copies of the operative report should be received in a timely fashion by the follow-up clinic and physicians. Further documentation includes manufacturer's registration form and hospital registry or log as required by the US Food and Drug Administration. It is important to have multiple sources for retrieving device implant data. It is important also to obtain a chest radiograph. This will document the procedure and/or the electrode's position, should it become necessary. In the case of percutaneous procedure, the chest radiograph is mandatory to rule out pneumothorax. It is advisable to obtain an overpenetrated film in the expiratory phase of respiration. This helps visualize the electrodes, as well as exclude pneumothorax. A postoperative 12-lead electrocardiogram is essential in documenting initial pacemaker and ICD function.

Timing of Discharge

There has been considerable change in the timing of discharge. In the early days of cardiac pacing and ICD therapy, the patient's postoperative stay was prolonged. Today, with the limited surgery and reliable lead systems, the hospital stay has been dramatically foreshortened. As a rule, with respect to pacemaker procedures, approximately 70% to 75% of all procedures can be conducted on am ambulatory basis. Early activity in the monitored postoperative period helps to detect potential problems. This also holds for any patient who is considered to be at high risk of developing a complication.

There are very few patient instructions. In the case of patients discharged 24 h prior to the next clinic visit, they are instructed to remove their dressing on the morning following the procedure. The wound should be left open to air and remain uncovered. The patient may bathe within 48 h, provided a dry eschar has formed. If prophylactic antibiotics are to be used, prescription with dosing instruction is important. It is also helpful to give instructions as to where to seek help should complications occur. If major symptoms occur, the patient is usually advised to report to the nearest emergency room. This also holds for any change in the surgical site. Sudden swelling or increased pain may suggest hematoma formation. Hematoma should be evacuated and drained early.

Special Situations

Use of the Coronary Sinus for Cardiac Pacing

The coronary sinus has been used for pacing both by design and misadventure (105,106). Recently the coronary sinus has been used for multisite pacing. In the past, this has proven to be an extremely unreliable site for ventricular pacing and has been avoided. In the case of a desired atrial pacing, coronary sinus has proven to be an ideal location. The major problem with coronary sinus pacing has been access and lead stability. Prior to the development of reliable atrial electrodes, the coronary sinus was a popular site for lead placement for atrial pacing. The best position for atrial pacing is the proximal coronary sinus. Special coronary sinus leads have been developed to enhance position stability. When simultaneous right and left atrial pacing is desired, a distal coronary sinus location has been used. Primary coronary sinus catheterization requires experience with a growing number of implanting electrophysiologists who routinely use the coronary sinus for diagnostic studies; this experience has become somewhat of a moot point. As a rule, placement of a coronary sinus lead is much easier from the left. A generous curve is required in the lead. Coronary sinus placement is confirmed by the posterior lead position on fluoroscopy in the lateral or left anterior oblique projections (107). In addition, lead placement is not associated with ventricular ectopy. As a popular approach for atrial pacing, the coronary sinus is used infrequently today. As biatrial pacing becomes more important for control of atrial arrhythmias and four-chamber pacing desired for management of cardiomyopathy, there has been resurgence in the use of the coronary sinus.

Electrode Placement via Anomalous Venous Structures

Occasionally a patient will have a persistent left superior vena cava. Embryologically, the normal left superior vena cava becomes atretic. In approximately 0.5% of the population, this structure persists. The persistent left superior vena cava connects directly to the coronary sinus. The persistent left superior vena cava actually represents failure in the development of the left innominate vein. This vein is normally formed by communication of the right and left anterior cardinal veins. In this situation, the left anterior cardinal vein persists and continues to drain to the brachiocephalic veins and sinus venosus. This ultimately develops into a left superior vena cava, which enters directly into the coronary sinus (Fig.4.60). Normally, the left innominate vein develops as an anastomosis between the left and right anterior cardinal veins. It should be noted that frequently with persistent left superior vena cava, there is also associated atresia and complete absence of the right superior vena caval system (Fig. 4.61). In this situation, venous access for pacing from the right is virtually impossible. Placement of electrodes via persistent left superior vena cava can prove extremely challenging, if not impossible (108–113). It is important to appreciate that the lead or leads are actually advanced into the coronary sinus and out its ostium into the right atrium. If right ventricular apical positions are to be achieved, the lead must then negotiate at an acute angle to cross the tricuspid valve. This is best accomplished by having a lead form a loop on itself using the lateral right atrial wall for support (Fig. 4.62). This maneuver can prove extremely challenging. Depending on anatomy, occasionally such efforts will prove unsuccessful, and changing the site of venous access must be considered. At this point it is prudent to assess the patency of the right venous system with contrast materials (114). If one encounters a persistent left superior vena cava, an assessment of the right superior vena cava via contrast injection may prove helpful. Advancing the standard endhole catheter from the left superior vena cava to the vicinity of the right superior vena cava can carry this out. Occasionally, such communication does not exist. If the right supe-

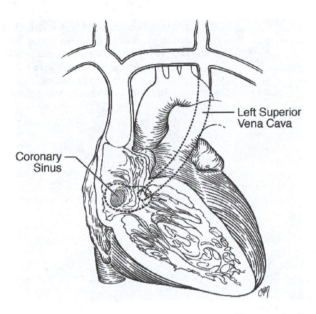

Fig. 4.60 Persistent left superior vena cava. (Belott PH. Unusual access sites for permanent cardiac pacing. In: Barold SS, Mugica J, eds. Recent advances in cardiac pacing: goals for the 21st century. Armonk, NY: Futura Publishing, 1997, with permission.)

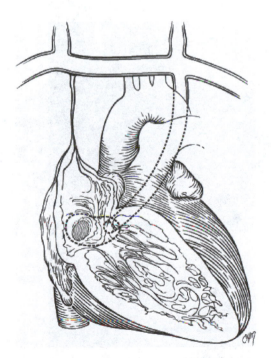

Fig. 4.61 Persistent left superior vena cava with absent right superior vena cava. (From Belott PH, Reynolds DW. Permanent pacemaker and cardioverter defibrillation implantation. In: Ellenbogen KA, Kay N, Wilkoff BL, eds. Clinical cardiac pacing and defibrillation, 2nd ed. Philadelphia: WB Saunders, 2000, with permission.)

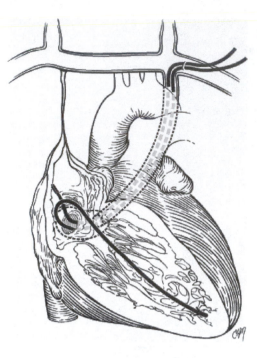

Fig. 4.62 Placement of an atrial and ventricular electrode via persistent left superior vena cava. (From Belott PH, Reynolds DW. Permanent pacemaker and cardioverter defibrillation implantation. In: Ellenbogen KA, Kay N, Wilkoff BL, eds. Clinical cardiac pacing and defibrillation, 2nd ed. Philadelphia: WB Saunders, 2000, with permission.)

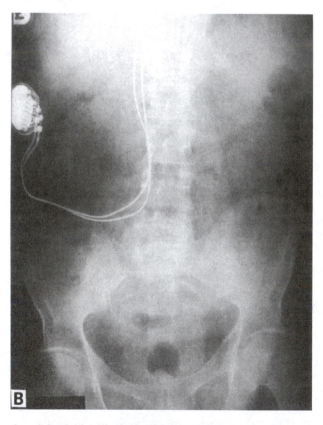

Fig. 4.63 Posterior–anterior abdominal radiograph showing the position of a pacemaker and generator lead inserted into the inferior vena cava using a retroperitoneal approach. (West JN, Shearmann CP, Gammage MD. Permanent pacemaker positioning via the inferior vena cava in a case of single ventricle with loss of right atrial-vena cava continuity. Pacing Clin Electrophysiol 1993;16(8):1753–1755, with permission.)

rior vena cava is absent, the iliac vein approach should be considered. Atrial electrode placement in the case of a persistent left superior vena cava is also challenging. It is recommended that positive fixation screw-in electrodes be used (115,116). The use of a preformed atrial J will prove difficult, if not impossible. Dislodgment of the preformed J is also a concern.

Permanent pacemakers have also been implanted using the inferior vena cava via a retroperitoneal approach (Fig. 4.63) (117). This is usually in the setting of complex congenital anomalies and subsequent corrective procedures. Venous access to the right atrium and ventricle is complicated by loss of continuity between the right atrium and the superior vena cava. Bipolar active fixation screw-in electrodes are used for both the atrium and ventricle. The pulse generator is usually implanted in a subcutaneous pocket formed on the anterior abdominal wall.

In a similar approach, pacemaker leads have been placed via transhepatic cannulation (Fig. 4.64) (118). Venous access is achieved percutaneously; with the guidewire passed transhepatically, the sheath set is applied, allowing the subsequent introduction of a permanent pacing electrode. Once again, this procedure has been reserved for complex congenital anomalies that preclude venous access via a superior vein.

Inframammary Implantation

The use of the principles of plastic surgery for standard pacemaker implantation can be adopted for optimal cosmetic effect (119). This technique involves more surgery and is best performed under modified or complete general anesthesia. Because of more postoperative wound pain, an overnight stay is advised. Venous access is achieved percutaneously for both single- and dual-chambered pacing. After the subclavian vein has been accessed, a limited 1- to 2-cm initial incision is made. This is carried to the surface of the pectoralis muscle. After the electrode(s) is placed, a second incision is made under the breast along the breast fold. A standard pocket is created under the breast (Fig. 4.65). The pacemaker lead(s) are tunneled to the inframammary pocket. The pulse generator and electrodes are connected and the incision closed. It is recommended that active fixation screw-in electrodes be employed for both the atrium and ventricle. It is also recommended that a Parsonnet pouch be used to avoid pulse generator migration and a Twiddler syndrome. An alternate approach calls for a second incision made in the axilla with the arm in abduction. The incision is carried to the depths that expose the muscular fascia. In this case the pulse generator is placed subpectorally. As previously noted Roelke and associates had described a submammary pacemaker implantation technique using unique tunneling (81). Venous access is achieved either percutaneously or by cephalic vein cutdown. The electrodes are positioned and anchored. A horizontal incision is made in the inframammary fold. A long 20-cm #18 gauge pericardiocentesis needle is directed from the inframammary pocket to the infraclavicular incision. A J wire is passed down the needle to the infraclavicular incision. The needle is removed and, using a retained-guidewire technique, two 10 French introducer dilators are passed consecutively over the guidewire. The free ends of the atrial and ventricular electrodes from the infraclavicular incision are placed in the sheaths and secured with a tie. The sheaths are then withdrawn to the inframammary pocket. A retropectoral transaxillary percutaneous tech-

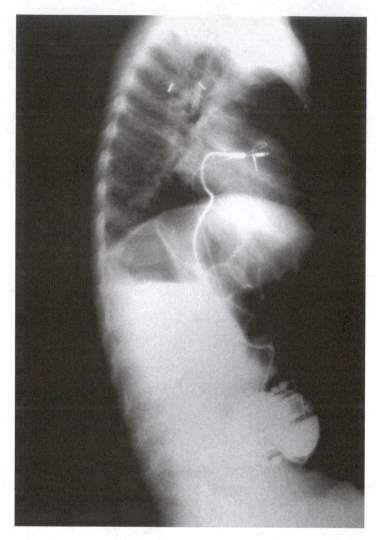

Fig. 4.64 Lateral view demonstrating transhepatic lead placement. (Fishberger SB, Camunas J, Rodriguez-Fernandez H, et al. Permanent pacemaker lead implantation via the transhepatic route. Pacing Clin Electrophysiol 1996;19(7):1124–1125, with permission.)

nique has also been used for optimal cosmetic effect (120). This technique is performed under local anesthesia and conscious sedation. Venography is used to confirm the relationship of the axillary vein to the surface anatomy. A marker is placed in the axillary vein via the antecubital fossa (Fig. 4.66). This marker may be either a temporary transvenous pacing wire or a standard 0.032-mm guidewire. Using the marker as a guide the axillary vein is punctured. A longitudinal incision is made along the posterior border of the pectoralis major muscle in the axilla. A standard retropectoral pocket is created. One or two pacing electrodes can then be placed by conventional techniques. The electrodes are secured by their suture sleeve to the pectoralis fascia. The leads are then connected to the pacemaker and inserted into the retropectoral pocket.

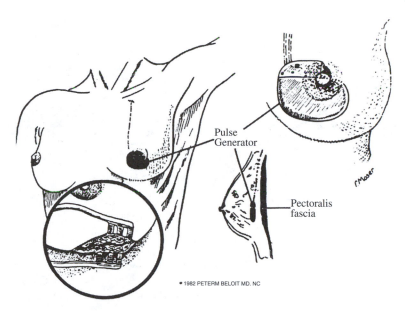

Fig. 4.65 Inframammary incision and placement of pulse generator with tunneled electrodes. (Belott PH, Bucko D. Inframammary pulse generator placement for maximizing cosmetic effect. Pacing Clin Electrophysiol 1983;6(6):1241–1244, with permission.)

This technique offers optimal cosmetic results, and there have been no restrictions in physical activity or movement of the shoulder joint (Fig. 4.67).

Transthoracic Endocardial Lead Placement

Occasionally, transvenous endocardial lead placement is impractical, impossible, or contraindicated. Endocardial leads may be placed transthoracically under general anesthesia and via a limited thoracotomy (121). The pacemaker electrodes are passed and positioned transatrially through a limited thoracotomy in the sixth intercostal space. The right atrium is identified and the electrode is passed transatrially through an incision or by using a sheath set. A pursestring suture about the entry site achieves hemostasis. Fluoroscopy can be used for ventricular placement of a tined or screw-in electrode. All electrodes are then secured to the endocardial surface. Sutures placed under the tines secure the electrode. The electrodes are then driven through an atriotomy into the atrial cavity and out the atrial muscle at a point of desired endocardial fixation. The electrodes are pulled through the incision and snugged to the endocardium by pulling and tying the double-ended suture (Fig. 4.68). This approach is recommended over the epicardial approach because of the excellent thresholds that can be achieved. Hayes and associates have described a similar technique of endocardial electrode placement at the time of corrective cardiac surgery (122). In this procedure, epicardial pacing was avoided because of poor pacing and sensing thresholds. Traditionally, at the time of surgery, the patient requiring a dual-chambered pacing system would receive epicardial ventricular electrodes. The atrial electrode was placed transvenously later during the hospitalization. In the postoperative period, a dual-chambered system appeared crucial for opti-

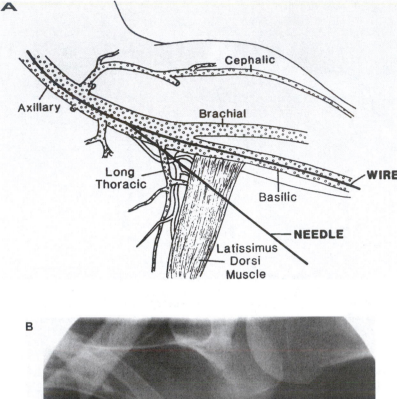

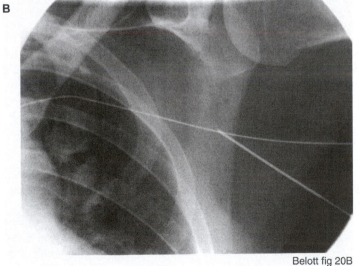

Belott fig 20B

Fig. 4.66 A: Stylized illustration of axillary venipuncture using the guidewire as a landmark. B: Radiograph of needle accessing the axillary vein using the guidewire as a landmark. (Shefer A, Lewis BS, Gang ES. The retropectoral transaxillary permanent pacemaker: description of a technique for percutaneous implantation of an "invisible" device. Pacing Clin Electrophysiol 1996;19(11 Pt 1):1646–1651, with permission.)

mal hemodynamics. In the Hayes and associates technique, a dual-chambered pacemaker patient with severe tricuspid regurgitation and chronic endocardial electrodes required removal of all endocardial electrodes and then placement of a prosthetic tricuspid valve. New epicardial electrodes were placed in the ventricle. Stable atrial pacing and sensing was achieved by transatrial endocardial placement of the atrial appendage (Fig. 4.69). Pursestring ligatures about the

Fig. 4.67 Lateral view of a patient after transaxillary retropectoral pacemaker implantation using the Shefer approach. (Shefer A, Lewis BS, Gang ES. The retropectoral transaxillary permanent pacemaker: description of a technique for percutaneous implanation of an "invisible" device. Pacing Clin Electrophysiol 1996;19(11 Pt 1):1646–1651, with permission.)

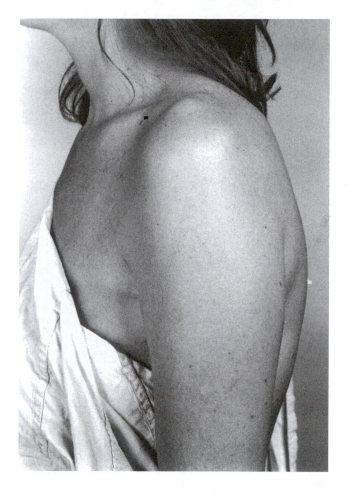

incision secured the lead. A third transthoracic endocardial approach has been described by Byrd (123). This technique allows for conventional transvenous electrodes to be implanted in patients requiring an epicardial approach. It has been used in patients with superior vena cava syndrome, anomalous pulmonary venous drainage, or in younger patients with innominate vein thrombosis. The technique involves a limited surgical approach under general anesthesia. A small incision is made in the third or fourth intercostal space. The third and fourth costal cartilages are excised and the atrial appendage exposed. An atriotomy is performed and an introducer placed inside an atrial pursestring suture and secured in a vertical position. The atrial and ventricular electrodes are passed down a standard sheath set into the atrium (Fig. 4.70). Using standard techniques, including fluoroscopy, the electrodes are positioned. Once the electrodes are positioned, the introducer is removed and the pursestring suture is used to close the atriotomy and secure the electrodes. The pacemaker is placed in a pocket adjacent to the incision on the right anterior chest wall. The advantage of this technique is minimal morbidity compared to the standard epicardial approach. The chest is never entered and the time required for such procedures is similar to the transvenous approach. The technique, however, requires general anesthesia, violation of the epicardium, and an obligatory right atriotomy.

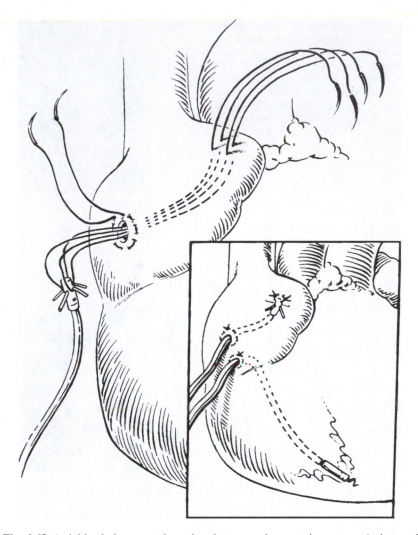

Fig. 4.68 Atrial lead placement through atriotomy and pursestring suture. Atrium and ventricular electrodes are positioned and the atriotomy is secured. (Westerman GR, Van Devanter SH. Transthoracic transatrial endocardial lead placement for permanent pacing. Ann Thorac Surg 1987;43(4):445–446, with permission.)

Implantation Techniques for Cardiac Resynchronization Therapy

Cardiac resynchronization therapy has clearly demonstrated hemodynamic benefit in patients with advanced CHF (124–130). Successful stimulation of the Left ventricular (LV) is critical to this new therapeutic pacing modality. This can be accomplished by either an epicardial or endocardial approach. The endocardial approach involves access to the LV endocardium transatrially through a patent foramen ovale or a direct transseptal puncture. This approach is considered potentially dangerous because of the risk of thromboembolism and stroke (131). The epicardium of the LV can be accesses by direct placement

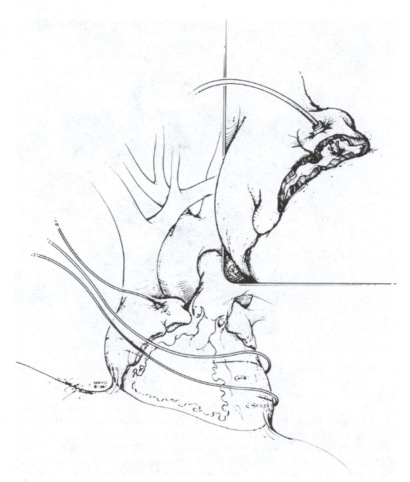

Fig. 4.69 Atrial lead placement. Insert in the upper right shows atrial endocardial lead being placed through the wall of the right atrial appendage with the tip of the pacemaker lead abutting the endocardial surface. A pursestring suture is placed around the lead at the point of entry. The relationship of the atrial lead is also shown. (Hayes DL, Vlietstra RE, Puga FJ, et al. A novel approach to atrial endocardial pacing. Pacing Clin Electrophysiol 1989;12(1 Pt 1):125–130, with permission.)

of pacing leads via thoracic surgery or a thoracoscopic approach. The direct placement of electrodes via thoracotomy in patients with advanced congestive heart failure (CHF) is a relatively high-risk procedure. The LV epicardium may also be accessed transvenously by passing a wire via the coronary sinus to a posterolateral branch of the coronary sinus on the left ventricular free wall (132). The coronary sinus has been used for cardiac pacing of both the ventricle and atrium for many years (133–137). Permanent LV pacing via the great cardiac vein was initially reported by Bai et al., in an unusual situation where there was no RV access (138). In 1994, Bakker reported the benefits of biventricular pacing in CHF by placing an endocardial right ventricular (RV) lead and an epicardial LV lead, both connected to the ventricular channel of a pacemaker (139). In that same year, Cazeau and co-workers reported the benefit of four-chamber pacing in a patient with end-stage dilated cardiomyopathy (140). Leads were placed transvenously to the left atrium, right atrium

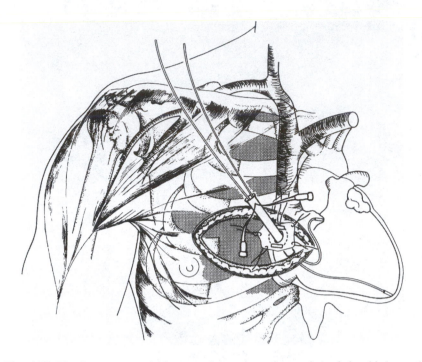

Fig. 4.70 The Lemmon surgical approach consists of resection of the third costal cartilage through a small incision, reflection of the pleura, and opening of the pericardium. Introducer and transvenous sleeve are inserted through a right atrial pursestring suture. The leads are positioned in the right ventricle and right atrium using standard fluoroscopic techniques. Through the incision, the subcutaneous pocket is constructed over the pectoralis muscle on the anterior chest wall in its normal position. The leads are connected to the pacemaker without the need for an adapter or tunneling. (Byrd CL, Schwartz SJ. Transatrial implantation of transvenous pacing leads as an alternative to implantation of epicardial leads. Pacing Clin Electrophysiol 1990;13(12 Pt 2):1856–1859, with permission.)

and RV apex, with the LV lead placed on the epicardium via thoracotomy. Subsequently, Daubert and co-workers have clearly demonstrated acute and long-term feasibility as well as safety of permanent LV pacing using leads inserted transvenously into coronary veins over the LV free wall (132). The transvenous approach is now favored and biventricular pacing can be accomplished using conventional pacing hardware with only minor adaptations compared to the thoracotomy approach associated with poor lead reliability (sensing and chronic pacing thresholds), as well as increased morbidity and mortality.

Anatomical Considerations

A complete understanding of the gross and radiographic cardiac anatomy is essential for successful cardiac resynchronization. Appreciation of the right atrial anatomy is necessary for coronary sinus cannulation. It is also important to understand that the right atrial and coronary sinus anatomy can be quite variable, especially in patients with advanced CHF. These hearts are usually extremely dilated and the normal cardiac anatomical structures are distorted.

Right Atrium

In the frontal plane, the right atrial cavity is located to the right and anteriorly. The left atrium is located to the left and mainly posteriorly in the intraatrial septum. When viewed in the transverse plane, it runs obliquely from a left anterior position to a right posterior position. The right atrium is somewhat larger than the left but its walls are somewhat thinner. Traditionally, the right atrium is considered to consist of two parts, a posterior smooth-walled part into which the superior and inferior vena cavae enter, and a very thin-walled, trabeculated part located anterolaterally (141). The two parts of the atrium are separated by a muscular ridge called the crista terminalis. This ridge consists of muscle which is more prominent superiorly and tapers as it moves in an inferolateral direction. Externally, the crista terminalis corresponds to a seam known as the sulcus terminalis. The pectinate muscles run laterally in a parallel fashion from the crista terminalis along the right atrial free wall. The atrial wall between the muscle bundles between the pectinate muscle bundles is almost paper thin and translucent. The right atrial appendage is the triangular-shaped superior portion of the right atrium. It is filled with pectinate muscles. The eustachian valve is a fold of tissue that guards the anterior border of the inferior vena caval ostium. In man it demonstrates considerable variability and may even be absent. Occasionally, it is perforated and even fenestrated, forming a lace-like network known as the network of Chiari. Anterior and medial to the eustachian valve, the coronary sinus enters the right atrium. The thebesian valve is a valve-like fold of tissue that guards the orifice of the coronary sinus. The intraatrial septum forms the posterior medial wall of the right atrium. Its central, ovoid portion is thin and fibrous and forms a shallow depression known as the fossa ovalis. The remainder of the septum is muscular, forming a ridge known as the limbus fossa ovalis (Fig. 4.71).

The recent developments in interventional electrophysiology techniques, as well as resynchronization therapy mandate a better understanding of atrial anatomy to improve therapeutic results. Contemporary anatomists Ho and Anderson have led the way to a better understanding of anatomy as it relates to cardiac electrophysiologic interventions (142,143). Ho considers the right atrium as consisting of three components, the appendage, a venous part, and the vestibule (Fig. 4.72 A,B). The intraatrial septum, a fourth component, is shared by the right and left atrium. Viewed from the epicardium, the atrial appendage is a triangular-shaped structure located anterior and lateral. The sulcus terminalis, corresponding to the crista terminalis, can be seen running along the lateral wall as a fat-filled groove. Epicardially, the sinus node is located in this groove adjacent to the superior-vena-cava-atrial junction. The right atrial musculature extends from the superior vena cava externally and terminates at the entrance of the inferior vena cava. When viewed externally, the pectinate muscles, as previously noted, can be seen radiating from the terminal crest. The pectinate muscles spread throughout the entire wall of the atrial appendage, extending to the lateral and inferior walls of the atrium. The pectinate muscles never reach the orifice of the tricuspid valve. The vestibule is a smooth muscular rim that sur-

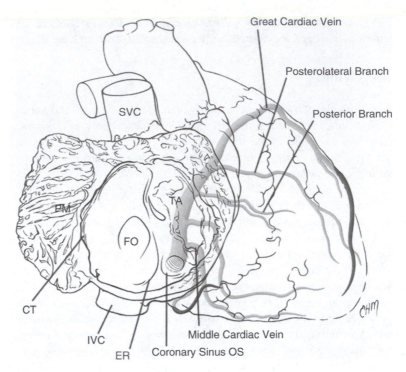

Fig. 4.71 Heart rotated into the RAO projection with the right atrial cavity exposed demonstrating the superfiscial and deep anatomy of the right heart in relationship to the coronary sinus and its branch tributaries. (from Belott PH: Implantation Techniques for Cardiac resynchronization Therapy Barold SS, Mugica J Fifth Decade of Cardiac Pacing. Armonk NY Futura. 2004 pp. 4)

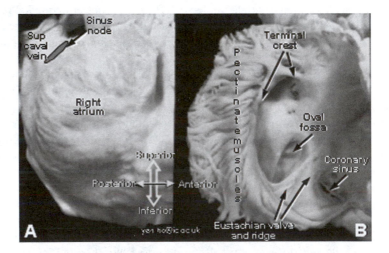

Fig. 4.72 A. Right anterior view of the right atrium from outside. Relationship of the superior vena cava and atrial appendage is seen the right atrium is thin walled with a rough texture. The relationship of the sinus node is shown. B. Inside of the right atrium as seen from the RAO view. The RA free wall is retracted posteriorly the septal aspect and venous component are seen. The pectinate muscles arise from the terminal arch of the crista terminalis. The Eustachian ridge and valve, and a fenestrated thesbesian valve are seen. (from Ho S: Understanding arial anatomy: Implications for atrial fibrillation ablation. In Cardiology International for a global perspective on cardiac care. London, Greycoat Publishing 2002. pp s17–s20)

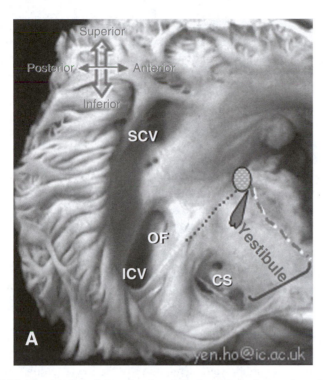

Fig. 4.73 The landmarks of the triangle of Koch are superimposed on the exposed right atrial cavity. The relationship of these structural landmarks to the coronary sinus is seen. (from Ho S: Understanding arial anatomy: Implications for atrial fibrillation ablation. In Cardiology International for a global perspective on cardiac care. London, Greycoat Publishing 2002. pp s17–s20)

rounds the tricuspid valve orifice (Fig. 4.73). The posterior smooth wall of the atrium composes the venous component. The terminal crest marks the division between the venous smooth and trabeculated parts of the atrium. The terminal crest is a muscular bundle that begins on the superior aspect of the medial wall and passes anterior and lateral to the orifice of the superior vena cava. It then descends obliquely along the lateral atrial wall. Its terminal portion consists of a number of smaller muscle bundles, extending to the vestibule and orifice of the inferior vena cava. As mentioned previously, the eustachian valve, a triangular flap of fibromuscular tissue, guards the entrance of the inferior vena cava. This valve inserts medially and forms the eustachian ridge or sinus septum, which is the border between the fossa ovalis and coronary sinus. The eustachian valve may at times be quite large and at other times fenestrated, perforated, and delicate. The free border of the eustachian valve extends as a tendon that runs into the musculature of the sinus septum, forming the posterolateral border of Koch's triangle. The anterior border is marked by the hinge of the septal leaflet of the tricuspid valve. The vestibular portion of the right atrium that surrounds the valvular orifice is the common location for slow-pathway ablations of AV node reentrant tachycardia. The thebesian valve is a small, flat, crescentic flap of fibrous tissue that guards the orifice of the coronary sinus. It also shows variability in size and thickness and is occasionally fenestrated. The atrial wall inferior to the coronary sinus os often forms a pouch known as the subeustachian sinus. The coronary sinus is the terminal portion of the great cardiac vein and is located posteriorly in the left atrioventricular groove. It is frequently covered by muscular fibers of the left atrium. The coronary sinus receives the veins draining the LV, including the great cardiac vein, posterior cardiac vein, left cardiac vein, and anterior cardiac veins. The coronary sinus terminates in the inferoposterior aspect of the right atrium and forms the inferior border of Koch's triangle.

The ostia of the veins draining into the coronary sinus may be guarded by unicuspid or bicuspid valves.

Angiographic Anatomy

In addition to understanding the gross anatomy of the right atrium and coronary sinus, an understanding of the radiologic and angiographic anatomy is crucial to success in cardiac resynchronization. There have been very few papers devoted to the angiographic anatomy of the coronary sinus and coronary veins (144,145). In an attempt to better define the angiographic anatomy of the coronary sinus, Guillard et al. studied 110 consecutive patients (146). The venous phase of left coronary angiography was analyzed in the right anterior oblique 30°, anteroposterior, AP, and the left anterior oblique 60° projections. The precise radio-anatomic descriptions of the number, dimensions, angulations, angulation, and tortuosity of tributaries of the coronary sinus were recorded. The diameter of the coronary sinus ostium was also measured. The tributaries of the coronary sinus were described as follows: The great cardiac vein, originating in the lower middle third of the interventricular sulcus, courses the sulcus and turns toward the left side of the atrioventricular groove, entering the coronary sinus at an approximately 180° angle. Frequently, the valve of Vieussens coincides with the great cardiac vein ostium. The middle cardiac vein has an origin at the cardiac apex and courses within the posterior interventricular groove and drains into the coronary sinus just prior to the coronary sinus ostium. The left posterior vein arises from the lateral and posterior aspects of the LV, draining into the great cardiac vein or coronary sinus. The left oblique vein of Marshall is a coronary vein that courses diagonally on the posterior surface of the left atrium and joins the great cardiac vein at a point where it becomes the coronary sinus. In the anteroposterior view, the coronary sinus has its ostium superimposed over the posterior portion of the thoracic vertebrae at the level of the diaphragm. Unfortunately, these landmarks are extremely variable and of little use in individual cases. Anatomically, the coronary sinus ends at the level of the thebesian valve and the great cardiac vein ends in the coronary sinus at the level of the Vieussens valve. The middle cardiac vein consistently arises in the coronary sinus perpendicular near the coronary sinus ostium at an angle of 60–90°, approximately 1 cm from the coronary sinus ostium. The great cardiac vein in the anteroposterior view demonstrates considerable variability, curving toward the atrioventricular groove. Past the curve, the great cardiac vein maintains an axis parallel to the coronary sinus. There is considerable variability with respect to tortuosity and diameter. The posterior veins originate from the posterior and lateral aspects of the LV and join the coronary sinus or great cardiac vein. The posterior veins are highly variable in number, size, and angulation. In general, this study demonstrated wide variation in the number and size of the left posterior veins. Occasionally, these veins were quite diminutive and even absent. In

RAO Projection

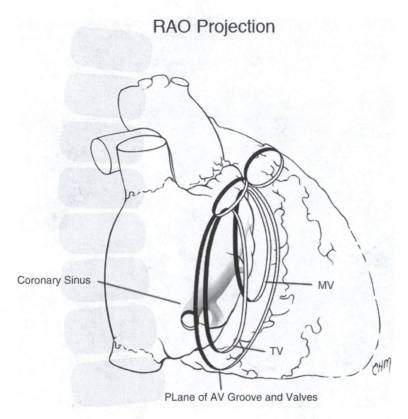

Coronary Sinus

MV

TV

PLane of AV Groove and Valves

Fig. 4.74 A Heart rotated in the right anterior oblique view. The relationship of the AV groove and spine is seen. (from Belott PH: Implantation Techniques for Cardiac resynchronization Therapy Barold SS, Mugica J Fifth Decade of Cardiac Pacing. Armonk NY Futura. 2004 pp 6)

the frontal plane, the right ventricle occupies most of the cardiac silhouette as an anterior structure. The upper half of the right heart border is formed by the superior vena cava, while the lower portion is formed by the lateral wall of the right atrium. The plane of the lateral valve is sandwiched between the anterior right ventricle and posterior LV. It can be conceptualized as an oval ring tipped somewhat to the left. The coronary sinus is located at the inferior aspect of the cardiac silhouette at the level of the diaphragms, approximately in the midline. Cannulation of the coronary sinus in this view can be somewhat difficult. The 30–60° right anterior oblique projection, however, rolls the right ventricle to the left. In this projection, the superior and inferior vena cavae and right atrium become an anterior structure. The plane of the tricuspid and mitral valves becomes more vertical and perpendicular to the anteroposterior plane. The right ventricle is thrown to the left. In the frontal projection, the coronary sinus runs obliquely from a right inferior position to a left superior position in the cardiac silhouette. As the heart is rotated to the right anterior oblique projection, the coronary sinus is tipped more superiorly (Fig. 4.74). In the left anterior oblique projection, the plane of the tricuspid and mitral valves becomes frontal with the coronary sinus tipped in a more horizontal position, crossing over the spine as it courses to the left, crossing over the spine

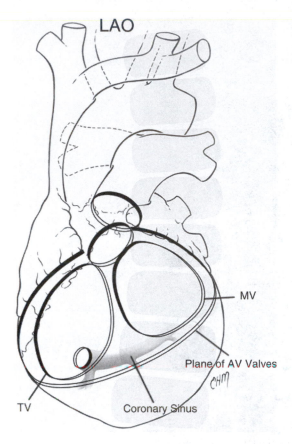

LAO

MV

Plane of AV Valves

CHM

TV

Coronary Sinus

Fig. 4.75 Heart rotated in the left anterior oblique view. The AV groove is tipped horizontally. (from Belott PH: Implantation Techniques for Cardiac resynchronization Therapy Barold SS, Mugica J Fifth Decade of Cardiac Pacing. Armonk NY Futura. 2004 pp 6)

from right to left and turning superiorly along the left heart border (Fig. 4.75). In the right and left anterior oblique projections, the os of the coronary sinus can be found at the inferior aspect of the cardiac silhouette at the level of the diaphragms just to the right of the spine. Rotating from the right anterior oblique to the left anterior oblique projection and back becomes extremely important when trying to cannulate the coronary sinus os. As a simple example, when in the frontal projection, the catheter may appear to be in the vicinity of the coronary sinus os with a trajectory pointing inferiorly and to the left, but when the image is rotated to the left anterior oblique projection, the catheter actually is 180° away from the coronary sinus os, pointing anterior and to the right. After adjusting the catheter to a posterior and leftward position, the right anterior oblique projection may show the catheter pointing laterally to the right, away from the coronary sinus os. Thus, the use of multiple views becomes essential for coronary sinus os cannulation.

Use of the left anterior oblique projection is extremely important in defining the tributaries of the coronary sinus (Fig. 4.76). In the frontal and right anterior oblique projections, tributaries of the coronary sinus appear to run perpendicular to the coronary sinus obliquely from a superior to an inferior direction (Fig. 4.77). The branches appear to be parallel, and differentiation of anteroseptal, lateral, and posterolateral branches is almost impossible. For simplicity and for the purpose of this discussion, branches or tributaries of the coronary sinus are described from their ostia in the coronary sinus. In the LAO projection, the great cardiac vein or anterior cardiac vein comes off of the coronary sinus superiorly into the right. It then turns acutely, descending inferiorly

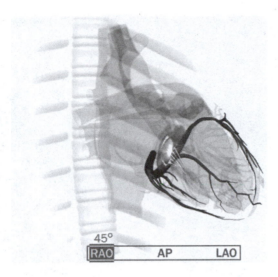

Fig. 4.76 Coronary sinus seen in the RAO projection. The plane of the CS is vertical with the branch tributaries at a right angle. In this view all the branches come of the CS at nearly a right angle and are directed slightly inferior and to the left. (from Belott PH: Implantation Techniques for Cardiac resynchronization Therapy Barold SS, Mugica J Fifth Decade of Cardiac Pacing. Armonk NY Futura. 2004 Plate 1.3)

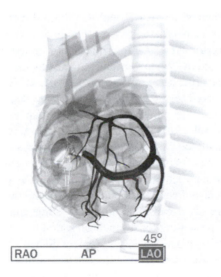

Fig. 4.77 Coronary sinus seen in the LAO projection. The plane of the CS is more horizontal and posterior. The posterior and lateral branches are directed inferiorly and to the left while the anterior branches are directed superiorly and to the right. (from Belott PH: Implantation Techniques for Cardiac resynchronization Therapy Barold SS, Mugica J Fifth Decade of Cardiac Pacing. Armonk NY Futura. 2004 Plate 1.4)

and to the right in the interventricular septum. The lateral and posterolateral branches of the coronary sinus generally come off the superior aspect, but arc superiorly and inferiorly to the left, crossing over to the left of the spine. The posterior branches generally come off the coronary sinus at right or acute angles, directed inferiorly and to the left of the spine. Reporting on his cardiac resynchronization experience, Niazi has noted the importance of understanding the right atrial anatomy and pointed out the variations in the right atrium as well

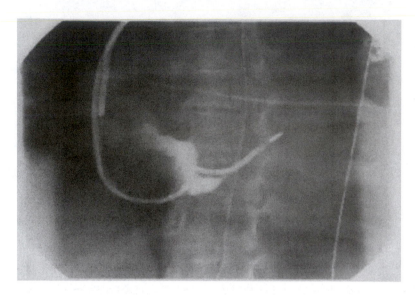

Fig. 4.78 Puffs of contrast through the guiding catheter defining the CS os and lower RA anatomy. Image courtesy of Imran Nazi MD (from Belott PH: Implantation Techniques for Cardiac resynchronization Therapy Barold SS, Mugica J Fifth Decade of Cardiac Pacing. Armonk NY Futura. 2004 Page 7)

as coronary sinus angulations. It is noted that these directly relate to guiding catheter selection for catheterizing the coronary sinus os. In addition, further analysis of the coronary sinus anatomy has demonstrated considerable variation in the branch anatomy. When viewed from the outside, Niazi considers the right atrium a tubular structure as opposed to a simple sac joined by the inferior and superior vena cavae. The synchronization experience demonstrates the importance of understanding the presence of the Thebesian valve, the eustachian valve, as well as the valve of Vieussens. Valvular structures and fossae of the right atrium can usually be demonstrated by simple puffs of contrast from the guiding catheter. The puffs of contrast are extremely useful in distinguishing fossae from the coronary sinus os itself (Fig 4.78). It is important to distinguish the subeustachian fossa, the pouch beneath the eustachian ridge and the eustachian valve, as it can make coronary sinus cannulation extremely difficult. In patients presenting for resynchronization therapy, it was noted that the annulus of the tricuspid valve was extremely dilated. It was noted that the right atrial anatomy was considerably distorted. The tricuspid valve annulus was dilated, as well as the various fossae, and occasional muscular ridges were encountered. These distortions and alterations in the right atrium rendered coronary sinus ostial cannulation extremely difficult. Niazi's study of 82 patients with heart failure noted that the right atrial size varied between 20 and 53 mm (147). Approximately 70% of the right atria were dilated and there was a 75% incidence of mild to moderate tricuspid regurgitation. As well as variations in the right atrial anatomy, coronary sinus os size, height of origin, shape, diameter, and angulation as well as the presence of valves were also noted. The coronary sinus angulation varied from shallow to extreme superior angulation. The coronary sinus varied from very small size to large, in addition to variations in angulation. Coronary sinus os variations were noted to vary from extremely wide and funnel-shaped to small coronary sinus os occasionally covered with

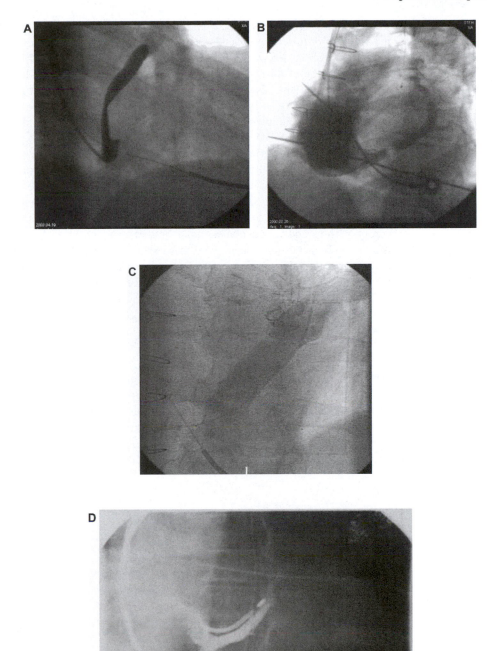

Fig. 4.79 A. Flat vertical CS. (From Niazi with permission.) B. Funnel shaped CS. C Large superiorly angulated CS. D Small superiorly angulated CS. (from Belott PH: Implantation Techniques for Cardiac resynchronization Therapy Barold SS, Mugica J Fifth Decade of Cardiac Pacing. Armonk NY Futura. 2004 pp 8) Image courtesy of Imran Nazi MD

the Thebesian valve. Niazi studied 52 patients with heart failure and noted that the diameter of the coronary sinus ranged between 2 and 22 mm. The shape of the coronary sinus also varied from tubular to wafer or funnel (Fig. 4.79 A–D). In an evaluation of 48 patients, Niazi noted that 20% of the coronary sinus angulations were sharp superior, 40% moderately superior, 15% horizontal, and 25% inferior (147). It appears that the angulation of the coronary sinus directly relates to the planes of the tricuspid and mitral valves. If the mitral valve is in a higher plane than the tricuspid, coronary sinus angulation will generally be upwards. In addition, coronary sinus angulation is also related to the size of the mitral valve annulus. The larger the mitral valve annulus, the more posterior displaced the coronary sinus is from its origin. In the case of a small mitral valve annulus, the degree of curvature posteriorly of the coronary sinus generally appears to be somewhat less. In addition to variations to the coronary sinus and its os, considerable branch variation was also noted by Niazi. The branches have been noted to vary in angle of branch takeoff, size, the presence of valves, and extreme tortuosity. The experience of Niazi and others has underscored the need to be prepared for considerable variation in the coronary sinus os and coronary sinus vein anatomy. Transverse branches of the coronary sinus have been noted to have considerable variations, from shallow takeoff to acute takeoff.

Implantation

LV pacing has undergone considerable evolution in its short history. Initially, pacemaker electrodes were placed in the coronary sinus using a stylet-driven technique. This has evolved to the currently acceptable use of a guiding catheter contrast venography for either a stylet-driven or some form of guidewire-assisted placement.

Preoperative Planning

In general, the support personnel required to carry out biventricular pacing are essentially identical to those utilized for a permanent pacemaker or ICD procedure (148). These would include a registered nurse who can administer drugs and deliver surgical supplies to the surgical field, a scrub nurse or technician familiar with all the particular needs of the implanting physician, and a cardiovascular technician familiar with the operation of the sophisticated radiologic equipment. The same individual can assist with the electrophysiologic recording of measurements required for biventricular threshold measurements. Unlike a simple pacemaker procedure, it is recommended that an anesthesiologist be present to administer conscious sedation or general anesthesia. Patients requiring cardiac resynchronization are extremely ill and require airway support that can only be administered by an anesthesiologist. Biventricular pacing systems from any manufacturer are extremely complex with many components unique to any particular manufacturer. A highly trained manufacturer's representative can be invaluable in the biventricular procedure. In addition, as the newer coronary sinus lead delivery systems incorporate the tools of interventional cardiology, it is recommended that the support cardiovascular

Table 4.13 Components of delivery system for coronary sinus cannulation.

I. Percutaneous introducer kit: sheath with hemostatic valve: multiple sizes
II. Guide catheters: multiple shapes and lengths
III. Hemostatic valves with optional flush system
IV. Balloon catheters
V. Angiographic contrast material
VI. Guidewires
VII. Lead stylets
VIII. Interventional guidewires
IX. Electrophysiologic catheters, preformed and deflectable
X. Angioplasty guidewires

technician assisting at the biventricular insertion be completely familiar with the tools and techniques utilized by interventional cardiology.

The cardiac catheterization laboratory is the ideal place for performing cardiac resynchronization procedures. It offers high-quality images for precise and easily achieved multiple projections that are required for coronary sinus lead placement. The cardiac catheterization laboratory is also the resource for any type of catheter, guidewires, sheaths, or angiographic material that may be required in any given situation. It is also the location of sophisticated physiologic recording and monitoring equipment essential for cardiac resynchronization therapy.

The placement of 12-lead electrocardiographic monitoring is often useful in determining left ventricular capture. In addition, patient monitoring equipment should include an automated blood pressure cuff, the presence of continuous oxygen saturation monitoring, as well as intravascular pressure monitoring, both arterial and venous.

The cardiac resynchronization procedure usually merely requires a minor surgical tray with a limited number of instruments. A simple pacemaker or ICD surgical tray is more than adequate (149). The usual pacemaker supplies and spare parts should be readily available. Today, since transvenous cardiac resynchronization therapy involves the placement of a coronary sinus lead, most manufacturers offer a complete delivery system for placement of their leads. These systems generally include a percutaneous lead introduction kit with needles, syringe and guidewire, peel-away introducers, an assortment of guiding catheters, adjustable hemostatic valve systems, coronary sinus lead, and an assortment of lead stylets. In the case of the over-the-wire lead system, multiple angioplasty stylets are available. An example of lead delivery system components is shown in Table 4.13. Many patients for cardiac resynchronization therapy have compromised renal function. Coronary sinus lead placement frequently requires contrast venography to locate the coronary sinus and the coronary sinus ostium. It is therefore important to check the blood urea nitrogen and creatinine levels prior to the procedure. If renal function is impaired, an attempt should be made to minimize the volume of contrast used, have the patient optimally hydrated, and consider dilution of the contrast material. In instances of extremely advanced renal failure, premedication with flumazicon has proven to be helpful. Careful attention should be paid to the patient's fluid status, as these compromised patients can easily be tripped into severe CHF and pulmonary edema. The biventricular procedure may be performed either with general anesthesia or conscious sedation. Most centers recommend conscious sedation due to the risks associated with general anesthesia. There is a diversion of opinion with respect to the use of general anesthesia, as some groups consistently use general anesthesia with very favorable results and no untoward complications. An echocardiogram can be extremely helpful in defining extreme structural changes that are associated with advanced heart failure. Marked left ventricular hypertrophy, dilatation of tricuspid and mitral annuli, as well as extreme right atrial dilatation may help one anticipate the structural changes in the coronary sinus os, its location and size. If a resynchronization patient is to undergo coronary angiography, every attempt should be made to encourage the operator to perform a forward angiogram demonstrating the venous or levo phase to localize the coronary sinus. In addition, in anticipation of performing coronary angiography during the resynchronization procedure, in the case of extreme difficulty in cannulating the coronary sinus, the right groin should be prepped and draped in anticipation of coronary angiography. The coronary venous anatomy is visualized during the levo phase after injection of the left main coronary artery in both the left anterior and right anterior oblique projections. Cineangiogram is continued through the visualization of the coronary system and then continued through the venous system, delineating the great cardiac vein, all major tributaries, and the coronary sinus with its os.

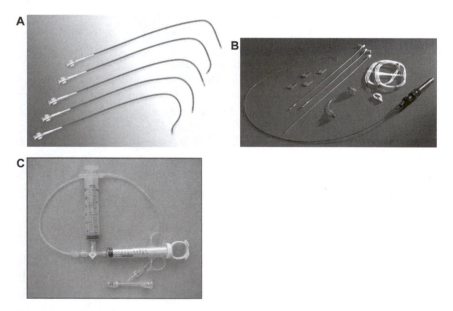

Fig. 4.80 A. Lead delivery system with guide catheters, Hemostatic valve, guide wires and EP catheter. Courtesy Guidant/Boston Scientific. B. Family of guide catheters with multiple distal tip curves. Courtesy Medtronic Corporation. C. Hemostatic valve and flush system. Courtesy Guidant/Boston Scientific. (from Belott PH: Implantation Techniques for Cardiac resynchronization Therapy Barold SS, Mugica J Fifth Decade of Cardiac Pacing. Armonk NY Futura. 2004 pp 10)

Equipment and Delivery Systems

The initial placement of permanent pacemaker electrodes in tributaries of the coronary sinus was performed by a simple stylet-driven approach. This approach proved to be quite difficult because of the altered anatomy of large dilated hearts and the variability in the coronary sinus anatomy. This has led to the development of a number of delivery systems to expedite location, cannulation and coronary sinus lead placement (150). Each manufacturer has developed a delivery system unique to its particular coronary sinus electrode (Fig. 4.80 A–C). Most systems consist of an introducer kit for venous acces, hemostatic valves, and an assortment of guiding catheters and guidewires. The guiding catheters are preformed in a number of shapes for rapid coronary sinus access. A number of sheaths with hemostatic valves are also used for guiding catheter stabilization and ease of manipulation. The delivery system also consists of a balloon catheter for the performance of venography within the coronary sinus. Hemostatic valve components of the delivery system is important, not only to prevent back-bleeding but also the aspiration of air and prevention of air embolization.

Implantation Procedure

The transvenous route is ideally performed in the cardiac catheterization laboratory. Although the operating room offers optimal sterility, the cardiac catheterization laboratory has all of the tools and equipment for both pacemaker and angioplastic procedures. The fluoroscopy should offer storage capability and there should be cineangiography readily available. A 12-lead electrocardiogram is essential so that proper left ventricular lead placement and capture can be documented. The patient should have a surgical prep that includes access to the right groin as well as both pectoral areas. A flush system should also be set up to allow for flush of the delivery system as well as ease of delivery of contrast.

Table 4.14 Endocardial approaches for coronary sinus left ventricular lead placement.

I. Free lead – stylet driven.
II. Guiding catheter assisted with free lead – stylet driven
III. Free over-the-wire – guidewire driven without the use of a guide catheter
IV. Guiding catheter-assisted, over-the-wire

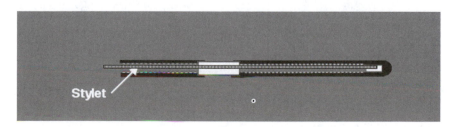

Fig. 4.81 A diagram of a stylet-driven lead. Courtesy Guidant/Boston Scientific. (from Belott PH: Implantation Techniques for Cardiac resynchronization Therapy Barold SS, Mugica J Fifth Decade of Cardiac Pacing. Armonk NY Futura. 2004 pp 11)

Table 4.14 lists the endocardial approaches developed for the positioning of a pacemaker electrode in a tributary vein of the coronary sinus for pacing of the left ventricular free wall. The simplest approach for positioning an electrode in a tributary of the coronary sinus is to employ the basic pacemaker lead that is stylet driven. This can be extremely problematic. This has led to a more desirable approach, employing a guiding catheter with a stylet-driven pacemaker lead. Even with a guiding catheter for localization and cannulation of the coronary sinus os, the stylet-driven approach has proven to be somewhat difficult. Drawing on interventional and angioplasty techniques, pacemaker wires have been adapted for an over-the-wire and side-wire approach (151). The conventional stylet-driven approach for lead placement precludes the accessibility of distal coronary sinus branches, often necessary for successful left ventricular pacing. An example of a simple stylet-driven electrode is shown in Fig. 4.81, preformed for operator-shaped stylet and is used to deliver the electrode to the appropriate branch in the coronary sinus. A number of electrode designs have been developed that incorporate different tip shapes and angulations for coronary sinus branch fixation. These have met with variable success. The monorail design or side-wire has has largely been abandoned because a tortuous anatomy requiring frequent wire exchanges made repositioning the wire in the loop difficult. The over-the-wire design appears ideal at this time. Using angioplastic guidewires, distal tortuous branches of the coronary sinus can now be accessed with lead placement in a desired coronary sinus tributary (Fig. 4.82).

Venous Access

A number of standard venous access techniques have been used for insertion of the multiple leads for biventricular pacing (Table 4.15). Venous access is

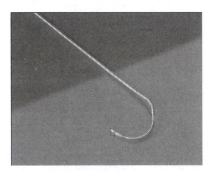

Fig. 4.82 Stylet-driven lead with preformed tip for support in the CS. Courtesy Medtronic Corporation. (from Belott PH: Implantation Techniques for Cardiac resynchronization Therapy Barold SS, Mugica J Fifth Decade of Cardiac Pacing. Armonk NY Futura. 2004 pp 11)

Table 4.15 Venous access for biventricular pacing.

I. Three separate percutaneous sticks – multiple venous entry sites

II. Combination of percutaneous sticks and cut-down with or without retaining the guidewire resulting in multiple venous entry sites

III. Single stick retaining the guidewire – single venous entry site

IV. Cut-down and percutaneous stick retaining the guidewire resulting in a single venous entry site

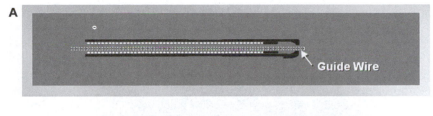

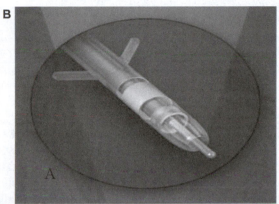

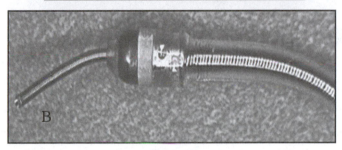

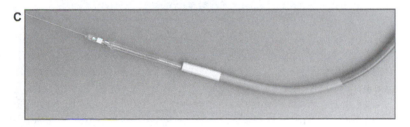

Fig. 4.83 a. Stylized drawing of over the wire lead design. b. Two over the wire lead s A: the EASY trak by Guidant Corporation and B the Attain OTW by Medtronic. c. Lead exiting the guiding sheath over the wire. (from Belott PH: Implantation Techniques for Cardiac resynchronization Therapy Barold SS, Mugica J Fifth Decade of Cardiac Pacing. Armonk NY Futura. 2004 pp 12)

required for three electrodes: The coronary sinus lead and its delivery system, a RV lead and right atrial lead. This can be accomplished by a number of approaches. The standard approach places up to three sheaths percutaneously with three separate percutaneous venous access sites. Accessing the subclavian or axillary vein multiple times carries the increased risk of pneumothorax and venous access failure. A combination of the cut-down and percutaneous approach has also been recommended with a separate cutdown and placement of the dual-chamber system or percutaneous venous access for the coronary sinus lead and delivery system. Two percutaneous punctures have also been employed for RV and atrial electrode insertion, and a second for the coronary sinus lead and delivery system. More recently, a single axillary venous stick has been carried out using the principles of the retained guidewire. (152,53) for successful placement of all three electrodes.

A 4 or 5 French sheath is passed over the guidewire. The dilator is removed and the initial guidewire retained. A second 037 guidewire is passed down the sheath. The sheath is removed. This results in two guidewires exiting the venous puncture. One of the guidewires is secured to the drape for future use. A hemostatic sheath is then passed over the initial guidewire. Through this hemostatic sheath, the coronary sinus lead that is stylet-driven may be passed and positioned in a branch of the coronary sinus, or a delivery system may be employed using the guiding catheter and a coronary sinus lead, stylet-driven, or an over-the-wire approach (Fig. 4.83).

After venous access, some consideration should be given to the sequence of lead placement. Some operators prefer to place the RV electrode first for emergency RV pacing, should heart block ensue because the heart failure patients commonly have a left bundle branch block and any trauma to the conduction system or right bundle may result in complete heart block. Other operators choose to place the coronary sinus lead first and, if necessary, depend on heart rate support via a temporary transvenous pacemaker placed via the femoral vein. The issue of failure speaks for placing the coronary sinus lead first. Should the procedure fail with unsuccessful left-sided left ventricular lead placement and the patient has already received right-sided electrodes, a pacing system may be left without an indication unless a future second attempt is considered. As more and more systems are placed for a primary prevention indication like MADIT II, this has become less problematic (153).

Locating and Cannulating the Coronary Sinus Os

Locating the coronary sinus os can be quite problematic, given the heart failure patient's distorted anatomy. Table 4.16 outlines the techniques devised to cannulate the coronary sinus. If a simple stylet-driven lead coronary sinus placement is undertaken, then coronary sinus access is dependent on the operator's skill, knowledge of the coronary sinus anatomy, and favorable tributaries for safe, reliable placement. Coronary sinus os localization is much easier with a guiding catheter delivery system. The operator simply selects the guiding

Table 4.16 Locating the coronary sinus os.

I.	Puffs of contrast material in the right atrium through guiding catheter
II.	Direct cannulation with guiding catheter
III.	Electrophysiologic catheter through guiding catheter
IV.	0.35 guidewire through guiding catheter
V.	Levophase coronary angiogram
VI.	Femoral vein coronary sinus cannulation

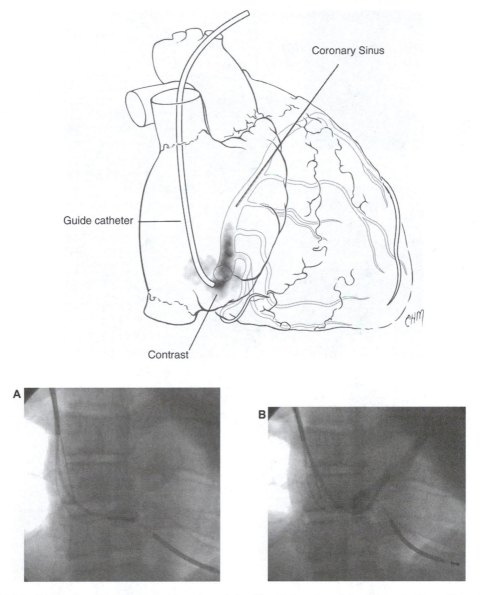

Fig. 4.84 Puff of contrast through the guide catheter helps identify location of the CS os. A. The guide catheter is in the low RA. The contrast defines fossa near CS os. B. the guide catheter is now in the CS. C. Guide catheter in CS. (from Belott PH: Implantation Techniques for Cardiac resynchronization Therapy Barold SS, Mugica J Fifth Decade of Cardiac Pacing. Armonk NY Futura. 2004 pp 14)

catheter that is felt to be ideal for any given patient's anatomy and attaches a hemostatic valve. A flush system is also incorporated for delivery of contrast. As the guide catheter is positioned in the low right atrium, puffs of contrast may be employed to define the anatomy of the vicinity of the eustachian valve and even the location of the coronary sinus os (Fig. 4.84). The most popular technique for coronary sinus os location and cannulation uses an electrophysiologic catheter specifically designed for coronary sinus cannulation (Fig. 4.85 A–E). This catheter may have a preformed or deflectable tip. An alternate approach utilizes a 0.035-in. guidewire passed via the guide catheter in an

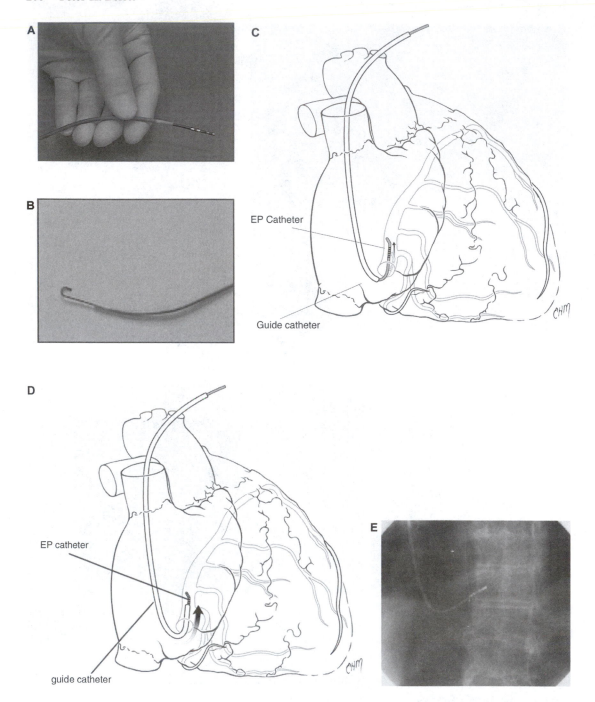

Fig. 4.85 A. Electrophysiology catheter to be passed down guide sheath. B. Alternate method:.037 guide wire down guide catheter. C. EP catheter passed down the guide sheath engaging the CS. D. Guide catheter advanced over the EP catheter into the CS. E. Radiogrph of EP catheter in the CS, through the guide catheter. (from Belott PH: Implantation Techniques for Cardiac resynchronization Therapy Barold SS, Mugica J Fifth Decade of Cardiac Pacing. Armonk NY Futura. 2004 pp 15)

attempt to locate and cannulate the coronary sinus os. The guidewire technique has been very successful and is extremely safe. The use of a deflectable EP catheter offers the ability to adjust catheter shape to the atrium. It can also provide electrical confirmation of successful coronary sinus placement. Since the EP catheter has more consistency than a guidewire, it provides excellent support for the guide catheter. The EP catheter's only disadvantage is the potential risk of a dissection. When the guide catheter is used for coronary sinus os localization, the use of contrast puffs in the right atrium frequently demonstrates retrograde flow from the coronary sinus os, assisting in its localization. Occasionally, the guiding catheter itself will directly pass into the coronary sinus. This directly relates to favorable anatomy and selection of the correct deflecting catheter tip curve. Once the coronary sinus os has been located, the guide catheter may be simply advanced directly into the coronary sinus. More often, the guide catheter is gently passed over the guidewire or deflectable-tip EP catheter, stabilizing its position in the coronary sinus. Once the guiding catheter is positioned some distance in the coronary sinus, the guidewire or the EP catheter are removed. Puffs of contrast through the guide catheter confirm its location within the coronary sinus.

Occasionally spasm as a result of irritation may cause coronary sinus constriction. In this case, coronary sinus cannulation should be attempted with an 035-in. guidewire instead of the deflectable electrophysiology catheter.

The coronary sinus may be guarded or contain valves that may interfere with coronary sinus cannulation. In extreme circumstances, the coronary sinus may be catheterized via the femoral vein. Once the coronary sinus is cannulated with the femoral catheter, this catheter may be used to hold the valve open while the guiding catheter is introduced into the coronary sinus from above.

Finally, as a general rule, if coronary sinus os cannulation proves to be extremely difficult, it is important to consider alternative catheters and methodology within a reasonable period of time. No more than 15 or 20 min. should be wasted on any given approach. In extreme instances, if a left-sided approach proves unsuccessful, one might consider right-sided venous access in coronary sinus cannulation.

Contrast Venography

Contrast venography is performed to visualize the coronary venous system, identifying its vascular anatomy, tributaries, and target branch (154). An effort should be made to limit the use of contrast, particularly in the heart failure patient with advanced renal failure. A venogram is usually obtained by using an occlusive balloon catheter to prevent washout of contrast caused by venous flow into the right atrium. The occlusive venogram provides better quality distal vein branch visualization. Caution should be used when using the occlusive balloon catheter to prevent overinflation and possible vascular dissection. Small puffs of contrast should be used for balloon tip localization. As a general safety precaution, the initial balloon inflation should be approximately half to assess what level of inflation is required for total occlusion. Visualization also ensures that the balloon catheter tip is not

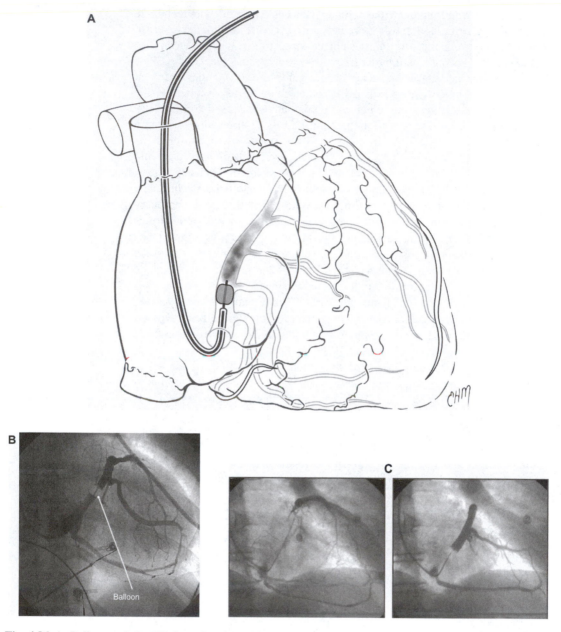

Fig. 4.86 A. Balloon catheter CS through guide catheter. B. Contrast venography using inflated ballon catheter. C. The right panel venogram with the balloon catheter to distal concealing the more desirable proximal postero-lateral branches. In the left panel the ballon catheter has been positioned more proximal revealing the lateral branches. (from Belott PH: Implantation Techniques for Cardiac resynchronization Therapy Barold SS, Mugica J Fifth Decade of Cardiac Pacing. Armonk NY Futura. 2004 pp 16)

against a vessel wall or in a tributary. The balloon catheter should be positioned in the middle of the coronary sinus so as to optimize branch definition. If the balloon catheter is advanced too distally, contrast may be injected beyond the desirable lateral or posterior branches, precluding their visualization (Fig. 4.86 A–C). Once optimal balloon position has been achieved, venograms should be performed in both the right anterior oblique and left

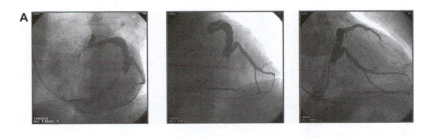

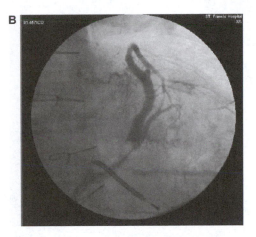

Fig. 4.87 A. Venogram of the CS, From rightto left in the LAO, AP and RAO projections. B. Venogram of the CS demonstrating as previously mentioned the tremendous variability of the CS. In this example there are no true left lateral or posterolateral branches. (from Belott PH: Implantation Techniques for Cardiac resynchronization Therapy Barold SS, Mugica J Fifth Decade of Cardiac Pacing. Armonk NY Futura. 2004 pp 16)

anterior oblique projections (Fig. 4.87 A,B). It is extremely important that the operator is completely familiar with the fluoroscopic coronary venous anatomy as it appears in multiple projections. The AP projection is least helpful in defining the coronary sinus branch anatomy. Occasionally, a minor dissection may occur. This is usually caused by a forceful injection of contrast into the vessel wall. A minor dissection will appear as transient staining. If a persistent large area of staining occurs, this may indicate a larger dissection and the physician may choose to discontinue the procedure. Minor dissections are considered to be benign and of no clinical consequence and the procedure should be continued.

Right-sided Lead Placement

The RV and right atrial leads are placed using standard implant techniques. In addition to offering pacing in the setting of complete AV block, initial right-sided lead placement also provides further assistance in locating the coronary sinus os and precludes potential dislodgement of the coronary sinus lead. On the other hand, initially placed right heart leads are vulnerable to dislodgement during cannulation of the coronary sinus and localization and cannulation of the coronary sinus with guidewire and EP catheters.

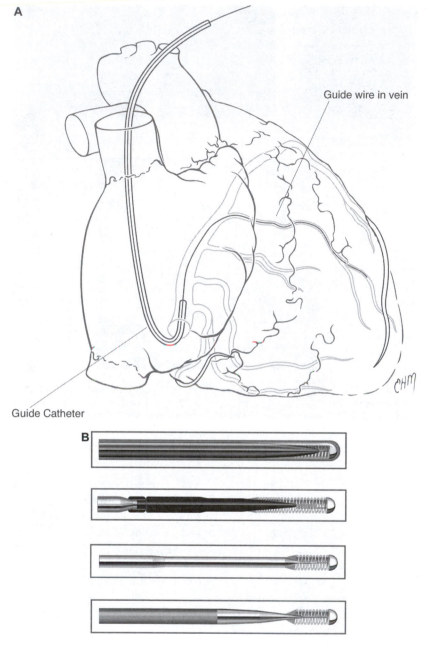

Fig. 4.88 A. Guide wire passed into a posterolateral branch of the CS. B. Example of the various angioplasty guide wires for use in over the wire lead placement. (from Belott PH: Implantation Techniques for Cardiac resynchronization Therapy Barold SS, Mugica J Fifth Decade of Cardiac Pacing. Armonk NY Futura. 2004 pp 18)

Lead Positioning

With the guide catheter safely positioned in the coronary sinus and the target coronary sinus tributary identified, the coronary sinus lead can be placed. If a stylet-driven approach is used, success depends on operator experience, skill, coronary sinus anatomy, lead stylet selection and stylet management. Stylet management relates to the configuration or shape that the distal stylet is formed to and the firmness of the stylet itself. Most manufacturers offer a spectrum of stylet flexibility, but even in the best of circumstances, successful positioning is directly related to any given patient's coronary sinus anatomy. Relating to the correct lead selection and correct stylet selection and curve configuration, precise lead placement is always a symphony of lead and stylet management. If the over-the-wire approach is utilized, appropriate guidewire selection and handling are essential for appropriate coronary sinus and left ventricular lead placement. The operator should become completely familiar with guidewire design and selection, the indications for use, and the benefits of each type of guidewire. This becomes problematic as these skills are currently possessed by the interventional cardiologist and now are essential to the electrophysiologist. The variations in the coronary sinus anatomy make it necessary to utilize guidewires of different designs to navigate the vasculature and reach desirable locations. Today, there is a constellation of guidewires available for the over-the-wire technique (Fig. 4.88 A,B). In essence, they range from extremely flexible to less flexible or rigid. The tips of the guidewires can be curved and shaped to negotiate the turns of the desired tributary of the coronary sinus. These guidewires allow the lead to easily move to the coronary sinus branches. Appropriate guidewire selection offers support for lead delivery and strengthens the force of the lead through the desired branch vein. The curve applied to the tip of the guidewire enables the wire to navigate acute angles and prolapse across coronary sinus venous valves. Both the over-the-wire and guidewire-directed coronary sinus leads are passed through the guiding catheter through a hemostatic valve. In the over-the-wire technique, the lead is advanced over the guidewire and lodged into the desired tributary branch vein of the coronary sinus. When the over-the-wire technique is employed, a torquing device on the guidewire assists in selection and entry into the appropriate branch vein. Occasionally, when advancing the guidewire and/or lead, the guiding catheter can be dislodged from the coronary sinus. It is important to simultaneously observe the movement of the lead, stability of the guidewire, and position of the guiding catheter in the process of positioning a lead. If the guiding catheter is observed to retract, forward pressure and lead advancement should be halted. The guidewire should always be positioned in the most distal possible position in the desired vein branch before advancing the lead over the wire. Just as the use of the stylet and lead in the stylet-driven system is a learned skill, similarly, with the over-the-wire technique, the operator will develop his own technique for appropriate lead advancement, and guidewire management is needed to negotiate the curves in a specific tributary. In both the stylet-driven and over-the-wire techniques, lead position is ultimately dependent on the patient's coronary sinus venous anatomy. Initial placement calls for a posterolateral position. Early acute data suggest that best hemodynamic benefit with posterolateral coronary sinus lead placement, and only if a left lateral position proves unachievable, should placement in an alternate branch be attempted (Fig. 4.89 A–D). Adequate lead position, as verified by electrical performance, should be undertaken with partial withdrawal of the guidewire back into the lead.

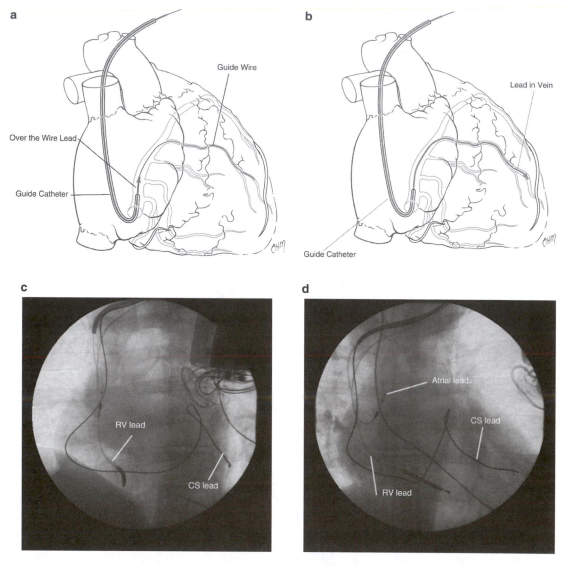

Fig. 4.89 A With the guide catheter supported in the CS os, The LV pacing is advanced over the guide wire. B. Over the wire LV lead placed in the distal aspect of the posterolateral branch of the CS. Radiograph of the CS lead in the RAO (A) and LAO (B) projections. (from Belott PH: Implantation Techniques for Cardiac resynchronization Therapy Barold SS, Mugica J Fifth Decade of Cardiac Pacing. Armonk NY Futura. 2004 pp 19)

Threshold Testing

The initial biventricular systems incorporated dual unipolar pacing. In this configuration, unipolar leads were placed either endocardially or epicardially. Using a Y adapter, one lead was connected to the anode and the other to the cathode. The bipolar Y adapter was then connected to a bipolar device with a single ventricular port. This system has been called "dual unipolar pacing" or split bipolar pacing. These systems have been abandoned because of the high-threshold problems. Dual site cathodal stimulation is now commonly used. This arrangement stimulates LV and RV cathodes simultaneously through an

Ventricular Lead Polarity

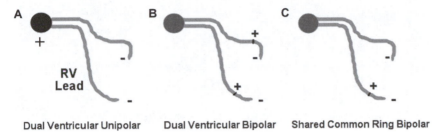

Shared Common Ring Bipolar Sensing/Pacing

Dual Ventricular Unipolar   Dual Ventricular Bipolar   Shared Common Ring Bipolar

Fig. 4.90 Diagramatic representation of the three ventricular lead polarity configurations. A. Dual ventricular unipolar. B. Shared common ring bipolar. C. Dual ventricular bipolar. (from Belott PH: Implantation Techniques for Cardiac resynchronization Theraphy Barold SS, Mugica J Fifth Decade of Cardiac Pacing. Armonk NY Futura. 2004 Page 20)

internal or external Y adapter with a connection between the two cathodes and anodes, respectively. Dual cathodal ventricular stimulation can have several configurations: (1). Two unipolar leads with a Y adapter connected to the negative pole of a unipolar pacemaker and the positive pacemaker. (2). The "shared common-ring bipolar" or "extended bipolar" system, which is presently the most commonly used system. The RV lead is bipolar and the LV lead is unipolar. The LV lead shares the ring or anode of the RV lead. This configuration allows for extended bipolar pacing of the LV lead and limits sensing to the heart, thereby avoiding myopotential oversensing or muscle stimulation seen with configuration #1. (3). The "dual ventricular bipolar" is the most desirable configuration of the future, in which both the RV and LV leads are bipolar and are independently programmable, enabling easy and precise determinations of acute and chronic BiV, RV, and LV threshold and sensing (Fig. 4.90).

Today biventricular systems are dual cathodal systems where the outputs to both chambers and sensing are common and simultaneous. The absence of independent outputs for separate pacing of each ventricle makes determination of the individual RV and LV threshold problematic. There is no problem testing the RV and LV independently using standard threshold testing techniques. Yet, when testing as a biventricular system through the Y adapter configuration, defining biventricular, RV, and LV thresholds can be difficult and frustrating. Occasionally, the RV and LV are nearly identical, and loss of capture can be challenging. Usually, the threshold is determined by reducing the pulse amplitude or pulse duration until there is loss of capture in the chamber with the highest threshold.

Threshold testing is a two-step process. First the LV threshold is determined. If unacceptable or complicated by diaphragmatic stimulation, the lead requires adjustment or repositioning. If the LV threshold is acceptable, the biventricular threshold is then determined. Unless dual bipolar leads are used, threshold testing is carried out in the unipolar configuration. Threshold testing

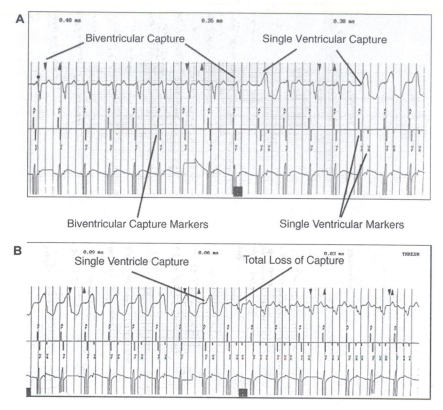

Fig. 4.91 A. Biventricular thres hold testing: the left side of the strip show biventricular capture as the threshold is decreased intermittent capture of either the RV or LV occurs as indicated by a change in morphology. B. With continued decrease in output total loss of ventricular occurs. (from Belott PH: Implantation Techniques for Cardiac resynchronization Therapy Barold SS, Mugica J Fifth Decade of Cardiac Pacing. Armonk NY Futura. 2004 pp 22)

Table 4.17 Acceptable biventricular pacing and sensing thresholds.

  I. Voltage threshold ≤ 3.0 V at 0.5 ms pulse duration
 II. R-wave amplitude ≥ 5.0 mV
III. Pacing impedance 300–1000 ohms

requires identification of loss of capture in one ventricle, then both (Fig. 4.91 A,B). This requires monitoring surface ECG, markers, and the ventricular electrogram. The measured lead impedance is the combination of both ventricles and is less than the individual impedance for pacing. The sensing threshold is a combination of sensing from both ventricles. Testing is performed in the extended-bipole configuration initially and then in the biventricular configuration. One should attempt to achieve a position that results in a threshold less than or equal to 3.0 V and endocardial R-wave signals greater to or equal to 5 mV. Impedance should range between 300 and 1000 ohms (Table 4.17). Should lead thresholds prove unacceptable, or extracardiac and diaphragmatic stimulation occur, lead repositioning will be necessary. An attempt at placement of the electrode in a different tributary of the coronary sinus should be attempted. If electrodes are still unacceptable, or diaphragmatic stimulation persists, alternate branch anatomy or tributary selection will become necessary. Extracardiac stimulation can be extremely problematic. Phrenic nerve or diaphragmatic stimulation has been observed. This is usually associated with the more posterior branches of the coronary sinus. To exclude the possibility of extracardiac stimulation, lead threshold testing should be carried out in the unipolar or extended bipolar configurations at outputs of 10 V or greater. Extracardiac stimulation may be avoided by increasing pulse width and decreasing voltage output. Most situations of extracardiac stimulation require reposition of the coronary sinus electrode into a new tributary or an extreme new coronary sinus branch tributary.

Removing the Guiding Catheter

Once the coronary sinus lead has been successfully positioned, if the right-sided leads have not been placed, the delivery system sheath and guiding catheter should be left in place. If the right-sided leads have yet to be positioned, the guiding catheter and sheath offer stability to prevent dislodgement of the coronary sinus lead. If the right-sided system has been previously positioned, then it is time to remove the delivery system, the lead, stylet, guidewire, guiding sheath and, if utilized, initial entry hemostatic sheath. This is a critical point in the placement of a coronary sinus lead, as removal of guidewires and sheaths can easily dislodge the coronary sinus lead. The guiding catheter and introducer sheaths must be peeled or slid away without dislodging the electrode. This procedure requires lead stabilization within the patient while guiding catheters and sheaths are removed. Guiding catheters can be removed by two techniques. One technique involves sliding the guiding sheath while stabilizing the lead in a simultaneous maneuver. A second technique utilizes careful retraction of the guiding catheter over the coronary sinus lead, stabilizing the lead with a stylet. Both techniques require an acquired skill and require operator experience. Both techniques require extreme patience and care. If an outer peel-away sheath is used, its prior removal requires skill in maintaining lead and guide catheter stability. Once the guiding catheter has been successfully removed and stable lead position has been confirmed, then all supporting guidewires or stylets may finally be removed. The lead is secured, finally tied down by use of the suture sleeve.

Table 4.18 Complications.

I. Air embolization
II. Minor coronary sinus dissection
III. Major coronary sinus dissection
IV. Coronary sinus perforation
V. Cardiac tamponade
VI. Diaphragmatic stimulation
VII. Arrhythmias such as far-field atrial sensing

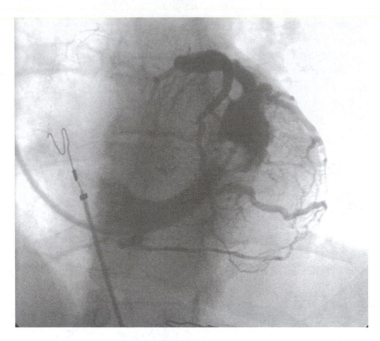

Fig. 4.92 Angiogram demonstrating a dissection of the coronary sinus. (from Belott PH: Implantation Techniques for Cardiac resynchronization Therapy Barold SS, Mugica J Fifth Decade of Cardiac Pacing. Armonk NY Futura. 2004 pp 21)

Complications

Although extremely safe, epicardial left ventricular electrode placement via the coronary sinus is associated with some potential life-threatening complications. The major ones are listed in Table 4.18.

There is potential for aspiration of large quantities of air causing air embolization with conscious sedation. This problem has been obviated by adequate patient preparation and utilization of sheaths incorporating hemostatic valves and guiding catheters equipped with hemostatic mechanisms.

In the process of introducing the guiding catheter, EP catheter, as well as balloon angiography, major dissection may take place in the coronary sinus, either from trauma or over-expansion of the balloon catheter (Fig. 4.92). A major dissection requires termination of the procedure, careful monitoring, and a repeat attempt postponed for several weeks.

Occasionally, the guiding catheter and EP guiding catheter, EP electrode or lead may cause a coronary sinus perforation, which is a true medical emergency. Its presence can be documented with contrast venography. The patient should be evaluated with echocardiography, close hemodynamic monitoring, and management in a critical care unit.

Extracardiac stimulation is not life-threatening but can be extremely problematic. Diaphragmatic stimulation is more common with posterolateral coronary sinus branch placement. At time of implant, this problem should always be sought in the unipolar or extended bipolar configurations, testing at 10 V. If extracardiac stimulation is encountered, the lead should be repo-

Table 4.19 Upgrading techniques for biventricular pacing and ICD systems.

I. Add coronary sinus lead ipsilaterally
II. Add coronary sinus lead contralaterally with tunneling
III. Add coronary sinus lead plus endocardial pacing and shocking electrode ipsilaterally
IV. Add coronary sinus lead ipsilaterally plus contralateral endocardial pacing and shocking electrode placement
V. Add coronary sinus lead, extract chronic ventricular electrode, add endocardial pacing and shocking electrode ipsilaterally
VI. Add coronary sinus lead and endocardial pacing and shocking electrode contralaterally with extraction of chronic lead system ipsilaterally

sitioned in a new tributary or a completely new branch. Occasionally, this problem may be resolved by programming, utilizing increased pulse duration and diminished voltage output.

Upgrading

A patient with a preexisting pacemaker system may require ventricular resynchronization. This can be simply performed by the addition of a coronary sinus lead adapted to a dedicated pacemaker for biventricular pacing. Although there are issues of venous access, this can usually be very easily accomplished. In many cases, the patient with advanced heart failure and a low ejection fraction should be considered for system upgrade to an implantable cardioverter defibrillator. This is particularly true in considering the results of MADIT-II in patients with advanced structural heart disease on an ischemic basis and ejection fractions less than 30%. In this situation, the patient will require the addition of a new ventricular lead that offers both pacing and shocking capabilities as well as the coronary sinus lead. If the patient is to receive two new additional leads, issues with respect to lead extraction of the abandoned ventricular electrode as well as venous access must be addressed. If lead extraction capability is available using conventional tools, such as laser or electrosurgical dissection sheaths, the removal of extemporaneous leads should be strongly considered. Clinical experience has shown that this is not absolutely necessary as the addition of a pacing and shocking electrode and coronary sinus lead to a preexisting dual-chamber system is usually accommodated without complication. In terms of venous access, should one re-access the venous circulation with a single or multiple punctures? Once again, using the principle of the retained guidewire has proven to be extremely successful in this operator's hands. In extreme instances, one can consider using the contralateral subclavian or axillary vein, and tunneling techniques to advance the additional leads back to the original pocket (86). Upgrade approaches are shown in Table 4.19.

Epicardial Approach

Recently, thoracoscopic approaches, less risky than thoracotomy, have been developed for the placement of left ventricular leads (155–157). Still to be resolved are the issues of lead instability and unreliable sensing and pacing characteristics. On the horizon, with respect to an epicardial approach, is a percutaneous technique utilizing robotics for left-sided lead placement.

Conclusions

In conclusion, left ventricular lead implantation for cardiac resynchronization therapy call upon the skills of pacing and cardioverter defibrillator implantation techniques, electrophysiologic techniques for cannulating the coronary sinus os, and the interventional and angioplasty techniques, utilizing angiography of the coronary venous system and angioplastic techniques for over-the-wire left ventricular lead placement. A thorough knowledge of both the gross and radiologic anatomy is essential for the success of any resynchronization procedure. The tools for cardiac resynchronization continue to undergo evolution (158). Even at this writing, they are still quite inadequate for swift left ventricular lead placement. With the development of tools for rapid access of the coronary sinus os and precise sites in the coronary venous system, the procedure will become shorter and safer. In addition, it is quite possible that the development of an improved epicardial approach using modern robotics may prove to be the ultimate reliable way to place left ventricular leads. At present, given the current tools and techniques, the operator reqires extreme patience and persistence when attempting cardiac resynchronization.

Selective Site Pacing

The preceding traditional implantation techniques describe positioning the transvenous leads in the right ventricular apex or right atrial appendage. Historically these techniques have evolved unproven and unscientific, largely driven by available techniques and technology. A clear example is the transition from epicardial to the endocardial approach and right ventricular apex. This is because the right ventricular apex is readily available, reliable, and proven to be stable over time. In addition, it is easily achieved. More recently, the conventional sites for placement of right atrial and ventricular leads have been challenged as inadequate and nonphysiologic (159,160). Right ventricular apical pacing has been demonstrated to cause left ventricular dysfunction. The resultant contraction from right ventricular apical pacing has been shown to produce abnormalities in regional systolic fiber shortening, mechanical work, blood flow, and oxygen consumption (161,162). Right ventricular apical pacing has also been shown to result in an increased incidence of atrial fibrillation (163). This has been underscored by the recent experience of cardiac resynchronization therapy. Atrial pacing has been shown to have a beneficial effect with respect to preventing atrial fibrillation (164–167). It is felt that the prolonged conduction times from high to low atrium that can occur with pacing from the atrial appendage may play an important role in the induction of atrial fibrillation. Recently, low atrial selective and multisite atrial pacing have been shown to reduce the incidence of atrial fibrillation (168–172).

As a result, the conventional approach to cardiac pacing has been challenged. The term "alternative sites" has entered the cardiac pacing literature. In an attempt to optimize cardiac function, right ventricular leads are no longer simply placed in the right ventricular apex but are being positioned along the intraventricular septum and outflow tract (173). The atrial leads are no longer simply placed in the high right atrium or atrial appendage but are now being positioned in one or more sites in the right and sometimes left atrium in an attempt to suppress atrial fibrillation (174). These concepts have resulted in the term "selective site pacing" as the preferred site of cardiac stimulation in any given patient.

Selective site pacing has resulted in new challenges of implantation from venous access to final lead position. A thorough knowledge of cardiac anatomy and, more specifically, radiographic cardiac anatomy is essential. In addition, the tools and techniques for achieving a selective site are evolving. There are also many problems to be solved and questions to be answered if selective site pacing is to become the standard of care. First the scientific community must define the best sites to pace in the heart. At present, the suggested selective sites include the intraatrial septum, right ventricular septum and outflow tract, the HIS bundle and coronary sinus ostium. Precise lead placement requires identification of locations that will result in optimal clinical benefit. The following section reviews the current state of the art of selective site pacing with respect to lead location, implantation techniques and tools. Left ventricular pacing implantation techniques are reviewed and in a separate chapter.

Selective Site Pacing: General Considerations

For the most part, the general considerations are identical to those of permanent pacemaker implantation. There are, however, several important considerations. The recommended location for the procedure is the cardiac catheterization or electrophysiology laboratory. This is because selective site pacing requires high-quality imaging equipment and the ability to easily achieved multiple radiographic projections. In addition, a physiologic recorder capable of obtaining high-quality electrograms for mapping is essential. Once again, the choice of anesthesia is related to operator preference. Most procedures can be conducted under conscious sedation on an outpatient basis.

Venous access for selective site pacing is essentially the same as previously discussed for conventional pacing techniques. The challenges involve the addition of multiple electrodes. This is best achieved by using the retained-guide-wire technique (54). By simply retaining the guide wire, multiple additional pacing leads may be introduced into the central circulation. This becomes important with multiple site atrial pacing and biventricular pacing, where three or more leads are introduced into the venous system. If one anticipates the addition of multiple electrodes after venous access is achieved, a 6 French sheath set can be placed over the guide wire and additional guide wires, corresponding to the number of required leads, can be passed down the sheath and retained. The extra guide wires are then pinned to the drape for future use.

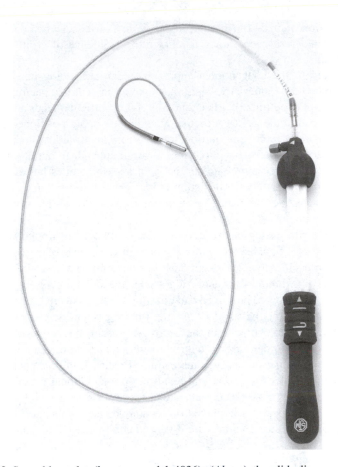

Fig. 4.93 Steerable stylet (locator, model 4036). (*Above*) the slide lies next to the clamp and the tip of the stylet is straight. (*Below*) the slide is moved from the clamp toward the handle resulting in the tip of the stylet being curved. PACE 27: 891, 2004. (from Mond HG, Grenz D: Implantable Transvenous pacing leads: The shape of the things to come. PACE 27: 891, 2004)

If multisite atrial pacing is to be performed, this usually requires lead Y adapters to connect the atrial leads to the pacemaker. An assortment of adapters for any given situation should be kept on hand at all times. Selective site pacing requires the use of active fixation leads, either extendable, retractable, or with a fixed extended helix. Positioning the lead depending on the selected site can be quite challenging. At times, with conventional leads a selected site is almost inaccessible. This is particularly true when trying to position the lead in the atrial septum or for direct His-Bundle pacing. Special J-shaped stylets are often required. Two types of delivery systems are now available for such difficult clinical situations. The first is a steerable stylet (Fig. 4.93). In its current design, the curves achieved by the stylet preclude access to some selective sites. A steerable stylet is connected to a handle with a slide bar. This activates and adjusts the curve. The stylet is actually inside a 0.0016 mm tube that is attached to the slide bar on the handle. The tube is passed down the pacing lead to be inserted. The lead is slipped over the tube and attached to the handle and the desired curve is made with the lead in the heart. The handle is also used to turn the lead around its axis, maneuvering

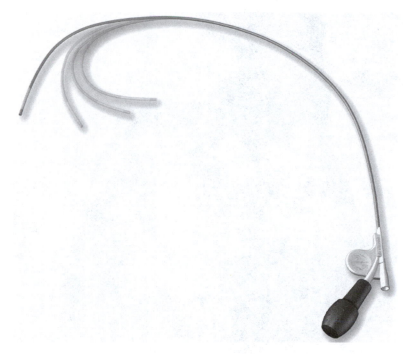

Fig. 4.94 (*Above*) The select site steerable catheter (model 10634, Medtronic Inc.).
PACE 27: 892, 2004. (from Mond HG, Grenz D: Implantable Transvenous pacing
leads: The shape of the things to come. PACE 27: 892, 2004

the curve clockwise or counterclockwise. The stylet can also be manually
curved to achieve desired secondary curves. The secondary curves can help
achieve stability of the lead in the superior vena cava. The stylet curves the
distal 4 cm of the pacing lead. The second system builds on the concept of a
catheter delivery system. Unlike the catheter delivery systems for resynchronization therapy that had fixed curves, a family of steerable catheters (Selectsite,
models 10634–39 and 10635–49, Medtronics, Inc.) had been developed to
guide pacing leads to selective sites (Fig. 4.94) the 4 French active fixation
lead that is passed down the steerable catheter to the desired position for fixation. This lead is a simple cable and has no guiding stylet. The lead is purely
a guide catheter delivered.

Anatomic Considerations

A complete understanding of the gross and radiographic cardiac anatomy
is essential for successful selective site pacing. An appreciation of the right
atrial anatomy is necessary for targeting the low atrial septum, and cannulation of the coronary sinus. An appreciation of the right ventricular spatial
orientation is important for direct His bundle, right ventricular septal, and
outflow tract pacing.

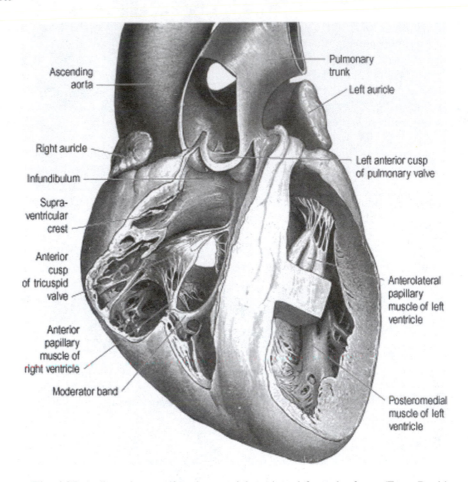

Ascending aorta

Pulmonary trunk

Left auricle

Right auricle

Left anterior cusp of pulmonary valve

Infundibulum

Supra-ventricular crest

Anterior cusp of tricuspid valve

Anterolateral papillary muscle of left ventricle

Anterior papillary muscle of right ventricle

Moderator band

Posteromedial muscle of left ventricle

Fig. 4.95 A dissection opening the ventricles, viewed from the front. (From David Johnson: Heart and great vessels. Standring S. Gray's anatomy the anatomical basis of clinical practice. Elsevier 2005p 1002.) From David Johnson: Heart and Great Vessels. In Standring S: Grays Anatomy: The Anatomical Basis of Clinical Practice. Philadelphia, Elsevier, 2005 page 1002.

Right Atrium

The anatomy of the right atrium has been previously described above under resynchronization therapy. (141–1413).

Right Ventricle

As previously stated, a right ventricle is anterior mediastinal structure, extending from the right atrial ventricular orifice to the cardiac apex (Fig. 4.95). It ascends leftward to become the infundibulum or conus arteriosus, reaching the pulmonic valve. The right ventricle consists of an inlet component supporting the tricuspid valve, and apical component that is a coarsely trabeculated and muscular infundibulum or outlet that attaches to the pulmonic valve. The anterior surface of the right ventricle is convex and comprises the majority of the heart under the anterior thoracic wall. Its inferior aspect is flat, resting on the diaphragm. A right ventricular left and posterior wall comprise the ventricular septum. The structure is slightly curved and bulges into the ventricular chamber. The right ventricular inlet and outlet components that support the tricuspid and pulmonic valves are separated and covered by the roof of the right ventricle. These are separated in the roof of the right ventricle by a prominent supraventricular crest called the crista supraventricularis. This is a thick muscular structure that extends obliquely forward and to the right from a septal extension on the interventricular septal wall to a mural or parietal extension on the anterolateral right ventricular wall. The inlet and outlet regions extend apically into the ventricle. The inlet component is trabeculated, whereas the outlet is predominantly smooth walled. It is the myriad of irregular muscular ridges and protrusions that are responsible for the trabeculated appearance. The protrusions and grooves result in great variation in wall thickness. The papillary muscles are prominent protrusions from the ventricular wall. The septal marginal trabecula or septal band is a prominent protrusion in the right ventricular chamber. It supports the septal surface at its base and divides into limbs embracing the supraventricular crest. The apex of the septal band supports the anterior papillary muscle. At this point it crosses to the parietal wall of the ventricle and is called the moderator band. The infundibulum or outflow tract is smooth walled and extends leftward below the arch of the supraventricular crest to the pulmonary orifice.

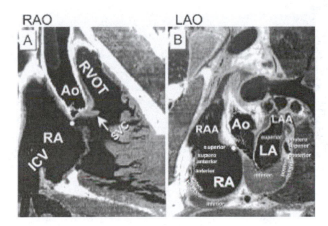

Fig. 4.96 Right anterior oblique (RAO) (panel A) and left anterior oblique (LAO) (panel B) sections of the male heart obtained from the EPFL's visible human surface server, EPFL 1998. Panel A shows the inferior caval vein (ICV), the inferior isthmus (CTI), the supraventricular crest (SVC), the aorta (Ao), and right ventricular outflow tract (RVOT). The white dot signals the site corresponding to the membranous septum or the maximal His-Bundle potential is usually recorded. In the LAO projection, the right atrial appendage (RAA) and the right and left atria at the level of the atrial ventricular junction's are depicted. The white dot also signals the area were the his bundle is recorded. The left atrial appendage (LAA) is superior. (from Farre J, Anderson RH, Cabrera JA, et al: Fluorscopic cardiac anatomy for catheter ablation of tachycardia. PACE 25: 88, 2002)

Radiographic Anatomy

In addition to understanding the gross anatomy of the right atrium, coronary sinus and right ventricle, a thorough knowledge of the radiologic and angiographic anatomy is crucial to success in selective site pacing and resynchronization therapy. Previously there were very few papers devoted to the angiographic anatomy of the right heart. With the recent popularity of resynchronization therapy, the coronary sinus angiographic anatomy has been extensively described. Recently, Farre has elegantly described the gross and fluoroscopic cardiac anatomy for interventional electrophysiology. He recommends use of the visible human slice and surface server developed by Hersch for understanding and correlating the cardiac anatomy to the fluoroscopic projections (175). It is important to understand the fluoroscopic anatomy in the frontal and oblique projections when implanting leads. The frontal view is generally used for introduction and positioning of leads in the right ventricular apex and high right atrium. When undertaking selective site pacing, it is difficult to locate with certainty the position of the lead using a single fluoroscopic projection. This is where oblique views are very important and help position the pacemaker lead within the three dimensions of the heart. The RAO and LAO projections define what is anterior, posterior, inferior, and superior in cardiac planes that are parallel to the input of the image intensifier (Fig. 4.96). In the frontal plane, the right ventricle occupies most of the cardiac silhouette as an anterior structure. The upper half of the right heart border is formed by the superior vena cava, while the lower portion is formed by the lateral wall of the right atrium. The plane of the lateral valve is sandwiched between the anterior right ventricle and posterior left ventricle. It can be conceptualized as an oval, ring tipped somewhat to the left. The coronary sinus is located at the inferior aspect of the cardiac silhouette at the level of the diaphragms, approximately in the midline. The RAO projection rolls the right ventricle to the left. In this view, the superior and inferior vena cave and right atrium become an anterior structure. The plane of the tricuspid and mitral valves becomes more vertical and perpendicular to the anteroposterior plane (Fig. 4.74). The right ventricle is pushed to the left. In the left anterior oblique projection, the plane of the tricuspid and mitral valves becomes frontal, with the coronary sinus tipped in a horizontal position crossing over the spine as it courses to the left, crossing over the spine from right to left and turning superiorly along the left heart border (Fig. 4.75). When placing a pacemaker lead in the right atrial appendage, the frontal projection is preferred. The tip of the right atrial appendage is superior and anterior. When the lead tip is placed in the apex of the atrial appendage, it moves back and forth from right to left. In the right anterior oblique projection, the tip points to the right, and in the left anterior oblique projection, it points to the left. The triangle of Koch is in the inferior paraseptal right atrial region. This region is important for right atrial septal and His bundle selective site pacing. In the RAO projection, the plane of Koch's triangle is parallel to the image intensifier. The LAO projection helps differentiate paraseptal lead positions from inferior to superior. The region of the His bundle is located superiorly and the coronary sinus os inferiorly. In the right and left anterior oblique projections, the os of the coronary sinus can be found at the inferior aspect of the cardiac silhouette at the level of the diaphragms just to the right of the spine. Rotating from the right anterior oblique to the left

Fig. 4.97 Axial section of the heart obtained from the visible human surface server. Right superior pulmonary vein (RSPV), left superior pulmonary vein (LSPV) and left atrial appendage (LAA). PACE 25: 88, 2002. (from Farre J, Anderson RH, Cabrera JA, et al: Fluorscopic cardiac anatomy for catheter ablation of tachycardia. PACE 25: 88, 2002)

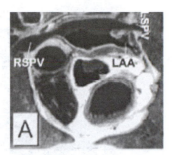

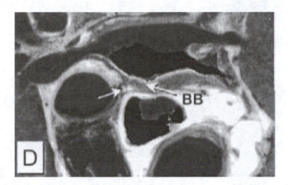

Fig. 4.98 Axial section of the heart and magnification of figure 106 depicting the area of Bachman's bundle (BB). PACE 25: 88, 2002. (from Farre J, Anderson RH, Cabrera JA, et al: Fluorscopic cardiac anatomy for catheter ablation of tachycardia. PACE 25: 88, 2002)

anterior oblique projection and back becomes important in trying to cannulate the coronary sinus os. As a simple example, when in the frontal projection, the catheter may appear to be in the vicinity of the coronary sinus os with the trajectory pointing inferiorly and to the left, but when the image is rotated to the left anterior oblique projection, the catheter is actually 180° away from the coronary sinus os pointing anteriorly and to the right. After adjusting the catheter to a posterior and leftward position, the right anterior oblique projection may show the catheter pointing laterally to the right, away from the coronary sinus os. This simple example points to the importance of multiple views in trying to achieve a selected site. With respect to the coronary sinus the left anterior oblique projection is extremely important in distinguishing anterior and posterior tributaries of the coronary sinus (Fig. 4.76). In the frontal and right anterior oblique projections, tributaries of the coronary sinus appear to run perpendicular to the coronary sinus obliquely from a superior to an inferior direction (Fig. 4.77). The branches appear to be parallel, making differentiation of anteroseptal, lateral, and posterolateral branches almost impossible.

Atrial Septal Pacing

Atrial fibrillation is the most common sustained tachycardia arrhythmia in clinical practice. It is associated with considerable morbidity and mortality. It is felt that atrial pacing might help prevent the onset of atrial fibrillation by a variety of mechanisms. Atrial pacing should prevent relative brady-

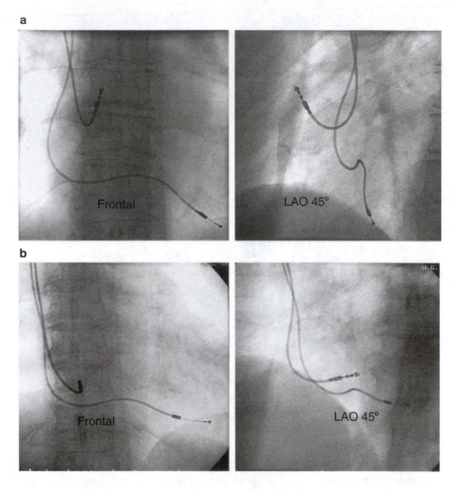

Fig. 4.99 A. Fluoroscopic image is of the position of the right atrial appendage (RAA) lead. The frontal view in the left panel and a left anterior oblique, 45° angulation in the right panel where the RAA lead is directed superior and anterior. B. Fluoroscopic images of the position of the low atrial septum(LAS) lead. The frontal view in the left panel and a left anterior oblique 45° angulation in the right panel, where the LAS lead is directed at 90° angles at the inter-atrial septum. EUROPACE 7: 62, 2005. (from de Voogt WG, van Mechelen R van den Bos AA, et al: Electrical characteristics of low atrial pacing compared with right atrial appendage pacing. Europace 7: 62, 2005

cardia that is oftentimes a trigger for atrial fibrillation. In addition, atrial pacing should suppress bradycardia-induced dispersion of refractoriness in the atrium as well as escape atrial ectopy that are potential causes of atrial fibrillation.

Bachman in 1916 described a distinct band of muscle tissue extending from the base of the left atrial appendage, called the anterior interatrial band (176). Bachman's bundle was later defined as a band of fibers traversing the left atrium, curving posteriorly within the intraatrial septum, reaching the crest of the AV node (177). Right atrial activation mapping, when pacing from the left atrium and coronary sinus, has demonstrated preferential sites of the transseptal conduction (Figs. 4.97 and 4.98). The earliest right atrial activation has been found to be near the insertion of Bachman's bundle (178–181). Electroanatomical mapping has confirmed the role of Bachman's bundle in intraatrial propagation and, as such, Bachmann's bundle may be an ideal selective site for prevention of atrial fibrillation.

The right atrial selective sites include the high right atrial septum and the low right atrial septum in the vicinity of the coronary sinus os. The area of the high right atrial septum involves the crista terminalis, and Bachman's bundle is particularly difficult to pace with conventional tools. The selective site low right atrial septum is the mouth or os of the coronary sinus. The usual target for lead attachment is just superior to the coronary sinus os. Atrial septal pacing from this position will result in negative P-waves in leads II III and aVF.

Atrial septal pacing is achieved by placing a permanent pacing lead in the posterior right atrial septal wall. To achieve a selective site, an active fixation lead is mandatory. The triangle of Koch is situated in the lower aspect of the interatrial septum. It is confined by the borders of the tricuspid valve annulus and the eustachian ridge superiorly. The base of the triangle, as mentioned previously, is formed by the coronary sinus. The posterior aspect of the triangle is the muscular part of the interatrial septum. The 45° left anterior oblique fluoroscopic projection is used to guide the pacing lead at a right angle into the intraatrial septum. The interatrial septum is oriented at about 45° from the right posterior to the left anterior. The 45° left anterior oblique projection will help confirm lead fixation to the triangle of Koch (Fig. 4.99). Selective site atrial septal lead placement in the frontal or right anterior oblique projection is next to impossible. These views can only be used for secondary confirmation of appropriate lead position. In the frontal plane, the lead will appear in the neutral position, or somewhat directed to the left depending on the contraction phase of the atrium. Unlike the fluoroscopic movement of the lead tip in the right atrial appendage, that is to and fro, the right atrial septal lead tip moves up and down. If the ventricular lead has been implanted prior to the atrial lead, its undulation over the tricuspid valve marks the position of the structure. The ventricular lead marks the inferior part of the tricuspid ostium. The coronary sinus ostium has also been used to locate the interatrial septum with active fixation leads placed just superior to the coronary sinus os. This site is recommended when approaching patients for dual site right atrial pacing (182). The second lead is usually placed in the atrial appendage. Achieving the desired location is directly related to stylet management and skill of the operator.

Local electrogram and stimulation analysis is important for the recognition of far-field R-wave detection. This is important because far-field R-wave detection can cause inappropriate mode switching. It is therefore important to measure the height of any far-field R-wave recorded on the atrial channel. During an implant, far-field R-wave analysis in sinus rhythm and normal AV conduction can be masked by the current of injury caused by the active fixation of the atrial septal lead. Far field R-wave signals become superimposed on the current of injury. To avoid this problem, far field R-waves can be measured during VVI pacing where the far-field R-wave can be seen to precede the atrial complex when VA conduction is present or can be seen between beats during VA dissociation. Far-field R-wave voltages should be less than the P-wave voltage. If high far-field R-wave voltages are found, lead repositioning should be considered. In addition, high far-field R-waves may also mean that the screw-in mechanism of the atrial lead is protruding into the ventricular myocardium. This can be evaluated with high output pacing from the atrium that results in simultaneous atrial and ventricular stimulation.

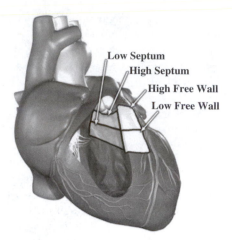

Fig. 4.100 Anteroposterior view of the right ventricle. The right ventricular outflow tract has been divided into four segments; two on the septum and two on the free wall. PACE 27: 884, 2004 part II. (from Lieberman R, Grenz D, Mond HG et al: Selective site pacing: defining and reaching the selected site. PACE 27: 884, 2004)

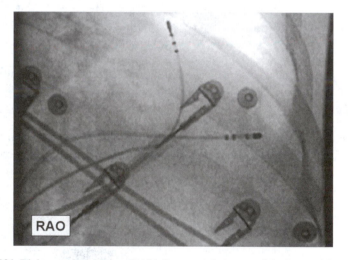

Fig. 4.101 Right anterior oblique (RAO) fluoroscopic image of the heart with two catheters in the right ventricle to define the upper and lower limits of the right ventricular outflow tract. PACE 27: 885, 2004. (from Lieberman R, Grenz D, Mond HG et al: Selective site pacing: defining and reaching the selected site. PACE 27: 884, 2004)

To do a malpositioned atrial septal lead can be deleterious, possibly causing pacemaker syndrome or, if high-rate atrial tachyarrhythmia therapy pacing is used, may result in inappropriate, dangerously high ventricular rates.

Right Ventricular Selective Site Pacing

The search for an alternative right ventricular pacing sites has gone on for many years. The results of a recent quantitative review suggest the right ventricular outflow tract is the ideal site (183). Yet the variability of anatomic, electrocardiographic, and functional criteria used to describe specific locations

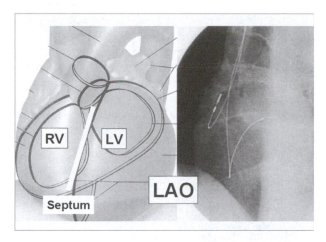

Fig. 4.102 Left anterior oblique (LAO) views of the heart. (*Left*) anatomic diagram to show the position of the right ventricle and septum. (*Right*) fluoroscopic image to show the pacing lead in the low septum. (from Lieberman R, Grenz D, Mond HG et al: Selective site pacing: defining and reaching the selected site. PACE 27: 884, 2004)

of the right ventricular pacing lead in many studies is huge and conflicting (184). The heterogenicity of selective site right ventricular pacing studies does not allow the definition of a single beneficial site. It may be that the single hemodynamically best site in any given patient must be searched for individually. Some studies have suggested that the width of the paced QRS complex could indicate the most favorable site. This concept has been questioned.

At present the selected site for right ventricular pacing is in the right ventricular outflow tract. In a recent review, Lieberman, et al., defined the right ventricular outflow tract as a broad area of the right ventricle that is poorly defined and encompasses all areas except the apex (185). In the frontal projection the lower border of the right ventricular outflow tract is a line extending from the apex of the tricuspid valve to the border of the right ventricle (Fig. 4.100). The right ventricular outflow tract's superior limit is the pulmonic valve. Fluoroscopic images and associated ECG patterns are used to define the right ventricular outflow tract. The lower border can be defined by extending an electrophysiologic catheter parallel to the right ventricular inferior border from the tricuspid valve apex to the lateral right ventricular border in the frontal or right anterior oblique projection (Fig. 4.101). The superior border of the right ventricular outflow tract is determined by positioning the catheter across the pulmonic valve. By monitoring electrograms, the right-ventricular-outflow-tract-pulmonic-valve junction can be identified. Once the right ventricular outflow tract boundaries have been defined, the selective site needs to be identified. This is done by dividing the RVOT into four quadrants. The RVOT is divided horizontally by a line midway between the pulmonic valve and the lower border, defining an upper and lower half. These halves are divided vertically by a line that connects the pulmonic valve to the RVOT lower border, thus dividing the RVOT into a septal and free wall. Thus the RVOT can be divided into four quadrants, high infundibular and low (outflow) septal RVOT, and high infundibular and low (outflow) free wall RVOT. The right anterior oblique fluoroscopic projection is used in determining high and low positions.

The 40° left anterior oblique projection is used to differentiate right ventricular outflow tract, septal, and free wall positions (Fig. 4.102).

The ECG is used to confirm pacing from the right ventricular septum. In this position the QRS in lead I is negative. When he right ventricular free wall is paced, the QRS in lead I is positive. Lead aVF may be used to differentiate high and low positions. Ventricular pacing in the high position will result in an upright QRS in lead aVF. Lower positions will result in a less positive QRS.

Direct His-Bundle Pacing

The normal His-Purkinje activation of the myocardium results in a rapid sequential depolarization of myocardial cells and efficient ventricular contraction. Because of this, it is felt that the His bundle would be an ideal target for selective site pacing. This site should prevent ventricular dyssynchrony and maintain normal ventricular activation sequence. There is very little human clinical experience with direct His-bundle pacing. In 1992, Karpawich et al. (186), described a permanent approach to His-Bundle pacing in open chests of canines. They used a specifically designed screw-in lead passed through a mapping introducer. The introducer was delivered through a right atriotomy. When using an entirely transvenous approach, considerable difficulty was encountered directing the lead tip into the desired target. In 2004, Deshmukh et al. reported attempted direct His-bundle pacing in 54 patient's (187). All patient's had a narrow QRS complex, < 120 ms, persistent atrial fibrillation requiring AV node ablation and a dilated cardiomyopathy. A hexapolar catheter introduced via the femoral vein was used to map and localize the His bundle. The right anterior oblique projection was used. Once localized the His bundle was paced. Criteria of His-bundle capture included (1) His-Purkinje mediated cardiac activation and repolarization, as evidenced by electrocardiographic concordance of the QRS and T-wave complexes; (2) the paced ventricular interval identical to that as ventricular interval; and (3) His-bundle capture in an all-or-none fashion. This means the QRS did not widen at a lower pacing output. This was critical in differentiating para-Hisian pacing or indirect capture of the His bundle from direct His-bundle pacing. Once the His bundle was localized, an active fixation pacing lead was advanced into the septum. Conventional lead placement was difficult and required a specially modified, J-shaped stylet with a secondary distal curve orthogonal to the J plane, which allowed the lead to be positioned medially toward the AV septum. An attempt was made to position the lead near the mapping catheter. Once in position, an electrophysiologic study was carried out measuring His ventricular and paced ventricular intervals. Occasionally, because of rapid ventricular rates, radio frequency ablation was performed. Deshmukh reported successful direct His-bundle pacing in 39 patients. It is clear from this experience that direct His-bundle pacing is feasible. Electrophysiologic mapping is critical to the procedure. Precise placement of a permanent pacing lead is extremely difficult, requiring special stylets for lead manipulation; and, in the future, some form of catheter delivery system will need to be developed for this selective site.

Selective Site Pacing: The Future

It is clear that selective site pacing in the atria and ventricles is evolving. There are many papers supporting this approach in either chamber. Unfortunately, most of these studies have been small and reflect conflicting and confusing data. The long-term harmful effects of right ventricular apical pacing have been well catalogued and accepted. Unfortunately there is a paucity of long-term data from carefully designed long-term studies. It is clear that patients with compromised LV function are at the greatest risk from RVA pacing. But the incidence of harm caused by RVA pacing in patients with normal LV function is unknown. There are no large, carefully designed studies. The large landmark studies, such as DAVID, most instruct us to minimize RVA pacing and use atrial-based modes that promote AV conduction.

But what about the patient that requires ventricular pacing? The results from alternative sites have been disappointing. There is no sound basis to do so from any other site than the RV apex. There are problems defining the ideal alternate selective site as well as accurate, reliable, and stable lead placement. The RVOT is a poorly defined, broad area that needs definition of boundaries, both fluoroscopically and electrocardiographically. The scientific community must define the best site to pace the heart, identify the location that provides optimal hemodynamic benefit, and create the tools to meet the challenge. There are also issues of training necessary for the implanting physician to let go of the old and embrace new techniques. If selective site pacing proves to be better, there is a need to develop safe, user-friendly, and cost effective tools that require a minimum of advanced training.

With the above considerations, there is need for long-term, randomized studies that include a well-defined patient population and multiple well-defined pacing sites that evaluate functional hemodynamics, lead stability, extractability, and complication data. Until such time, the right atrial appendage and right ventricular apex, with proven reliability, stability, and simplicity, should not be abandoned.

Complications

Fortunately with today's modern pacemaker systems, the complications from pacing very rarely lead to a patient's demise. With the advent of the transvenous approach to cardiac pacing, many of the major complications associated with general anesthesia and thoracotomy have been eliminated. Complications can be divided into acute, those complications occurring during the intraoperative and immediate postoperative periods; and chronic, those occurring much later (17). The complications associated with the transvenous approach occur rarely but can be grouped into those associated with venous access and those related to the placement of a lead. The implanting physician's skill and experience level are extremely important in reducing the incidence of complications. The experienced operator is fully aware of all the potential risks as well as the appropriate management of complications. The importance of physician skill level has been pointed out by Parsonnet and associates (188). In analyzing pacemaker implantation complication rates with respect to contributing factors, Parsonnet reviewed 632 consecutive implants over a 5-year

Table 4.20 Percutaneous complications.

Pneumothorax	Nerve injury
Hemothorax	Thoracic duct injury
Hemopneumothorax	Cheilothorax
Laceration, subclavian artery	Lymphatic fistula
Arteriovenous fistula	

period performed by 29 different implanting physicians at a single institution. There were 37 perioperative complications. The complications were analyzed together with the experience of the implanting physician. Percutaneous venous access was associated with the highest complication rate and contributed significantly to a 5.7% overall complication rate. If complications related to percutaneous approach were excluded, the complication rate dropped to more than 3.5%. The highest complication rate was among the physicians implanting fewer than 12 pacemakers per year with the least pacing experience. The following section reviews pacemaker complications with respect to venous access and entry, lead placement, and the pulse generator pocket.

Venous Access

Complications of venous access are largely associated with the Seldinger percutaneous sheath-set technique (189–191). Such access has been associated with pneumothorax, hemopneumothorax, as well as air embolization and perforation of the innominate vein. In addition, the percutaneous needle can inadvertently damage or puncture the lung, subclavian artery, thoracic duct, and nerves. A pneumothorax may be asymptomatic and discovered on routine postoperative chest radiograph. In almost every instance, an alert operator can suspect the presence of a pneumothorax when air is withdrawn into the probing percutaneous needle and syringe. The presence of pneumothorax may also be suspected by the patient's complaint of pleuritic pain, dyspnea, and a cough. In rare circumstances, the patient may develop a tension pneumothorax. This can result in profound respiratory distress, hypoxemia, and cardiovascular collapse. Tension pneumothorax may be potentiated by the use of general anesthesia and its positive-pressure ventilation. The management of pneumothorax depends on the severity and symptoms. In the case of a tension pneumothorax, emergent chest tube insertion is mandatory. Whether a small asymptomatic pneumothorax should be managed with a chest tube or Heimlich valve is a matter of debate. As a rule, a pneumothorax greater than 10% should be managed with a chest tube.

Hemopneumothorax or hemothorax is extremely rare. It is usually secondary to subclavian artery puncture and dissection. This occasionally occurs when the artery is punctured and a sheath is applied to this vascular structure. Most hemopneumothoraces and hemothoraces require drainage. In rare instances, a chronic hemothorax will require a decortication procedure.

There is an ongoing debate with respect to the safety and efficacy of blind subclavian puncture. Furman has demonstrated remarkable efficiency of the cutdown approach for dual-chambered pacing, particularly with unipolar leads. The cutdown technique was less successful for bipolar leads via a single

Table 4.21 Prevention of air embolism during permanent pacemaker procedures.

Awareness of the potential problem
Well-hydrated patient, avoiding long periods of NPO
Awareness of when patient is at greatest risk – open sheath in vein
Assess hydration: take a peak
High-risk patient
Increased hydration/wide-open Ivs
An awake, cooperative patient
Elevate lower extremities/wedge
Trendelenburg position (if available)
Expeditious lead placement and sheath removal
Check for introduction of air
Continuous monitoring (vital signs, oxygen saturation, blood pressure)
In an extremely high-risk, uncooperative patient, intubation and temporary loss of consciousness may be required

cephalic vein. Furman recorded no vascular or pleural complications in a series of 3500 cases using the cutdown approach for single- and dual-chambered pacing implants. Furman has emphasized that the complication rate of a blind subclavian puncture technique has probably been underestimated. A list of common complications associated with the percutaneous approach is shown in Table 4.20.

Air embolism is a complication associated with the use of the Seldinger technique with a percutaneous sheath set. Air embolism is a well-known, well-documented complication of the percutaneous approach. To avoid this problem, it has been recommended that the patient be well hydrated and placed in the Trendelenburg position. The most important step in prevention is awareness on the part of the implanting physician for the risk of air embolization. There are many steps that may be taken to avoid this complication (Table 4.21) (192). The time of greatest risk is when the dilator is removed from the sheath set. In patients with a volume-overload state, there is little or no risk. On the other hand, an elderly dehydrated patient who has been NPO for many hours is at risk for serious air embolization. It is recommended that prior to any percutaneous pacemaker or ICD procedure, the patient be maintained in a mild state of overhydration. The patient's state of hydration should be assessed just prior to removal of the dilator.

By careful withdrawal of the dilator from the sheath, one can assess the patient's state of hydration and venous pressure with the cycles of respiration. In a patient who is well hydrated or with a high venous pressure, there is a continuous flash of blood from the sheath despite the cycles of respiration. On the other hand, a dehydrated patient manifests with no blood meniscus or flash of blood and, with each inspiration, retraction of the meniscus. If the blood meniscus is observed to move inward, the dilator is rapidly readvanced back into the sheath to avoid air embolism during this assessment. If the patient

Table 4.22 Complications of pacemaker insertion.

Subclavian vein puncture leading to pneumothorax	1.0%
Subclavian artery puncture	3.0%
Wound/pocket hematoma	5.0%
Hematoma requiring reoperation	0.1–0.5%
Failure of wound healing	0.1%
Infection	1.0%

From Sutton R, Bourgeois I. The foundations of cardiac pacing: an illustrated practical guide to basic pacing. Bakken Research Center Series, vol 1, part 1. Armonk, NY: Futura Publishing, 1991, with permission.

Table 4.23 Complications of the pacing lead.

Perforation of right ventricle	0.1%
Ventricular lead displacement	0.5–2.0%
Atrial lead displacement	1.5–5.0%
Ventricular exit block (>5 years)	>1.0%
Conductor fracture (>10 years)	0.1%
Insulation fracture (>10 years)	0–0.15%
Undersensing (ventricular)	Rare
Undersensing (atrial)	1–10%
Oversensing (unipolar)	20–80%
Oversensing (bipolar)	0%
Diaphragmatic pacing	1%

From Sutton R, Bourgeois I. The foundations of cardiac pacing: an illustrated practical guide to basic pacing. Bakken Research Center Series, vol 1, part 1. Armonk, NY: Futura Publishing, 1991, with permission.

is deemed to be at high risk for air embolism, several precautions should be instituted. First, the lower extremities can be elevated to increase venous return. This is carried out by the insertion of a wedge. Second, if the patient is sleeping or oversedated, it is important to arouse the patient and achieve total patient cooperation with respect to the cycles of respiration. Third, in addition, increased hydration can be initiated by increasing administration of intravenous fluids. Measures such as pinching the sheath with the lead have proven to be completely ineffective. Expeditious lead insertion is extremely important. The lead should be inserted rapidly and the sheath totally removed. The practice of slowly peeling the sheath away in situ should be totally avoided. The pacemaker electrode should never be positioned with the sheath set left in place.

More recently, a peel-away sheath with a hemostatic valve has been developed that completely avoids the problem of air embolization.

A review of the incidence of complications associated with venous access suggests a 1% incidence of pneumothorax. Arterial puncture, somewhat more common, occurs at a rate of 3%. A list of pacemaker complications associated with insertion proposed by Sutton and Bourgeois is found in Table 4.22 (17).

Complications Associated with the Pacing Lead and Its Placement

The introduction and manipulation of pacing leads are frequently associated with both tachyarrhythmias and bradyarrhythmias as a lead negotiates the chambers of the right heart. Ventricular tachycardia is extremely common as the pacing electrode or guidewire contacts the right ventricular myocardium. Simple withdrawal of these objects usually terminates the arrhythmia. In extreme cases, sustained monomorphic ventricular tachycardia and even ventricular fibrillation may occur. Some institutions have instituted a policy of placing external defibrillation pads prophylactically in anticipation of required cardioversion.

Perforation

The pacing lead, during the process of placement, may perforate the right ventricular free wall. The incidence of this complication is relatively low, occurring at a rate of approximately 0.1%. It is suspected that right ventricular perforation may be somewhat more common than reported, as many patients remain clinically asymptomatic. This is because most perforations are self-sealing when the lead is withdrawn. Should a life-threatening tamponade occur, the implanting physician should be prepared to perform an emergency pericardiocentesis tray readily available should such a drainage procedure be required. Nonclinical perforations may be suspected by the presence of a friction rub and documented by two-dimensional echocardiography.

Sutton and Bourgeois have compiled a list of complications associated with the pacing lead as well as their incidence (Table 4.23) (17). Lead dislodgment, once the commonest lead complication, has declined to between 0.5% to 2% for the ventricular electrode and 1.5% to 5% for the atrial lead. This is largely owing to the genesis of fixation devices. Lead dislodgment is generally managed by reoperation and the lead repositioned. In rare instances, an electrode will require replacement, exchanging a passive fixation for an active fixation device.

Occasionally, the ventricular lead can be inadvertently placed in the left ventricle. This usually occurs if a lead is passed from the right atrium through a patent foramen ovale into the left atrium and then advanced into the left ventricle across the mitral valve. The radiographic appearance can be extremely deceptive in the anteroposterior projection. A lateral radiographic projection is extremely telling. The electrocardiogram is also characteristic with a right bundle-branch QRS pattern during ventricular pacing. Acute left ventricular lead placement requires repositioning within the first 24h to avoid the potential complication of thromboembolic phenomenon. Chronic left ventricular lead placement usually requires longterm anticoagulant therapy because lead reposition is inadvisable and extremely hazardous.

Occasionally, the permanent pacing lead may be damaged in the process of implantation. This may occur acutely or on a chronic basis from crush wear. Depending on the lead, atrial or ventricular, this may present with sensing

Table 4.24 Complications of the vein used for pacing.

Axillary vein thrombosis	0.5%–1.0%
Partial great vein obstruction	Up to 100%
Pulmonary embolism	Very rare

From Sutton R, Bourgeois I. The foundations of cardiac pacing: an illustrated practical guide to basic pacing. Bakken Research Center Series, vol 1, part 1. Armonk, NY: Futura Publishing, 1991, with permission.

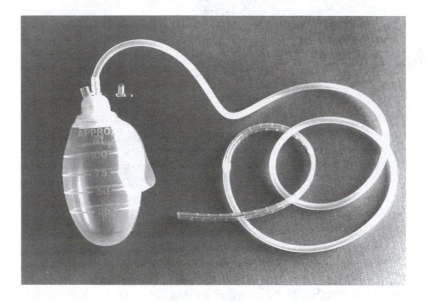

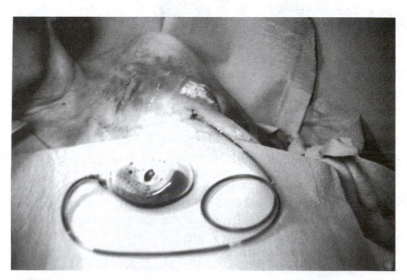

Fig. 4.103 A: Jackson–Pratt drain closed dural drainage system. B: Postoperative evacuation of wound hematoma using the Jackson–Pratt continuous drainage system.

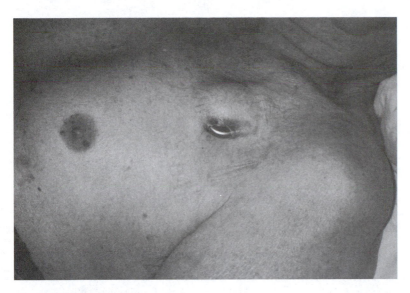

Fig. 4.104 Pacemaker pocket erosion.

problems, inappropriate sensing and capture, and even premature battery depletion.

Intravascular Complications

Complications of the vein used for pacing usually involve thrombosis. Clinical pulmonary embolism is rare. Although some degree of thrombosis along the vein–lead route is common, symptomatic thrombosis is rare. Axillary venous thrombosis may result in an edematous upper extremity. This usually occurs several weeks after implant. With the development of collaterals, most axillary vein thromboses resolve spontaneously. Some centers have used thrombolytic and heparin therapy with modest success. As mentioned previously, most thromboses resolve without therapy. The use of chronic aspirin and oral anticoagulant therapy is usually unnecessary. However, in extremely rare situations, a superior mediastinal syndrome has been reported. This is generally owing to progressive thrombosis and fibrosis. The superior vena cava syndrome usually requires balloon dilatation and stent placement. Complications of the vein used for pacing as stated by Sutton are shown in Table 4.24 (17). Complications can occur with respect to the connector between pacing leads and the pulse generator. This usually results from failure to tighten the lead connector block or a failure to adequately seat the connector pin in the pulse generator. In this modern era of dual-chambered pacing, the atrial and ventricular electrodes may occasionally be switched. Fortunately, these complications are extremely uncommon and occur in less than 1%. These complications require reoperation to correct the problem.

Complications of the Pacemaker Pocket

Infection is the major complication associated with the pacemaker pocket. This may occur acutely, several days to weeks after implantation, or chroni-

Table 4.25 Complications of the pulse generator pocket.

Infection	1.0%
Ulceration	<1.0% pa
Pain	<0.5%
Pacemaker migration requiring intervention	0.1%
Pacemaker twiddler	0.2%

From Sutton R, Bourgeois I. The foundations of cardiac pacing: an illustrated practical guide to basic pacing. Bakken Research Center Series, vol 1, part 1. Armonk, NY: Futura Publishing, 1991, with permission.

cally many years later. Pacemaker pocket infection is frequently associated with large postoperative wound hematomas. This is because the avascular collection of blood acts as an excellent culture medium. The incidence of infection is approximately 1%. Once a pacemaker pocket becomes infected, all hardware must be removed. The incidence of pocket hematoma requiring reoperation is between 0.1% and 0.5%. Although unknown with the increased use of prophylactic platelet inhibitors, the incidence of pocket hematoma is suspected to be much higher. Pacemaker pocket infection may be avoided by scrupulous sterile technique as well as prophylactic antibiotic and antiseptic therapy. It is also recommended that symptomatic hematomas of any size associated with pain should be immediately evacuated and some form of drainage procedure performed.

One should consider some form of drainage procedure in a pocket that continues to ooze profusely. The use of topically applied thrombin or a weak solution of epinephrine has been somewhat effective. The drainage procedure should always be considered in patients on anticoagulants who demonstrate a "wet" pocket. Wound drainage is usually carried out by using either a Jackson-Pratt or Hemovac system (Fig. 4.103). The drainage system should be removed within 24 h because the risk of introducing retrograde infection increases with time. In the case of copious continuous drainage, strong consideration should be given to wound reexploration. In such circumstances, usually an arterial bleeder that requires some form of ligation or cauterization is encountered.

In the case of pacemaker pocket infection, whether acute or chronic, all hardware must be removed.

The migration of the pulse generator today is extremely uncommon. The earlier large pulse generators by their sheer weight would frequently migrate into the axilla. The modern small pulse generator rarely exerts enough pressure to cause migration.

Pacemaker pocket erosion continues to be a problem (Fig. 4.104). This is best avoided by creating a pacemaker pocket that has maximum optimal tissue thickness. Occasionally, in extremely asthenic individuals, subpectoralis major muscle pulse generator placement should be considered to afford optimal tissue thickness. Patients can also present with preerosion secondary to pressure necrosis of the overlying tissue. Such situations represent a quasiemergency if one is to avoid complete erosion and wound infection. The patient should be reoperated, the old pocket abandoned, and new pacemaker pocket created away from the involved site. Sutton and Bourgeois' incidence of pacemaker pocket complications are shown in Table 4.25 (17).

References

1. Schecter DC. Modern era of artificial cardiac pacemakers. In Schecter DC. Electrical cardiac stimulation. Minneapolis: Medtronic, 1983:110–134.

2. Furman S, Schwedel JB. An intracardiac pacemaker for Stokes-Adams seizures. N Engl J Med 1959;261:948.

3. Senning A. Discussion of a paper by Stephenson SE Jr, Edwards WH, Jolly PC, et al. Physiologic P-wave stimulator. J Thorac Cardiovasc Surg 1959;38:639.

4. Mirowski M, Reid PR, Mower MM, et al. Termination of malignant ventricular arrhythmias with an implantable automatic defibrillator in human beings. N Engl J Med 1980;303:322–324.

5. Smyth NPD. Techniques of implantation: atrial and ventricular, thoracotomy and transvenous. Prog Cardiovasc Dis 1981;23:435.

6. Smyth NPD. Pacemaker implantation: surgical techniques. Cardiovasc Clin 1983;14:31.

7. Littleford PO, Spector SD. Device for the rapid insertion of permanent endocardial pacing electrode through the subclavian vein: preliminary report. Ann Thorac Surg 1979;27:265.

8. Parsonnet V, Furman S, Smyth NP, et al. Optimal resources for implantable cardiac pacemakers. Pacemaker Study Group. Circulation 1983;68(1):226A.

9. Harthorne JW, Parsonett V. Seventeenth Bethesda Conference: Adult Cardiac Training. Task Force VI: training in cardiac pacing. J Am Coll Cardiol 1986;7:1213.

10. Parsonnet V, Bernstein AD. Pacing in perspective: concepts and controversies. Circulation 1986;73:1087.

11. Parsonnet V, Bernstein AD, Galasso D. Cardiac pacing practices in the United States in 1985. Am J Cardiol 1988;62:71.

12. Hayes DL, Naccarelli GV, Furman S, et al. Training requirements for permanent pacemaker selection, implantation, and follow-up. PACE 1994;17:6.

13. Bernstein AD, Parsonnet V. Survey of cardiac pacing in the United States in 1989. Am J Cardiol 1992;69:331.

14. Stamato NJ, O'Toole MF, Enger EL. Permanent pacemaker implantation in the cardiac catheterization laboratory versus the operating room: an analysis of hospital charges and complications. PACE 1992;15:2236.

15. Hess DS, Gertz EW, Morady F, et al. Permanent pacemaker implantation in the cardiac catheterization laboratory: the subclavian approach. Cathet Cardiovasc Diagn 1982;8:453.

16. Anderson FH, Alexander MB. Use of a three-channel electrocardiographic recorder for limited intracardiac electrocardiography during single- and double-chamber pacemaker implantation. Ann Thorac Surg 1985;39:485.

17. Sutton R, Bourgeois I. Techniques of implantation. In: Sutton R, Bourgeois I, eds. The foundations of cardiac pacing: an illustrated practical guide to basic pacing, vol 1, pt 1. Mount Kisco, NY: Futura Publishing, 1991.

18. Levine PA, Balady GJ, Lazar HL, et al. Electrocautery and pacemakers: management of the paced patient subject to electrocautery. Ann Thorac Surg 1986;41:313.

19. Belott PH, Sands S, Warren J. Resetting of DDD pacemakers due to EMI. PACE 1984;7:169.

20. Chauvin M, Crenner F, Brechenmacher C. Interaction between permanent cardiac pacing and electrocautery: the significance of electrode position. PACE 1992;15:2028.

21. Hauser RG, Edwards LM, Guiffe VW. Limitation of pacemaker system analyzers for evaluation of implantable pulse generators. PACE 1981;4:650.

22. Dreifus LS, Fisch C, Griffin JC, et al, eds. Guidelines for implantation of cardiac pacemakers and antiarrhythmic devices: a report of the ACC/AHA task force on assessment of diagnostic and therapeutic cardiovascular procedures. Circulation 1991;84:455.

23. Zegelman M, Kreyzer J, Wagner R. Ambulatory pacemaker surgery: medical and economical advantages. PACE 1986;9:1299.
24. Belott PH. Outpatient pacemaker procedures. Int J Cardiol 1987;17:169.
25. Dalvi B. Insertion of permanent pacemakers as a day case procedure. Br Med J 1990;300(6717):119.
26. Hayes DL, Vliestra RE, Trusty JM, et al. Can pacemaker implantation be done as an outpatient? J Am Coll Cardiol 1986;7:199.
27. Hayes DL, Vliestra RE, Trusty JM, et al. A shorter hospital stay after cardiac pacemaker implantation. Mayo Clin Proc 1988;63:236.
28. Haywood GA, Jones SM, Camm AJ, et al. Day case permanent pacing. PACE 1991;14:773.
29. Belott PH. Ambulatory pacemaker procedures: a 13-year experience. PACE 1996;19:69.
30. Belott PH. Ambulatory pacemaker procedures. Mayo Clin Proc 1988;63:301.
31. Goldstin DJ, Losquadro W, Spotnitz HM. Outpatient pacemaker procedures in orally anticoagulated patients. PACE 1998;21:1730.
32. Giudici MC, Barold SS, Paul DL. Pacemaker and implantable cardioverter defibrillator implantation without reversal of warfarin therapy. PACE 27:358, 2004.
33. Philip BK, Corvino BG. Local and regional anesthesia. In Wetchler BV, ed. Anesthesia for ambulatory surgery, 2nd ed. Philadelphia: JB Lippincott, 1991:309–334.
34. Bubien RS, Fisher JD, Gentzel JA, et al. NASPE expert consensus document: Use of IV (conscious) sedation/analgesia by nonanesthesia personnel in patients undergoing arrhythmia-specific diagnostic, therapeutic, and surgical procedures. PACE 1998;21:375.
35. Page CP, Bohnen JMA, Fletcher R, et al. Antimicrobial prophylaxis for surgical wounds: guidelines for clinical care. Arch Surg 1993;128:79.
36. Muers MF, Arnold AG, Sleight P. Prophylactic antibiotics for cardiac pacemaker implantation: a prospective trial. Br Heart J 1981;46:539.
37. Ramsdale DR, Charles RG, Rowlands DB. Antibiotic prophylaxis for pacemaker implantation: a prospective randomized trial. PACE 1984;7:844.
38. Bluhm G, Jacobson B, Ransjo U. Antibiotic prophylaxis in pacemaker surgery: a prospective trial with local and systemic administration of antibiotics at pulse generator replacement. PACE 1985;8:661.
39. Antimicrobial prophylaxis in surgery. Med Lett 1992;34(862):5–8.
40. Golightly LK, Branigan T. Surgical antibiotic irrigations. Hosp Pharm 1989;24:116.
41. Netter FH. Atlas of human anatomy. West Caldwell, NJ: Ciba-Geigy Medical Education, 1992:174–176, 186, 200, 201.
42. Gray H, Pick TP, Howden RE. Anatomy, descriptive and surgical, 1901 ed. Philadelphia: Running Press, 1974:609.
43. Netter FH. The Ciba Collection of Medical Illustrations, vol 5. Heart. Summit, NJ: Ciba Medical Education Division, 1981:22–26.
44. Byrd C. Current clinical applications of dual-chamber pacing. In Zipes DP, ed. Proceedings of a symposium. Minneapolis: Medtronics, 1981:71.
45. Furman S. Venous cutdown for pacemaker implantation. Ann Thorac Surg 1986;41:438.
46. Feiesen A, Kelin GJ, Kostuck WJ, et al. Percutaneous insertion of a permanent transvenous pacemaker electrode through the subclavian vein. Can J Surg 1977;10:131.
47. Littleford PO, Spector SD. Device for the rapid insertion of permanent endocardial pacing electrodes through the subclavian vein: preliminary report. Ann Thorac Surg 1979;27:265.
48. Littleford PO, Parsonnet V, Spector SD. Method for rapid and atraumatic insertion of permanent endocardial electrodes through the subclavian vein. Am J Cardiol 1979;43:980.
49. Miller FA Jr, Homes DR Jr, Gersh BJ, et al. Permanent transvenous pacemaker implantation via the subclavian vein. Mayo Clinic Proc 1980;55:309.

50. Parsonnet V, Werres R, Atherly T, et al. Transvenous insertion of double sets of permanent electrodes. JAMA 1980;243:62.

51. Bognolo PA, Vijayanagar RR, Eckstein PR, et al. Two leads in one introducer technique for A-V sequential implantation. PACE 1982;5:217.

52. Vandersalm TJ, Haffajee CI, Okike ON. Transvenous insertion of double sets of permanent electrodes through a single introducer: clinical application. Ann Thorac Surg 1981;32:307.

53. Belott PH. A variation on the introducer technique for unlimited access to the subclavian vein. PACE 1981;4:43.

54. Gessman LJ, Gallagher JD, MacMillan RM, et al. Emergency guidewire pacing: new methods for rapid conversion of a cardiac catheter into a pacemaker. PACE 1984;7:917.

55. Belott PH. Retained guidewire introducer technique, for unlimited access to the central circulation: a review. Clin Prog Electrophysiol Pacing 1981;1:59.

56. Ong LS, Barold S, Lederman M, et al. Cephalic vein guidewire technique for implantation of permanent pacemakers. Am Heart J 1987;114:753.

57. Belott PH, Byrd CL. Recent developments in pacemaker implantation and lead retrieval. In Barold SS, Mugica J, eds. New perspectives in cardiac pacing, 2nd ed. Mount Kisco, NY: Futura Publishing, 1991:105–131.

58. Belott PH. Implantation techniques: new developments. In: Barold SS, Mugica J, eds. New perspectives in cardiac pacing. Mount Kisco, NY: Futura Publishing, 1988:258–259.

59. Stokes K, Staffeson D, Lessar J, et al. A possible new complication of the subclavian stick: conductor fracture. PACE 1987;10:748.

60. Fyke FE III. Simultaneous insulation deterioration associated with side by side subclavian placement of two polyurethane leads. PACE 1988;11:1571.

61. Fyke FE III. Infraclavicular lead failure: tarnish on a golden route. PACE 1993;16:445.

62. Jacobs DM, Fink AS, Miller RP, et al. Anatomic and morphological evaluation of pacemaker lead compression. PACE 1993;16:373.

63. Magney JE, Flynn DM, Parsons JA, et al. Anatomic mechanisms explaining damage to pacemaker leads, defibrillator leads, and failure of central venous catheters adjacent to the sternoclavicular joint. PACE 1993;16:445.

64. Subclavian venipuncture reconsidered as a means of implanting endocardial pacing leads. Angleton, TX: Issues Intermedics, 1987:1–2.

65. Subclavian puncture may result in lead conductor fracture. Medtronic News 1986–1987;16:27.

66. Byrd CL. Safe introducer technique for pacemaker lead implantation. PACE 1992;15:262.

67. Nichalls RWD. A new percutaneous infraclavicular approach to the axillary vein. Anesthesia 1987;42:151.

68. Taylor BL, Yellowlees I. Central venous cannulation using the infraclavicular axillary vein. Anesthesiology 1990;72:55.

69. Byrd CL. Clinical experience with the extrathoracic introducer insertion technique. PACE 1993;16:1781.

70. Magney JE, Staplin DH, Flynn DM, et al. A new approach to percutaneous subclavian needle puncture to avoid lead fracture or central venous catheter occlusion. PACE 1993;16:2133.

71. Belott PH. Blind percutaneous axillary venous access. PACE 1998;21:873.

72. Belott PH. Blind axillary venous access. PACE 1999;22:1085.

73. Varnagy G, Velasquez R, Navarro D. New technique for cephalic vein approach in pacemaker implants. PACE 1995;18:1807a.

74. Higano ST, Hayes DL, Spittell PC. Facilitation of the subclavian-introducer technique with contrast venography. PACE 1992;15:731.

75. Spencer W III, Kirkpatrick C, Zhu DWX. The value of venogram-guided percutaneous extrathoracic subclavian venipuncture for lead implantation. PACE 1996;19:700.

76. Spencer W III, Zhu DWX, Kirkpatrick C, et al. Subclavian venogram as a guide to lead implantation. PACE 1998;21:499.

77. Ramza BM, Rosenthal L, Hui R, et al. Safety and effectiveness of placement of pacemaker and defibrillator leads in the axillary vein guided by contrast venography. Am J Cardiol 1997;80:892.

78. Fyke FE III. Doppler-guided extrathoracic introducer insertion. PACE 1995;18:1017.

79. Gayle DD, Bailey JR, Haistey WK, et al. A novel ultrasound-guided approach to the puncture of the extrathoracic subclavian vein for surgical lead placement. PACE 1996;19:700.

80. Nash A, Burrell CJ, Ring NJ, et al. Evaluation of an ultrasonically guided venipuncture technique for the placement of permanent pacing electrodes. PACE 1998;21:452.

81. Said SA, Bucx JJ, Stassen CM. Failure of subclavian venipuncture: the internal jugular vein as a useful alternative. Int J Cardiol 1992;35:275.

82. Roelke M, Jackson G, Hawthorne JW. Submammary pacemaker implantation. A unique tunneling technique. PACE 1994;17:1793.

83. Elletad MH, French J. Iliac vein approach to permanent pacemaker implantation. PACE 1989;12:1030.

84. Antonelli D, Freedberg NA, Rosenfeld T. Transiliac vein approach to a rate-responsive permanent pacemaker implantation. PACE 1993;16:1637.

85. Bognolo DA, Vijayanagar RR, Eckstein PF, et al. Method for reintroduction of permanent endocardial pacing electrodes. PACE 1982;5:546.

86. Bognolo DA, Vijay R, Eckstein P, et al. Technical aspects of pacemaker system upgrading procedures. Clin Prog Pacing Electrophysiol 1983;1:269.

87. Belott PH. Use of the contralateral subclavian vein for placement of atrial electrodes in chronically VVI paced patients. PACE 1983;6:781.

88. Hayes DL, Holmes R Jr, Furman S. A Practice of Cardiac Pacing, 3rd ed. Mount Kisco, NY: Futura Publishing, 1993:271–274.

89. Belott PH. Retained guide wire introducer technique, for unlimited access to the central circulation: a review. Clin Prog Electrophysiol Pacing 1981;1:59.

90. Bognolo DA, Vijayanagar R, Ekstein PF, et al. Anatomic suitability of the right atrial appendage for atrial J lead electrodes. In: Proceedings of the Second European Pacing Symposium, Florence, Italy. Cardiac pacing. Padova, Italy: Piccin Medical Book, 1982:639.

91. Bognolo DA, Vijayanagar R, Ekstein PF, et al. Implantation of permanent atrial J lead using lateral fluoroscopy. Ann Thorac Surg 1981;316:574.

92. Thurer RJ. Technique of insertion of transvenous atrial pacing leads: the value of lateral fluoroscopy. PACE 1981;4:525.

93. Jamidar H, Goli V, Reynolds DW. The right atrial free wall: an alternative pacing site. PACE 1993;16:959.

94. Shepard RB, Goldin MD, Lawrie GM, et al. Automatic implantable cardioverter defibrillator: surgical approaches for implantation. J Cardiol Surg 1992;7(3):208–224.

95. Watkins L Jr, Taylor E Jr. The surgical aspects of automatic implantable cardioverter-defibrillator implantation. PACE 1991;14(5 Pt 2):953–960.

96. Watkins L Jr, Guarnieri T, Griffith LS, et al. Implantation of the automatic implantable cardioverter defibrillator. J Cardiol Surg 1998;3(1):1–7.

97. Shahian DM, Williamson WA, Streitz JM Jr, et al. Subfascial implantation of implantable cardioverter defibrillator generator. Ann Thorac Surg 1992;54(1):173–174.

98. O'Neill PG, Lawrie GM, Kaushik RR, et al. Late results of the left subcostal approach for automatic implantable cardioverter. Am J Cardiol 1991;67(5):387–390.

99. Lawrie GM, Kaushik RR, Pacifico A. Right minithoracotomy: an adjunct to left subcostal automatic implantable cardioverter defibrillator implantation. Ann Thorac Surg 1989;47(5):780–781.

100. Damiano RJ Jr, Foster AH, Ellenbogen KA, et al. Implantation of cardioverter defibrillators in the post-sternotomy patient. Ann Thorac Surg 1992;53(6): 978–983.

101. Frumin H, Goodman GR, Pleatman M. ICD implantation via thoracoscopy without the need for sternotomy or thoracotomy. PACE 1993;16(2):257–260.

102. Krasna MJ, Buser GA, Flowers JL, et al. Thoracoscopic versus laparoscopic placement of defibrillator patches. Surg Laparosc Endosc 1996;6(2):91–97.

103. Bardy GH, Yee R, The International Active Can Investigators. World wide experience with the Jewel 7219C unipolar, single lead active can implantable pacer-cardioverter/defibrillator. PACE 1995;18(II):806.

104. Brooks R, Garan H, Torchiana, et al. Determinants of successful nonthoracotomy cardioverter-defibrillator implantation: experience in 101 patients using two different lead systems. J Am Coll Cardiol 1993;22:1835–1842.

105. Moss AJ, Rivers RJ Jr. Atrial pacing from the coronary vein: ten-year experience in 50 patients with implanted pervenous pacemakers. Circulation 1978;57:103.

106. Greenberg P, Castellanet M, Messenger J, et al. Coronary sinus pacing. Circulation 1978;57:98.

107. Hewitt MJ, Chen JTT, Ravin CE, et al. Coronary sinus atrial pacing: radiographic considerations. Am J Radiol 1981;136:323.

108. Dosios T, Gorgogiannis D, Sakorafas G, et al. Persistent left superior vena cava: a problem in transvenous pacing of the heart. PACE 1991;14:389.

109. Hussaine SA, Chalcravarty S, Chaikhouni A. Congenital absence of superior vena cava: unusual anomaly of superior systemic veins complicating pacemaker placement. PACE 1981;4:328.

110. Ronnevik PK, Abrahamsen AM, Tollefsen J. Transvenous pacemaker implantation via a unilateral left superior vena cava. PACE 1982;5:808.

111. Cha EM, Khoury GH. Persistent left superior vena cava. Radiology 1972;103:375.

112. Colman AL. Diagnosis of left superior vena cava by clinical inspection: a new physical sign. Am Heart J 1967;73:115.

113. Dirix LY, Kersscochot IE, Fiernen SH, et al. Implantation of a dual-chambered pacemaker in a patient with persistent left superior vena cava. PACE 1988;11:343.

114. Giovanni QV, Piepoli N, Pietro Q, et al. Cardiac pacing in unilateral left superior vena cava: evaluation by digital angiography. PACE 1991;14:1567.

115. Robbens EJ, Ruiter JH. Atrial pacing by unilateral persistent left superior vena cava. PACE 1986;9:594.

116. Hellestrand KJ, Ward DE, Bexton RS, et al. The use of active fixation electrodes for permanent endocardial pacing via a persistent left superior vena cava. PACE 1982;5:180.

117. West JNW, Shearmann CP, Gammange MD. Permanent pacemaker positioning via the inferior vena cava in a case of single ventricle with loss of right atrial to vena caval continuity. PACE 1993;16:1753.

118. Fishberger SB, Cammanas J, Rodriguez-Fernandez H, et al. Permanent pacemaker lead implantation via the transhepatic route. PACE 1996;19:1124.

119. Belott PH, Bucko D. Inframammary pulse generator placement for maximizing optimal cosmetic effect. PACE 1983;6:1241.

120. Shefer A, Lewis SB, Gang ES. The retropectoral transaxillary permanent pacemaker: description of a technique for percutaneous implantation of an invisible device. PACE 1996;16:1646.

121. Westerman GR, Van Devanter SH. Transthoracic transatrial endocardial lead placement for permanent pacing. Ann Thorac Surg 1987;43:445.

122. Hayes DL, Vliestra RE, Puga FJ, et al. A novel approach to atrial endocardial pacing. PACE 1989;12:125.

123. Byrd CL, Schwartz SJ. Transatrial implantation of transvenous pacing leads as an alternative to implantation of epicardial leads. PACE 1990;13:1856.

124. Abraham WT, Fisher WG, Smith AL et al. Cardiac resynchronization in chronic heart failure. New Engl J Med 2002;346:1845–1853.

125. Saxon LA, DeMarco T. Cardiac Resynchronization: A cornerstone in the foundation of device therapy for heart failure. J Am J Cardiol 2001;38:1971–1973.

126. Stellbrink C, Breithardt AO, Franke A et al. Impact of cardiac resynchronization therapy using hemodynamically optimized pacing of left ventricular remodeling in patients with congestive heart failure and ventricular conduction disturbances. J Am Coll Cardiol 2002;38:1957–1965.

127. Grass D, Leclercq C, Tang AS et al. Cardiac resynchronization therapy in advanced heart failure, the Multicenter Insync clinical study. Eur J Heart Fail 2002;4:311–320.

128. Auricchio A, Stellbrink C, Sack S. Long-term clinical effect of hemodynamically optimized cardiac resynchronization therapy in patients with heart failure and ventricular conduction delay. J Am Coll Cardiol 2002;39:12:2026–2033.

129. Auricchio H, Kloss M, Trautmann SL et al. Exercise performance following cardiac resynchronization therapy in patients with heart failure and ventricular conduction delay. Am J Cardiol 2002;89:198–203.

130. Linde C, Leclercq C, Rex S et al. Long-term benefits of biventricular pacing in congestive heart failure, results from the multisite stimulation in cardiomyopathy (MUSTIC) study. J Am Coll Cardiol 2002;40:111–118.

131. Leporte V, Pizzarelli G, Dernevik L. Inadvertent transatrial pacemaker insertion: An unusual complication. PACE 1987;10:951–954.

132. Daubert JC, Ritter P, Le Breton H et al. Permanent left ventricular pacing with transvenous leads inserted into the coronary veins. PACE 1998;21:239–245.

133. Greenberg P, Castellanett M, Messenger J, et al. Coronary sinus pacing. Circulation 1978;57:98–103.

134. Hunt D, Sloman G. Long-term electrode catheter placement from coronary sinus. Br Med J 1968;4:495–496.

135. Spitzberg JW, Milstoc M, Wertheim AR. An unusual site for ventricular pacing occurring during the use of the transvenous catheter pacemaker. Am Heart J1969; 77:529–533.

136. Kemp A, Johansen JK, Kjaergaard E. Malplacement of endocardial pacemaker electrodes in the middle cardiac vein. Acta Med Scand 1976;199:7–11.

137. Shattigar UR, Loungani RR, Smith CA. Inadvertent permanent ventricular pacing from the cardiac vein: An electrocardiographic roentgenographic and echocardiographic assessment. Clin Cardiol 1989;12:267–264.

138. Bai Y, Strathmore N, Mond H et al. Permanent ventricular pacing via the great cardiac vein. PACE 1994;17:678–683.

139. Bakker PF, Meijburg H, de Jonge N, et al. Beneficial effects of biventricular pacing in congestive heart failure (Abstract). PACE 1994;17:820.

140. Cazeau S, Ritter P, Bakdach S et al. Four-chamber pacing in dilated cardiomyopathy. PACE 1994;17:1974–1979.

141. Netter FH. In: Yonkman FF, ed. Ciba Collection of Medical Illustrations, Vol 5 Heart 1969:A.

142. Yen Ho S, Anderson RH, Sanchez-Quintana D. Gross structure of the atriums: More than an anatomical curiosity. Pacing Clin Electrophysiol 25: 842, 2002.

143. Ho S. Understanding atrial anatomy: implications for atrial fibrillation ablation. Cardiology International for a Global Perspective on Cardiac Care. Greco Publishing Ltd., S17 through S20, 2002.

144. Cabrera JA, Sanchez-Quintana D, Ho Sy, et al. Angiographic anatomy of the inferior right atrial isthmus in patients with and without history of common atrial flutter. Circulation 1999;99:3017–3023.

145. Jansens JL,Jottrand M, Preumont N et al. Cardiac resynchronization therapy with robotic thoracoscopy (abstract). Europace 2002;3;92

146. Gilard M, Mansourati J, EtienneY et al. Angiograhic anatomy of the coronary sinus and its tributaries. PACE 1998;21:2280–2284.

147. Niazi I. Power Point presentation on Cardiac anatomy St Paul MN Guidant 2002.

148. Belott PH, Reynolds DW. Permanent pacemaker and implantable cardioverter defibrillator implantation. In Ellenbogen, Kay, Wilkoff (eds): Clinical Cardiac Pacing and Defibrillation, Second Edition. WB Saunders Company, Philadelphia, Pennsylvania 2000:578.

149. Belott PH, Reynolds DW. Permanent pacemaker and implantable cardioverter defibrillator implantation. In Ellenbogen, Kay, Wilkoff (eds): Clinical Cardiac Pacing and Defibrillation, Second Edition. WB Saunders Company, Philadelphia, Pennsylvania 2000:576.

150. Blanc JJ, Benditt D, Gilard M et al. A method for permanent transvenous left ventricular pacing. PACE 1998;21:2021–2024.

151. Auricchio A, Klein H, Tockman B et al. Transvenous biventricular pacing for heart failure: Can the obstacles be overcome? Am J Cardiol 1999;83:136–142.

152. Belott PH. Retained-guidewire-introducer technique for unlimited access to the central circulation: A review. Clin Progr Electrophysiol and Pacing 1983;1:59 Last page.

153. Moss AJ, Zareba W, Hall WJ et al. Prophylactic implantation of a defibrillator in patients with myocardial infarction and reduced ejection fraction. N Engl J Med 2002;346:877–883.

154. Meisel E, Pfeiffer D Engelmann L et al. Investigation of the coronary venous anatomy by retrograde venography in patients with malignant ventricular tachycardia. Circulation 2001;104:442–7.

155. Kleine P, Grönefeld G, Dogan S et al. Robotically enhanced placement of left ventricular epicardial electrodes during implantation of a biventricular implantable cardioverter defibrillator system. PACE 2002;25:989–991.

156. McVenes R. The future of left ventricular stimulation: Transvenous, endocardial or epicardial? (Abstract). Europace 2002;3:A13.

157. SantAnna J, Prates P, Kalil R. Robotically assisted implantation for biventricular stimulation (abstract). Europace 2002;3:A92.

158. Daoud E, Kalbfleisch S, Hummel J et al. Implantation techniques and chronic lead parameters of biventricular pacing dual –chamber defibrillators. J Cardiovasc Electrophsiol 2002;13:971–979.

159. Ingus B David Trial Investigators. Dual chamber pacing or ventricular backup pacing in patients with an implantable defibrillator. The dual chamber and VVI implantable defibrillator (DAVID) trial. JAMA 2002;288:315.

160. Nielson JC, Kristensen L, Anderson HR, et al. A randomized comparison of atrial and dual-chambered pacing in 177 consecutive patients with sick sinus syndrome. J Am Coll Cardiol 2003;42:614.

161. Prinzen FW, Peschar M. Relationship between the pacing-induced sequence of activation and left ventricular pump function in animals. PACE 2002;25:484.

162. Rosenqvist M, Isaaz K, Botvinick EH, et al. Relative importance of activation sequence compared to atrial ventricular synchrony in left ventricular function. Am J Cardiol 1991;67:148.

163. Rosenqvist M, Brandt J, Schuller H. Long-term pacing in sinus node disease: effects of stimulation mode on cardiovascular morbidity and mortality. Am Heart J 1998;116:16.

164. Stangl K, Seitz K, Wirtzfeld A, et al. Differences between atrial single-chamber pacing (AAI) and ventricular single-chamber pacing (VVI) with respect to prognosis and antiarrhythmic effect in patients with sick sinus syndrome. Pacing Clin Electrophysiol 1990;13:2080.

165. Brandt J, Anderson H, Fahraeus, et al. Natural history of sinus node disease treated with atrial pacing in 213 patients: implications for selection of stimulation mode. J Am Coll Cardiol 1992;20:633.

166. Anderson HR, Thuesen L, Bagger JP, et al. Prospective randomized trial of atrial versus ventricular pacing in sick sinus syndrome. Lancet 1994;344:1523.

167. Daubert C, Gras D, Berger D, Leclercq C. Permanent atrial resynchronization by synchronous biatrial pacing in the preventive treatment of atrial flutter associated with high degree of intraatrial block. Arch Mal Coeur Vaiss 1994;87:1535.

168. Saksena S, Prakash A, Hill M, et al. Prevention of recurrent atrial fibrillation with chronic dual-site right atrial pacing. J Am Coll Cardiol 1996;28:687.

169. Levy T, Walker S, Rochelle J, Ball V. Evaluation of biatrial pacing, right atrial pacing, and no pacing in patients with drug-refractory atrial fibrillation. Am J Cardiol 1999;84:426.

170. Levy T, Walker S, Rex S, et al. No incremental benefit of multisite atrial pacing compared to right atrial pacing in patients with drug-refractory atrial fibrillation. Heart 2001;85:48.

171. Leclercq JF, DeSisti A, Fiorello P, et al. Is dual site better than single site atrial pacing in the prevention of atrial fibrillation? Pacing Clin Electrophysiol 2000;23:2101.

172. Padeletti L, Porciani MC, Michelucci A, et al. Intraatrial septum pacing: a new approach to prevent recurrent atrial fibrillation. J Interventional Card Electrophysiol 1999;3:35.

173. Frohlig G, Schwaab B, Kindermann M. Selective site pacing: the right ventricularA approach. PACE 2004;27:855.

174. Padeletti L, Michelucci A, Pieragnoli P, et al. Atrial septal pacing: a new approach to prevent atrial fibrillation. J Intervent Cardiac Electrophysiol 1999;3:35.

175. Farré J. Anderson RH, Cabrera JA, et al. Fluoroscopic cardiac anatomy for catheter ablation of tachycardia. Pacing Clin Electrophysiol 2002;25:76.

176. Bachmann G. The interauricular time interval. Am J Physiol 1907;1:1.

177. James TN, Sherf L. Specialized tissues and preferential conduction in the atria of the heart. Am J Cardiol 1971;28:414.

178. Roithinger FX, Cheng J, Sippens A, et al. Use of electroanatomical mapping to delineate transseptal atrial conduction in humans. Circulation 1999;100:1791.

179. Anderson RH, Ho SY. The architecture of the sinus node, the atrioventricular conduction axis in the intranodal atrial myocardium. J Cardiovasc Electrophysiol 1998;9:1233.

180. Chauvin M, Shah DC, Hauissaguerre M, et al. The anatomic basis of connections between the coronary sinus musculature and the left atrium in humans. Circulation 2000;101:647.

181. DePonti R, Ho SY, Salerno-Uriarte JA, et al. Electroanatomical analysis of sinus impulse propagation in normal human atria. J Cardiovasc Electrophysiol 2002;13:1.

182. Saksena S, Prakash A, Hill M, et al. Prevention of recurrent atrial fibrillation with chronic dual-site right atrial pacing. J Am Coll Cardiol 1996;28:687.

183. deCock CC, Giudici MC, Twisk JW. Comparison of the hemodynamic effects of right ventricular outflow tract pacing with right ventricular apex pacing: a quantt. Woitative review. Europace 2003;5:275.

184. Stambler BS, Ellenbogen KA, Zhang X, et al. Right ventricular outflow versus apical pacing in pacemaker patients with congestive heart failure and atrial fibrillation. J Cardiovas Electrophysiol 2003;14:1180.

185. Lieberman R, Grenz D, Mond HG, et al. Selective site pacing: defining and reaching the selected site. PACE 2004;27:883.

186. Karpawich P, Gates J, Stokes K. Septal His-Purkinje ventricular pacing in canines: a new endocardial electrode approach. PACE 1992;15:2011.

187. Deshmukh PM, Romanyshyn M. Direct His-bundle pacing, present and future. PACE 2004;27:862.

188. Parsonnet V, Bernstein AD, Lindsay B. Pacemaker implantation complication rates: an analysis of some contributing factors. J Am Coll Cardiol 1989;13:917.

189. Parsonnet V, Roelke M. The cephalic vein cutdown versus subclavian puncture for pacemaker/ICD lead implantation. PACE 1999;22:695.

190. Furman S. Venous cutdown for pacemaker implantation. Ann Thorac Surg 1986;41:438.

191. Furman S. Subclavian puncture for pacemaker lead placement. PACE 1986;9:467.

192. Belott PH. A practical approach to permanent pacemaker implantation. Mount Kisco, NY: Futura Publishing, 1995:59–63.TABLES

Transvenous Left Ventricular Lead Implantation

Westby G. Fisher

Introduction

With the publications of the Miracle (1), Miracle ICD (2), COMPANION (3) and CARE-HF (4) trials, biventricular pacing is now an undisputed adjunctive therapy for heart failure, demonstrating an additive symptom and survival benefit over pharmacological therapies alone. Its wider application has been hampered, in part, by the technical challenges of left ventricular lead implantation encountered by the operating physician. (Table 5.1)

Inroads to successful LV lead implantation have been achieved through collective sharing of implant experiences (5). New sheath delivery systems, catheters, and guide wires continue to improve LV lead implantation success. It is hoped that this chapter will serve as a useful springboard to improving outcomes with LV lead implantation.

Anatomy

Successful and safe transvenous placement of left ventricular leads requires a thorough understanding of the anatomy of the coronary sinus (CS), triangle of Koch, and surrounding structures. Significant anatomic variability regarding the size, morphology, and course of the coronary sinus exists. In addition, cardiac chamber enlargement, particularly right atrial enlargement, can increase the complexity of localizing the coronary sinus.

The coronary sinus is bounded posteriorly by the Thebesian valve joining with the Eustacian ridge from the inferior vena cava to become the tendon of Todoro, anteriorly by the tricuspid annulus, and inferiorly by the inferior vena cava (Fig. 5.1). The coronary sinus typically courses posteriorly and parallelly to the mitral annulus. The diameter of the coronary sinus can be quite variable and commonly has a prominent Thebesian valve over its orifice. This venous valve is often fenestrated and can occasionally impede placement of long sheaths deeply within the main body of the coronary sinus. Additionally, within the mid-body if the coronary sinus, venous valves are often present, the most prominent is the venous valve of Vieussens, located at the junction of the vestigial remnant of the vein of Marshall and the origin of the great cardiac

Table 5.1 Representative Coronary Sinus lead implantation success rates.

	MIRACLE trial	MIRACLE-ICD trial	Insync III trial	Total
Number of patients attempted	591	421	334	1346
Unable to access the CS	8 (1.4%)	16 (3.8%)	7 (2.1%)	31 (2.3%)
Implant success rate	92%	88%	95%	92%

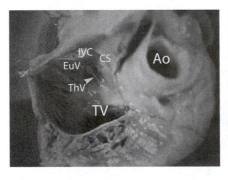 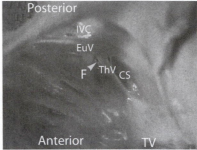

Fig. 5.1 Anatomy of the Medial Floor of the Right Atrium. To view the medial aspect of the floor of the right atrium, the anterosuperior portion of the tricuspid valve (TV) was resected. The Thebesian valve (ThV) of the coronary sinus (CS), joins posteriorly with the Eustacian valve (EuV) of the inferior vena cava (IVC). In the close-up view, small fenestrations (F) can be seen within the ThV. These fenestrations can impede placement of a long vascular sheath within the coronary sinus if a guide wire were placed through them.

vein as it connects to the coronary sinus. Other venous anomalies must also be considered and anticipated during the implant process, particularly such anatomic variants as a persistent left superior vena cava, dual osteal coronary sinuses, and a prominent vein of Marshall (anatomically in the same location as a persistent left superior vena cava) that courses posterolaterally to the true body of the coronary sinus and great cardiac vein. Identification of these anatomic variants, as well as planning the left ventricular lead implant procedure, is facilitated greatly by coronary sinus venography.

Importantly, the right coronary artery is surrounded by a layer of fat as it courses along the epicardial surface of the tricuspid valve. This fat layer provides a radiographic marker of the location of the tricuspid annulus when viewed in real-time fluoroscopy in the 20–30° right anterior oblique (RAO) projection, and is noted by a radiographic vertical lucency that moves anteriorly and posteriorly during the cardiac contraction cycle. Since the coronary sinus is reliably located approximately 1 cm posterior to and at the inferior aspect of this radiographically lucent line, this radiographic marker has proven remarkably helpful at coronary sinus localization during the left ventricular lead implant process, especially in patients with marked right atrial enlargement.

The anatomy of the coronary sinus venous branches warrants review (Fig. 5.2). The coronary sinus typically joins with the great cardiac vein

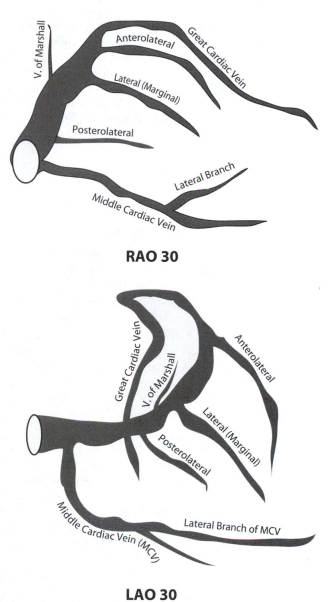

RAO 30

LAO 30

Fig. 5.2 The Schematic of the Anatomy of Coronary Sinus Venous Branches. Appropriate coronary sinus branch vessel targets for left ventricular lead implantation include those supplying the lateral wall of the left ventricle. These include the anterolateral, lateral (or marginal), posterolateral branches, as well as lateral branches of the middle cardiac vein or great cardiac vein. Individual patients rarely have all of these branches, so techniques to implant at any of these locations during difficult cases should be attempted if one target branch is unacceptable.

where the Vein of Marshall joins the coronary sinus. The great cardiac vein courses laterally and posteriorly and extends anteriorly along the interventricular septum. Posterolateral and lateral (or true marginal) branches from the great cardiac vein arise in its course along the lateral aspect of the mitral annulus in 55–65% of patients. In approximately 35–40% of patients, these lateral branches arise from very near the origin of the coronary sinus from branches of a large posterolateral branch. This posterolateral branch should be differentiated from the middle cardiac vein which courses adjacent to the posterior descending artery in the posterior interventricular groove. Occasionally, the middle cardiac vein will drain a lateral branch that extends to the posterolateral aspect of the left ventricle and may be a suitable target vessel for left ventricular lead implantation when other venous branches do not suffice.

Procedural Issues

Patient Preparation

Although outside the scope of this chapter, appropriate patient selection for cardiac resynchronization therapy is pivotal to assuring the best results with left ventricular lead implantation. Patients in whom resynchronization therapy is not likely to be of value include patients with unstable coronary artery disease, severe aortic stenosis, severe mitral stenosis or mitral insufficiency due to structural abnormalities of the mitral valve, or patients with advanced right ventricular dysfunction from severe pulmonary disease. Additionally, patients with severe congestive heart failure must be able to lie relatively flat long enough to tolerate the implant procedure. Pharmacologic optimization of left ventricular hemodynamics prior to the implant procedure will greatly improve the patient's and physician's comfort during the implant process and permit the safest possible milieu for device implantation.

Additionally, all patients should have backup external defibrillation and pacing patches applied should these be required during the implant process. Patients should receive prophylactic antibiotics within 1 hour of the beginning of the implant procedure with antibiotics typically effective against staphylococcal species, usually cefazolin or vancomycin (4). Skin preparation with 0.4% chlorhexidine or povidone iodine scrub for 5 min before implantation is also recommended, along with fastidious sterile technique.

Laboratory Preparation

Transvenous implantation of left ventricular leads demands acceptable fluoroscopy facilities. Catheterization laboratories used routinely for coronary angiography or electrophysiology studies offer the best visualization of coronary venous anatomy. Biplane fluoroscopic facilities are not required, but the ability to image in multiple fluoroscopic projections, especially the RAO and left anterior oblique (LAO) projections, coupled with the ability to capture images for later recall and analysis, are mandatory. The use of older 9-in. image-intensifier c-arms used in many operating rooms limits one's ability to image the entire cardiac silhouette due to magnification issues, requires an additional x-ray technician to move the camera from RAO to LAO projections, and are unable to perform image capture and recall to limit contrast injections. Newer vascular fluoroscopic c-arms equipped with 16-in. image intensifiers provide enhancements overcoming many of these limitations and are acceptable for left ventricular implantation.

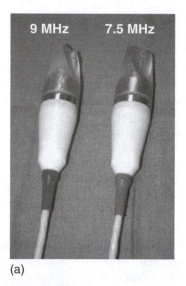

(a)

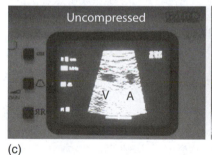
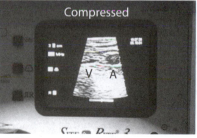

(b)

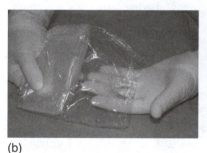
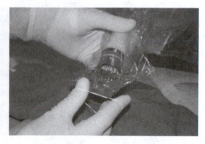

(c)

Fig. 5.3 Intracardiac Ultrasound for Vascular Access. Use of vascular ultrasound to gain access to the axillary vein can greatly facilitate left ventricular lead implantation by improving vascular access at the beginning of the procedure. Typical ultrasound probes have frequencies of 7.5 or 9 MHz (a). The higher frequency probes are better for access for more superficial vascular structures like those in the neck, whereas the lower frequency 7.5 MHz transducers permit acceptable imaging of the axillary, cephalic and portions of the subclavian veins. Ultrasound gel must be placed inside the plastic probe cover to gain acceptable images (b, Panel A). The plastic cover is secured with sterile rubber bands (b, Panel B). To differentiate to the axillary vein (V) from artery (A), gentle compression is applied to the vessels, causing the vein to collapse while the artery does not (c).

The availability of additional angiographic guide wires and catheters can also greatly facilitate coronary sinus sheath cannulation and left ventricular lead implantation. Favorite diagnostic angiographic catheters used have included 5Fr catheters with varying tip configurations including JR4, multipurpose, and Amplatz catheters (AL1, AL2, and AL3). Hydrophilic guide wires are also very useful during the implant procedure. Additionally, many operators use a right-heart catheterization manifold and control syringe connected to a saline flush line and contrast bottle to permit repeated small contrast injections as necessary. Judicious use of contrast should be emphasized, however, since many heart failure patients have compromised renal function. A small stool for the operator to sit upon during left ventricular lead implantation has facilitated operator comfort, especially when the image intensifier is rotated to the ipsilateral implantation side for prolonged periods.

Vascular ultrasound has also greatly facilitated the implant process by easing axillary vein localization. Commercially available systems (Site Rite®, Bard Access Systems, Salt Lake City, UT) include either a 9 or 7.5 MHz ultrasound probe to localize the axillary artery and vein. Differentiating the vein from artery is easily accomplished by compressing the structures with probe and noting which collapses more easily (Fig. 5.3). In patients with elevated right heart pressures, this same effect can be facilitated by having the patient inspire forcefully.

Left Ventricular Lead Implantation

After venous access is achieved, successful left ventricular lead implantation requires several basic steps: (1) coronary sinus ostium localization, (2) coronary sinus venography and development of an implant strategy, and (3) placement of the left ventricular lead, and (4) confirmation of acceptable pacing characteristics. Should left ventricular lead pacing characteristics be unacceptable due to extracardiac stimulation or poor pacing thresholds, then earlier CS venography can facilitate placement of the left ventricular lead in an alternative coronary venous branch.

In patients with left bundle branch block, it is advised that right ventricular lead placement be secured before left ventricular lead implantation or coronary sinus osteal localization since traumatic interruption of right bundle branch conduction could lead to the development of catheter-induced complete heart block and the need for urgent ventricular pacing.

Long (45–50 cm) vascular sheaths have been developed to engage the coronary sinus. These sheaths are novel because they can be removed without removing the internal pacing lead by slitting or peeling the sheath from the lead after its placement. Such sheaths improve lead tracking and advancement into a target vessel by transmitting force through the longitudinal axis of the lead. Adequately seating the long sheath within the coronary sinus assures stable and repeatable lead access to branch vessels as well. Because of the large diameter of these sheaths and their single-planed curves, care must be exercised when placing these sheaths into the coronary sinus to avoid dissection of the intimal wall of the coronary sinus. Additional smaller diagnostic catheters first placed into the larger sheaths can facilitate their introduction deeper into the body of the coronary sinus by providing additional support and curvature

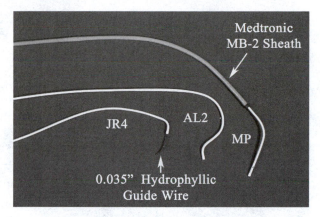

Fig. 5.4 Long Vascular Sheath with Internal Diagnostic Catheter and Hydrophilic Guide Wire to Facilitate Cannulation of the Coronary Sinus. Varying 5Fr diagnostic catheters of different tip shapes, including the Judkins right (JR4), Amplatz (AL2), or multipurpose (MP) variety placed through a long vascular sheath (e.g., a Medtronic MB-2) can greatly facilitate coronary sinus cannulation. Probing for the ostium of the coronary sinus with a soft, hydrophilic guide wire can avoid excessive contrast administration, preserving renal function in patients with diminished renal function. Once the guide wire enters the ostium, the diagnostic catheter can first be advanced over the guide wire to provide support for advancing the stiffer long vascular sheath over the diagnostic catheter into the coronary sinus. This "telescoping" technique also avoids damaging the intima of the coronary sinus.

to negotiate the CS ostium (Fig. 5.4). The routine use of such catheters within the long sheath, coupled with the placement of an internal hydrophilic guide wire within the internal catheter, provides an excellent platform with which to locate and engage the coronary sinus. Companies are now equipping their implant tools with inner pre-curved dilators that mimic the curvatures of the more conventional diagnostic catheters to facilitate the placement of the long sheath (Fig. 5.5).

Localization of the Coronary Sinus Ostium

The long sheath, diagnostic catheter (either a 5Fr JR4, AL2 or multipurpose catheter), and hydrophilic guide wire assembly (Fig. 5.6) is first placed into the inferior right atrium. Localization of the coronary sinus ostium can be reliably obtained by first placing a long sheath equipped with a diagnostic catheter into the right ventricle. This is denoted by the development of premature ventricular complexes during the sheath implant process. The fluoroscopic camera is then rotated to the 20–30° RAO position. Real-time identification of the tricuspid annular fat pad is then attempted. Once localized, the sheath assembly is withdrawn just into the right atrium and rotated in the counterclockwise direction (when implanting from the left side) to a point just proximal to the tricuspid annulus. The inner Jr-4 catheter is then rotated in very fine increments anteriorly and posteriorly while advancing the hydrophilic guide wire. When the guide wire is seen coursing horizontally and to the left, confirmation of its placement is made by rotating the fluoroscopy image to the LAO orientation. The diagnostic catheter is then carefully advanced into

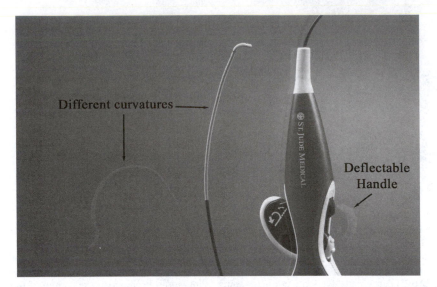

Fig. 5.5 An Alternative to Multiple Diagnostic Catheters in Fig. 5.4. This catheter with a deflectable tip permits multiple curvatures of the internal catheter within a long vascular sheath to facilitate cannulation of the coronary sinus. Once the long sheath is positioned into the coronary sinus, this catheter must then be removed before the left ventricular lead can be implanted.

the coronary sinus over the guide wire. The catheter and guide wire are then anchored in place while the sheath is advanced over them into the coronary sinus. If difficulty is encountered passing the sheath over the catheter, the fluoroscopy is rotated back to the RAO projection to assure the sheath is being advanced in the anatomic plane of the coronary sinus. If the sheath still cannot be advanced, the guide wire and catheter can be exchanged for introducing sheath with a more graduated tip. An example of such a deflectable catheter is Medtronic's Prevail catheter with its tapered tip (Fig. 5.7). We have found this to be effective at gaining access to the coronary sinus in patients in whom we suspected we may have had the guide wire passing through a fenestration of the Thebesian valve of the coronary sinus.

Fig. 5.6 (continued) the JR4 catheter. (Note: *Before inflating the balloon on a balloon-tipped catheter for occlusive venography, it is important to re-confirm that the tip of the balloon catheter has not engaged a smaller branch vessel by injecting a small amount of contrast prior to balloon inflation. This will avoid rupture of a venous branch with balloon inflation.*) Panel H: A second venogram again performed in the 25° LAO projection. Panel I: The JR4 catheter was removed and replaced with a 6Fr bipolar left ventricular pacing lead equipped with a straight 0.014 in. stylet. The larger lead was used because of the large diameter of the branch vessel. Note the lead is placed distal to expected location of the posterolateral branch. Panel J: The stylet is then withdrawn slightly (approx 0.5 cm) to develop a more pronounced curvature to the distal lead tip. The lead is then withdrawn and rotated clockwise until the tip of the lead engages the targeted posterolateral vessel. Panel K: The lead is then carefully advanced distally into the vessel. Pacing thresholds and maximum output pacing from the lead confirmed excellent capture thresholds and no evidence of extracardiac stimulation.

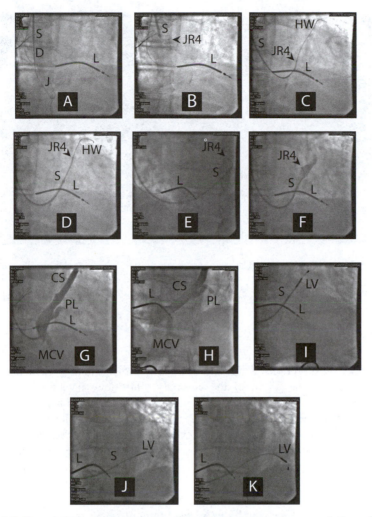

Fig. 5.6 Cannulation of the Coronary Sinus Ostium. Stepwise cannulation of the coronary sinus is demonstrated. Panel A: Initially, a long sheath (S) and its dilator (D) are passed over a 0.035 in. J-wire (J) to access the right atrium. An active-fixation defibrillator (L) was positioned previously in the right ventricle. Panel B: The dilator and guide wire were removed and replaced with a 5Fr JR4 angiographic catheter through the long sheath. (Other labels as in Panel A). Panel C: A hydrophilic guide wire (HW) was then passed through the JR4 catheter, and the catheter and guide wire assembly advanced initially to the tricuspid valve, then torqued counterclockwise slightly while probing with the guide wire until the wire passed freely posterolaterally into the coronary sinus. The JR4 catheter was then advanced over the hydrophilic guide wire. Note the sheath (S) is still well back in the right atrium. Panel D: The long sheath (S) is then passed over the JR4 and hydrophilic guide wire assembly safely into the coronary sinus. Panel E: Confirmation of the leftward location of the JR4 catheter is made by imaging in the LAO (25°) projection. Panel F: A small puff of contrast is placed through the JR4 catheter to assure it has not engaged a branch vessel like the Vein of Marshall. Note the camera is now back to the RAO view. Panel G: A more forceful injection of a 50:50 mix of contrast and saline (approximately 7–8 cc) is then placed into the coronary sinus in an attempt to image the venous branches. Note that adequate visualization of the proximal portion of an obtusely-angled posterolateral branch (PL) was identified, as was the origin of the middle cardiac vein (MCV). If a branch vessel had not been seen, a 1 cm balloon-tipped catheter would have replaced

(legend continues on preceding page)

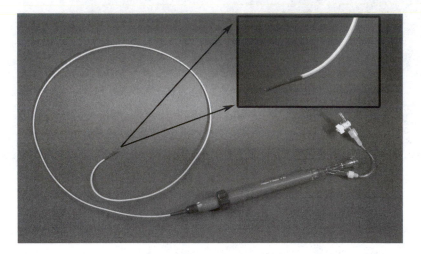

Fig. 5.7 An Attain Prevail Catheter (Medtronic, Inc), This deflectable 7Fr catheter has a tapered (to 4Fr) soft tip (inset) that can be placed over a 0.035 in. guidewire and facilitate passage of a larger sheath through a stenosis or fenestration of the Thebesian valve (as seen in Fig. 5.1).

Special Considerations: Difficulty in Locating the Coronary Sinus Ostium
In rare cases, the origin of the coronary sinus may be sufficiently mal-positioned with a vertical origin or unusual cardiac rotation prohibiting its identification. In these cases, one may resort to having a colleague perform a coronary artery angiogram. Imaging levophase will identify the coronary sinus origin. A capable angiographer can be summoned during the procedure in an appropriately equipped laboratory to perform coronary angiography in these circumstances via the contralateral femoral arterial approach.

Coronary Sinus Venography and Development of Lead Implant Strategy

Once the long sheath is successfully seated within the coronary sinus, contrast venography is typically used to identify target coronary venous branches in which to place the left ventricular pacing lead. This is accomplished through small hand injections of contrast into the diagnostic catheter, sheath itself, or ide-ally with the use of a small balloon-tipped catheter to provide temporary venous occlusion. Retrograde occlusive coronary sinus venography has the advantage of opacifying all available coronary venous vessels with a single injection.

The importance of coronary sinus venography cannot be overstated. Examples where venography has proven invaluable include situations with coronary sinus venous branches near parallel to the coronary sinus (Fig. 5.8) or in the case of an unusually large vein of Marshall or post-operative patients (Fig. 5.9).

Occlusive Retrograde Coronary Sinus Venography

If occlusive coronary sinus venography is performed, care must be exercised to assure the relatively stiff tip of the balloon catheter does not engage a small lateral branch vessel or dissect the wall of the coronary sinus before balloon

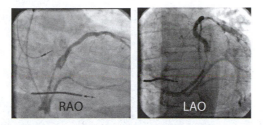

Fig. 5.8 RAO and LAO images of a coronary sinus occlusive venogram demonstrating a near parallel orientation of a lateral venous branch that originates close to the ostium of the coronary sinus (seen best in the LAO projection).

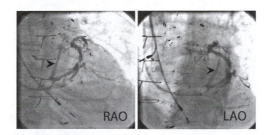

Fig. 5.9 RAO and LAO images of a coronary sinus occlusive venogram in a post-operative patient demonstrating a large vein of Marshall (arrow) that could have easily been mistaken for the true coronary sinus. Note the complex lateral venous anatomy. Successful lead implantation was achieved in a lateral venous branch.

inflation. This is accomplished by injecting a small 0.5–1 cc contrast injection prior to balloon inflation to assure the body of the balloon catheter is free in the lumen of the coronary sinus. Careful inflation of the balloon catheter with 1.0–1.5 cc of air is then performed. Distal injection of approximately 5–8 cc of contrast (typically diluted with 50% saline first to spare dye load) is gently but rapidly injected distal to the balloon to retrogradely fill the coronary venous branches. Coronary vein cineangiograms are then obtained in the RAO and LAO projections and stored for later recall. Review of these images permits selection of vessels of adequate caliber and orientation to accommodate the left ventricular lead. Vessels that are as lateral as possible from the interventricular septum are ideal for implantation.

Special Consideration: What to Do When No Lateral Venous Branch is Identified

In some cases, identification of a lateral venous branch in which to place a left ventricular lead is not immediately visualized. Most commonly, this is because either an insufficient mount of dye retrogradely filled all venous branches due to poor balloon occlusion, the balloon itself occluded the proximal aspect of an eligible lateral vessel, or another more proximal branch was not visualized due to distal balloon or angiographic catheter placement. In these cases, withdrawing the sheath to the ostium of the coronary sinus and performing a hand injection at this location will often identify a vessel supplying the lateral wall when none was previously seen.

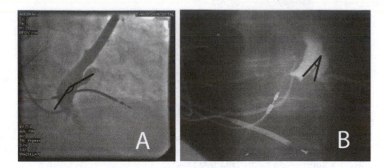

Fig. 5.10 An example of an obtusely angled coronary sinus venous branch (**Panel A**) and an acutely angled (and more challenging) venous branch. Note the black angle symbols were added for effect.

Placement of the Left Ventricular Lead

Once the appropriate target vessel for left ventricular lead implantation is identified, the balloon-tipped catheter is removed and replaced with an appropriate left ventricular lead. Most LV leads come in a shorter (typically 75–78 cm) length or longer (85–88 cm) length. Implants via the right axillary or subclavian approaches often accommodate the shorter lead length, while implants procedures via the left axillary or subclavian approaches might require longer lead lengths especially if anterolateral lead implant locations are required. *The longer leads are always required if it is anticipated that a dual slittable sheath approach (see below) is required.*

Venous branches arise at varying angulations to the plane of the main coronary sinus body. Typically more obtusely-angled vessels provide easier implant targets than those that are acutely angled. (Fig. 5.10) Leads can be manipulated into obliquely-angled vessels using a stylet-driven approach or an over-the-wire approach. The availability of over-the-wire implant leads have greatly facilitated placement of the lead tip into secondary branches of the targeted vessel. This can be particularly important when attempting to avoid phrenic nerve or direct diaphragmatic stimulation.

Special Considerations: Acutely Angled Coronary Sinus Branches

By far an away, the most consistently challenging left ventricular lead implant cases are those with acutely angled branch vessel origins. Several approaches have been found useful in these circumstances:

Fig. 5.11 (continued) IMA catheter, two 280-cm 0.014 in. Ironman guide wires were passed distally into the targeted branch vessel. The IMA catheter was removed. Panel E: A unipolar LV pacing lead was "back-loaded" and passed over one of the guide wires to the branch vessel. Using the alternate guidewire to straighten the branch vessel, the LV lead could then be manipulated past the branch vessel's origin a fair distance to permit stable lead placement. Panels F and G: Both guide wires were removed after threshold testing demonstrated excellent pacing thresholds and no evidence of extra-cardiac stimulation. RAO (Panel F) and LAO (Panel G) projections of the final lead placement is demonstrated.

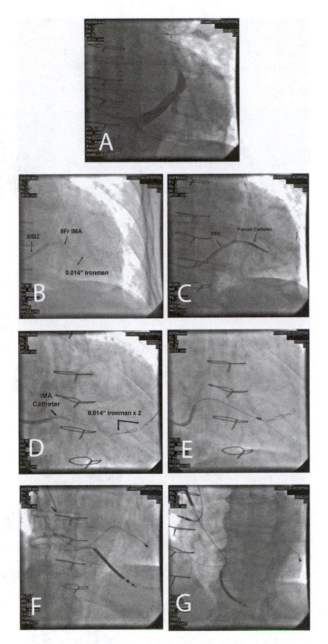

Fig. 5.11 Use of a "Buddy Wire" Approach for LV Lead Implantation in an Acutely Angled Coronary Sinus Venous Branch. Panel A: A non-occlusive venogram through a JR4 catheter (not seen) demonstrating the acutely angled nature of the target vessel. Panel B: A 5Fr internal mammary artery (IMA) diagnostic catheter was used to sub-select the acutely angled branch vessel from within the coronary sinus. Initially, a single 0.014 in. exchange-length (280 cm) Ironman (Guidant) guide wire was passed distally into the targeted vessel. The IMA catheter was then removed and a 4Fr unipolar lead passed over the guide wire but could not be negotiated past the origin of the branch vessel. Panel C: The LV lead was removed (but the guide wire retained) and an Attain Prevail catheter was passed over the 0.014 in. guide wire in hopes of straightening the branch vessel to permit the long sheath to sub-select the branch vessel. This was unsuccessful. Panel D: Next, the original Ironman guide wire was removed, and the IMA catheter again used to engage the coronary sinus branch vessel. Through the

(legend continues on preceding page)

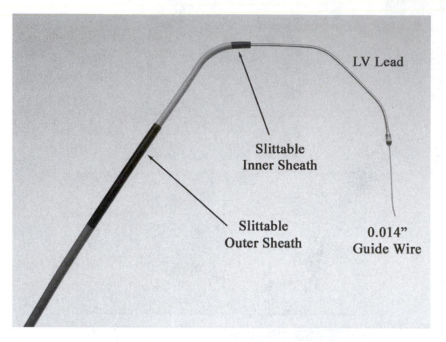

Fig. 5.12 The "Slittable Sheath Within a Slittable Sheath" System to Place a Left Ventricular Lead Into an Acutely-Angled Branch Vessel. Note that a 7Fr slittable inner sheath is passed through the 9Fr larger slittable sheath. Thorough both, an LV lead is passed, usually over a 0.014 in. guide wire.

1. In some cases, a "buddy wire" approach (Fig. 5.11) with two 0.014 in. guide wires can be used to facilitate lead delivery in acutely angled vessels.
2. Alternatively, an acutely angled lead (such as the Medtronic Model 2187 unipolar lead) might be able to be manipulated into the proximal portion of the CS branch.
3. More recently, a dual slittable sheath strategy has become available that has greatly facilitated the implant process. The outer sheath is a conventional 9Fr outer-diameter slittable sheath, through which is placed a second 7Fr slittable sheath with either a 90° or 130° angled soft tip to engage the target branch vessel. (Fig. 5.12). Once engaged, the LV lead can be easily advanced over a guidewire since acceptable support at the origin of the branch vessel is provided by the inner sheath. (Fig. 5.13 – example). Once positioned, the inner sheath is slit off the lead, followed by the outer sheath, leaving the LV lead seated well within the tortuous branch vessel.

Verification of Left Ventricular Lead Pacing Characteristics

After placing a left ventricular lead as laterally as anatomically feasible from the interventricular septum, pacing thresholds should be evaluated. In newer pacing systems, thresholds of 3.5–5 V at 0.5 ms pulse width are the maximum tolerable one should accept, though. At such threshold levels, extending the pulse width can improve the voltage required to achieve acceptable pacing safety margins, but battery longevity will be adversely affected. Every attempt should be made to also avoid extracardiac stimulation from phrenic nerve stimulation, diaphragmatic pacing, or direct intercostal muscle stimulation.

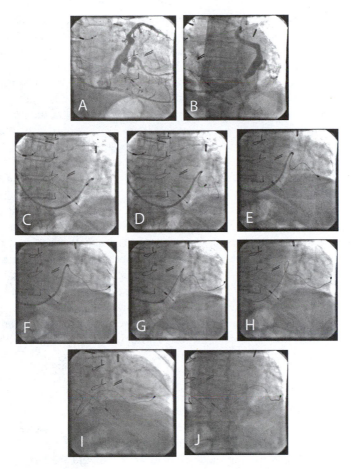

Fig. 5.13 Placement of an LV lead through a very tortuous, acutely angled lateral branc of the coronary sinus. Panels A and B: RAO and LAO images (respectively) of the venous anatomy encountered. Panel C: Using an assembly similar to that seen in Fig. 5.12, the inner sheath is engaged into the branch vessel and position confirmed with a small injection of contrast (1 cc). Panel D: Once in place, a 0.014 in. guidewire was passed distally into the targeted vessel, and the left ventricular pacing lead passed over the guide wire. Panels E and F: Because of initial diaphragmatic stimulation with the lead in a more medial position, the guide wire was repositioned laterally into another portion of the vessel. The lead was then placed laterally with resolution of the diaphragmatic pacing. Acceptable pacing thresholds of 2.5 V at 0.5 ms pulse width were obtained. Panel G: The guide wire was removed and a straight 0.014 in. stylet was passed into the left ventricular lead, but was not advanced passed the origin of the lateral vessel. The inner sheath is then slit off the lead. Panel H: With the straight stylet still within the portion of the left ventricular lead within the body of the coronary sinus, the outer sheath is also slit from the left ventricular lead. Panels I and J: Final fluoroscopic images of the 20° RAO and 25° LAO projections (respectively) demonstrating the final lead length and course of the lateral venous branch.

Special Considerations: Diaphragmatic or Other Extracardiac Stimulation

With transvenous epicardial left ventricular lead implantation, one of the most common reasons a particular implantation is unsuccessful is not the inability to place the lead in an appropriate vessel. Rather, the extracardiac stimulation of structures outside the heart can cause significant discomfort and concern for the patient, and often requires repositioning of the pacing lead. In these cases, even small 0.5 cm movements either distally or proximately of the pacing lead tip within the targeted vessel can have profound differences in extracardiac pacing thresholds. Even so, there are occasional patients where ANY location in a targeted branch vessel can cause extracardiac stimulation, and there is no other option than to attempt implant in another branch vessel. One should attempt to find a location where no extracardiac stimulation occurs at pacing thresholds exceeding the maximum output of the implanted device. In instances where no other pacing location exists, a site with at least a three to one differential between pacing capture threshold and extracardiac stimulation threshold will suffice but require careful programming postoperatively. Unfortunately, because the heart tends to migrate inferiorly within the thorax with upright postures, extracardiac stimulation thresholds often are significantly lower postoperatively in clinical practice than those seen intraoperatively when the patient is in a recumbent position. In very rare cases where no suitable implantable vessel exists, transvenous implant of the left ventricular lead must be abandoned in favor of a transthoracic epicardial approach.

Removal of the Long Vascular Sheath after Left Ventricular Lead Placement

For the implanting surgeon, removal of the long sheath that facilitated delivery of the left ventricular lead to its acceptable branch remains an area for potent psychological and physical disappointment should the left ventricular lead dislodge. Some operators prefer a long sheath that can be manually split and pealed from the LV lead, while others prefer a mechanical slitting (cutting) of the long sheath because they can hold the lead directly within the slitting tool, making adjustments to lead length (if needed) during the slitting process. Irrespective of the removal technique used, several points have proven to minimize dislodgement during long sheath removal:

First, be sure all other required leads are implanted successfully before attempting to remove the long vascular sheath over the left ventricular lead. Placing the left ventricular lead first in patients without left bundle branch block can be accomplished, but the long sheath within the coronary sinus should only be removed after the other leads are implanted to afford a final chance to adjust left ventricular lead length after the implant of the other leads and affords the best chance to maintain left ventricular lead stability following the slitting process.

Secondly, before attempting to remove the long sheath, place a small stylet inside the lead that extends well into the main body of the coronary sinus. This stylet provides support to the long sheath to prevent the sheath from straightening upon leaving the coronary sinus ostium and avoids pulling upon the existing lead.

Thirdly, secure the slitting hand (either against the shoulder or the operator's abdomen) before slitting the long sheath to assure the lead is not dislodged by retraction of the slitting hand during the slitting process. It can be helpful to image the lead during the slitting process to avoid accidental tugging on the LV lead.

After the long sheath is removed, the stylet also must be removed. Not uncommonly, the stylet can also tug on the lead as it retracts proximal to the portion of the lead within the coronary sinus. Also, excessive lead length might coil the lead within the right atrium after the stylet is removed, requiring retraction of the redundant lead before it is drawn into the right ventricle. Careful adjustment of left ventricular lead length (short enough to avoid the redundant lead from being drawn into the right ventricle and long enough to assure adequate CS lead length to assure left ventricular capture) can be made as the stylet is withdrawn if imaged using fluoroscopy.

After the stylet is removed and the left ventricular lead appears stable, securing the lead by tying the lead over its sewing sleeve before other manipulations is also advised.

Conclusions

With careful understanding of the anatomy of the right atrium and coronary sinus, proper preparation of the implanting laboratory, and careful planning of the lead implantation following coronary sinus venography, left ventricular lead implantation success is facilitated. Coronary sinus venography should be routinely considered during the implant process in most cases, due to unexpected anatomic variants, post-operative alterations in underlying anatomy, and for planning alternate pacing sites should the initial targeted vein be unacceptable for lead implantation due to extracardiac stimulation or poor pacing thresholds.

Acknowledgments: The author is forever indebted to his staff in the EP Laboratory at Evanston Hospital, whose patience and tireless devotion to our patients made this manuscript possible. In addition, the expert photography of Jon Hillenbrand of the Multimedia Services Department of Evanston Northwestern Healthcare is greatly appreciated.

References

1. Abraham WT, Fisher WG, Smith AL, et al., Cardiac Resynchronization in Chronic Heart Failure, New Engl J Med 2002; 346:1845–1853.
2. Young JB, Abraham WT, Smith AL, et al., Combined Cardiac Resynchronization and Implantable Cardioversion Defibrillation in Advanced Chronic Heart Failure, JAMA 2003; 289:2685–2694.
3. Bristow MR, Saxon LA, Boehmer J, et al. Cardiac-Resynchronization Therapy with or without an Implantable Defibrillator in Advanced Chronic Heart Failure, New Engl J Med 2004; 350:2140–2150.
4. Cleland JGF, Daubert J-C, Erdmann E, et al. The Effect of Cardiac Resynchronization on Morbidity and Mortality in Heart Failure, New Engl J Med 2005; 352:1539–1549.
5. Gras D, Leon AR, Fisher WG. The Road to Successful CRT Implantation: A Step-by-step Approach. Blackwell Futura 2004.
6. Da Costa A, Kirkorian G, Cucherat M, et al. Antibiotic Prophylaxis for Permanent Pacemaker Implantation: A Meta Analysis, Circulation 1998; 97:1796–1801.

6

Endocardial Lead Extraction

Peter H. Belott

There is an ever-increasing need to manage complications in this era of implantable antiarrhythmic devices. Infections, sepsis, and the threat of mechanical trauma can necessitate partial or complete removal of an antiarrhythmic system, including device and leads. Such removal comes with the potential risk of significant morbidity and even mortality. The management of device complications has become a subspecialty of cardiology and cardiovascular surgery (1–5). It requires special training to acquire the skills for successful results.

Intravascular lead extraction is a relatively new technique in cardiac pacing. With the ever-expanding number of implanted leads and the change in lead requirements resulting from upgraded and incompatible systems, it has become desirable to remove unwanted, abandoned, and malfunctioning leads. Such intravascular "junk" is perceived as a potential cause of increased morbidity from a variety of causes (4,6,7). Increased bulk and unnecessary debris can interfere with valve function, propagate thromboembolisms, and welcome infection. Traditionally, lead extraction has been reserved for life-threatening situations, such as infection and sepsis. This is because the early conventional extraction techniques were potentially dangerous. The challenge is to safely free the lead from encapsulating fibrous scar tissue at fixation sites along venous structures and on the myocardial wall (8,9). Early techniques ranged from simple traction to an open-heart surgical procedure. These methods were associated with significant morbidity and potential mortality (10–13). More recently, safer and more expeditious intravascular tools and techniques have been developed, and the indications for lead extraction are no longer confined to strictly life-threatening mandatory situations. In the past, electrode failure usually involved capping the defunct electrode and introducing a new one. A local retrieval was occasionally required because of infection. Simple traction techniques were generally successful, and only in rare cases was thoracotomy required.

The most primitive and least complicated method of lead removal was simple, gentle traction. If this was unsuccessful, weighted traction was used. An exposed lead was grasped by a hemostat and attached to Buck's traction, which applied continuous traction until the lead fell out of the heart (Fig. 6.1). The weight applied to Buck's traction was increased progressively until premature ventricular contractions occurred. This technique carried the

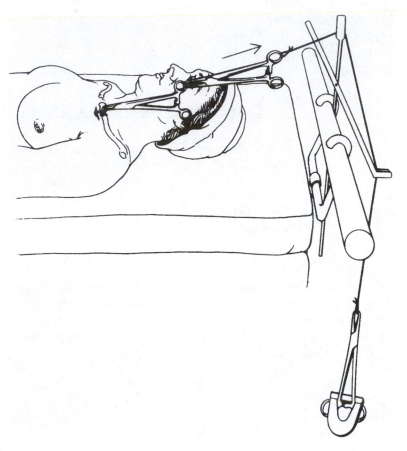

Fig. 6.1 Chronically implanted lead removed by Buck's traction. This is accomplished by slow progressive and gentle traction. The weight is increased progressively over time until the lead is removed. Figure courtesy of Dr S Furman.

risk of life-threatening arrhythmias, eversion of the right ventricular apex, and cardiac tamponade. The sound of the weights crashing to the floor signaled successful lead removal.

Scar tissue formation is directly responsible for the difficulty and morbidity associated with lead extraction (14–16). The difficulty in extraction is further enhanced by the use of passive fixation devices, longer implant durations, and the greater number of leads implanted in any given patient. The passive fixation devices promoted exuberant encapsulating fibrous scar formation at the myocardial electrode interface (Fig. 6.2). Scar tissue forms at the contact sites along vascular walls and, in the case of multiple electrodes, scarring can completely encompass multiple leads. In extreme cases, the scar tissue may completely obliterate the venous channel. One of the most common locations of scar formation is at the lead venous entry site. Leads implanted more than 8 years are the most difficult to remove.

The retrieval of intravascular foreign bodies by transluminal catheter techniques dates back to the 1960s. Portsmann reported in the radiology literature successful removal of a guide string that was literally passed across a

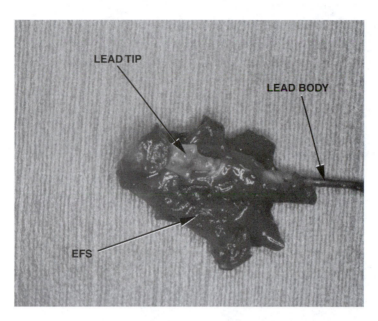

Fig. 6.2 Passive fixation lead tip completely encased in encapsulating fibrous scar. (From Belott PH. *Endocardial lead extraction: A videotape and manual.* Armonk, NY: Futura Publishing, 1998, with permission.)

patient's ductus into the right heart (17). At the same time, Massumi described techniques for removal of broken catheters from within the cardiac cavities (18). In general, early intravascular foreign body retrieval involved the use of wire loop snares, hook-tipped guidewires and catheters, basket retrievers, and grasping forceps. Once again, it is undesirable and next to impossible to remove conventional leads with fixation mechanisms by use of simple traction. This frequently results in uncoiling of the wire and disruption of the insulation. Traction may also result in low-cardiac-output syndromes from traction on the right ventricular apex and cardiac tamponade from tearing of the myocardium.

Charles Byrd is responsible for most of the pioneering work in endocardial lead extraction over the past two decades (19–26). Byrd developed an intravascular extraction system that incorporates telescoping countertraction sheaths. Elongated sheaths that could reach the apex of the right ventricle were passed over the electrode. The lead could be freed up because of the leverage applied by the sheath and direct application of forces at the electrode–myocardial interface. In the case of extreme fibrosis, Byrd developed metal sheaths to strip away densely adherent, encapsulating fibrous scar. An innovative "locking stylet" developed by the Cook Pacemaker Corp. (Cook Vascular, Inc., Beachberg, PA) solved the problem of grasping and supporting a lead without stretching and uncoiling it when retrieving from the implant vein (Fig. 6.3) (27,28). This special stylet is passed to the tip of the lead to be retrieved by counterclockwise rotation of the stylet; a locking mechanism is activated, binding the stylet to the lead coil.

Byrd developed retrieval techniques for removal of the lead via the femoral vein in the case of broken electrodes, free floating in the right heart (29–34). These techniques involve the snaring of the electrode by use of the Masumi

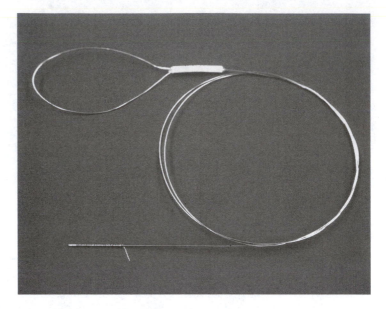

Fig. 6.3 The locking stylet. This is a 60 cm, relatively stiff stylet, with a wire-loop handle and a fine wire wound clockwise at the distal tip. The stylet is advanced to the tip of the lead, where the stylet is locked in place with counterclockwise rotation. (Photograph courtesy of Cook Pacemaker Corp., Beachberg, PA.)

technique and the subsequent application of traction. The femoral retrieval system for free-floating electrodes incorporates a large 16 French long sheath through which the lead is removed. This system is designated the "Byrd Femoral Work Station."

More recently, Byrd, working in collaboration with the Spectronetics Corp., has developed a laser lead extraction system for safer and more expeditious lead retrieval. This section reviews contemporary lead extraction techniques.

Personnel

Endocardial lead extraction poses the risk of vascular catastrophe from multiple points of view. There is a risk of tearing the innominate vein, the superior vena cava, and the right ventricular apex during the process of extracting endocardial leads. The cardiothoracic surgeon ideally manages such vascular catastrophes by immediate thoracotomy. Given this potential, it appears that a cardiac surgeon should be either directly or indirectly involved with every lead extraction. This should not, however, preclude experienced cardiologists from performing lead extractions. Individuals performing lead extractions should have some basic skills in the management of wound complications and infections because lead extractions are frequently associated with some form of wound complication. The individuals should be able to perform wound debridement, pocket revision, and drainage procedures. The assistance of a general surgeon or plastic surgeon may be necessary in the case of large open wounds where skin grafting may be required. It has been proposed that anyone requesting such privileges should have complete rights for permanent pacemaker insertion in an attempt to design privileging criteria for extraction of endocardial pacing and ICD leads. It is also recommended that such a person be experienced in all aspects of cardiac pacing. The individual should demonstrate participation or direct experience with a minimum of 10 pacemaker endocardial lead extractions by the implant vein, including lead identification, preparation, locking stylet application, and countertraction sheath implementation. In addition, the individual should have participated in 10 lead extractions by the femoral approach and should be familiar with the application of the femoral workstation and the use of deflecting wire and assorted snares. In the case of laser endocardial lead extraction, the individual should demonstrate formal in-service in the use of the laser and should have participated in a minimum of two endocardial lead extractions using the laser. Once privileges have been granted for permanent lead extraction, it should be pointed out that there is a certain currency requirement with respect to maintaining competency. The precise annual number of cases to maintain competency has never been addressed because endocardial lead extraction is a relatively new venue in cardiac pacing. Endocardial lead extraction involves every aspect of pacemaker implantation. There is frequently the requirement for temporary pacing once a lead has been retrieved. This is also a requirement for reinsertion of a new lead system and appropriate wound care. An individual performing endocardial lead extraction obviously should demonstrate adequate surgical skills with respect to all modes of venous access, as well as proficiency in postoperative wound care and pacemaker follow-up.

Support Personnel

Endocardial lead extraction is ideally performed in the operating room. The procedure should be performed with a cardiac surgical team as a dedicated support staff for this procedure to avoid inconsistencies (Table 6.1).

Table 6.1 Cardiac surgical team.

Support personnel – operating room
Anesthesiologist
Nursing personnel
Surgical nurse or technician
Circulating nurse or technician
Perfusionist
Radiology technician
Manufacturer's representative
Cardiac surgeon
Support personnel—catheterization laboratory
Cardiovascular technician
Cardiac catheterization nurse
Anesthesiologist
Radiology technician
Heart team
Cardiac surgeon
Manufacturer's representative

Table 6.2 Extraction team.

Cardiovascular technicians

Radiology technicians

Catheterization laboratory nurse

Heart team/perfusionist

Cardiac surgeon

Anesthesiologist

Extraction coordinator

It is frequently desired to perform permanent pacemaker lead extractions in the cardiac catheterization laboratory, where special imaging requirements are necessary. In this case, in addition to the regular staff of the cardiac catheterization laboratory, there is an additional requirement for backup from the cardiothoracic surgical team. Support personnel for endocardial lead extraction, no matter where it is performed, should essentially include an anesthesiologist for delivery of general anesthesia and/or conscious sedation; a registered nurse; a scrub nurse or technician who is familiar with all the needs of any extracting physician; a cardiovascular technician who is familiar with the operation of sophisticated radiologic equipment; and the cardiac surgery team, including staff who are familiar with open-heart surgical procedures. A cardiothoracic surgeon should be immediately available or present when a cardiologist performs the procedure. As a general rule, general anesthesia is used when the procedure is performed in the operating room. It is extremely important to designate one individual from the cardiothoracic surgical team or from the cardiac catheterization laboratory as an "extraction coordinator" who is responsible for the maintenance of the extraction equipment. An extraction procedure can involve the use of multiple disposable extraction tools that must be replaced. The problem of inadequate supplies can be avoided by designating personnel responsible for the extraction supplies and equipment. Nothing is more disconcerting than undertaking an extraction procedure only to find that at a crucial moment the appropriate locking stylet, countertraction sheaths, dilators, and deflecting wires are not available.

It is worthwhile to consider creation of a formal extraction team, considering the complexities and the serious nature of pacemaker and lead extraction (Table 6.2).

Extraction Facility and Required Equipment

There are many who think that endocardial lead extractions should only be performed in an operating room and under general anesthesia. This is because, under these circumstances, such a procedure can be performed safely and expeditiously if a thoracotomy or even circulatory bypass is required. The operating room is ideally suited for such a situation if a more extensive surgical procedure becomes necessary. The ideal location in the operating room is the cardiothoracic surgical suite. The cardiothoracic surgical suite offers optimal hemodynamic monitoring, electrophysiologic equipment, and supplies for cardiothoracic surgery, including appropriate anesthesia machines and bypass equipment.

Endocardial lead extraction can be safely carried out in the cardiac catheterization laboratory. The cardiac catheterization laboratory can prove to be an ideal place for extracting endocardial leads because it offers optimal radiologic capabilities. The high-quality images can facilitate endocardial lead extraction.

The monitoring requirements for endocardial lead extraction are somewhat more demanding than those for a permanent pacemaker procedure. In addition to reliable electrocardiographic monitoring, it is recommended that intra-arterial monitoring also be carried out. This helps to readily detect any sudden change or drop in blood pressure caused by a vascular tear or tamponade.

The surgical instruments for endocardial lead extraction are identical to those for a permanent pacemaker procedure, which merely requires a minor surgical tray with a limited number of instruments. A standard thoracotomy tray should be readily available in addition to a minor surgical set. A pneumatic thoracotomy saw and/or sternotomy saw should be available in the operating room and even in the catheterization laboratory, in case a thoracotomy or sternotomy is required. Unlike the permanent pacemaker procedure, lead extraction should have a source of reliable suction readily available.

Standard two-dimensional and transesophageal echocardiography should also be readily available. Two-dimensional echocardiography can assist in rapid diagnosis of tamponade and assist in the location of a tear. Transesophageal echocardiography can prove invaluable for lead identification and guidance during extraction in a high-risk case of multiple endocardial leads with dense encapsulating fibrous scar.

Even when one is prepared to perform an emergency thoracotomy, precious time can be saved and the patient stabilized by performing an emergency pericardiocentesis. It is recommended that a pericardiocentesis tray also be available in the operating room or catheterization laboratory during an endocardial lead extraction procedure. A checklist of required equipment for endocardial lead extraction is shown in Table 6.3.

Tools of Endocardial Lead Extraction

The tools of endocardial lead extraction have evolved from the crude pulley-and-weight system of Buck's traction to modern excimer laser sheaths. Today, there is a complete armamentarium of tools designed to make endocardial lead extraction safe and expeditious. Each tool has its place and can play an integral part in any challenging lead extraction case.

The common angiographic catheter is an important tool for lead extraction. One such catheter is the common angled pigtail catheter. This catheter can be used to retrieve and position electrodes by the femoral approach. Other catheters used to assist in lead extraction include a right Judkin's coronary catheter, multi-purpose coronary catheter, and Amplatz catheter (Microvena Corp., White Bear Lake, MN). The catheters are usually passed femorally through a sheath.

The common guidewire, in addition to angiographic catheters, is an essential tool for lead extraction. The guidewire can be used in combination with the catheter to form a wire loop to retrieve free ends and free-floating lead remnants. The tip-deflecting guidewire is a special form of guidewire that is passed down a guiding sheath. A screw to a three-ringed handle connects this guidewire. When this is activated, the tip of the deflecting wire becomes hooked, enabling it to grab the pacemaker lead.

Table 6.3 Monitoring, pacemaker/ICD, and surgical instruments for lead extraction.

Physiologic recording and monitoring
Electrocardiographic monitor/oscilloscope
Arterial line
Oximetry
End-expiratory CO_2
Pacemaker and ICD equipment
Pacemaker systems analyzer
Pacemaker/ICD programmers
Miscellaneous pacemaker ICD supplies and spare parts
Surgical instruments
Minor surgical set
Thoracotomy tray
Pneumatic sternal saw
Electrocautery
Drainage system
Pericardiocentesis set
Temporary pacing tray and leads
Special diagnostics
Echocardiography
Transesophageal echocardiography

A variety of snares have been used for endocardial lead extraction. The snare is usually passed down a guiding catheter, which directs it toward the object to be removed. The most common snare consists of a long guidewire, folded in half and passed through a catheter. The Curry snare is an example of such a wire-loop catheter system (Fig. 6.4). The Amplatz gooseneck snare is a variation of the loop snare catheter. The loop of this snare is at a right angle to the guidewire.

The basket retrieval catheter has been used to retrieve endocardial leads. This device was initially developed for urologic use. The Dotter intravascular retriever is an example of such a device (Fig. 6.5). This system consists of a catheter with a helical loop basket and introducer sheath. With this system, the object to be retrieved becomes entangled in the helical basket. There is little or no reversibility once an object is entangled. The Dormia basket may also be used to retrieve free-floating remnants or loose lead ends.

The Needle's Eye snare is a new snare developed by Cook Vascular (Cook Vascular, Inc., Leachburg, PA). This consists of a hoop-shaped loop called the Needle's Eye for grasping and a sliding threader for locking. The Needle's Eye is looped over the lead body to be retrieved. The threader is then passed through the "Needle's Eye." The Needle's Eye and threader are preloaded in a 16 French inner sheath that is passed down the Byrd Femoral Work Station. A handle that extends and retracts the threader controls this system. This system is reversible; objects grabbed by the Needle's Eye can be released by retracting the threader.

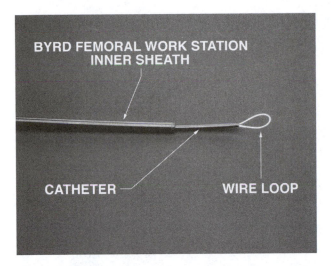

Fig. 6.4 The Curry snare. This is a simple wire loop snare created with use of a guidewire and catheter. The catheter is passed down the inner sheath of a Byrd workstation. (Photograph courtesy of Cook Pacemaker Corp.)

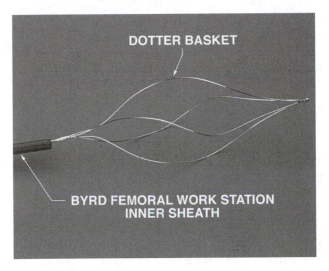

Fig. 6.5 A Dotter retriever consists of a wire basket, which is passed down the Byrd femoral workstation inner sheath. (Photograph courtesy of Cook Pacemaker Corp.)

Grasping forceps have also been used for retrieval of pacemaker leads. An alligator forceps, either 12 or 14 French, is passed down an appropriate-sized sheath. Grasping alligator forceps, similar to those used for rigid bronchoscopy, have also been used. The common myocardial bicep forceps has also been used for retrieval of lead remnants.

The problem of grasping and supporting a lead without stretching or uncoiling during retrieval has been solved with the innovative locking stylet developed by the Cook Pacemaker Corp. This special stylet is passed down the lead coil to the lead tip. The locking mechanism is activated with counterclockwise rotation of the stylet, binding the stylet to the coil. The locking stylet serves to increase tensile strength of the lead and deliver the extraction

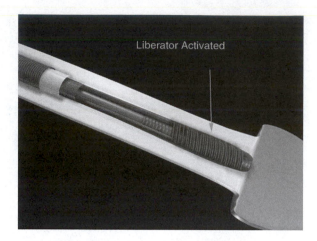

Fig. 6.6 The liberator locking stylet engaging the distal aspect of the inner coil.

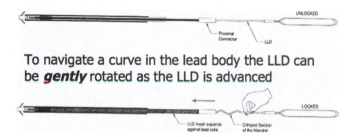

To navigate a curve in the lead body the LLD can be *gently* rotated as the LLD is advanced

Fig. 6.7 The LLD locking stylet within the inner coil of the lead to be extracted.

forces directly to the tip of the lead. The locking stylet functions as a lead extender and handle for the application of traction. The locking mechanism is a small wire attached to the stylet tip. It is wrapped counterclockwise. Counterclockwise motion of the locking stylet causes the small wire to bundle together, binding the stylet to the conductor coil. The locking stylet can be reversed by clockwise rotation.

The locking stylet has continued to evolve; today the original locking stylet has been replaced by the liberator stylet (Cook Vascular, Inc., PA) and the Spectranetics LLD (Colorado Springs, CO). The Liberator locking stylet (Fig. 6.6) uses a spring at the end of the stylet that is compressed, locking it in the lead lumen. The Liberator has the advantage of one size fits all. The Spectranetics LLD locking stylet (Fig. 6.7) uses a wire mesh stretched over a stylet. By expanding, the mesh locks the stylet in the lead lumen. The LLD has the advantage of locking the entire length of the lead to be removed and not just the tip. This gives more support and the lead is less likely to break apart.

Byrd Dilator Sheaths

It is essential that a sheath pass over a lead down to the distal aspect of the electrode when removing a lead via the implant vein. The sheath disrupts the encapsulating fibrous scar at binding sites and ultimately allows for countertraction. Byrd developed telescoping stainless steel sheaths that are

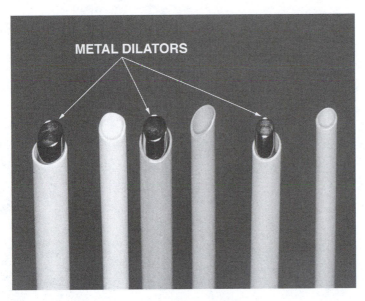

Fig. 6.8 Flexible telescoping sheaths mounted on inner metal dilator sheaths. Sheaths 1, 3, and 5 from the left are seen applied over the metal dilator. (Photograph courtesy of Cook Pacemaker Corp.)

passed over the lead and used to break through the tissue at the venous entry site. The telescoping metal dilators are exchanged for telescoping flexible plastic sheaths once venous entry has been achieved. The initial metal dilating sheaths were long and curved; these have been replaced by shorter, telescoping metal sheaths. The metal sheaths are exchanged for flexible telescoping sheaths. These are used to maneuver around curves and force a way through thick, encapsulating fibrous scar tissue (Fig. 6.8). The flexible sheaths are made of either polypropylene or Teflon.

Powered Sheaths

Powered sheaths have replaced the telescoping metal, polypropylene, and Teflon sheaths. There are now two powered sheaths available for clinical use for lead extraction. Powered sheaths use an energy source to cut through and vaporize the encapsulating fibrous scar that has grown around the endocardial lead. The first commercially available and FDA approved power sheath is the Spectranetics excimer laser sheath. The second and more recently available is the Cook Vascular Electrosurgical Dissection Sheath. The powered sheaths are available in multiple sizes between 12 and 16 French (Fig. 6.9). The power sheaths are also complemented with outer Teflon sheaths for counterpressure and countertraction.

Tools for Lead Preparation

A number of tools are essential when preparing a lead for extraction. There should be a variety of stylets available for sizing and measuring the precise length of the lead to be extracted as well as for assessing patency. In addition,

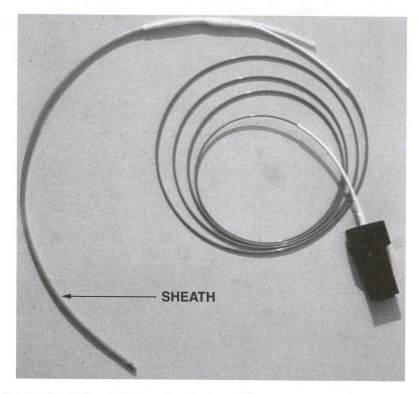

Fig. 6.9 The 12 French Excimer laser lead extraction sheath. (Photograph courtesy of Cook Pacemaker Corp.)

when supporting the electrode, a pair of soft-grip hemostats is required to hold the lead without destroying the inner coil. When a lead is to be extracted, a pair of lead clippers must be available to sacrifice the pin. A coil expander should be available to free the inner coil of wire burs (Fig. 6.10). Selection of the appropriate sized locking stylet is accomplished with a series of gauge pins (Fig. 6.11).

The Byrd Femoral Work Station

The Byrd Femoral Work Station is a special sheath that was developed for retrieving leads by the femoral approach. The sheath can function as an introducer and guide catheter for the manipulation of snares and guidewires. It also functions as a countertraction sheath. The Byrd Femoral Work Station is available as a set consisting of a #18 gauge introducer needle, guidewire, and 16 French workstation with an 11 French tapered dilator and an 11 French telescoping inner sheath, preloaded with a Cook deflecting wire and a Dotter retriever. The deflecting wire is activated by a metal deflecting handle. The Byrd Femoral Work Station is equipped with a check-flow valve for continuous irrigation. Its length is approximately 30 cm.

Indications for Endocardial Lead Extraction

The indications for endocardial lead extraction have increased over the past several years (5, 25,35). It is important to note that previously, there were

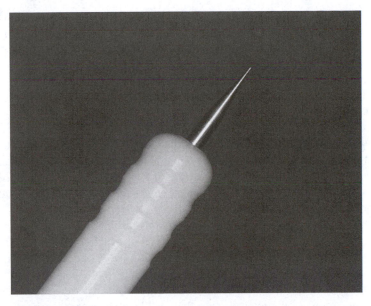

Fig. 6.10 The coil expander. (Photograph courtesy of Cook Pacemaker Corp.)

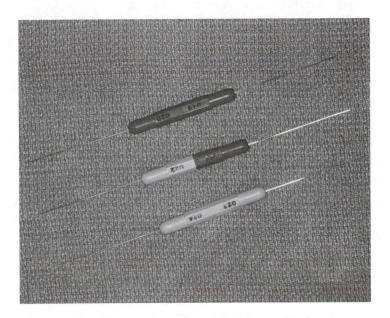

Fig. 6.11 Gauge pins. (Photograph courtesy of Cook Pacemaker Corp.)

no formal American College of Cardiology or American Heart Association guidelines for the extraction of endocardial leads. Initially, the only indications for lead extraction were life-threatening situations, such as septicemia. Today, leads are extracted for a variety of reasons. Byrd has proposed three broad categories or conditions for endocardial lead extraction: mandatory, necessary, and discretionary.

Mandatory indications mean that a lead must be removed. Generally, this is because of a life-threatening or disabling situation. Septicemia and endocarditis are mandatory conditions for lead removal. The migration of a lead remnant resulting in life-threatening arrhythmias and/or embolization is another example of a mandatory indication. Lead perforation also constitutes a mandatory indication for lead extraction. Other mandatory indications include the obliteration of all usable veins, broken or free-floating lead remnants, and trauma to a lead vein site. More recently, device–device interactions resulting in interference have represented a mandatory indication.

Necessary conditions comprise the second broad category of endocardial lead removal indications. These generally represent situations in which a lead is removed to directly prevent the development of a potential life-threatening problem. Examples of necessary indications are pacemaker pocket infection, chronic draining sinuses, erosions, venous thromboses, lead migration, device–device interference, and the necessity for lead replacement in the case of supernumerary leads in the setting of venous thrombosis.

Discretionary indications represent situations in which it is preferable that a lead be removed but the actual removal is not a medical necessity. Examples of discretionary indications or conditions include pain at a pacing site, malignancy, and lead replacement. Today, with increasing experience, experts are extracting more discretionary leads that would otherwise have been abandoned. These are leads that are not routinely extracted, that are not infected and that have been in place for more than 10 years.

In 1998, the north American Society of Pacing and Electrophysiology (NASPE), now the Heart Rhythm Society (HRS), convened a policy conference that confirmed the Byrd clinical indication scheme. This scheme has evolved into the familiar three classes of categories (Table 6.4). The policy conference recommendations for extraction of chronically implanted pacing and defibrillator leads with respect to indications, training, and facilities were formerly published in 2000 (36).

Preparation

Preparation is an important part of any endocardial lead extraction procedure. Because there are many components of an extraction procedure that must be prearranged, it is extremely helpful to establish a checklist. The procedure is either scheduled in the cardiac catheterization laboratory or in the open-heart room in the OR. If it is scheduled in the cardiac catheterization laboratory, the open-heart room should be scheduled for standby. The thoracic surgical backup should also be set up. In addition, as the case should always have an anesthetist, anesthesiology arrangements must be made for an anesthetist to be present for the procedure. Arrangements must also be made for all of the tools and equipments for extraction. All of the manufacturer's representatives that will be involved in the case must also be scheduled. The pericardiocentesis tray, pneumatic sternal saw, and temporary transvenous pacing tray must be available. The equipment for physiologic recording and monitoring must be in readiness and ordered. This also includes the pacemaker system analyzer, the pacemaker, and ICD programmers as well as all of the miscellaneous spare pacemaker and ICD supplies and spare parts. Special diagnostics, such as transesophageal echocardiography, need to be prearranged. Since there are many components of an extraction procedure that must be prearranged, it would be extremely helpful to establish a formal checklist. Such a checklist is shown in Table 6.5.

Table 6.4 Indications for lead removal using transvenous techniques.

Class I (conditions for which there is general agreement that leads should be removed)

   a. Sepsis (including endocarditis) as a result of documented infection of any intravascular part of the pacing system, or as a result of a pacemaker pocket infection when the intravascular portion of the lead system cannot be aseptically separated from the pocket

   b. Life-threatening arrhythmias secondary to a retained lead fragment

   c. A retained lead, lead fragment, or extraction hardware that poses an immediate or imminent physical threat to the patient

   d. Clinically significant thromboembolic events caused by a retained lead or lead fragment

   e. Obliteration or occlusion of all useable veins with the need to implant a new transvenous pacing system

   f. A lead that interferes with the operation of another implanted device (e.g., pacemaker or defibrillator)

Class II (conditions for which leads are often removed, but there is some divergence of opinion with respect to the benefit versus risk of removal)

   a. Localized pocket infection, erosion, or chronic draining sinus that does not involve the transvenous portion of the lead system, when the lead can be cut through a clean incision that is totally separate from the infected area.[a]

   b. An occult infection for which no source can be found, and for which the pacing system is suspected

   c. Chronic pain at the pocket or lead insertion site that causes significant discomfort for the patient, is not manageable by medical or surgical technique without lead removal, and for which there is no acceptable alternative

   d. A lead that, due to its design or its failure, may pose a threat to the patient, though is not immediate or imminent if left in place

   e. A lead that interferes with the treatment of a malignancy

   f. A traumatic injury to the entry site of the lead for which the lead may interfere with reconstruction or the site

   g. Leads preventing access to the venous circulation for newly required implantable devices

   h. Nonfunctional leads in a young patient

Class III (conditions for which there is general agreement that removal of leads is unnecessary)

   a. Any situation where the risk posed by removal of the lead is significantly higher than the benefit of removing the lead

   b. A single nonfunctioning transvenous lead in an older patient

   c. Any normally functioning lead that may be reused at the time of pulse generator replacement, provided the lead has a reliable performance history

[a] The lead can be cut and the incision closed; then the infected area can be opened, the clean distal portion of the lead pulled into the infected area, and that portion removed. This allows a total separation of the retained lead fragment from the infected area.

Lead Extraction

The patient is connected to electrocardiographic monitoring, pulse oximetry, and other monitoring apparatus on arrival to the procedure room. An intra-arterial line is established. Continuous oxygen is administered. If it is determined that a temporary transvenous pacing system is in order, the patient is prepped and

Table 6.5 Lead extraction checklist.

Schedule catheterization laboratory

Schedule operating room standby

Schedule thoracic surgical backup

Arrange anesthesia

Arrange extraction equipment

Manufacturer's representative

Pacemaker ICD programmer and spare parts

Pericardiocentesis tray

Consider temporary pacing

Consider arterial line

draped either about the right groin or right supraclavicular area. Using the Seldinger sheath-set technique, a temporary transvenous electrode can be expeditiously placed. The patient should be prepped and shaved in anticipation of a potential thoracotomy. The prep should start at the angle of the jaw and include the neck, thorax, and abdomen, and extend to the midthigh bilaterally.

Anatomic Approach

There are three fundamental anatomic approaches for lead extraction (23,24,37). The first is retrieval by the implant vein, frequently called the superior approach. This approach can include simple traction, Buck's traction, the use of locking stylets with traction, or the use of locking stylets with countertraction sheaths. The second approach is transfemoral, frequently called the inferior approach. This approach may involve several distinct techniques. When this involves entangling a lead with a pigtail catheter, the catheter is passed from below. When free open ends present themselves, a wire-loop system may be used with traction. Both the Dotter retriever and Dormia basket may also be applied for traction from below. Finally, the lead to be removed may be extracted by the Byrd Femoral Work Station with the use of a combination of snares and wire loops. The third and final approach is retrieval of leads by a limited thoracotomy.

Extraction Using the Implant Vein

Lead Preparation

After this site has been appropriately draped and prepped, the patient's pacemaker and/or ICD pocket is opened with a scalpel. The pulse generator is exposed, freed up, and disconnected from the lead system. All sutures or tie-down materials should be removed and the leads freed of all encapsulating fibrous scar. Once totally freed up, the leads are again identified. Model and serial numbers are recorded. The dissection should be carried down to the venous entry point. At this location, it is recommended that a figure-of-eight stitch be placed about the leads at the venous entry site. This serves for hemostasis after the leads are removed. The leads are then checked for patency with the passage of a standard stylet. This stylet can also gauge the length to the distal tip and the distance to

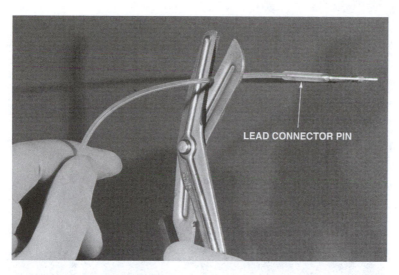

Fig. 6.12 The lead connector pin is sacrificed using the lead clippers. (Photograph courtesy of Cook Pacemaker Corp.)

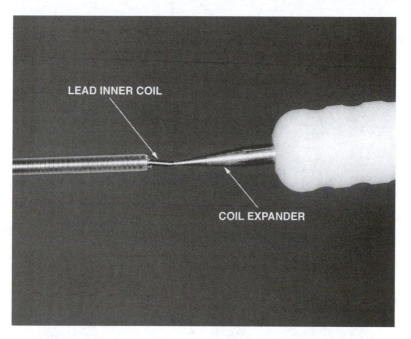

Fig. 6.13 The lead inner coil is freed of wire burs with the coil expander. (Photograph courtesy of Cook Pacemaker Corp.)

any obstruction. The proximal pin of the lead to be removed is sacrificed and the insulation removed, exposing 1 cm of coil (Fig. 6.12). The coil expander is used to free the inner coil of any wire burs and ensure luminal patency (Fig. 6.13). In the case of a bipolar coaxial lead, the outer insulation must be stripped, the outer or anodal coil unwound and cut free for a short segment, and the inner insulation must be stripped to expose the inner coil. The lead is continuously supported

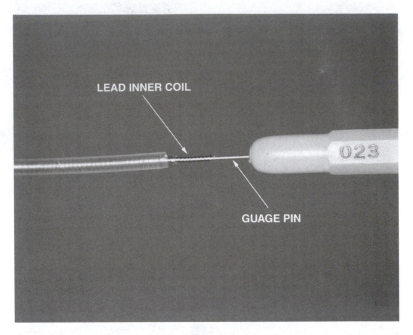

Fig. 6.14 The lead inner coil is sized with a gauge pin, in this case a 0.023-gauge pin has been selected. (Photograph courtesy of Cook Pacemaker Corp.)

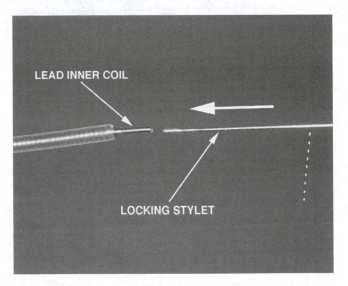

Fig. 6.15 A locking stylet is inserted into the lead inner coil. (Photograph courtesy of Cook Pacemaker Corp.)

with a soft-grip hemostat. The inner coil is then sized by the use of the gauge pins for the selection of the appropriate locking stylet (Fig. 6.14).

After the lead has been sized and the appropriate locking stylet selected, the locking stylet is then advanced down the inner coil (Fig. 6.15). Successful distal locking of the locking stylet can be frustrating at times. Once the locking stylet has reached the distal tip, the stylet is rotated counterclockwise multiple times to engage the locking mechanism (Fig. 6.16). After successful engagement

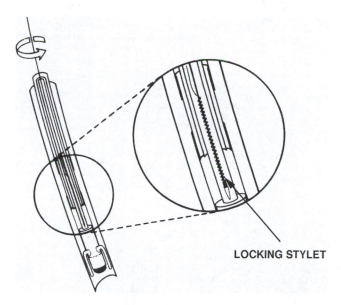

LOCKING STYLET

Fig. 6.16 The locking stylet engaging the lead by counterclockwise rotation. The insert shows the fine-coiled wire at the tip of the locking stylet. (From Belott PH, Byrd CL. Recent developments in pacemaker and lead retrieval. In: Belott PH. *New perspectives in cardiac pacing implantation techniques,* 2nd ed. Armonk, NY: Futura Publishing, 1991, with permission.)

of the locking stylet, a tie is applied to the proximal aspect of the outer insulation. The tie serves to support the outer insulation during advancement of the sheaths. Occasionally, with simple traction, a lead may be pulled free and completely removed from the venous system using the locking stylet alone. If any resistance is encountered, the operator should stop and prepare to apply the sheaths.

Sheath Application

The application of a sheath over the lead is essential for applying countertraction. Counterpressure is the pressure applied by the sheath to tissue at a binding site. The tissue resistance counters this. The tissue resistance countering this pressure is a combination of the strength of the encapsulating fibrous scar tissue binding the lead and the strength of the vascular structure. Once the lead is supported with the locking stylet for countertraction, the stainless steel sheaths are applied. Telescoping stainless steel sheaths are passed over the lead and advanced to the venous entry site; they are used only to break through the encapsulating fibrous scar tissue and to just enter the vein (Fig. 6.17). Once in the vein, the sheaths are exchanged for the more flexible plastic sheaths. Only the plastic sheath is advanced farther into the venous system (Fig. 6.18). With continuous traction applied to the locking stylet, the flexible telescoping sheaths are maneuvered around curves, forcing their way through encapsulating fibrous scar tissue toward the distal tip of the lead. It is important to apply continuous traction on the locking stylet. This avoids the creation of a false passage by the sheath or inadvertent puncture of the superior vena cava or innominate vein (Fig. 6.19). Continuous fluoroscopic visualization is imperative. By use of counterpressure and countertraction, the lead tip is pulled free

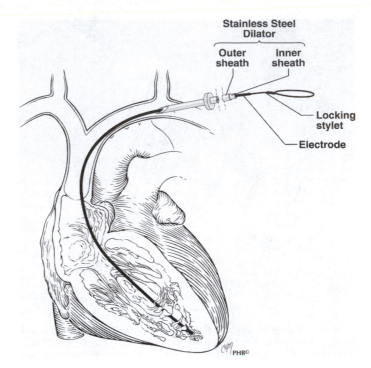

Fig. 6.17 Application of the stainless steel telescoping dilators. (From Belott PH. *Endocardial lead extraction: A videotape and manual*. Armonk, NY: Futura Publishing, 1998, with permission.)

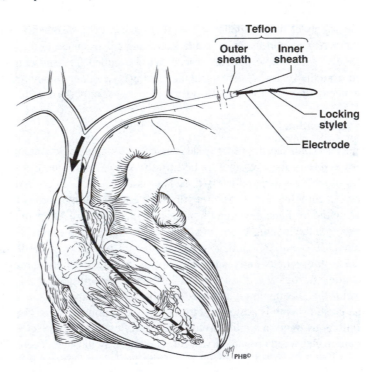

Fig. 6.18 The stainless steel sheaths have been exchanged for the flexible Teflon sheaths, which are advanced over the lead. (From Belott PH. *Endocardial lead extraction: A videotape and manual*. Armonk, NY: Futura Publishing, 1998, with permission.)

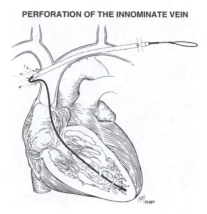

PERFORATION OF THE INNOMINATE VEIN

Fig. 6.19 Catastrophic puncture of the superior vena cava owing to inadequate continuous traction on the lead and locking stylet while advancing the flexible sheaths. (From Belott PH. *Endocardial lead extraction: A videotape and manual*. Armonk, NY: Futura Publishing, 1998, with permission.)

and removed from the central circulation (Fig. 6.20). If, after successful application of the telescoping sheaths, the lead fails to free up, it may be necessary to abandon this approach for an alternate method of extraction.

Extraction Using the Femoral Vein

Extraction using the femoral vein is a much more versatile approach. In reality, extraction via the femoral vein may be used as a primary approach and is the procedure of choice for extraction of broken or cut leads that are free-floating in the venous system, heart, or pulmonary artery. It is also the technique of choice in situations of grossly contaminated venous entry sites where there is risk of pushing contaminated debris into the central circulation by the superior approach. There are a variety of techniques for extracting leads by the femoral vein approach (Table 6.6).

Extraction via the femoral vein uses two fundamental extraction principles. First, wire loops are used to gently snare free ends or a looped lead. Second, if there are no free ends to snare, techniques have to be employed to create a loop around the lead that must be removed. One of the early methods of extracting leads via the femoral approach used a Dotter retriever and pigtail catheter (35,38–41). The pigtail catheter is advanced via the femoral vein to the heart. The pigtail catheter is used to grab the lead. The pigtail catheter is rotated multiple times until it is securely entwined around the pacing lead (Fig. 6.21). Once the pacing lead is entwined in the pigtail catheter, traction is applied to pull it from the heart. The pigtail catheter is positioned as close to the lead tip as possible in order to limit stretching, tearing, or uncoiling of the lead. The Dotter retriever may finally be used to grasp the lead in the inferior vena cava and remove it from the central circulation (Fig. 6.22). Once the Dotter retriever has grasped the lead, it is slowly removed by withdrawing the Dotter apparatus through the femoral vein.

There are other approaches that use a variation of this theme; an example is the use of the common wire loop snare (42). This snare may be used to

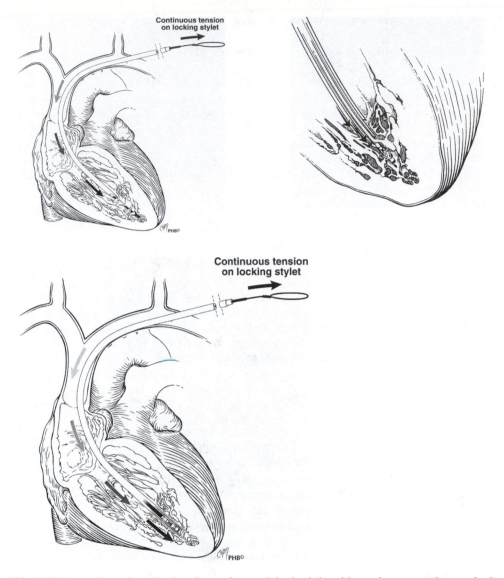

Fig. 6.20 (**a**) Flexion telescoping sheaths advanced toward the lead tip with continuous traction on the locking stylet. (**b**) Close up of advancing telescoping flexible sheaths cutting encapsulating fibrous scar through the lead tip. (**c**) Telescoping sheaths have advanced to the lead tip, with continuous countertraction and counterpressure the lead tip has been pulled into the inner telescoping sheath. (From Belott PH. *Endocardial lead extraction: A videotape and manual.* Armonk, NY: Futura Publishing, 1998, with permission.)

Table 6.6 Femoral lead extraction techniques.

Byrd femoral sheath
Inner sheath plus deflecting wire plus Dotter retriever
Curry snare
Inner sheath plus wire loop
Amplatz snare
Amplatz snare plus deflecting wire
"The Needle's Eye"

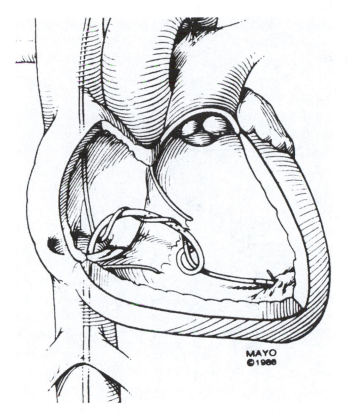

Fig. 6.21 Femoral lead extraction using a pigtail catheter to remove the lead. (From Espinosa RE, Hayes DL, Vlietstra RE, et al. The Dotter retriever and pigtail catheter: efficacy in extraction of chronic transvenous pacemaker leads. *Pacing Clin Electrophysiol* 1993;16(12):2337–2342, with permission.)

grab free ends or knuckles of catheters. Gentle traction is employed to extract the leads via the femoral vein. The most common procedure for extracting leads via the femoral approach is performed by using the Byrd Femoral Work Station. With this system, leads are extracted through a large sheath with the use of a combination of snares. Some operators feel that the femoral approach offers less risk of perforation, innominate vein tear, or right ventricular avulsion. In addition, the operator is always in control with this approach. One of the most important principles to be followed with this approach is reversibility. Whenever a lead is grasped, the potential must exist to reverse the process and release the lead. This is extremely important when working with the Byrd Femoral Work Station. If, through the use of the Byrd Femoral Work Station, a lead or leads are grabbed and the situation cannot be reversed, the only solution is a trip to the operating room and an open chest procedure.

Femoral Lead Extraction: Lead Preparation

Of course, all femoral lead extractions proceed via the superior approach or implant vein. The lead must be prepared in an identical manner as described for extraction via the implant vein. The lead must be dissected free and all tie-downs removed. Once the lead is freed up, some consideration should be given to the application of a locking stylet, even though the lead is to be removed

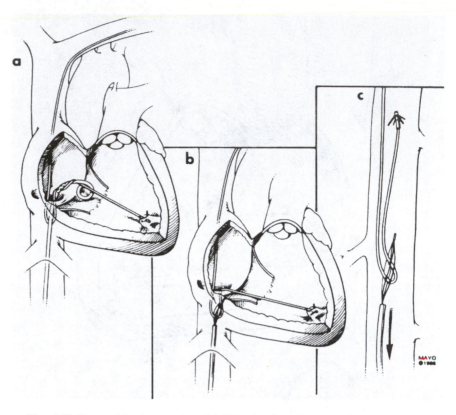

Fig. 6.22 Femoral lead extraction. (**a**) The pigtail catheter entwines the lead to be removed. (**b**) Redundant loop of lead is grabbed with the Dotter retriever. (**c**) The Dotter basket removing the lead by the inferior vena cava. (From Espinosa RE, Hayes DL, Vlietstra RE, et al. The Dotter retriever and pigtail catheter: efficacy in extraction of chronic transvenous pacemaker leads. *Pacing Clin Electrophysiol* 1993;16(12):2337 –2342, with permission.)

from below. The locking stylet can lend support to the lead when countertraction is applied from below.

The Byrd Femoral Work Station

The Byrd Femoral Work Station is a special sheath that has become essential to the removal of leads via the femoral vein. The workstation acts as a countertraction sheath. The femoral workstation consists of a #18 gauge introducer needle, guidewire, 16 French sheath workstation, 11 French tapered dilator, 11 French telescoping sheath, a Cook deflecting snare, and a Dotter basket retriever (Fig. 6.23). The Byrd Femoral Work Station is inserted by using the Seldinger sheath-set technique via the femoral vein (Fig. 6.24). The distal end of the sheath is positioned in the lower right atrium or inferior vena cava. Once positioned, there are several femoral lead extraction techniques that may be employed (Fig. 6.25).

Deflecting Wire and Dotter Retriever

The use of a deflecting wire and Dotter retriever is ideal when the lead to be removed has no free end. This system enables the creation of a loop around the lead to be extracted and, ultimately, retraction of the lead into the femo-

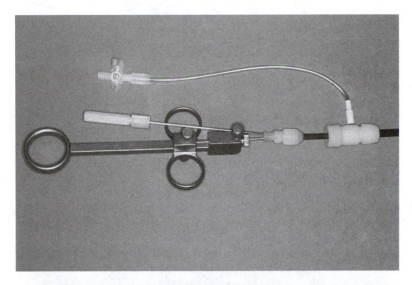

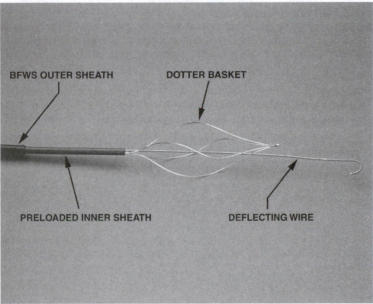

Fig. 6.23 The Byrd Femoral Work Station. (**a**) The sheath is seen with its preloaded inner sheath containing a deflecting wire with wire-deflecting handle and Dotter retriever. The Check-Flo valve and side-port are also shown. (**b**) The distal end of the Byrd Femoral Work Station showing the outer sheath, preloaded inner sheath, Dotter basket, and tip-deflecting wire. (Photographs courtesy of Cook Pacemaker Corp.)

ral workstation. This approach has the potential for irreversibility. The Byrd Femoral Work Station comes prepackaged with an inner sheath that is preloaded with the deflecting wire and the Dotter retriever. The preloaded inner sheath with Dotter and deflecting wire is advanced down the femoral workstation. The deflecting handle is attached to the proximal end of the deflecting wire. The lead to be removed is encircled by the deflecting wire (Fig. 6.26). The Dotter retriever is then advanced to grab the tip of the deflecting wire, thus

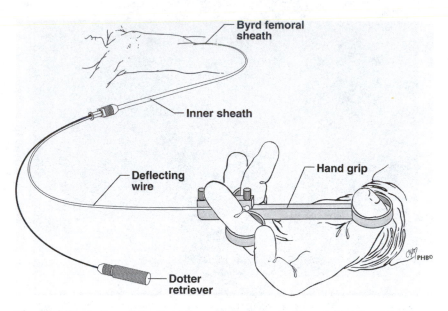

Fig. 6.24 Illustration of the Byrd Femoral Work Station inserted by the right femoral vein. The relationship of the Byrd femoral sheath, preloaded inner sheath with its Dotter retriever, and handle-activated deflecting wire are shown. (From Belott PH. *Endocardial lead extraction: A videotape and manual.* Armonk, NY: Futura Publishing, 1998, with permission.)

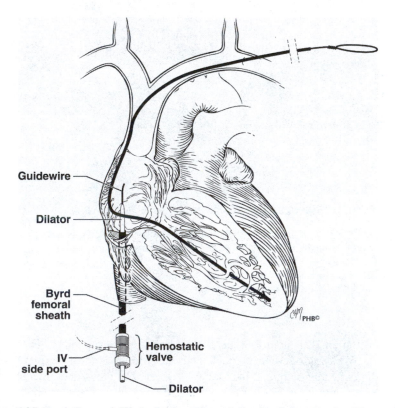

Fig. 6.25 Byrd Femoral Work Station inserted by the femoral vein dilator and guidewire advanced to the right atrium. (From Belott PH. *Endocardial lead extraction: A videotape and manual.* Armonk, NY: Futura Publishing, 1998, with permission.)

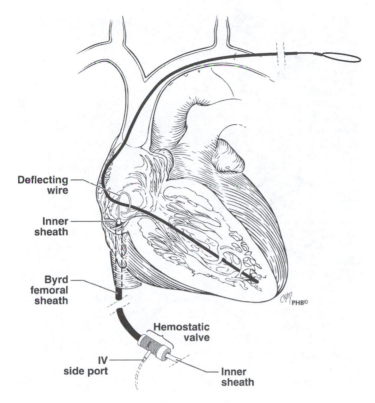

Fig. 6.26 The guidewire and rubber dilator have been removed. The deflecting wire encircles the lead to be removed. (From Belott PH. *Endocardial lead extraction: A videotape and manual*. Armonk, NY: Futura Publishing, 1998, with permission.) 5.27

creating a continuous loop (Fig. 6.27). The deflecting wire grasped by the Dotter basket is then pulled into the Byrd Femoral Work Station. The lead encircled by the deflecting wire and trapped in the mouth of the inner sheath is then retracted into the Byrd Femoral Work Station, pulling the lead with it. With continuous traction on the sheath, the lead is pulled into the worksta-tion. The Byrd Femoral Work Station is advanced over the lead to the lead tip (Fig. 6.28). Using the principles of countertraction and counterpressure, the lead tip is freed from the endocardium and removed femorally through the Byrd Femoral Work Station. The process of grabbing the lead with the deflecting wire may be expedited by bowing the lead into the inferior vena cava (Fig. 6.29). It is important to realize that the Dotter retriever offers the poten-tial for irreversibility. Once the deflecting wire is caught in the apex of the Dotter basket, there is little reversibility. If the lead cannot be pulled free from its encapsulating fibrous scar tissue and withdrawn into the Byrd Femoral Work Station, release of the loop around the lead and removal of the workstation may prove impossible. Ultimate removal may require an atriotomy.

Curry Wire Loop Snare

The Curry Wire Loop Snare is generally reserved for retrieval of a lead that has a free end (43). These are usually lead remnants that are free-floating in the venous structures, right atrium, and right ventricle. The fundamental

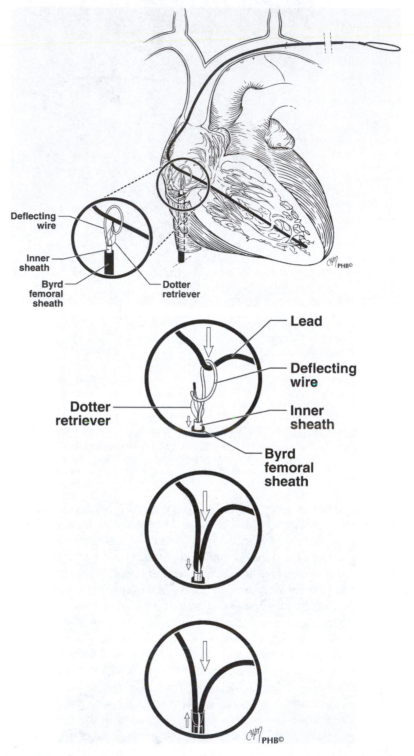

Fig. 6.27 (**a**) The lead to be removed has been grabbed by the deflecting wire and the deflecting wire tip hooked by the Dotter retriever. (**b**) The union of the deflecting wire and Dotter retriever has created the continuous loop. This loop is closed by application of traction to the Dotter retriever and the deflecting wire, thus locking the lead to the tip of the inner sheath. The inner sheath is then retracted into the outer larger sheath of the Byrd Femoral Work Station. (From Belott PH. *Endocardial lead extraction: A videotape and manual*. Armonk, NY: Futura Publishing, 1998, with permission.)

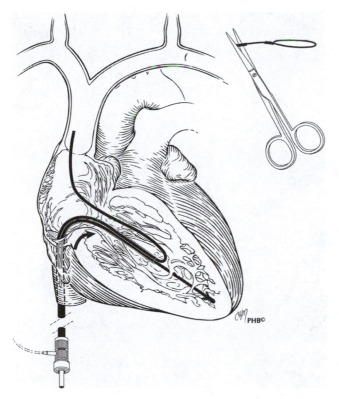

Fig. 6.28 With continuous retraction of the inner sheath into the outer sheath, the outer sheath is advanced over the lead toward the lead tip. The locking stylet has also been cut free proximally. (From Belott PH. *Endocardial lead extraction: A videotape and manual*. Armonk, NY: Futura Publishing, 1998, with permission.)

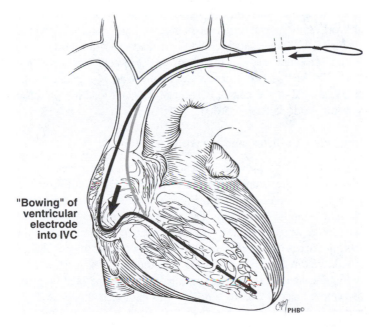

"Bowing" of
ventricular
electrode
into IVC

Fig. 6.29 With locking stylet in place, the lead is advanced and bowed into the inferior vena cava. This facilitates grabbing the lead with the deflecting wire. (From Belott PH. *Endocardial lead extraction: A videotape and manual*. Armonk, NY: Futura Publishing, 1998, with permission.)

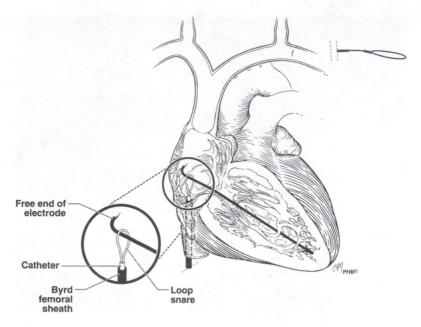

Fig. 6.30 The Curry wire loop encircling the free end of an electrode. (From Belott PH. *Endocardial lead extraction: A videotape and manual.* Armonk, NY: Futura Publishing, 1998, with permission.)

wire loop consists of a large end-hole catheter through which a folded long exchange wire has been passed, creating a loop at the distal end. The Curry snare is no more than a prepackaged catheter-and-wire-loop system.

If a free end is encountered, the wire loop snare is passed down the Byrd Femoral Work Station. The wire loop is enlarged and manipulated around the free end (Fig. 6.30). Once the free end is grasped, the wire loop is closed and the free end retracted into the mouth of the catheter, locking it into place (Fig. 6.31). The lead is held tight by the application of a clamp to the wires at the proximal end of the catheter. The catheter and lead are pulled into the Byrd Femoral Work Station.

Deflecting Wire, Catheter, and the Amplatz Snare

A variation on the two previously described themes involves the use of a deflecting wire and the Amplatz gooseneck snare (44,45). The Amplatz snare, when used in combination with a 6 French catheter, can grasp free-floating lead ends. The Amplatz snare may also be used in combination with a deflecting wire to create a reversible loop around the lead to be removed. In this case, the deflecting wire is removed from its prepackaged inner sheath and is passed separately down the Byrd Femoral Work Station (Fig. 6.32). After application of the deflecting handle, the deflecting handle grasps the lead body as previously described. Once the deflecting wire has encircled the lead, an Amplatz snare loaded in its 6 French catheter is advanced to just beneath the deflecting wire. The Amplatz gooseneck snare is then used to grasp the tip of the deflecting wire (Fig. 6.33). At this point, the loop is closed and the tip of the deflecting wire held tightly (Fig. 6.34). The proximal end of the deflecting

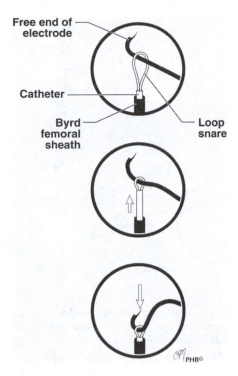

Fig. 6.31 The wire loop has encircled the lead. The loop is closed and the lead bound to the catheter. The catheter is then withdrawn to the Byrd Femoral Work Station. With continuous traction, the sheath is advanced over the lead all the way to the lead tip, freeing it from the endocardial attachment. (From Belott PH. *Endocardial lead extraction: A videotape and manual*. Armonk, NY: Futura Publishing, 1998, with permission.)

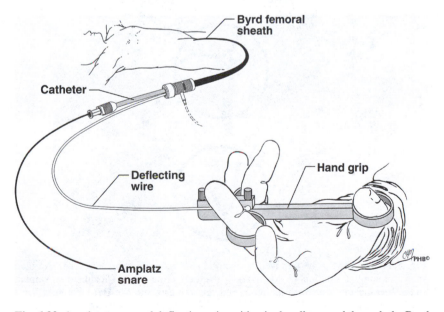

Fig. 6.32 Amplatz snare and deflecting wire with wire handle passed through the Byrd Femoral Work Station. (From Belott PH. *Endocardial lead extraction: A videotape and manual*. Armonk, NY: Futura Publishing, 1998, with permission.)

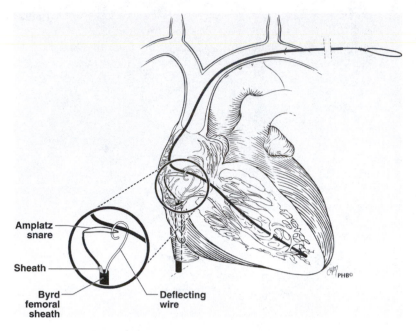

Fig. 6.33 The deflecting wire has encircled the lead. The Amplatz gooseneck snare then snares the deflecting wire. (From Belott PH. *Endocardial lead extraction: A videotape and manual.* Armonk, NY: Futura Publishing, 1998, with permission.)

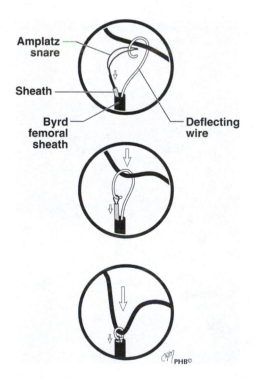

Fig. 6.34 The lead to be removed is encircled by the deflecting wire. The Amplatz snare, creating a continuous loop, grabs the deflecting wire. Closing the Amplatz snare, locking the loop with a clamp, and retracting it into the Byrd Femoral Work Station closes the loop. The Byrd Femoral Work Station is advanced over the lead all the way to the lead tip, freeing it from the endocardial attachment. (From Belott PH. *Endocardial lead extraction: A videotape and manual.* Armonk, NY: Futura Publishing, 1998, with permission.)

wire is then pushed forward, creating a large loop while the Amplatz snare is retracted. The Amplatz-snare-deflecting-wire junction is retracted into the Byrd Femoral Work Station. The deflecting-wire-Amplatz-snare junction is positioned in the middle of the Byrd Femoral Work Station. With this junction in the middle of the Byrd Femoral Work Station, optimal reversibility is achieved, as only the release of the Amplatz snare is necessary to free the deflecting wire. Once the loop has been created, it is closed by application of simultaneous traction on the deflecting wire and Amplatz snare catheter, which pulls the lead into the Byrd Femoral Work Station. The Byrd Femoral Work Station is advanced to the lead tip using the principles of countertraction and counterpressure. This system offers optimum reversibility.

The Needle's Eye

Cook Pacemaker Corp. has developed the Needle's Eye in an attempt to facilitate grasping and locking leads to be retrieved. This system offers total reversibility. The system consists of a catheter that is preloaded with a large curved loop for grabbing the lead and an elongated, narrow loop or tongue called the Needle's Eye. When used in combination, the loop grasps the lead and the Needle's Eye locks it to the base of the catheter. This system is controlled with a handle that extends and retracts the loop in the Needle's Eye for locking. The preloaded Needle's Eye catheter is used with the Byrd Femoral Work Station. The Needle's Eye catheter is passed down the femoral work-station. The Needle's Eye loop is extended to grasp the lead (Fig. 6.35). Once the loop is created, the Needle's Eye is extended through the loop and lead. The loop is then closed, locking the

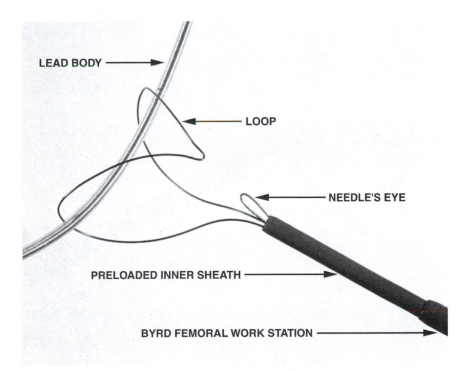

Fig. 6.35 The Needle's Eye. The Needle's Eye loop is extended around the lead to be removed. (Photograph courtesy of Cook Pacemaker Corp.)

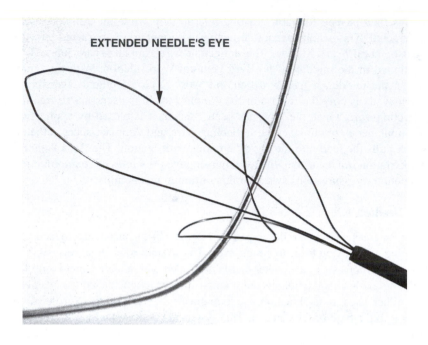

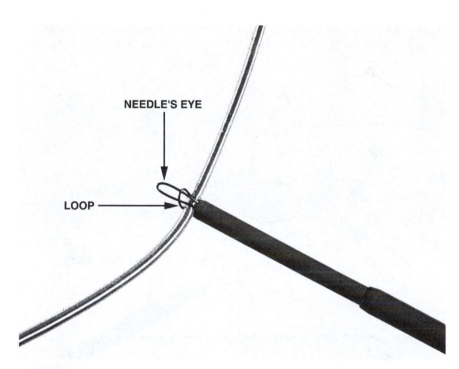

Fig. 6.36 (**a**) Extended Needle's Eye. (**b**) Needle's Eye loop closed, locking the lead tip to the catheter. (Photographs courtesy of Cook Pacemaker Corp.)

lead to the catheter tip (Fig. 6.36). The Needle's Eye may be extended and the bond released if reversibility is required. Once grasped, the catheter and lead are retracted into the Byrd Femoral Work Station. The workstation is then advanced once again. The Byrd Femoral Work Station is advanced to the lead tip using the principles of both countertraction and counterpressure.

Extraction Using a Limited Thoracotomy

Transatrial Approach

A limited thoracotomy should be considered if both the superior (implant vein) and inferior (femoral) approaches fail to extract the lead. In 1985, Byrd and associates described a limited surgical approach for extracting chronic pacing leads that were unsuccessfully removed by transvenous techniques (46). A limited thoracotomy with low morbidity has been developed that totally avoids an extensive thoracotomy, as well as median sternotomy. This approach generally has been used as a primary approach in patients with uninfected lead systems that require removal. The transatrial approach allows for removal of leads that are inaccessible by the superior vena cava or inferior vena cava approach. This approach also affords ease of replacement of endocardial lead systems by the same technique. This is why it is most amenable to patients who are not infected. The transatrial approach with a limited thoracotomy has also been used for replacement of endocardial lead systems when all available veins have been obliterated after a superior vena caval or inferior vena caval extraction procedure.

The transatrial approach involves the removal of the third or fourth right costal cartilage. The pericardium is visualized, exposed, opened, and suspended. A purse-string suture is placed on the right atrium. The right atrium is opened and, using fluoroscopy, the lead body is grasped with a surgical instrument in most instances. The lead body is grasped and the lead is pulled free (Fig. 6.37). The proximal aspect of the lead is cut and then gently extracted by traction through the implant vein. In the case of extremely dense encapsulating fibrous scar tissue, the use of a locking stylet and countertraction sheath may be required. Once again, the principles of counterpressure and countertraction are used. The transatrial approach with limited thoracotomy should also be considered in the presence of large vegetations that are connected to the endocardial leads to be removed. Standard use of traction and sheaths will shear the vegetations free and cause a large pulmonary embolus. It should be pointed out that the transatrial approach with limited thoracotomy usually requires some form of pericardial drainage as well as insertion of a chest tube. At the end of the case, the atriotomy incision is closed with a purse-string suture.

Use of Powered Sheaths for Lead Extraction

Excimer Laser Lead Extraction

The excimer laser now has a lead extraction application (47–54). This laser, which once held much promise in angioplasty, is now used in endocardial lead extraction. Byrd, working with Spectranetics, developed a laser sheath to assist lead removal. The sheath was designed to work in conjunction with the Spectranetics CVX-300 excimer laser system (Fig. 6.38). The laser sheath consists of circumferentially arranged laser fiber bundles (Fig. 6.39).

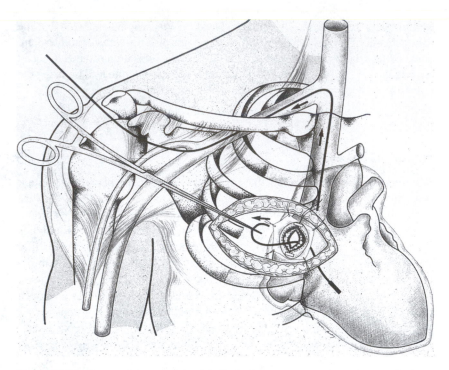

Fig. 6.37 The transatrial approach with limited thoracotomy. An atriotomy incision is made. For an atrial lead, the entire lead is removed retrograde. The ventricular lead is pulled up through the atriotomy with forceps. The lead is grasped and transected. The proximal end is then removed retrograde. A locking stylet is inserted into the remaining distal portion of the lead, which is then removed using the countertraction technique. (From Byrd CL, Schwartz SJ, Sivina M, et al. Technique for the surgical extraction of permanent pacing leads and electrodes. *J Thorac Cardiovasc Surg* 1985;89(1):142–144, with permission.)

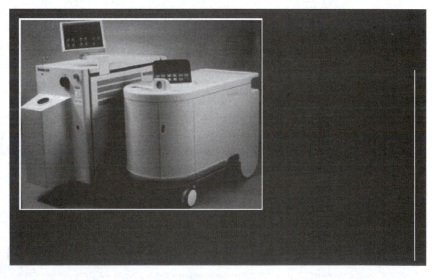

Fig. 6.38 The Spectronetics eximer laser console.

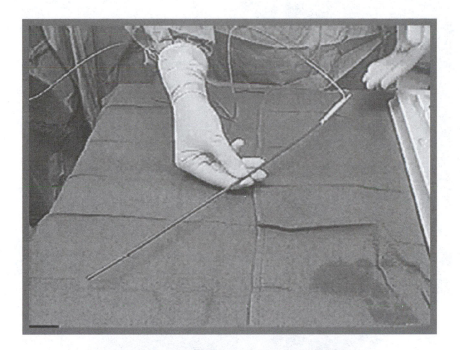

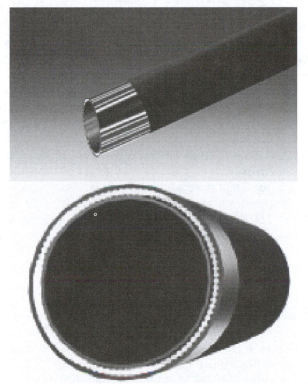

Fig. 6.39 (**a**) The excimer laser sheath. (**b**) The tip of the laser sheath and cross-sectional view of the laser sheath demonstrating the circumferentially arranged fiber bundles.

(continued)

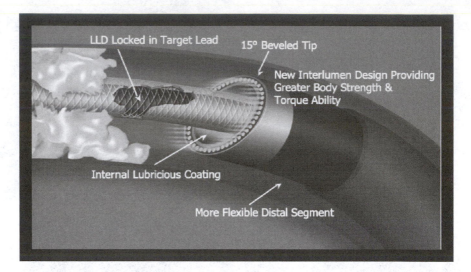

Fig. 6.39 (continued) (**c**) Illustration of the laser sheath passing over the lead and approaching an area of encapsulating fibrous scar. Note the laser sheath is advancing through an outer Teflon sheath. The tip of the laser sheath is beveled 15°. The LLD locking stylet is seen within the lead lumen.

In essence, the laser sheath is passed over the lead intended for extraction. When an obstruction by encapsulating fibrous scar tissue is encountered, pulses of ultraviolet laser light emitted from a ring of optical fibers at the distal tip of the sheath vaporize the encapsulating fibrous scar tissue. The excimer laser was chosen for lead extraction and vaporization of fibrous encapsulating scar because of its extremely short depth of ablation, approximately 50 μm. This laser makes very precise, clean cuts with low lateral tissue damage, charring, and vacuolization. There is very little residual damage to tissue after vaporization. The laser is considered a cool laser because its laser tissue temperature is in the range of approximately 44°C. The excimer laser ablates tissue by using photons of light to disrupt molecular bonds of the tissue, reducing it to a gas and water. It is important to note that the excimer laser has little or no effect on calcified tissue. This is frequently encountered in extremely old lead systems. Today, there are three laser sheaths available, 12, 14, and 16 French. The laser sheath, with its circumferentially arranged fiber bundles, replaces the Byrd telescoping and plastic sheaths. The intention is laser vaporization of fibrous encapsulating scar tissue versus blunt tissue tearing and cutting.

Extraction of leads with use of the excimer laser sheath requires proximal support of the lead to be removed. The identical lead preparation must be carried out as described for extraction by the implant vein. The placement of a locking stylet is preferred. Sometimes a simple tie about the proximal aspect of the lead will suffice because a laser sheath requires very little pressure. This is necessary in the case of damaged leads that fail to accept a locking stylet. Selection of the appropriate laser sheath size requires knowledge of the lead body diameter and tip size. The laser sheath is used with an outer telescoping Teflon sheath. Teflon sheaths assist in cutting and distal counterpressure. After the lead has been prepared and the appropriate laser sheath size selected, the laser sheath is applied to the lead by use of a hook stylet. The hook stylet is used to grab the proximal end of the locking stylet and loop of ligature that is supporting the proximal end of the lead. With traction on the hook stylet, the laser sheath is passed over the proximal aspect of the lead to be extracted. The laser sheath is advanced to the lead venous entry site. The laser sheath is aligned with the lead with the use of fluoroscopy. With gentle countertraction and counterpressure, the laser is activated and the laser sheath advanced. The laser will deliver continuous pulses for 10 s and then shut off automatically. The laser sheath can be observed under continuous fluoroscopy to move slowly forward into the central circulation. Using a process of laser application and sheath advancement with continuous countertraction, the sheath is advanced to the distal lead tip. Once the lead tip is freed up, the laser sheath can be withdrawn into the outer Teflon sheath and removed from the central circulation. The outer Teflon sheath offers an excellent conduit for introduction of a guidewire or, if one so chooses, a second lead. It is recommended that one preplace a large figure-of-eight suture stitch about the lead to be extracted at the venous entry point. Once the leads have been extracted and the sheaths removed, a rather sizable hole is made at the venous entry site that may be anywhere between 12 and 16 French in size. Traction on a preplaced figure-of-eight suture stitch allows for effective hemostasis. The excimer laser sheath appears to have dramatically reduced the time required to extract a lead. In addition, it appears that the lead extraction morbidity and mortality have similarly been reduced.

Electrosurgical (Radiofrequency) Lead Extraction

The electrosurgical technique is identical to the laser technique except for the use of an electrosurgical dissection sheath (EDS). The electrosurgical sheath has two bipolar tungsten electrodes that run the length of the sheath. The electrodes are exposed at the distal end of the sheath (Fig. 6.40). Radiofrequency

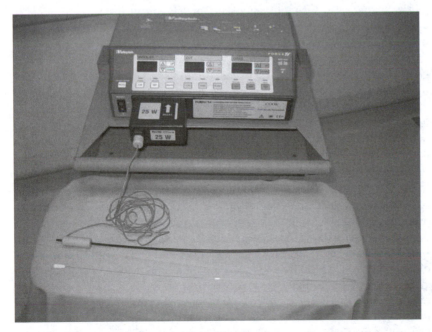

Fig. 6.40 The Valley labs electrocautery unit with the Cook electrosurgical faceplate modification.

energy identical to that used for electrocautery is used to disrupt the encapsulating fibrous scar. The energy is delivered using a modified conventional Valleylab's electrocautery unit (Fig. 6.41). Like the laser sheath, an outer Teflon sheath is used to apply countertraction and counterpressure as the sheath is advanced to the lead tip. The EDS is more supple than the laser sheath, offering greater maneuverability around bends and tortuous veins. It is also felt that the radiofrequency energy allows for more careful dissection of tissue, reducing the risk of vascular injury. An additional important consideration is the fact that the EDS is much less expensive. Generally the electrosurgical sheath is used as the sheath of choice for leads with shorter implant durations in patients who are at high risk for complications. For leads with longer implant durations that are risks for calcification, the laser sheath is a better selection.

Special Considerations and Situations

In the course of a lead extraction, there are certain issues that deserve special consideration, as well as clinical situations that are worthy of note. These include the timing of pacemaker replacement, the question of how to deal with grossly infected pacemaker pockets or large vegetations, and the unique problems presented by the Telectronics Accufix 801 and 854 leads.

Timing of Replacements

The timing of pacemaker system replacement is generally not a problem. In the case of an extraction that does not involve infection, replacement is generally carried out immediately. If the lead is being removed via the implant vein or superior approach, the sheaths offer an excellent opportunity for direct lead reinsertion or replacement of a guidewire for subsequent sheath application. If a lead is removed via the femoral vein, lead reintroduction and system replacement generally involve standard venous-access techniques. A more innovative approach in a situation of femoral lead extraction calls for the attachment of a guidewire to the proximal aspect of the lead to be removed. This can be done by using an 18 French thin-walled needle and a standard sheath set guidewire. The #18 gauge thin-walled needle is used to puncture the proximal aspect of the insulation. A guidewire is inserted between the insulation and inner coil. When the lead to be removed is extracted via the femoral approach, the guidewire is pulled into the central circulation. Continuous traction on the lead to be removed from below will disengage the proximal aspect of the extracted lead from the guidewire. The guidewire is left in place for subsequent application of the sheath. In the case of an infected system, some time should be allowed prior to reinsertion of a new system. The new system should be inserted on the contralateral side. In the case of superficial infection, an afebrile period should be documented for at least 24 h prior to system replacement. In the case of endocarditis, much longer periods are required prior to replacement of the system. Generally speaking, a 6-week period with all hardware removed is recommended. This becomes a challenge in cases of totally pacemaker-dependent patients. In this case Byrd recommends the use of an active fixation permanent pacemaker lead position in the right ventricle. The lead is connected to the

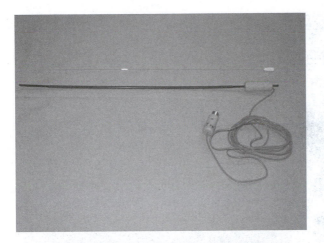

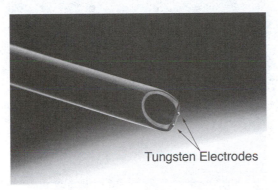

Tungsten Electrodes

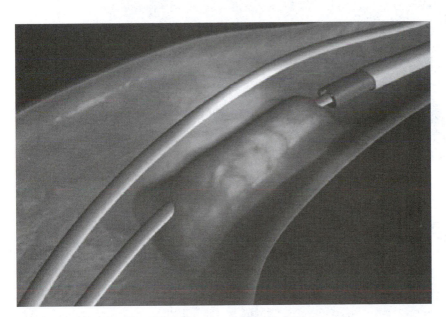

Fig. 6.41 (**a**) The electrosurgical dissection sheath. (**b**) The tip of the electrosurgical dissection sheath showing the tungsten electrodes. (**c**) EDS advancing over the lead approaching an area of dense encapsulating fibrous scar. Traction is maintained at the lead tip by the Liberator locking stylet.

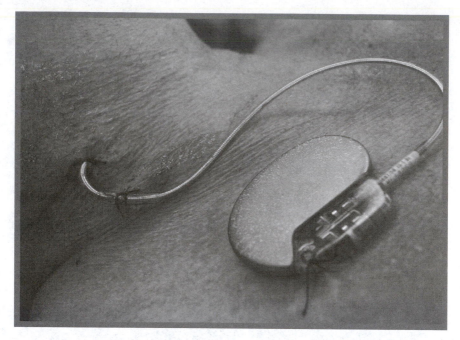

Fig. 6.42 Permanent active-fixation pacing electrode placed via the right internal jugular vein. Suture sleeve securing the lead to the neck. Lead connected to the explanted pulse generator, which is sutured to the anterior chest.

recently explanted pulse generator. The lead is usually placed via the internal jugular vein. The lead is secured with a suture sleeve to the neck. Hemostasis is effected by application of a figure-of-eight stitch at the puncture site. The pulse generator and lead are then secured to the anterior chest (Fig. 6.42). Such a system is extremely reliable and can be used for an extended period of time.

Large Vegetations

Occasionally, large vegetations are found attached to the pacing lead as well as the tricuspid valve. In this situation, some consideration should be given to lead removal via a limited thoracotomy. By definition, in most lead extractions, there is some embolization of either fibrous encapsulating scar tissue and/or infected material to the lung. The procedure may be monitored by the use of transesophageal echocardiography in the presence of large vegetations. It is the general consensus of most physicians involved with extraction that leads with vegetations up to 10 mm can be removed with standard extraction techniques. In the case of larger vegetations, an open thoracotomy should be considered.

Telectronics Model 801 and 854 Leads

Much has been written concerning these two Telectronics leads. They pose unique problems with respect to the best approach to their extraction (55–58). The retention wire of the Telectronics 801 electrode is imbedded in the outer insulation. The 854 electrode has its retention wire welded to the distal aspect of the inner coil. The Telectronics 801 electrode can be extracted by either the implant vein or femoral approach if there is no extrusion. In the case of a proximal extrusion of the retention wire, extraction by the implant vein with sheaths may result in embolization of the retention wire. This is less likely to occur with the distal extrusion of the retention wire. Whether there is a proximal or distal extrusion, the femoral approach appears to be ideal for removing Telectronics 801 leads. This is because use of the femoral approach causes the lead and retention wire to be folded into the Byrd Femoral Work Station. This is less likely to result in embolization of the retention wire.

The Telectronics 854 lead, with its retention wire located in the inner coil, also poses risks during extraction via the implant vein. This is especially true if the insulation and inner coil are broken between the anode and distal tip. The very process of inserting a locking stylet may embolize the retention wire (Fig. 6.43). Once again, the femoral approach appears to be ideal because it causes folding and crimping of the retention wire as it is drawn into the Byrd Femoral Work Station. Any traction on the 854 lead will usually result in a retained lead tip and, in extreme cases, lead tip embolization, because this lead is frequently associated with a fracture between the anode and cathode (Fig. 6.44). The use of endocardial biopsy forceps has also been described for the retrieval of the retention wire. Telectronics Pacing Systems initially

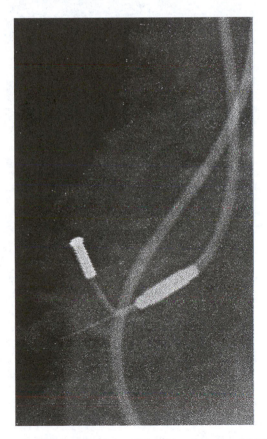

Fig. 6.43 Protrusion of the retention wire of the Telectronics model 854. The retention wire has been dislodged and advanced by application of the locking stylet. (From Belott PH. *Endocardial lead extraction: A videotape and manual.* Armonk, NY: Futura Publishing, 1998, with permission.)

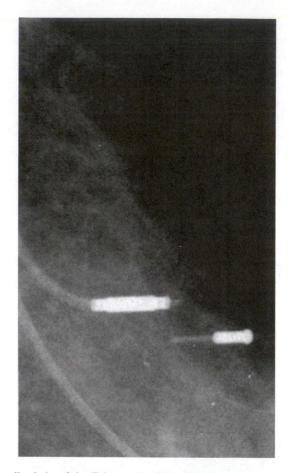

Fig. 6.44 The distal tip of the Telectronics 804 atrial electrode has been completely separated from the proximal aspect of the lead. With advancement of a locking stylet or lead stylet, the retention wire is free to embolize. (From Belott PH. *Endocardial lead extraction: A videotape and manual.* Armonk, NY: Futura Publishing, 1998, with permission.)

handled the management of patients with the Telectronics Accufix Model 801 and Model 854 atrial electrodes. They are responsible for accumulation of data for making recommendations with respect to the Accufix 801 and 854 leads. At present, the Accufix Institute now handles management of patients with these leads. The present fluoroscopic classification of patients with the 801 Accufix atrial J lead is shown in Table 6.7. Patient management guidelines now relate to patient-projected life expectancy and are shown in Table 6.8. Lead fluoroscopic classification for the Encor 854 lead is shown in Table 6.9. Patient management for Models 330–854 and 033–856 is as follows: All patients with these leads should undergo a one-time fluoroscopic examination to determine the current physical condition of their leads. A patient who has kinked or fractured leads should be monitored with the use of fluoroscopy every 6 months. The patient should be strongly encouraged to comply with the requested screening. If the initial fluoroscopic screening identifies a protruding J wire or a severed lead, the patient should be

Table 6.7 Accufix atrial J lead.

Definition of fracture classification	
Class I	No fracture suspected
Class II	Fracture suspected, but wire does not protrude through the outer insulation
Class III	Fracture suspected, and wire does protrude through the outer insulation
Class IV	Fracture suspected, and fragment of wire has migrated free from the lead

Table 6.8 Patient management guidelines[a].

Life expectancy	
Longer: Younger or with no comorbidities	
Class I	Monitor/consider extraction
Class II	Strongly consider extraction
Class III	Strongly consider extraction
Class IV	Case-by-case basis
Shorter: Very elderly or with comorbidities	
Class I	Monitor
Class II	Monitor/consider extraction
Class III	Case-by-case basis
Class IV	Case-by-case basis

[a]By projected life expectancy for the Accufix 801 atrial J lead.

Table 6.9 Lead fluoroscopic classification for Encore atrial J lead.

Fluoroscopic classification	
Class A	Fracture of the J retention wire not suspected
Class B	Fracture of J retention wire suspected, but not visualized
Class C	Fracture of J retention wire visualized, but J wire does not protrude from lead
Class D	The J retention wire protrudes from lead
Class E	Fragment of J retention wire has migrated away from lead

considered a candidate for lead extraction. The Accufix Institute continues to update physicians on the management recommendations for the Accufix 801, atrial J electrode, and the Encor 854 atrial electrode.

Defibrillator Lead Extraction

Defibrillator lead extraction is much more challenging when compared to pacemaker leads. This is because defibrillator leads are larger in diameter and have coils that can result in exuberant encapsulating fibrous scar attachment to endovascular structures. The defibrillator coils tend to promote dense fibrosis and fibrous bands that can attach to venous and myocardial structures. The extraction of such leads call for the use of larger extraction sheaths and increase the risk of vascular injury and avulsion. Generally defibrillator lead extractions are associated with a longer procedure and fluoroscopy times.

Lead Extraction from the Coronary Sinus

Cardiac resynchronization therapy calls for the placement of leads in distal branches of the coronary sinus. These leads are generally smaller in size and have no fixation mechanisms. Nonetheless they are prone to the formation of encapsulating fibrous scar attachments to the delicate coronary sinus wall. As the number of left ventricular leads increases there will be an increasing need to remove these left ventricular leads. The coronary sinus and its branches are thin and fragile. The passage of extraction sheaths as well as traction techniques will increase the risk of dissection rupture. Thus the removal of pacing and/or defibrillator leads placed in the coronary sinus is problematic and raises many concerns. The prospect of passing power sheaths into a delicate, fragile coronary sinus is of major concern. At present, the experience of extracting leads from the coronary sinus is early. There is very little data regarding results. In small series of very young leads there has been a 100% success rate with no complications and short procedure and fluoroscopy times (59). These leads have been removed by traction alone, not requiring locking stylets or power sheaths. In addition, most of these leads have been of short implant duration, generally less than 6 months. We require further data with respect to risks and complications. If in the future left ventricular leads become larger or utilize shocking coils, the situation will be extremely problematic.

Lead Extraction Database

In 1988, a voluntary database was established to track removal of intracardiac leads by intravascular techniques (60–64). The database was funded by, although not directed or controlled by, Cook Vascular, Inc. The database is designed to track the removal of intracardiac leads using any intravascular techniques, independent of what devices may be used to aid removal of the leads. Several abstracts, papers, and technical bulletins describing the results from database are available. In May 1997, the experience from December 1988 through February 1997 was presented at the North American Society of Pacing and Electrophysiology's annual meeting.

As of February 1997, 507 physicians had participated in the database, reporting attempted intravascular extraction of some 7,015 leads from 4,431 patients. The initial data were analyzed in three distinct periods (Table 6.10)

Table 6.10 Distribution of cases.

	12/88–12/93	1/94–12/95	1/96–2/97
Patients	1,255	1,995	1,181
Leads	2,118	2,978	1,919
Months implanted	56 ± 45	48 ± 41	56 ± 45

From experience to date: The Extraction Registry NASPE 5/97.

Table 6.11 Indications for lead extraction.

Mandatory (life threatening)

    Septicemia

    Endocarditis

    Lead migration (preparation, causing arrhythmia, causing emboli)

    Device interference (abandoned implantable defibrillator lead)

    Obliteration of all usable veins

Necessary (significant morbidity)

    Pocket infection

    Chronic draining sinus

    Erosion

    Vein thrombosis

    Lead migration (not presently causing life-threatening problem)

    Potential device interference

    Lead replacement (supernumerary, extraction, and implant
      thrombosed vein)

Discretionary (optional)

    Pain

    Malignancy

    Lead replacement (abandoned lead for less than 3–4 years)

From experience to date: The Extraction Registry NASPE 5/97.

– from December 1988 to December 1993 (a period that represents technological development of the extraction tools); from January 1994 to December 1995 (a stable period); and a final period from January 1996 to February 1997. The indications for lead extraction in the initial period were 10% for sepsis and endocarditis, 44% for other infection, and 42% for nonfunctional or failed leads (Table 6.11). Approximately 48% of the extraction procedures in the mid-period, 1994–1995, were for the Accufix lead. In the last period, the Accufix indication appears to have dropped off.

The predominant extraction approach was via the implant vein in all three periods. The major method of extraction via the superior approach was by use of the locking stylets and sheaths together. In the third period, during which several centers participated in the clinical trial for the excimer laser sheath, laser sheaths were used in combination with locking stylets and mechanical sheaths for 30% of the leads.

The outcomes with the use of intravascular techniques have been quite favorable (Table 6.12). Complete removal in the first period was 86%, whereas in the second period this increased to 93%. It is believed that this mid-period represents increased familiarity with the tools and techniques.

It became difficult to assess completeness of reporting as the number of centers voluntarily reporting increased. Therefore, participating centers with at least 20 cases reported were asked to verify whether they had completely reported all extraction procedures and complications since 1994. As of April 1997, 23 physicians had certified complete reporting of extraction procedures during the period from January 1994 through February 1997. The data from

Table 6.12 Extraction outcome using intravascular approach.

	Percent of leads		
Indication	1988–1993	1994–1995	1996–1997
Complete	86	93	94
Partial	8	5	5
Failed	6	2	1
Complete or only tip in heart	90	95	95

From experience to date: The Extraction Registry NASPE 5/97.

Table 6.13 Complications by intervention and analysis record.

Only most serious event counted	12/88–12/93, 1,255 Patients (%)	1/94–12/95, 1,995 Patients (%)	1/96–2/97, 1,181 Patients (%)
Death	7 (0.6)	1 (0.05)	4 (0.3)
Thoracotomy repair	12 (1.0)	12 (0.6)	8 (0.7)
Drainage required	3 (0.2)	11 (0.6)	3 (0.3)
Transfusions	2 (0.2)	3 (0.2)	1 (0.1)
Other major	1 (0.1)	2 (0.1)	3 (0.3)
Total "major"	25 (2.0)	29 (1.5)	19 (1.6)
Minor	14 (1.1)	33 (1.7)	13 (1.1)
Total complications	39 (3.1)	62 (3.1)	32 (2.7)

Includes complications associated with reimplant during the same procedure.
From experience to date: The Extraction Registry NASPE 5/97.

fully reporting centers have been analyzed separately. This subgroup represents 1,895 patients with the attempted extraction of 3,040 leads. The results of this analysis suggested that incomplete or failed extractions increased with implant duration. The ventricular leads had the highest risk of incomplete or failed extraction. In addition, physicians whose experience included fewer than 50 procedures had the highest risk of incomplete or failed extraction.

Complications

The incidence of complications from all reporting centers during the three analysis periods was analyzed (Table 6.13). The total incidence of major complications, including death, tamponade, and thoracotomy for repair of tamponade or hemothorax drainage, was 2% for the first period, 1.5% for the second, and 1.6% for the third. Minor complications ranged between 1.1% and 1.7%. The incidence of major complications was also analyzed from fully reporting centers between January 1994 and February 1997. The list and incidence are shown in Table 6.14. A multivariant analysis of the complications from the fully reporting centers was also carried out. They now focused on complications with respect to patient age, gender, number of leads, indications, physician experience, and lead type. Some interesting results were uncovered. First, for unexplained reasons, female patients appeared to be at higher risk for major complications. This risk

Table 6.14 Major complications: fully reporting centers, January 1994 to February 1997.

Number	Percent	Description
3	(0.2)	Nontargeted lead damaged/dislodged
5	(0.3)	Arrhythmia requiring cardioversion
4	(0.2)	Hypotension treated with fluids/drugs
3	(0.2)	Migrating fragment
2	(0.1)	Minor pneumothorax
2	(0.1)	Air embolism
2	(0.1)	Hematoma
2	(0.1)	Pericardial effusion not requiring drainage
3	(0.2)	Other: minor thoracic effusion (no treatment), delayed infection, minor pulmonary embolism

Includes complications associated with reimplant during the same procedure. Minor complications may be underreported.

From experience to date: The Extraction Registry NASPE 5/97.

also increased with increasing number of leads to be removed. Analysis of the data for risk of any complication showed that this risk appeared to increase with increasing number of leads, physician experience with fewer than 50 patients and female gender. Analysis of complications with respect to the number of leads was also analyzed. Major complications increased from 0.9% for one lead to 1.5% for two leads and 4.2% for three to five leads. Minor complications increased from 0.9% for one lead to 1.8% for two leads and 2.5% for more than two leads. Analysis of data with respect to gender and number of leads reveals the following: Female incidence of major complications increased from 1.6% for one lead to 4.0% for two leads and 10% for more than two leads. This pattern was not present in the male population.

The results of analysis since January 1994 of lead extraction at the reporting centers has been highly successful. Factors associated with the high incidence of success include shorter implant duration, older patients, higher physician experience, and atrial leads. The factors that increase the risk of complications include the higher number of leads, female gender, and lower physician experience. Given the gratifying early results, it is felt that with continued development of new tools and techniques, one can expect lead extraction will soon become extremely safe and expeditious.

References

1. Wallace H, Sherafat M, Blakemore WS. The stubborn pacemaker catheter. *Surgery* 1970;68:914–915.
2. Bilgutay AM, Jensen NK, Schmidt WR, et al. Incarceration of transvenous pacemaker electrode. Removal by traction. *Am Heart J* 1969;77:377–379.
3. Imparato A, Kim GE. Electrode complications in patients with permanent cardiac pacemakers. *Arch Surg* 1972;105:705–710.
4. Myers MR, Parsonnet V, Bernstein AD. Extraction of implanted transvenous pacing leads: a review of a persistent clinical problem. *Am Heart J* 1991;121:881–888.
5. Byrd CL, Schwartz SJ, Hedin N. Lead extraction: indications and techniques. *Cardiol Clin* 1992;10:735–748.

6. Hayes DL. Extraction of permanent pacing leads: There are still controversies in (Editorial). *Heart* 1996;75(6):539.

7. Furman S, Behrens M, Andrews C, et al. Retained pacemaker leads. *J Thorac Cardiovasc Surg* 1987;94:770.

8. Myers MR, Parsonnet V, Bernstein AD. Extraction of implanted transvenous pacing leads: A review of a persistent clinical problem. *Am Heart J* 1991;121:881.

9. Belott PH, Introduction. In Endocardial head Extraction A Videotape and Manual Mount Kisco New York, Futura Publishing to page X1, 1998.

10. Garcia-Jimenez A, Alba CMB, Cortes JMG, et al. Myocardial rupture after pulling out a tined atrial electrode with continuous traction. *PACE* 1989;12:508.

11. Sonnhag C, Walfridsson H. Extraction of chronically infected pacemaker leads: two cases with serious complications. (Abstract) *PACE* 1989;12:1204.

12. Lee ME, Chaux A, Matloff JM. Avulsion of a tricuspid valve leaflet during traction on an infected, entrapped endocardial pacemaker electrode. *J Thorac Cardiovasc Surg* 1977;74:433–435.

13. Jarvinen A, Harjula A, Verkkala K. Intrathoracic surgery for retained endocardial electrodes. *J Thorac Cardiovasc Surg* 1986;34:94–97.

14. Madigan NP, Curtis JJ, Sanfelippo JF, et al. Difficulty of extraction of chronically implanted tined ventricular leads. *JACC* 1984;3:724–731.

15. Rettig G, Doenecke P, Sen S, et al. Complications with retained transvenous pacemaker electrodes. *Am Heart J* 1979;98:587–594.

16. Shennib H, Chiu R, Rosengarten M, et al. The non-extractable tined endocardial pacemaker lead. *Can J Cardiol* 1989;5:305–307.

17. Porstman NW, Wierny L, Warnke H. Closure of persistent ductus arteriosus without thoracotomy. *German Med Monthly* 1967;12:1.

18. Massumi RA, Ross AN. Atraumatic nonsurgical technique for removal of broken catheters from the cardiac cavities. *Med Intell* 1967;277:195.

19. Meibom J. A new method for transvenous electrode explantation. (Abstract) *PACE* 1985;8:A-54.

20. Byrd CL, Schwartz SJ, Sivina M, et al. Experience with 127 pacemaker lead extractions. (Abstract) *PACE* 1986;9:282.

21. Byrd CL, Schwartz SJ, Ciraldo RJ, et al. Update on transvenous countertraction lead extraction experience. (Abstract) *PACE* 1987;10:443.

22. Byrd CL, Schwartz SJ, Hedin NB, et al. Intravascular lead extraction using locking stylets and sheaths. *PACE* 1990;13:1871–1875.

23. Byrd CL, Schwartz SJ, Hedin N. Intravascular techniques for extraction of permanent pacemaker leads. *J Thorac Cardiovasc Surg* 1991;101:989–997.

24. Byrd CL, Schwartz SJ, Hedin NB. Lead extraction: techniques and indications. In: Barold SS, Mugica J, eds. *New perspectives in cardiac pacing*, vol. 3. Mount Kisco, NY: Futura Publishing, 1993:29–55.

25. Byrd CL. Management of implant complications. In: Ellenbogen KA, Kay GN, Wilkoff BL, eds. *Clinical cardiac pacing*. Philadelphia: WB Saunders, 1995:491–522.

26. Goode LB, Byrd CL, Wilkoff BL, et al. Development of a new technique for explantation of chronic transvenous pacemaker leads: five initial case studies. *Biomed Instrument Technol* 1991;25:50–53.

27. Fearnot NE, Smith HJ, Goode LB, et al. Intravascular lead extraction using locking stylets, sheaths, and other techniques. *PACE* 1990;13:1864–1875.

28. Love CJ, Nelson SD, Schaal SF. Extraction of permanent pacemaker leads using the Cook extraction set; initial clinical experience. (Abstract) *J Am Coll Cardiol* 1990;15(2):50A.

29. Byrd CL, Schwartz SJ, Hedin NB, et al. Inferior vena cava extraction technique. (Abstract) *PACE* 1992;15:571.

30. Foster CJ, Brownlee WC. Percutaneous removal of ventricular pacemaker electrodes using a Dormia basket. *Int J Cardiol* 1988;21:127–134.

31. Hayes DL, Vlietstra RE, Neubauer S. Snare retrieval of entrapped infected transvenous pacing leads to avoid thoracotomy. (Abstract) *PACE* 1987;10:686.
32. Taliercia CP, Vlietstra RE, Hayes DL. Pigtail catheter for extraction of pacemaker lead. (Letter) *J Am Coll Cardiol* 1985;5:1020.
33. Ramsdale DR, Arumugam N, Pidgeon JW. Removal of fractured pacemaker electrode tip using Dotter basket. *PACE* 1985;8:759–760.
34. Espinosa RE, Hayes DL, Vlietstra RE, et al. The Dotter retriever and pigtail catheter: efficacy in extraction of chronic transvenous pacemaker leads. *PACE* 1993;16:2337–2342.
35. Byrd CL, Schwartz SJ, Hedin NB. Lead extraction: techniques and indications. In: Barold SS, Mujica J, eds. *New Perspectives in Cardiac Pacing*, vol. 3. Mount Kisco, NY: Futura Publishing, 1993:9–55.
36. Love CJ, Wilkoff BL,Byrd CL et al. Recommendations for extraction of chronically implanted transvenous pacing and defibrillator leads: indications, facilities, training. North American Society of pacing electrophysiology lead extraction conference faculty. PACE 2000;23:544.
37. Smith CW, Messenger JC, Schanner SP, et al. Cardiac pacemaker electrodes: improved methods of extraction. Work in progress. *Radiology* 1994;193:739.
38. Cope C, LaRieu AJ, Isaacson CS, et al. Transfemoral removal of a chronically implanted pacemaker lead: report of a case. *Ann Thorac Surg* 1986;42:329.
39. Maisch B, Ertl G, Kurke H. Extraction of a chronically infected endocardial screw-in pacing lead by pigtail catheter and wire loop via the femoral vein. *PACE* 1983;8:230.
40. Maisch B, Ertl G. Transfemoral extraction of endocardial screw-in pacemaker leads. *J Electrophysiol* 1987;1:172.
41. Dotter CT, Rösch J, Bilbao MK. Transluminal extraction of catheter and guide fragments from the heart and great vessels: twenty-nine collected cases. *Am J Radiol* 1971;111:467.
42. Enge I, Flatmark A. Percutaneous removal of intravascular foreign bodies via the snare technique. *Acta Radiol* 1973;14:747.
43. Curry JA. Recovery of a detached intravascular catheter or guidewire fragments: a proposed method. *Am J Radiol* 1969;105:894.
44. Yedlicka JW Jr, Carlson JE, Hunter DW, et al. The Nitonol "Gooseneck" snare for foreign body removal: an experimental study and clinical evaluation. *Am J Radiol* 1991;156:1007.
45. McSweeney WJ, Schwarts DC. Retrieval of a catheter foreign body from the right side of the heart using a guidewire deflector system. *Radiology* 1971;100:61.
46. Byrd CL, Schwartz SJ, Sevina M, et al. Technique for surgical extraction of permanent pacemaker leads and electrodes. *J Thorac Cardiovasc Surg* 1985;89:142.
47. Byrd CL. Extracting chronically implanted pacemaker leads using the Spectranetics excimer laser: initial clinical experience. (Abstract) *PACE* 1996;19:567.
48. Byrd CL. Wilkoff BL, Love CJ, et al. Update of the PLEXES trial: two-year experience. (Abstract) *PACE* 1998;21:817.
49. Bracke FA, Meijer A, Van Gelder B. Learning curve characteristics of pacing lead extraction with a laser sheath. *PACE* 1998;21:2309–2313.
50. Al-Khadra AS, Wilkoff Bl, Byrd CL, et al. Extraction of nonthoracotomy defibrillator leads using the Spectranetics LASER sheath: the US experience. (Abstract) *PACE* 1998;21:889.
51. Krishnan S, Epstein L. Initial experience with a laser sheath to extract chronic transvenous implantable cardioverter-defibrillator leads. *Am J Cardiol* 1998;82: 1293–1295.
52. Reiser C, Taylor K, Lippincott R. Large laser sheaths for pacing and defibrillator lead removal. *Lasers Surg Med* 1998;22:42–45.

53. Varma N, Selke FW, Epstein LM. Chronic atrial lead explantation using a staged percutaneous laser and open surgical approach. *PACE* 1998;21:1483–1485.

54. Wilkoff BL, Byrd CL, Love CJ, et al. Pacemaker lead extraction with the laser sheath: results of pacing lead extraction with the excimer sheath (PLEXES) trial. *J Am Coll Cardiol* 1999;33(6):1671–1676.

55. Love C, Brinker J, Gross J, et al. Predictors of life-threatening and major intravascular extraction complications with an ACCUFIX atrial J lead. (Abstract) *PACE* 1998;21:817.

56. Hayes DL, Lloyd MA, Holmes DR Jr. Counseling and management of patients with Telectronics 330–801 Accufix leads. *PACE* 1995;18(8):1595.

57. Lloyd MA, Hayes DL, Stanson AW, et al. Snare removal of a Telectronics Accufix atrial J retention wire. *Mayo Clin Proc* 1995;70:376.

58. Sulke N, Chambers J, Blauth C. Life-threatening degeneration of the Accufix active fixation atrial pacing electrode. *Lancet* 1995;346:25.

59. Tyers GF, Clark J, Wang Y, Mills P, Bashir J. Coronary sinus lead extraction. PACE 2003;26:524–526.

60. Byrd CL, Wilkoff B, Love C, et al. Clinical study of the laser sheath: Results of the PLEXES Trial. *PACE* 1997;20(II):1053.

61. Smith HJ, Fearnot NE, Byrd CL, et al. Five-year experience with intravenous lead extraction. U.S. Lead Extraction Data Base. *PACE* 1994;17:2016.

62. Smith HJ, Fearnot NE, Byrd CL, et al. Intravascular extraction of chronic pacing leads: the effect of physician experience. (Abstract) *PACE* 1992;15:513.

63. Van Zandt HJ, on behalf of Extraction Database Participants. Experience to date: The Extraction Registry. Presented as part of the minicourse Lead Extraction: 1997. In: NASPE 18th Annual Scientific Sessions Highlights. New Orleans: NASPE; produced by Medical Support Systems, 1997.

64. Byrd CL, Wilkoff BL, Love CJ, et al. Intrvascular intravascular extraction of problematic or infected permanent pacemaker leads: 1994–1996 U.S. extraction database. Med Institute. *PACE* 1999;22:1348–1357.

Techniques for Temporary Pacing

Ejigayehu Abate, Fred M. Kusumoto, and Nora F. Goldschlager

Temporary pacing of the heart was first accomplished by Hyman in the early 1930s by a transthoracic approach using a clockwork-driven generator. In the early 1950s Zoll successfully resuscitated an asystolic patient using temporary transcutaneous pacing. Later in that decade, the feasibility of transvenous pacing and transesophageal pacing was demonstrated. Temporary pacing has become the standard method for providing immediate treatment of severe bradycardias and certain tachycardias for the past 20 years.

Temporary pacing of the heart can be achieved by several approaches: transcutaneous, transvenous, transesophageal, and transthoracic. The approach chosen for temporary pacing is generally based on factors such as urgency, likelihood of need for permanent pacing, patient-specific factors (body size, anatomy, available access), and potential complications. Perhaps the most critical of these factors is urgency. Many patients who require temporary pacing have hemodynamic instability (or impending instability) and need swift action to prevent or treat cardiovascular collapse. Frequently, several approaches for temporary pacing are required for an individual patient. For example, the patient presenting to the emergency room with profound bradycardia may be treated initially by transcutaneous pacing and once stabilized, by transvenous pacing. The advantages and disadvantages of the various temporary pacing methods are summarized in Table 7.1.

Transcutaneous Pacing

Of all the methods for temporary pacing, transcutaneous pacing is unique in its ability to be noninvasively applied and initiated within seconds after the recognition of a serious bradyarrhythmia. Although feasible since the early 1950s, transcutaneous pacing has been in widespread use for only the last 10–15 years after a series of technical improvements in the equipment (1). Transcutaneous pacing is now considered the pacing method of choice for rapid treatment of bradycardia (2). The complication rates are extremely low because transcutaneous pacing is noninvasive. There have been no published reports of skeletal muscle damage, skin damage, or other significant problems associated with transcutaneous pacing. The most serious drawback is its

Table 7.1 Methods for temporary pacing.

Method	Advantages	Disadvantages
Transcutaneous	Noninvasive	Uncomfortable
	Minimal complications	Cannot be used long term
	Usually reliable short term	
Transvenous	Most comfortable	Requires central venous access
	Reliable	
	Can be used for atrioventricular or P-synchronous pacing	
Transesophageal	Relatively noninvasive	Atrial pacing only
		Cannot be used long term
Transthoracic	Very rapidly initiated	Pacing wires are frequently not placed correctly
		Variable effectiveness for pacing (often because the patient is in extremis)
		High complication rate
Epicardial	Very effective short term after open heart surgery	Used only after open heart surgery
	Low complication rate	

variability for providing effective and reliable pacing. In early studies, effective capture had been demonstrated in 50–100% of healthy volunteers and between 70 and 80% of patients in a variety of clinical settings (3,4). Transcutaneous pacing is very effective (>90%) when pacing is initiated quickly for persistent bradycardia or asystolic arrest (within 5 min). Today, the majority of pacing failures with this systems occur in patients during prolonged cardiopulmonary arrest and terminal circulatory collapse. In these patients, myocardial capture may be more difficult because of underlying ischemia, hypoxia, and various electrolyte abnormalities (3,5,6).

In transcutaneous pacing the heart tissue is electrically stimulated by current passing through excitable myocardium lying between surface electrodes placed on the chest wall. Standard electrodes have a large surface area of 70–120 cm^2, which provide ample coverage of the thoracic window and reduce the current density at the skin–electrode interface, which, in turn, minimizes cutaneous nerve stimulation. Pediatric electrodes with a surface area of 30–50 cm^2 are also available. Initially, high impedance (500–1,000 Ω) electrodes that minimized the current density at the skin–electrode interface were used to improve patient comfort, but these electrodes could not be used for cardioversion or defibrillation. Newer electrodes use a low-impedance (50–100 Ω) design, which provides more effective pacing; they are relatively well tolerated and can also be used for cardioversion and defibrillation.

Proper electrode placement is the single most important factor for determining whether transcutaneous pacing will be effective. The proper position of the cathode (negative) electrode is directly over the cardiac apex or over the position of ECG chest leads V$_3$ (Fig. 7.1). The anode (positive) electrode is placed either posteriorly (recommended) on the back between the spine and the lower half of the left or right scapulae, or, alternatively, if the back is inaccessible, over the right upper chest centered approximately 6–10 cm above the

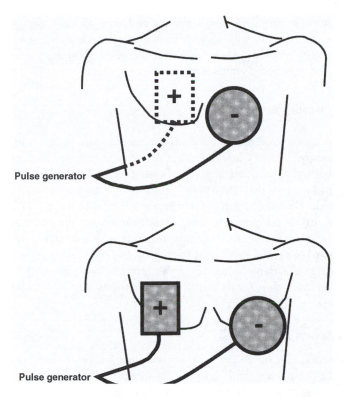

Fig. 7.1 Correct position of transcutaneous pacing electrodes. *Top*: Anteroposterior positioning with the cathode (circle) over the cardiac apex and the anode (rectangle) in the back between the spine and the right scapula (the space between the spine and left scapula can also be used). *Bottom*: Anterior-anterior position with the cathode over the cardiac apex and the anode on the right chest.

right nipple. The posterior electrode should not be placed directly on the spine or the scapula because of the increased impedance of bone. If the electrodes are inadvertently switched, the likelihood of capture is reduced to less than 10%; the increased threshold in this electrode configuration is probably due in part to the greater distance between the ventricles and the cathode (7).

The pulse generators used (in most instances a combined defibrillator/pacer unit) must generate high current at long pulse durations to capture myocardial tissue. Threshold values range between 20 and 140 mA (generally 40–70 mA) at pulse durations between 20 and 40 ms (3,8–10). Standard ECG strip recordings sometimes can be difficult to interpret because of significant artifact associated with the large and broad pacing stimuli. Modern transcutaneous pacing systems are equipped with special ECG monitor displays that provide 100-ms suppression with each pacing stimulus to reduce the effects of artifact. Capture must be confirmed once the electrodes are in place. Pacing should be maintained with a safety margin of between 5 and 20 mA as patient tolerance allows once capture is confirmed.

Complications from transcutaneous pacing are extremely rare (3,4). The primary reasons for intolerance by patients are pain and cough. Although newer designs have lowered the current densities delivered at the surface of the skin, thereby reducing the incidence of cutaneous nerve stimulation, skeletal muscle stimulation still occurs and can be very uncomfortable. Therefore, all patients who require prolonged transcutaneous pacing must be adequately sedated and once stabilized, they should be immediately prepared for transvenous temporary pacing.

Transvenous Pacing

Although transcutaneous pacing offers ease of use, rapid initiation of pacing therapy, and very low complication rates, it is by far more stable and better tolerated by patients if pacing is needed for longer than 20–30 min. First introduced in the late 1950s, transvenous approaches are now the most commonly used method for temporary cardiac pacing (11). Today, over 95% of all temporary pacing is accomplished via the transvenous route, usually performed by placing a catheter in the right ventricle. In rare cases where temporary atrial pacing is also required, a catheter can be positioned in the right atrium or in the proximal portion of the coronary sinus. The first step for instituting transvenous pacing is establishing central venous access.

Venous Access

Venous access can be obtained by several approaches. The internal jugular veins, subclavian veins, and femoral veins are all potential sites for introduction of the pacing catheter into the right heart (Table 7.2). The median basilic veins and basilic veins can also be used, but these sites are associated with a very high incidence of catheter dislodgment (because of arm motion) and are rarely, if ever, used today.

Before obtaining venous access, the existence of a bleeding diathesis or coagulopathy should be excluded or corrected if possible. If this is not possible, the femoral vein should be considered as the initial access site

Table 7.2 Potential sites for venous access.

Access site (rate of successful venous cannulation)	Advantages	Disadvantages
Internal jugular vein (80–94%)	Small chance of pneumothorax (<1–3%)	Uncomfortable
		Carotid artery puncture (rare)
		Easy access to the right heart chambers from the right internal jugular vein
Subclavian vein (85–98%)	Most comfortable	Higher incidence of pneumothorax and hemothorax (2–5%)
	Easy access to the right heart chambers from the left subclavian vein	May be required as a future site for a permanent pacing system
Femoral vein (89–95%)	Quickly and easily cannulated	Very uncomfortable; immobilization of leg required
		High rate of venous thrombosis (25–35% after 24 h)
		Fluoroscopy required for catheter placement

because it is easier to apply pressure and achieve hemostasis in this region if a complication occurs. The presence of a prosthetic tricuspid valve is a contraindication to right ventricular pacing. In this setting, left ventricular pacing can be performed by positioning the pacing catheter in the left ventricular veins via the coronary sinus. Other factors, such as the patient's pulmonary status, the location of dialysis shunts, and previous neck surgery or radiation therapy should be taken into account when considering the appropriate site for venous access.

Internal Jugular Vein

The venous access site of choice for most operators is the right internal jugular vein. This approach gives the most direct access into the right ventricle and a stable catheter position. Disadvantages include decreased neck mobility for the patient and difficulty in keeping the site sterile in intubated patients, particularly in patients with tracheostomies. The left internal jugular can also be used, but fluoroscopy is often required for satisfactory pacing catheter placement. In addition, the dome of the left lung is often higher than the right lung and the thoracic duct is located on the left side, making this site potentially more prone to complications. Several approaches to the internal jugular vein have been described. The two most widely utilized approaches are the middle and posterior approaches, referring to the access site relative to the sternocleidomastoid muscle (12–14).

The internal jugular vein emerges from the base of the skull and lies behind the sternocleidomastoid muscle within the carotid sheath. In the middle and lower portions of the neck, the internal jugular vein lies anterior and lateral to the carotid artery and vagus nerve (Fig. 7.2). Behind the sternal head of the clavicle the internal jugular vein joins the subclavian vein to form the innominate vein. In a general sense, the path of the internal jugular vein extends from the region of the pinna of the ear to 1–3 cm lateral to the sternoclavicular joint when the patient's head is turned approximately 45° to the contralateral side. Although a number of insertion techniques have been described, the two most commonly used entry points are (a) near the top of the triangle formed by the separation of the sternal and clavicular heads of the sternocleidomastoid muscle and the clavicle (middle approach), or (b) posteriorly behind the sternocleidomastoid muscle where the external jugular vein crosses the lateral border of the clavicular head of the sternocleidomastoid muscle (posterior approach) (Fig. 7.2). Having the patient tense the sternocleidomastoid muscle by lifting his or her head off the bed helps to define the neck anatomy.

The middle approach, which is sometimes called the anterior approach because its insertion point is anterior to the *clavicular* head of the sternocleidomastoid muscle, has a high rate of success and carries a relatively low risk of complications. After the patient has been positioned in a 20° to 25° Trendelenburg position (to distend the veins and reduce the risk of venous air embolism), the skin is sterilized, the neck is draped, and landmarks in the neck are identified. The carotid artery is palpated at the apex of the triangle formed by the sternocleidomastoid, and retracted slightly medially. Local anesthesia is accomplished with 1% lidocaine starting with a generous skin wheal at the insertion site near the apex. Deeper infiltration is then performed by inserting a #22 gauge needle ("finder" needle) from the wheal toward the ipsilateral

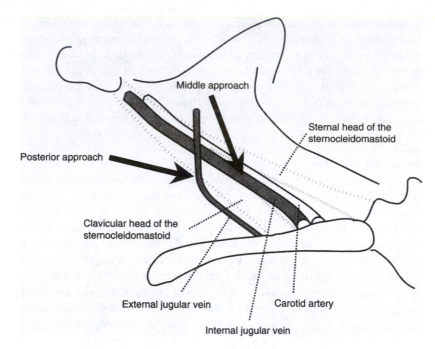

Fig. 7.2 Middle and posterior approaches for cannulating the internal jugular vein. Although there is significant individual variability, in general, the jugular vein travels from the pinna of the ear to the medial end of the clavicle and lies lateral to and above the carotid artery.

nipple at about a 30–40° angle from the body's frontal plane. The needle's path usually travels just under the clavicular head of the sternoclastomastoid muscle. The needle is advanced with continuous aspiration to ensure that the operator will observe a "flash" of blood when the vein is struck. As the needle is advanced, the operator should stop approximately every 0.5 cm to inject small boluses of lidocaine along the track, aspirating first, so that lidocaine is not being injected directly into a vessel. Usually, the internal jugular vein is found within 1–3 cm under the skin. If no blood return is noted after 3 cm, remove the needle with continuous aspiration, and at the same insertion site redirect the "finder" needle slightly laterally and repeat the steps just described. If lateral angulation fails, medial angulation can be tried, but this increases the risk of inadvertent puncture of the carotid artery, which lies just medial and deep to the internal jugular vein. If difficulty in finding the vein is encountered, having the patient perform a Valsalva maneuver or elevating the legs can distend the internal jugular vein, or the vein can be located with ultrasound.

Once the vein has been located, it is cannulated using a method initially described by Seldinger in 1953 (15). A 2-in. #18 gauge thin-wall needle is inserted bevel up along the same track as the "finder" needle with continuous aspiration using a 5- or 10-mL syringe filled with 2–3 mL of sterile saline. Some operators advocate leaving the "finder" needle in the skin for guiding the thin-wall needle. When free blood returns with *gentle* suction, the vein is cannulated. If the vein has not been cannulated when the thin-wall needle has been inserted to the depth indicated by the "finder" needle, the thin-wall needle should be gently retracted. In some cases the thin-wall needle has indented the jugular vein and cannulation occurs with gentle release of forward pressure. Once the vein is cannulated, the syringe is removed while stabilizing the needle. Blood should slowly drip out of the needle if the patient has normal right atrial pressure. While the syringe is removed, the patient, if possible, should hold his or her breath or hum to reduce the risk of venous air embolism. If blood spurts from the needle, the carotid artery has likely been inadvertently cannulated; the needle should be removed and the operator should hold pressure for 5–10 min to allow adequate hemostasis. Blood oxygen saturation can be measured if there is concern that the carotid artery may have been inadvertently punctured.

Once venous access is confirmed, a 45-cm 0.035-in. J guidewire is inserted through the needle and advanced smoothly. The guidewire should not be forcefully advanced if *any* resistance is met within the first 10 cm. Instead, the angle of the needle can be lowered slightly to obtain a more direct route into the vein. If resistance is still encountered, the wire should be removed and adequate venous return should be confirmed. If blood flow is adequate, proceed with wire placement again. If blood flow is not adequate, minor readjustment of the needle either forward or backward can be performed, but not side-to-side, because lateral movement can cause laceration of the vein. If these maneuvers are unsuccessful, it is necessary to repeat the procedure or move to another access site after holding pressure for 5–10 min to achieve hemostasis.

The wire is likely to be within a vascular structure if it has advanced *easily* for 10 cm. If resistance is met after this point (usually 15 cm), it is usually owing to the wire traveling down the subclavian vein into the arm rather than into the superior vena cava. The wire can be withdrawn 3–5 cm, rotated, and readvanced. Continuous ECG monitoring is required whenever the wire is advanced to observe for ventricular ectopy (which would suggest the guidewire is in the right ventricle). Once the wire has been inserted approximately 20–25 cm, the thin-wall needle is removed, a small skin nick is made using a #11 surgical scalpel, and the subcutaneous tissue under the skin nick is enlarged using small "mosquito" forceps. A sheath-dilator assembly is threaded over the guidewire; the guidewire should protrude more than 5 cm from the proximal hub of the sheath-dilator assembly. The sheath-dilator assembly is advanced into the vein over the guidewire and once in place the guidewire and dilator are removed. Finally, the sheath is aspirated and flushed with heparinized saline.

The posterior approach is another method for cannulating the internal jugular vein. In this approach, the insertion site is located posteriorly behind the lateral aspect of the sternocleidomastoid muscle just above the site where the external jugular vein crosses the sternocleidomastoid muscle obliquely. In the posterior approach, the "finder" needle is directed superiorly toward the suprasternal notch passing just underneath the sternocleidomastoid muscle. Once the internal jugular vein is located (usually within 5 cm of the insertion site), the vein is cannulated using the Seldinger technique previously discussed.

Ultrasound can be used to guide vascular access. Some authors have advocated routine use of ultrasound while a large retrospective study at one institution found no significant difference in complication rates between standard landmark approach and ultrasound guidance (16,17).

Subclavian Vein

The subclavian vein is a frequently used site for venous access. The major disadvantages of this site are a higher risk of pneumothorax when compared to other access sites, and inability to compress vascular structures should vein laceration or arterial puncture occur. The principal advantages are patient comfort and superior stability. The left subclavian approach is easier than the right because of the natural curve of the vessels leading into the right atrium; however, this is often the best site for insertion of a permanent pacemaker (if the patient is right-handed), and therefore should be avoided if permanent pacing is likely to be required. The right subclavian can also be successfully utilized, but as with the left internal jugular approach fluoroscopy may be necessary for pacing catheter placement once venous access is obtained. Anatomy and techniques for cannulating the subclavian vein are covered in detail in Chap. 4.

Femoral Vein

In certain situations the internal jugular or subclavian veins may be inaccessible or the patient may have uncorrectable thrombocytopenia or coagulopathy, which necessitates access to the central venous system by the femoral vein. When using this approach for temporary pacing, fluoroscopy is required for pacing catheter placement. In addition to the need for fluoroscopy, other disadvantages include patient comfort (because the leg cannot be bent at the hip), increased risk of infection, and poor catheter stability.

The landmarks used for cannulating the femoral vein are the inguinal ligament running between the pubic symphysis and the anterior superior iliac crest, and the femoral pulse (Fig. 7.3). The insertion site is found by palpating the femoral pulse approximately 2–3 cm below the inguinal ligament. This position normally falls within the inguinal crease but may be somewhat more superior to the inguinal crease in obese patients. The insertion site should be above the inferior border of the femoral head if fluoroscopy is being used. The femoral vein is usually located 1–2 cm medial and parallel to the femoral artery. A low insertion site should be avoided because distally the superficial femoral artery frequently travels above the femoral vein. Cannulation of the femoral vein through the superficial femoral artery can cause excessive bleeding and may lead to the formation of an arteriovenous fistula. An insertion point above the inguinal ligament is associated with a higher incidence of hematoma formation and retroperitoneal bleed because of inadequate compression when the sheath is removed. Cannulation of the femoral vein is performed using the Seldinger technique described in the preceding section, although the use of a "finder" needle is usually not required. The guidewire should never be advanced forcefully; if resistance is met, it may be due to the guidewire entering a lumbar vein. The guidewire should be withdrawn 2–3 cm, rotated, and then readvanced. If fluoroscopy is available, then injecting dye (diluted 1:1 with saline) through the needle may help delineate the anatomy. Finally, a Valsalva maneuver can be used to cause venous distension.

The femoral venous site can be used for only approximately 24–36 h because of the risk of infection and venous thrombosis (16–18). The femoral venous insertion site also necessitates that the patient remain in bed in the supine position with minimal bending at the waist. Usually, the femoral vein

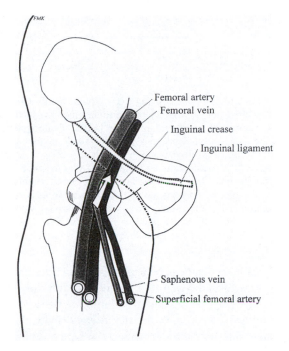

Fig. 7.3 Anatomy and landmarks for cannulating the femoral vein. The femoral vein should be cannulated at or just above the inguinal crease. A low cannulation point should be avoided because there is an increased risk of puncturing the superficial femoral artery.

is used for temporary pacing only in the cardiac catheterization laboratory during high-risk procedures.

Multiple Sheaths

In rare situations two sheaths may be needed; for example, in some patients separate atrial and ventricular pacing catheters may be necessary to maintain atrioventricular synchrony, and other patients may require both a Swan-Ganz catheter and a pacing catheter. One method for placing two sheaths is to initially place a single sheath as discussed in the preceding section, then place two guidewires into the sheath, remove the original sheath while keeping the wires in place, and advance two separate sheaths over the two guidewires. Alternatively, a second puncture site can be placed near the first site.

Pacing Catheter Insertion

Once venous access is obtained, the pacing catheter must be placed into the appropriate intracardiac position to begin pacing. A variety of leads that range from 3 to 6Fr in diameter can be used for transvenous temporary pacing. Balloon-tipped flotation electrode catheters use vascular and intracardiac blood flow to direct them into the right ventricle. Balloon-tipped pacing catheters are very pliable and are also available with preformed curvature to facilitate placement from the femoral vein. Traditional temporary electrode catheters are relatively stiff, and must be placed in the ventricle with the aid of fluoroscopy. Traditional electrode catheters come in a variety of shapes

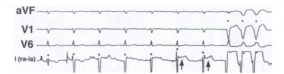

Fig. 7.4 Placement of a pacing catheter using electrograms. In this case a bipolar electrogram is recorded by attaching the distal electrode to the right arm lead and the proximal electrode to the left arm lead and recording ECG "lead I." Continuous ECG recording is performed as the pacing lead is inserted. In the left side of the strip, the atrial and ventricular(*) signals are equal in size suggesting the tip of the catheter is near the tricuspid annulus. As the pacing catheter is advanced into the right ventricle the ventricular electrogram becomes larger and the atrial electrogram smaller, and the catheter is advanced until an injury current (arrows) is recorded. A short burst of nonsustained ventricular tachycardia with left bundle branch block morphology and superior axis (which is probably produced by direct catheter irritation of ventricular tissue) suggests that the pacing catheter tip is properly located in the right ventricular apex.

and are the only catheters that can be used for pacing the right atrium and the coronary sinus. Specialized Swan-Ganz catheters with electrodes built into the catheter are available, but their use is limited by lack of stable and reliable contact with the endocardium. Another Swan-Ganz catheter design uses a right ventricular side port through which a separate 2.5Fr pacing wire is inserted. Finally, in some circumstances, a permanent pacing lead can be used for longer-term temporary pacing. Permanent pacing leads have active fixation mechanisms at the tip that allow for more stable positioning and are very pliable. However, they require fluoroscopy for placement.

Pacing catheters can be placed by fluoroscopy, electrogram monitoring, or documenting capture during continuous pacing. Whenever possible fluoroscopy should be used for catheter placement. Fluoroscopy allows direct visualization of the pacing catheter as it passes through the venous vascular structures, right atrium, and right ventricle. Fluoroscopic positioning of permanent pacing leads is discussed in Chap. 4; the same guidelines can be used for placing a temporary pacing catheter in the right ventricle. The correct and most stable position of a temporary ventricular pacing lead is at the apex of the right ventricle with the lead tip pointing "down" and to the left of the spine.

If fluoroscopy is not readily available, then electrogram monitoring can be used to place a balloon-tipped temporary pacing catheter (Fig. 7.4). Electrogram monitoring can be performed using two methods. To obtain a unipolar recording from the electrode tip, the four limb leads are connected to a standard electrocardiogram machine and the V_1 lead is connected to the terminal pin of the distal electrode using an alligator clip. To obtain a bipolar electrogram the leg leads are placed as usual and the distal and proximal electrodes from the pacing catheter are attached to the right arm and left arm leads of the ECG machine. Lead I is a bipolar electrogram generated from electrical activity recorded between the two pacing electrodes within the heart. The tip unipolar electrogram is best used to indicate the position of this electrode within the heart. The bipolar electrogram provides an assessment of the intracardiac signal amplitude, which is useful because most temporary pulse generators use the bipolar intracardiac signal for sensing.

The pacing catheter is advanced with the balloon inflated while continuously recording the surface ECG and intracardiac electrogram. A large atrial signal is observed when the catheter has reached the right atrium, and the atrial and ventricular signals have similar amplitude at the tricuspid annulus. The ventricular electrogram becomes larger and the atrial electrogram smaller as the catheter enters the right ventricle, and ST segment elevation ("injury" current) is observed when contact with the endocardium is made; premature ventricular depolarizations are also frequently noted. The atrial electrogram is not visible when the electrode tip is in the right ventricular apex. Once the "injury" current is observed, the balloon is deflated and pacing should be performed with a simultaneous surface ECG. Capture should be confirmed and the paced QRS complexes should be documented to have left bundle branch block morphology (because temporary pacing from the right ventricle causes initiation of ventricular depolarization from the right ventricle) and a superior mean frontal axis, because ventricular depolarization proceeds from apex to base if the catheter is placed in the apex.

Transcutaneous pacing should be attempted first during an asystolic arrest. Transvenous pacing can be tried if this fails. However, in this scenario, electrogram monitoring cannot be used because there is no intrinsic ventricular depolarization that can be sensed. In this case a balloon-tipped catheter is introduced from the right internal jugular vein. Once the catheter has been advanced past the sheath tip, the balloon is inflated and advanced to the region of the tricuspid annulus as estimated from measurements made on the body surface. The terminal pins of the catheter are then connected to an external pulse generator set to moderate output (5–10 mA), the balloon is deflated and the catheter is advanced 5–10 cm. Ventricular pacing is observed when the catheter has passed into the right ventricle. If ventricular ectopy is noted without sustained ventricular capture, the pacing output should be increased to the highest possible value. If atrial pacing is observed, the pacing catheter should be withdrawn 1–2 cm and readvanced with slight rotation. A 12-lead ECG should be obtained and catheter position confirmed by chest radiograph or fluoroscopy once ventricular capture is achieved. Unfortunately, pacing leads cannot be placed or are positioned incorrectly in up to 50% of cases of asystolic arrest where temporary transvenous pacing is attempted.

Atrioventricular synchrony may be necessary in certain conditions, such as right ventricular infarction. Temporary atrial pacing leads are available in which a preformed distal J shape allows the lead to be placed in the right atrial appendage when inserted from the internal jugular or subclavian veins. The atrial pacing catheter is advanced into the right atrium, then withdrawn back to the superior vena cava while rotating the catheter slightly anteriorly to facilitate advancement into the right atrial appendage (the most stable atrial position). Appropriate position can be confirmed by fluoroscopy or chest radiography, which demonstrates a J curve that points cranially to the left and slightly anterior.

Threshold Testing and Confirmation of Placement

Capture and sensing thresholds should be tested once the pacing catheter is placed. The pulse generator rate is set approximately 10–20 pulses/min above the patient's native ventricular rate (if present) to determine capture thresholds, while the output is gradually decreased until capture is lost. Alternatively, the output can be slowly increased until consistent ventricular capture is observed (Fig. 7.5). Temporary pulse generators designed for temporary pacing deliver an electrical

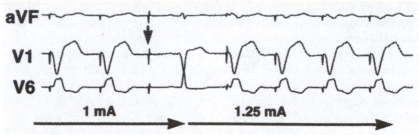

Fig. 7.5 Threshold testing. The first three stimuli are delivered with 1 mA output. The third pacing stimulus (arrow) does not result in ventricular depolarization. The output is increased slightly to 1.25 mA and consistent capture is observed.

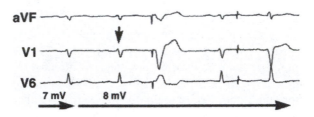

Fig. 7.6 Sensitivity testing. The pacing rate is set to a rate less than the intrinsic ventricular rate and the sensitivity dial is slowly adjusted. With the sensitivity set to 7 mV, the first QRS complex is sensed by the temporary pacemaker and causes inhibition of the pacing output. With the sensitivity set to 8 mV (which reduces sensitivity) the second QRS complex (arrow) is not sensed and the pacemaker delivers a pacing output at the programmed rate. The pacemaker then begins to output asynchronously; the second pacing stimulus does not result in ventricular capture because it is delivered during the ventricular refractory period. In this case the intrinsic ventricular electrogram has an amplitude between 7 and 8 mV. If no intrinsic ventricular rhythm is present, sensitivity testing cannot be performed.

stimulus that has a fixed pulse width (1–2 ms); thus, the stimulus output energy is reduced or increased by decreasing or increasing current. Ventricular capture thresholds should be less than 2 mA and ideally less than 1 mA (or <1 V) in stable lead positions, and should not change with coughing or deep breathing. Atrial leads are typically less stable, and capture thresholds around 2 mA (or 1–2 V) are acceptable. The presence of myocardial infarction, ischemia, flecainide, hyperkalemia, and other metabolic derangements can increase capture thresholds (Chap. 11) (19). The pulse generator output should then be set at two to three times the capture threshold for an adequate safety margin.

Sensing thresholds are determined by setting the pacing rate 10 pulses/min below the patient's native rate. The pulse generator sensitivity is progressively decreased (the sensitivity value is increased). When the sensitivity reaches a value greater than the amplitude of the intracardiac electrogram, the pulse generator begins to deliver pacing stimuli (Fig. 7.6). The sensitivity threshold represents the value at which the pacemaker no longer senses the native intracavitary potentials. The sensitivity should then be set at least one-half the value of the sensing threshold. The intrinsic intracardiac signal can be modified by myocardial ischemia or infarction, hyperkalemia, and Class IA antiarrhythmic agents, leading to undersensing. Ectopic ventricular depolarizations are often undersensed because of poor signal quality. These factors need to be borne in mind when setting the sensitivity of the pacemaker.

The lead must be repositioned until stable pacing is achieved if thresholds are not adequate for reliable pacing. Once stable capture and sensing thresholds are obtained, the pacing catheter should be secured to the skin with nonabsorbable suture both at the entry site and a site farther away with adequate slack between to ensure stability. The entry site is then sterilely dressed to prevent infection. A chest radiograph with both anterior, posterior, and lateral projections and a 12-lead ECG should be obtained to confirm appropriate positioning of the lead.

Daily Care

A daily chest radiograph and paced 12-lead ECG should be performed and compared to prior studies to check for possible pacing catheter migration (Fig. 7.7). Lead dislodgment ranges from 10% to 46% with higher rates when temporary transvnous pacing is required for extended periods (20,21). In situations where transvenous pacing is required for prolonged periods (symptomatic AV block in a patient with Lyme myocarditis or inferior wall myocardial infarction in which AV conduction will probably return or treatment of

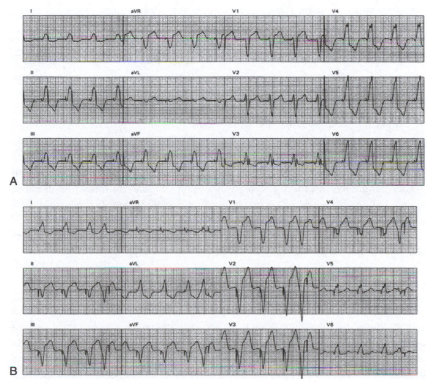

Fig. 7.7 (A) Twelve-lead ECG during pacing demonstrates left bundle-branch block morphology and inferiorly directed mean frontal plane axis, suggesting that the pacing electrode is in the right ventricular outflow tract. (B) Pacing lead placement in the right ventricular apex is indicated by the left bundle branch block morphology and the mean frontal plane superior axis. Notice that the pacemaker does not sense the premature ventricular depolarization (fourth QRS complex in all leads), which indicates that the sensitivity should be increased (by reducing the sensitivity value).

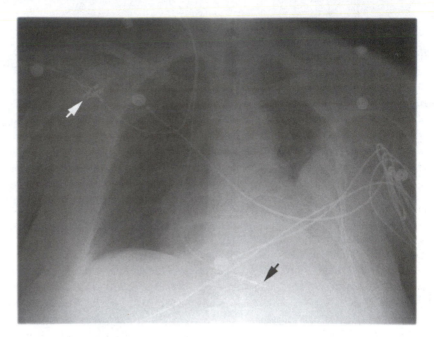

Fig. 7.8 Chest radiograph of a patient requiring long-term temporary pacing using an active fixation permanent pacing lead with the lead tip (black arrow) in the right ventricular apex and the proximal IS-1 lead connector (white arrow) seen outside the body attached to a temporary pacemaker.

infection in a pacemaker dependent patient) several investigators have used permanent active fixation pacing leads placed fluoroscopically attached to external temporary pacemakers or resterilized permanent pulse generators (Fig. 7.8) (22,23). In one study of 49 patients that required prolonged periods of temporary pacing due to infection (median duration: 8 days), lead dislodgment requiring repositioning occurred in 46% of patients with conventional temporary pacing lead and in 4% of patients with a percutaneously placed active fixation permanent pacing lead. Regardless of the pacing catheter/temporary pacing system used, pacing and sensing thresholds should be checked at least daily with any significant changes investigated for possible lead migration, lead disconnection from the pulse generator or change in the clinical status of the patient. Battery status should be monitored by the appropriate biomedical personnel and batteries replaced as needed.

Complications

Although transcutaneous temporary pacing is associated with few adverse effects, transvenous pacing does have the disadvantage of potentially serious complications. Complications rates range from 4% to 20%, and include pneumothorax, hemopneumothorax, arterial puncture, air embolism, serious bleeding, myocardial perforation, pericardial tamponade, nerve injury, thoracic duct injury, arrhythmias, infection, and thromboembolism (18,20). The risk of all complications is increased if pacing is initiated in emergent situations. To minimize risk, transvenous pacing should be accomplished when the patient is relatively hemodynamically stable. If emergent insertion is required, transcutaneous pacing should be initiated as a bridge to transvenous temporary pacing.

Most of the complications associated with transvenous pacing are related to obtaining venous access, and vary with insertion site. Subclavian vein access is associated with a higher rate of pneumothorax and hemopneumothorax (1–5%) (21). The internal jugular vein approach has a higher rate of carotid artery puncture (10%), and the femoral approach has a significantly higher rate of venous thrombosis (25–35%) and infection (5–10%) (21–23).

Myocardial perforation is a major complication that is not associated with the access site but is related to pacing wire insertion itself. This complication has a reported incidence of 1–10% (18,19,24). Fortunately, cardiac tamponade is uncommon even if perforation occurs. Myocardial perforation should be suspected if the patient complains of chest pain or a pericardial friction rub is heard after lead insertion. Other findings that suggest perforation are failure to (or loss of) sense or capture, diaphragmatic stimulation, or a change in morphology of paced QRS complexes. For example, although extremely rare, lead perforation into the left ventricle is associated with a change in paced QRS complexes from a left to a right bundle branch block pattern. Once perforation is suspected, the possibility should be investigated further by either recording electrograms from the electrode tip and ring or obtaining an echocardiogram. If perforation is present the tip electrogram is characterized by a Rs- or pure R-wave configuration, often resembling a surface lead V4, V5, or V6 appearance. Once the diagnosis of perforation is made, the catheter should be repositioned if pacing function is not stable or if the patient is experiencing chest pain. The catheter should be pulled back into the right atrium, then readvanced into the ventricle. Urgent pericardiocentesis is required if there is evidence of significant pericardial effusion or tamponade; otherwise, the patient can be followed expectantly with close hemodynamic and echocardiographic monitoring in addition to frequent physical examinations.

Transesophageal Pacing

Successful transesophageal pacing was first described in 1957. Although this method is effective for atrial sensing and stimulation, it is significantly less effective for ventricular pacing, which is achieved in only 3–6% of patients (25–28). The most common clinical use for transesophageal pacing is to terminate reentrant supraventricular tachycardias in children (29–38). Some investigators have also evaluated the use of transesophageal pacing as a stressor to evaluate for the presence of coronary artery disease (39).

Methods

Several esophageal electrode catheters are commercially available. The most popular is the "pill" electrode, which is comprised of a small-gauge flexible wire within a gelatin capsule that is swallowed by the patient; the gelatin capsule dissolves within 2–3 min and transesophageal pacing can be performed. Alternatively, new small diameter (4Fr and 5Fr) catheters can be used; these newer catheters have four electrodes so that pacing and recording can be performed simultaneously.

The catheters are usually placed via the nares to a depth of 40 cm in an adult. A standard ECG machine can be used to obtain a bipolar intracardiac electrical signal by placing the proximal and distal pacing catheter electrodes on the right and left arm electrodes and recording ECG "lead I." Because standard ECG machines use a high-pass filter of 0.5 Hz, the high-pass filter should be increased to 30 Hz if possible, which significantly reduces the artifact owing to respiration. A unipolar intracardiac signal is recorded by attaching the limb leads normally and the tip (or ring) electrode of the pacing lead to the V_1 terminal of the ECG machine.

In transesophageal atrial pacing, the lowest capture thresholds are observed at sites having the largest atrial electrograms; relatively long pulse durations of 10 ms are usually required. Specially designed pulse generators that are capable of providing pulse widths of 10 ms (and preferably 20 ms) and output of 30 mA (40–75 V) must be used; pulse generators designed for transvenous pacing rarely provide sufficient energy for effective transesophageal pacing.

Transesophageal pacing can be performed rapidly at the bedside because it requires neither vascular access nor fluoroscopy. The most common patient complaint is discomfort during pacing, which can be minimized by using lower energies. Long-term transesophageal pacing is not generally recommended because it has been associated with damage to the esophagus, albeit minimal.

Uses

Diagnosis and Treatment of Atrial Arrhythmias

The diagnosis of arrhythmias in pediatric patients is the most common use for transesophageal recording and pacing. The atrial electrogram recorded from within the esophagus reflects atrial activation just to the left of the interatrial septum. Atrial electrical signals can help differentiate atrial flutter, atrioventricular reentrant tachycardia owing to an accessory pathway, and junctional tachycardia.

Transesophageal pacing can be used to terminate reentrant atrial arrhythmias such as atrial flutter, atrioventricular reentrant tachycardia, and AV nodal reentrant tachycardia. If the pacing stimuli can enter a reentrant circuit in both the orthodromic and antidromic directions, the reentrant circuit can be terminated on cessation of pacing. Because atrioventricular tachycardia and AV nodal reentrant tachycardia often can be treated with vagal maneuvers or pharmacologic agents (adenosine, verapamil, diltiazem), the best use for transesophageal pacing is for termination of atrial flutter and other reentrant atrial tachycardias.

Typical atrial flutter is due to a reentrant circuit traveling around the tricuspid annulus. A number of different pacing protocols have been developed for terminating atrial flutter. Most protocols provide burst pacing at a rate slightly faster than the atrial rate, with progressive increases in rate until the patient develops atrial fibrillation or sinus rhythm returns. Short bursts (4–5 stimuli) are better tolerated and less likely to cause atrial fibrillation (29). In uncontrolled studies, transesophageal pacing has been successful in terminating atrial flutter in 43–86% of cases (30,31). Use of antiarrhythmic drugs such as propafenone may facilitate flutter termination by transesophageal pacing by slowing conduction velocity, which increases the "excitable gap." The larger excitable gap increases the chance that pacing stimuli will interact with the reentrant circuit and lead to flutter termination. Transesophageal pacing is also effective for treating patients with reentrant atrial tachycardias that occur after congenital heart surgery. In one study successful cardioversion was reported in 48 of 51 patients with atrial tachycardia after an atrial baffle procedure (Mustard or Senning) for transposition of the great arteries (32).

Stress Testing

Another potential use for transesophageal pacing is to increase the heart rate in patients who are unable to exercise and who require evaluation for coronary artery disease. In a recent study, stress echocardiography using both transesophageal atrial pacing and dobutamine was performed in 100 patients using a randomized crossover design (39). Both stress testing methods provided similar results for the evaluation of ischemia. Transesophageal atrial pacing stress echocardiography reduced the procedure time by 50%, and more than 50% of the patients preferred transesophageal atrial pacing or had no particular preference. Transesophageal atrial pacing may provide an alternative to pharmacologic stress (dipyridamole, adenosine, dobutamine) for evaluating patients who cannot exercise or are receiving negative chronotropic drugs.

Transthoracic Pacing

Transthoracic pacing is performed in two very different circumstances: during resuscitation from asystolic cardiac arrest and after open-heart surgery via epicardial wires placed by the surgeon (40–49).

Cardiac Arrest

The utility of transthoracic pacing in cardiac arrest is poorly defined. Transthoracic pacing is accomplished by insertion of a hooked pacing lead through the chest wall or epigastric area and adjacent ventricular wall to allow contact of the electrode with the ventricular endocardium. Because placement requires ventricular puncture with its associated risks of myocardial and coronary artery laceration, pericardial tamponade, and pneumothorax, its use has been limited to life-threatening situations where transcutaneous pacing is either not available or ineffective and when transvenous pacing cannot be accomplished rapidly. Capture rates are low (5–20%), probably because of the dire situations in which transthoracic pacing is usually used. In most studies very few if any patients survive resuscitative efforts (<5%) (40–42). No study has ever demonstrated improved survival with the use of transthoracic pacing.

Transthoracic pacing can be performed via a subxiphoid approach or parasternal approach (Fig. 7.9). For a subxiphoid approach, a 15-cm #18 gauge cannula is inserted in the subxiphoid area and advanced approximately 10 cm toward the left shoulder at a 30° angle. On free blood return, a 30- to 35-cm J-shaped pacing wire is advanced as far as possible through the cannula, and the cannula is removed. Pacing is attempted via the pacing wire. Thresholds usually range from 1 to 6 mA. If myocardial capture is not observed, then the pacing wire is slowly retracted while high output stimuli continue to be delivered. For the parasternal approach, the #18 gauge cannula is inserted in the left fifth intercostal space, 1–4 cm from the parasternal border, and directed toward

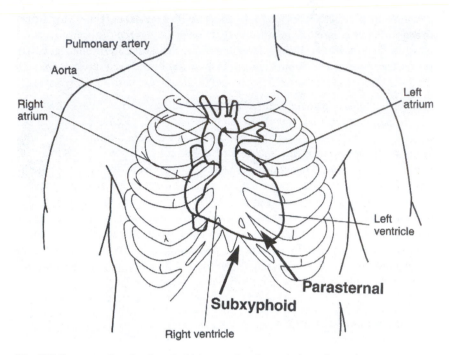

Fig. 7.9 Parasternal and subxyphoid approaches for transthoracic pacing.

the second right costochondral junction at a 30° angle. The cannula is advanced approximately 10 cm and the pacing wire is advanced as far as possible on free blood return. In a postmortem study, adequate pacing lead position was found in 80–90% of patients when the parasternal approach was used and 25–65% of patients when the subxiphoid approach was used (43). Transcutaneous pacing has rendered transmyocardial pacing virtually obsolete.

Epicardial Pacing

Epicardial pacing is employed after many types of cardiac surgery (44–47). At the time of operation, Teflon-coated leads with bare tips are sutured to the atrial and ventricular epicardium, exposed externally, and connected to a temporary pulse generator. These leads are usually placed prophylactically for use in the short-term management of bradycardias and tachycardias after major cardiac surgery. They can also be used to diagnose various tachycardias by simultaneously recording the atrial and ventricular electrograms with the surface ECG for comparison. Perhaps the most important use of this system is the maintenance or improvement of hemodynamic status in postoperative patients. The stroke volume and cardiac output can be optimized in hemodynamically compromised patients by maintaining or reestablishing an appropriate heart rate and AV synchrony. In addition perioperative cardiac resynchronization with temporary left ventricular and right ventricular epicardial leads has been used to improve hemodynamic function in selected patients with severely reduced left ventricular ejection fraction and widened QRS complex that do not have a permanent cardiac resynchronization device in place (50, 51). In a study of 70 consecutive patients undergoing open-heart surgery epicardial pacing wires were clinically useful for either therapeutic or diagnostic purposes in

80% of patients (52). The effects of epicardial biatrial pacing on the incidence of postoperative atrial fibrillation have also been studied. One study was prematurely stopped because of an increased incidence of atrial fibrillation in patients who received biatrial pacing (53).

Epicardial leads can be used in a standard bipolar or unipolar configuration. Pacing and sensing thresholds tend to deteriorate over several days. Epicardial leads with specially designed epicardial electrodes (as opposed to uninsulated braided wire) provide lower pacing thresholds (54, 55). The leads are removed by simple traction. The use of temporary epicardial wires is generally safe. In one series of more than 9,000 patients no complications were observed other than inability to remove the electrode in three patients; in all three patients the lead wire was simply clipped at the skin without sequelae. The effectiveness and safety of the epicardial system have led to widespread use.

References

1. Zoll PM. Resuscitation of the heart in ventricular standstill by external electric stimulation. *N Engl J Med* 1952;247:768–952.
2. Zoll PM. Noninvasive cardiac stimulation revisited. *PACE* 1990;13:2014.
3. Zoll PM, Zoll RH, Falk RH, et al. External noninvasive temporary cardiac pacing: clinical trials. *Circulation* 1985;71:937.
4. Falk RH, et al. Safety and efficacy of noninvasive cardiac pacing: a preliminary report. *N Engl J Med* 1988;17:27.
5. Talit IJ, et al. The effect of external cardiac pacing on stroke volume. *PACE* 1990;13:598.
6. Niemann JT, et al. External noninvasive cardiac pacing: a comparative hemodynamic study of two techniques with conventional endocardial pacing. *PACE* 1984;7:230–984.
7. Falk RH, et al. External cardiac pacing: influence of electrode placement on pacing threshold. *Crit Care Med* 1986;14:93.
8. Falk RH, et al. Cardiac activation during external cardiac pacing. *PACE* 1987;10:503.
9. Luck JC, et al. Clinical applications of external pacing: a renaissance? *PACE* 1991;14:1299.
10. Trigano JA, et al. Noninvasive transcutaneous cardiac pacing: modern instrumentation and new perspectives. *PACE* 1992;15:1937.
11. Furman S, et al. Intracardiac *PACE* maker for Stokes-Adams seizures. *N Engl J Med* 1959;261:943.
12. Marino PL. *The ICU book. Central venous access*. Philadelphia: Lea & Febiger, 1991:39.
13. Seneff MG. Central venous catheterization: a comprehensive review, Part 1. *Int Care Med* 1987;2:163.
14. Seneff MG. Central venous catheterization: a comprehensive review, Part 2. *Int Care Med* 1987;2:218.
15. Seldinger SI. Catheter replacement of the needle in percutaneous arteriography: a new technique. *Acta Radiol Diagn* 1953;89:368.
16. McGee DC, Gould MK. Preventing complications of central venous catheterization. *New Engl J Med* 2003;348:1123–1133.
17. Martin MJ, Husain FA, Piesman M, Mullenix PS, Steele SR, Andersen CA, Giacoppe GN. Is routine ultrasound guidance for central line placement beneficial? A prospective analysis. *Curr Surg* 2004;61:71–74.
18. Nolewajka J, et al. Temporary transvenous pacing and femoral vein thrombosis. *Circulation* 1980;62:646.

19. Pandian NG, et al. Transfemoral temporary pacing and deep venous thrombosis. *Am Heart J* 1980;100:847.
20. Austin JL, et al. Analysis of pacemaker malfunction and complications of temporary pacing in the coronary care unit. *Am J Cardiol* 1982;49:301.
21. Dohlma ML, et al. Myocardial stimulation threshold in patients with cardiac pacemakers: effect of physiologic variables, pharmacologic agents, and lead electrodes. *Cardiol Clin* 1985;3:527.
22. Murphy JJ. Current practice and complications of temporary transvenous pacing. *Br Med J* 1996;312:1134.
23. Braun MU, Rauwolf T, Bock M, Kappert U, Boscheri A, Schnabel A, Strasser RH. Percutaneous lead implantation connected to an external device in stimulation dependent patients with systemic infection – A prospective and controlled study. *Pacing Clin Electrophysiol* 2006;29:875–879.
24. Lever N, Ferguson JD, Bashir Y, Channon KM. Prolonged temporary pacing using subcutaneous tunneled axtive-fixation permanent pacing leads. *Heart* 2003;89:209–210.
25. Zei PC, Eckart RE, Epstein LM. Modified temporary cardiac pacing using transvenous active fixation leads and external resterilized pulse generators. *J Am Coll Cardiol* 2006;47:1487–1489.
26. Hynes JK, et al. Five-year experience with temporary pacemaker therapy in the coronary care unit. *Mayo Clin Proc* 1983;58:122.
27. Feliciano DV, et al. Major complications of percutaneous subclavian vein catheters. *Am J Surg* 1979;138:869.
28. Sznajder JI, et al. Central vein catheterization: failure and complication rates by three percutaneous approaches. *Arch Intern Med* 1986;146:259.
29. Kaiser CW, et al. Choice of route for central venous cannulation: subclavian or internal jugular vein: a prospective randomized study. *J Surg Oncol* 1981;17:345.
30. Morelli RL, et al. Temporary transvenous pacing: resolving postinsertion problems. *J Crit Illness* 1987;2(4):73.
31. Gallagher JJ, et al. Esophageal pacing: a diagnostic and therapeutic tool. *Circulation* 1982;65:336.
32. Benson DW Jr, et al. Transesophageal cardiac pacing: history, application, technique. *Clin Prog Pacing Electrophysiol* 1984;2:360.
33. Benson DW Jr, et al. Transesophageal atrial pacing threshold: role of interelectrode spacing, pulse width and catheter insertion depth. *Am J Cardiol* 1984;53:63.
34. Nishimura M, et al. Optimal mode of transesophageal atrial pacing. *Am J Cardiol* 1986;57:791.
35. Crawford W, Plumb VJ, Epstein AE, et al. Prospective evaluation of transesophageal pacing for interruption of atrial flutter. *Am J Med* 1989;86:663–667.
36. Falk RH, Werner M. Transesophageal atrial pacing using a pill electrode for termination of atrial flutter. *Chest* 1987;92:110–114.
37. Doni F, Della Bella P, Kheir A. Atrial flutter termination by overdrive transesophageal pacing and the facilitating effect of oral propafenone. *Am J Cardiol* 1995;76:1243–1246.
38. Butto F, Dunnigan A, Overholt E, et al. Transesophageal study of recurrent atrial tachycardia after atrial baffle procedures for complete transposition of the great arteries. *Am J Cardiol* 1986;57:1356–1362.
39. Montoyo J, et al. Cardioversion of tachycardias by transesophageal atrial pacing. *Am J Cardiol* 1973;32:85.
40. Benson DW Jr, et al. Transesophageal study of infant supraventricular tachycardia: electrophysiologic characteristics. *Am J Cardiol* 1983;52:1002.
41. Santini M, et al. Transesophageal pacing. *PACE* 1990;13:1298.

42. Blomstrom-Lundqvist C, et al. Transesophageal versus intracardiac atrial stimulation in assessing electrophysiologic parameters of the sinus and AV nodes and of the atrial myocardium. *PACE* 1987;10:1081.

43. Critelli G, et al. Transesophageal pacing for prognostic evaluation of pre-excitation syndrome and assessment of protective therapy. *Am J Cardiol* 1983;51:513.

44. Benson DW Jr, et al. Atrial pacing from the esophagus in the diagnosis and management of tachycardia and palpitations. *J Pediatr* 1983;102:40.

45. Lee CY, Pellikka PA, McCully RB, et al. Nonexercise stress transthoracic echocardiography: transesophageal atrial pacing vs. dobutamine stress. *J Am Coll Cardiol* 1999;33:506–511.

46. Edhag O, et al. Cardiac pacing through transthoracic electrode in acute myocardial infarction. *Acta Med Scand* 1972;192:145.

47. Tintinalli JE, et al. Transthoracic pacing during CPR. *Am J Emerg Med* 1981;10:113.

48. White JD, et al. Transthoracic pacing in cardiac asystole. *Am J Emerg Med* 1983;1:264.

49. Brown CG, et al. Placement accuracy of percutaneous transthoracic pacemakers. *Am J Emerg Med* 1985;3:193.

50. Del Nido P, et al. Temporary epicardial pacing after open heart surgery: complications and prevention. *J Cardiac Surg* 1989;4:99.

51. Dzemali O, Bakhtiary F, Dogan S, Wittlinger T, Moritz A, Kleine P. Perioperative biventricular pacing leads to improvement of hemodynamics in patients with reduced left-ventricular function–interim results. *Pacing Clin Electrophysiol.* 2006 Dec;29(12):1341–1345.

52. Waldo AL, et al. Use of temporarily placed epicardial atrial wire electrodes in the diagnosis and treatment of cardiac arrhythmias following open-heart surgery. *J Thorac Cardiovasc Surg* 1978;76:500.

53. Kurz DJ, Naegeli B, Kunz M, et al. Epicardial, biatrial synchronous pacing for prevention of atrial fibrillation after cardiac surgery. *PACE* 1999;22:721–726.

54. Waldo AL, MacLean WAH. *Diagnosis and treatment of cardiac arrhythmias following open heart surgery: Emphasis on the use of atrial and ventricular epicardial wire electrodes.* Mount Kisco, NY: Futura Publishing, 1980.

55. Kallis P, Batrick N, Bindi F, et al. Pacing thresholds of temporary epicardial electrodes: Variation with electrode type, time, and epicardial position. *Ann Thorac Surg* 1994;57:623–626.

8

Defibrillator Function and Implantation

Robert E. Eckart, Jane Chen, and Laurence M. Epstein

The development of the implantable cardioverter-defibrillator (ICD) is primarily the result of pioneering work by Michel Mirowski. First-generation devices consisted of a large generator placed in an abdominal pocket capable only of high-energy shocks. In the 25 years since the first implantation in humans (1), advances in technology have resulted in significantly smaller devices, with sophisticated detection algorithms and tiered therapies. Despite these advances, the primary goal of the ICD continues to be the rapid and effective treatment of ventricular arrhythmias.

Description of Defibrillation Systems

Today, all defibrillators contain many of the features found in pacemakers elsewhere. Similar to a pacemaker, the generator supplies low-energy current to power the basic functions of the device, but also is capable of delivering a high-energy current density for depolarizing the myocardium. The ICD lead has the ability to pace and sense intrinsic ventricular activity like a pacemaker, but also has one or two coils which act with the generator as additional electrodes. The first human implants used a titanium spring coil positioned in the subclavian vein along with an epicardial cup or patch sutured over the cardiac apex, via a left thoracotomy incision (1,2). The leads were tunneled under the skin to the generator, which was placed in the subcutaneous tissue overlying the abdominal wall. With advances in lead technology allowing transvenous implantation, and a reduction in generator size allowing for a pectoral implant, a nonthoracotomy approach was rapidly adopted (3). Continued advances now allow for nearly all contemporary ICD systems to be placed in the electrophysiology laboratory with the assistance of conscious sedation (4). The success of ICD technology has been well demonstrated and large trials continue to identify patient populations that may benefit from prophylactic implantation for the reduction of sudden cardiac death (5–8).

Although original indications for ICD implantation were in survivors of sudden cardiac death or known ventricular arrhythmia (9–11), prophylactic ICD implantation is now common to a population with less "high-risk." As Bayesian theory would suggest, the probability of successfully detecting and treating a potentially fatal ventricular arrhythmia is proportionate to the risk that the patient is of having a ventricular arrhythmia. As prophylactic therapy is pursued, enhanced algorithms to assist in the discrimination between ventricular and supraventricular arrhythmias (notably sinus tachycardia and atrial fibrillation) to reduce the burden of "inappropriate shocks" while maintaining a high sensitivity toward ventricular arrhythmia has become a focus of intense research (12–14). Research has demonstrated that early administration of rapid ventricular pacing (antitachycardia pacing, ATP) can be successful in the termination of many ventricular arrhythmias, which, when backed up by an ICD, has proven to be extremely successful in the reduction of discomforting, but appropriate, shocks (15,16). Lastly, widespread dissemination of this technology is costly, and the pursuit of lower cost, safe, "lead-less" systems is continuing.

Pulse Generators

First-generation devices were approximately twice the size of a modern personal digital assistant (PDA), or about four times the size of a modern ICD. The large size (~300 g, 250 cc) forced implantation in the abdomen. Evolving ICD technologies have focused on decreasing the size of the pulse generators, which would allow pectoral implantations, improve patient comfort, and decrease local pocket complications. The bulk of the pulse generator consists of the battery and the capacitor (Fig. 8.1). The battery serves as the energy storage reservoir, and charges the capacitor to a significantly greater voltage, which can then be discharged across the myocardium. The size of the devices is directly related to the maximum available energy output. The ability to manufacture smaller devices while maintaining adequate available energy is mainly limited by advances in battery and capacitor technology.

Besides the battery and the capacitors, the pulse generator also contains the operational circuitry of the device, which consists of low-power circuits (sensing, pacing, amplifiers, microprocessors) and high-power charging and output circuits. ICD generators must monitor electrical status through sense amplifiers, analyze waveforms for abnormal arrhythmias, deliver appropriate therapy, be reliable, and have a significant lifetime before battery depletion.

Battery

The power for the ICD system is supplied by the battery, which serves as the energy storage reservoir. ICDs use either a single-cell battery (~3 V) or two cells in series (~6.5 V) to charge a high-voltage capacitor up to 750–800 V for

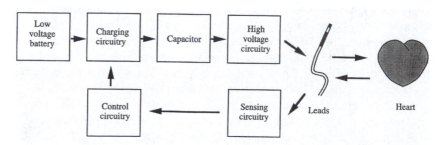

Fig. 8.1 Simplified diagram of major components of an ICD generator.

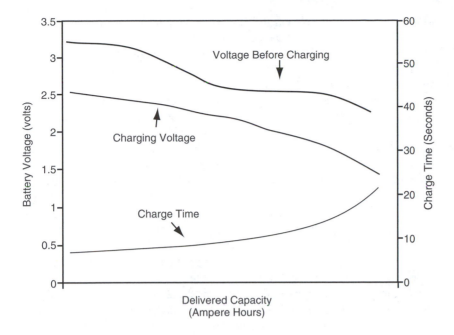

Fig. 8.2 Characteristics of a typical lithium silver vanadium oxide battery. See text for details. (From Mehra R, Cybulski Z. Tachyarrhythmia termination: lead systems and hardware design. In: Singer I, ed. *Implantable cardioverter defibrillator*. Armonk, NY: Futura Publishing, 1994:127, with permission.)

defibrillation with 25 to 40 J. It must be remembered that although the batteries do not directly supply the energy necessary for high-voltage defibrillation, frequent recharging of discharged capacitors will more rapidly deplete the battery voltage. The battery is used nearly continuously for the control of the microprocessors essential for function, as well as pacing functions that may be required. The ideal battery should be small, with high stored energy per unit volume, no internal resistance in order to facilitate charging the capacitor, and predictable end-of-life (EOL) characteristics. The lifetime of the battery is dependent on the number of shocks, percentage of time spent in monitoring and pacing, and battery capacity.

Unlike pacemakers, designed for a slow continuous discharge, ICD design mandates rapid charging of the capacitor with a high peak current. Conventional pacemaker batteries (lithium iodine, Li/I_2 and lithium carbon monofluoride, Li/CFx) have continuous microamperage drainage that is critical for sustainability of a low output, but may be inappropriate for transient high output needs. Most of the currently available ICDs use lithium silver vanadium oxide (Li/SVO) batteries (Fig. 8.2). Lithium/manganese dioxide batteries are occasionally used (e.g., Biotronik), although this formulation is usually reserved for automated external defibrillators. The Li/SVO battery has the advantage of a high charge density with resultant high peak currents (~2–3 A) needed to provide adequate defibrillation. A typical Li/SVO battery can store 1,800 J/cc. Therefore a 10 cc battery can store 18,000 J, allowing for about 500 shocks at 34 J each during its lifetime. Because the battery charges the capacitor, whether the capacitor delivers its charge for the purpose of defibrillation, or the charge is allowed to dissipate over time is of little relevance to the battery life. As will be discussed shortly, the capacitor is periodically charged and passively drained to allow for short charge times. The capacitor charge time is responsible for the critical delay between detection of ventricular arrhythmia and treatment with defibrillation. This capacitor charging, although programmable on many devices, is nominally performed every 1–3 months. With a set capacitor recharge of every 1–3 months, a conventional ICD can have an expected battery performance life of 5–8 years. To increase battery longevity, one can increase the interval between capacitor recharge, although this may come at the expense of marked prolongation in charge times, and thereby prolong delivery of life-sustaining therapy. More importantly, the converse is true, in that more frequent recharging of the capacitor leads to shorter charge times, but likewise at the expense of battery longevity.

The elective replacement indicator (ERI) signifies that the battery is approaching EOL, and that a generator change should be electively scheduled as soon as feasible. Although previously determined by prolonged capacitor charge time and residual battery voltage, most manufacturers rely strictly on battery voltage to determine ERI and EOL in conventional ICDs. Although generally designed for a 3 month delay (17–20), the time from ERI to EOL is dependent on the same features that are responsible for any battery depletion, most notably, low output pacing and high output capacitor charge. For standby ICDs reaching ERI was generally not problematic; however, cardiac resynchronization therapy-defibrillators (CRT-D) now require both continuous low output pacing and the high output necessary for capacitor charging. Clinically effective CRT-D requires near total biventricular pacing, and therefore the time from ERI to EOL may be markedly shorter than a conventional standby ICD and replacement should be pursued shortly after ERI. When a device reaches ERI, the time available for backup pacing and the number of shocks remaining is limited, but all other functions of the device operate as programmed until the battery reaches EOL. Although dependent on manufacturer, at EOL the device may be limited to bradycardia pacing and maximum energy shock therapy. All other functions, such as antitachycardia pacing and low energy cardioversion, are no longer available.

Current ICD batteries are limited in that the power capability is significantly less in the second-half of each discharge, and there can be a continual increase in internal battery impedance over the life of the device. Since internal battery impedance is the critical component determining charge time, that interval between detection and treatment with defibrillation, there can be prolongation of charge time as the battery ages, premature of anticipated performance (21). Current algorithms change the relationship of capacitor charging in an attempt to have a consistent charge time over the life of the device (22). A second problem with conventional Li/SVO batteries is the additional generator space required to accommodate battery swelling associated with the development of propylene gas as part of the reduction reaction. A combination lithium-limited silver vanadium oxide battery (Li/CSVO) has been described that is more consistent in delivery of power across a 7 year period without the development of propylene gas (23). The combination of a more reliable energy supply without the need for additional space may become the next standard in battery design.

Alternative battery sources will continue to be sought. The "nuclear pacemaker" of the 1970s, while expensive and unlikely to make a return, had a longevity of 99% at 15 years (24,25). Innovative thought will identify the next direction of battery development. Continued discussion of transforming finite energy sources to a principle of scavenging energy from the environment is a possible new chapter in battery design. In the same fashion that some hybrid electric vehicles attempt to recapture the energy dissipated when braking, microelectricomechanical systems are being designed to capture the small vibrations associated with body movement and transform this motion to energy (26). Although transcutaneous energy transforming systems are being actively pursued, some programs, such as recharging implantable systems through special shoes while walking on a customized floor, may be best left to a select group of patients (e.g., artificial heart recipients) (27). Infrared energy sources are of demonstrated value in recharging external batteries of those with artificial hearts (28), and research continues in miniaturization and subcutaneous implantation of these "solar panels" for infrared recharging of implantable medical devices (29).

Capacitors

Capacitors store charges drawn from the battery. The most common capacitors currently used in ICDs are aluminum and tantalum electrolytic capacitors. Capacitors are necessary because the battery itself cannot deliver a current fast enough for defibrillation, and it cannot deliver a voltage high enough for defibrillation. Energy cannot be chronically stored in a capacitor, however, because charges passively dissipate from a capacitor. Therefore, capacitors must be charged just before defibrillation. Current flows from the battery to the capacitor when an electronic switch between the battery and the capacitor is closed. A highly specialized and complex high-voltage circuitry converts the battery voltage (~3–6.5 V) to the 750–800 V in the capacitor. This process in devices available today takes approximately 3–10 s. When the switch between the battery and the capacitor is opened, the high voltage in the capacitor is then discharged via the leads across the myocardium in a matter of milliseconds. The total energy available for discharge (E_{Stored}) is proportional to the capacitance–voltage product ($C \cdot V$) stored in a capacitor, such that $E_{Stored} = \frac{1}{2} C \cdot V^2$.

The energy required for defibrillation should be with the lowest voltage necessary in order to minimize myocardial injury. According to the preceding equation, however, lower voltage would require larger capacitances (i.e., a larger capacitor) and subsequently a larger pulse generator. In practice, the design of the capacitor is a balance between delivering low energy and a reasonably small capacitance size. This is usually accomplished by using capacitances between 50 and 150 μF. The surface area of the capacitor is markedly increased by either etching small holes into the aluminum foil, or heating and solidifying the tantalum powder causing small cracks to appear, both of which can be used to hold a charge.

When voltage is discharged from capacitors after a shock, the dielectric within the capacitors slowly deteriorates, meaning that the alignment of molecules within the capacitor necessary for effective storage becomes random. The important clinical consequence of this behavior is that, if a device has not been used for a prolonged period, the time required for initially charging the capacitor can become excessive (more than 40 s in some older devices that had not been used for several years). Therefore, the capacitors must be periodically realigned by charging the capacitors and "dumping" the charge using a process called capacitor reformation. Earlier devices required capacitor recharging to be performed manually via the programmer at the time of clinic visits. Newer devices can usually be set to automatically perform this function several times throughout the year.

Sensing Circuitry

Before an arrhythmia can be treated, the electrodes must first sense it. First-generation devices used an algorithm called the "probability density function" or PDF to sense ventricular arrhythmias (30). PDF was based on the concept that sinus rhythm spends a significant amount of time at a point of myocardial isoelectricity while most fibrillatory rhythms spent a minimum amount of time at isoelectricity (31). This algorithm failed to reliably detect all life-threatening ventricular arrhythmias, and inappropriate defibrillation for faster supraventricular rhythms, to include sinus tachycardia limited its viability. Similarly, intracardiac pressure sensors identifying sustained myocardial stand-still were used as clues to indicate arrhythmia (32). Although a rate corrected PDF for identification was tried (33), modern systems use local bipolar electrograms (two distinct electrodes measuring change in electrical potential in tissue) and amplifying systems to permit accurate sensing of small electrograms such as seen in ventricular fibrillation (VF) (34,35). Local recordings of these electric signals are sensed from the electrodes and processed through the sensing circuitry (Fig. 8.3) (36). Similar to a pacemaker, the signals are amplified, and then filtered to reject low-frequency signals (e.g., skeletal myopotentials, electromagnetic interference) and high-frequency noise. Next, a rectifier transforms the signals to negate effect of polarity. Finally, the signal is compared to a threshold voltage, and an R wave is sensed when the signal exceeds the threshold. Both R-wave amplitude and voltage threshold are measured in millivolts. The sensitivity setting of a device refers to the voltage threshold against which the R waves are compared. The more sensitive the setting, the lower the threshold, therefore a setting of 2 mV is more sensitive than a setting of 8 mV.

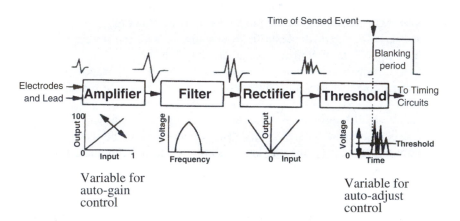

Fig. 8.3 Block diagram of an ICD sensing circuit. Raw signals are amplified, filtered to reject high and low frequency noises, rectified to eliminate polarity dependency, then compared to a voltage threshold. (From Olsen WH. Tachyarrhythmia sensing and detection. In: Singer I, ed. *Implantable cardioverter defibrillator*. Armonk, NY: Futura Publishing, 1994:75, with permission.)

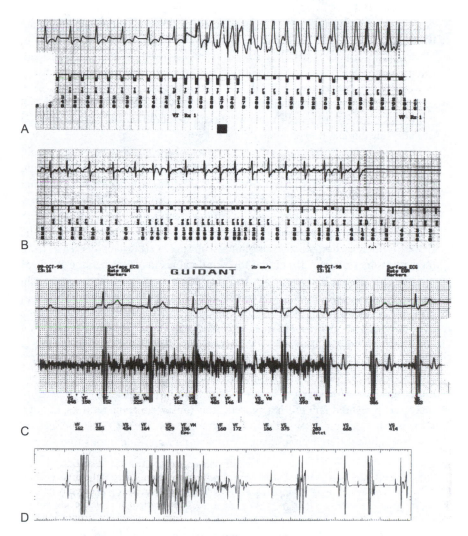

Fig. 8.4 Examples of ICD oversensing. **(A)** T-wave oversensing. During sinus rhythm, double counting of R and T waves led to VT detection (TD), triggering therapy with antitachycardic pacing (ATP). ATP resulted in true VF, which was detected and treated with a single shock. **(B)** Crosstalk. In this example, the ventricular lead is sensing not only R waves from the ventricle, but also activity in the right atrium. The patient is in atrial fibrillation, which is sensed by the device as VF. The patient subsequently received a shock. **(C)** Oversensing of diaphragmatic myopotentials. The patient in this example received multiple shocks while having a bowel movement. Interrogation showed sensing of diaphragmatic myopotentials with Valsalva maneuvers, sensed by the ICD as VF. **(D)** Lead fracture. Electrical noise (large, sharp spikes) was detected as VF. In this particular case, the shock was aborted when decreased noise at a later strip allowed for detection of sinus rhythm.

ICDs, like pacemakers, can be subject to oversensing or undersensing. Oversensing occurs when the device detects an event that either does not exist or is not owing to ventricular depolarization, and may result in inappropriate shocks. Examples of oversensing are T wave sensing, crosstalk (sensing electrical signals from another chamber, i.e., atrium), myopotential or diaphragmatic sensing, or lead fracture leading to electrical noise (Fig. 8.4). Undersensing occurs when the device fails to register an event. This occurs most often when the electrogram is smaller than the sensitivity setting of the device. Changes in electrograms can occur with lead dislodgment, infarction at the site of the lead, inflammation or fibrosis at the electrode site, and lead fracture. Undersensing is a particular concern with ICDs, because they must be able to sense not only normal R waves (which may be up to 20 mV in amplitude), but also VF (which can be less than 1 mV). Inappropriate withholding of therapy because of undersensing can be potentially catastrophic.

Because of the variations in the amplitudes of the electrograms, fixed gain and sensitivity settings, such as used in pacemakers, may result in undersensing of VF or oversensing of T waves. Some devices attempt to enhance VF sensing with autoamplifiers. The two most common types of amplifiers currently used in ICDs are the automatic gain control and autoadjustable threshold. With automatic gain control, the sensitivity threshold is fixed, and the gain of the EGMs is increased when the amplitudes of several R waves decrease from the large values of sinus rhythm to the small values in VF. When the R waves increase in amplitude during VF or after spontaneous termination, the gain automatically decreases (37). Oversensing of T waves, pacing spikes, and diaphragmatic activity may occur during this period of increased gain, and thus specificity may be reduced. An alternative that is more commonly used is an autoadjusting threshold, in which the amplifier gain is fixed, and the sensitivity threshold is increased for each beat to a fraction of the preceding R-wave electrogram (38). The threshold then decreases exponentially until it reaches the programmed sensitivity. T waves that follow fall under the temporarily increased threshold and are not sensed. The sensitivity then declines rapidly, allowing for detection of small electrograms seen in VF (39). As seen in Fig. 8.5 subtle differences in manufacturer programming demonstrate similar

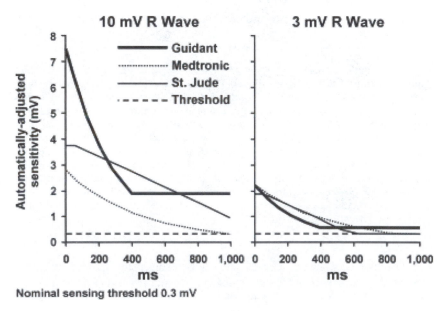

Fig. 8.5 Figure from Swerdlow and Friedman, Fig 19, comparing autoadjusting threshold by manufacturer. (Swerdlow CD, Friedman PA. Advanced ICD troubleshooting: Part I. *Pacing Clin Electrophysiol* 2005;28:1322–46.)

(A)

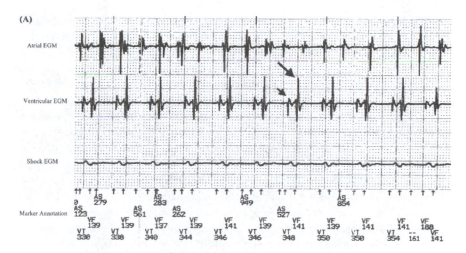

Fig. 8.6 Figure of irregular SVT, with stabilization at 125 bpm, and double counting (large and small arrows) leading to sensed rate of 250 bpm. 23 J delivered, terminates SVT (not shown). (Chugh A, Scharf C, Hall B, Cheung P, Good E, Horwood L, Oral H, Pelosi F, Jr., Morady F. Prevalence and management of inappropriate detection and therapies in patients with first-generation biventricular pacemaker-defibrillators. *Pacing Clin Electrophysiol* 2005;28:44–50.)

objective. With a set ventricular sensitivity of 0.3 mV, after a sensed event, the Medtronic ICD multiplies nominal sensitivity by eightfold to tenfold, up to a maximum of 75% of sensed R-wave amplitude with an exponential decay based on time constant and blanking period. The St. Jude Medical ICD starts at 62.5% of sensed R-wave (with range limitation from 1.875–3.75 mV), then remains constant for 60 ms, and then decays linearly at 3 mV/s. The Guidant ICD starts at 75% of the sensed R-wave and then decays over the next 290 ms to a predetermined minimal value based on the average R-wave.

Autoadjustment is critical not only to avoid T-wave oversensing but also to avoid double-counting associated with CRT-D therapy. When Y-adapters were used for left ventricular pacing, and prior to software upgrades, the sensed event in the left ventricle, by virtue of ventricular dyssynchrony, may be significantly later than the sensed right ventricular activation. As such, double-counting of sequential right and then left ventricular activity, commonly caused devices to meet detection criteria for arrhythmia management (Fig. 8.6) (40).

After an electrical signal is sensed, the device times the interval to the next sensed event. The time between two consecutively sensed signals is measured in milliseconds, and is known as the cycle length. Initial tachyarrhythmia detection in conventional devices is primarily based on rate, as is discussed in detail elsewhere is this chapter.

Leads

Although the pulse generator provides the power for defibrillation and vcontains circuitry for sensing and detection, the leads set up the current flow for defibrillation and provide the actual sensing of local electrograms. Current density is achieved when current flows between two electrodes, and density of the current decreases rapidly with distance away from the electrodes. Higher energy can be achieved with a larger electrode surface area, because they can distribute current density more evenly across the myocardium. The energy delivered is also directly proportional to the impedance of the electrodes, which in turn is inversely proportional to their surface areas.

Initial electrodes used for defibrillation were patches that were sewn onto the epicardium or pericardium. Patches come in a variety of sizes, and are either rectangular or oval in shape, flat, or contoured. They are made with either titanium or with platinum alloy helical coil, materials that are chosen because of their low impedance. The choice of patch location and number of patches used is based on heart size and the combination that can achieve the lowest defibrillation threshold (DFT), or the lowest energy at which defibrillation is achieved. The patches are usually placed with one at the posterolateral LV wall or at the apex, and a second one against either the right ventricle (RV) or right atrium (RA) (Fig. 8.7) (41,42). Early series with epicardial patches were complicated by high perioperative mortality (up to 5%), and long term by "crinkling" leading to unacceptably high DFTs (up to 30%) as well as patient discomfort and hemodynamically significant constrictive pericarditis (up to 10%) (43–45).

Initially, the high-voltage patch electrodes were also used for sensing. However, frequent oversensing prompted the use of a separate sensing lead, either epicardial or endocardial (46). Epicardial sensing and pacing was achieved using two distinct unipolar screw-in leads to generate a bipolar signal. Although the treated population was indeed at high-risk during early lead development, the high perioperative mortality, the discomfort associated with sternotomy and subsequent long-term complications spurred rapid development of an alternative nonthoracotomy approach.

Transvenous endocardial leads are made of high-voltage conductors. At least one conductor is used for the defibrillation coil, which is usually located near the tip of the lead and is meant to be placed along the posterior wall of the RV. Defibrillation leads can have either a single coil (one conductor) or two

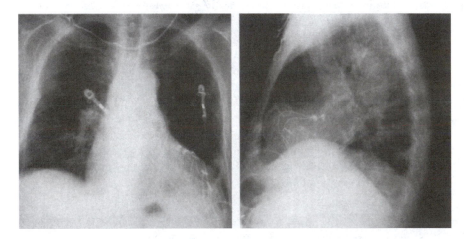

Fig. 8.7 Posterior–anterior and lateral plain film radiograph demonstrating defibrillation patches on the anterior and anterolateral left ventricle accompanied by multiple sensing leads. All of this is attached to an ICD pulse generator implanted in the abdomen. (From Eager G, Gutierrez FR, Gamache MC. Radiologic appearance of implantable cardiac defibrillators. *Am J Radiol* 1994;162:25–29.)

shocking coils (two conductors). The second coil is located more proximally to the distal coil. Because endocardial ICD leads have a fixed coil interspace, although the distal coil is placed in the RV the proximal coil will be anywhere from the subclavian vein to the RA, depending on the anatomy of the patient, most notably the degree of RV dilatation. Typically, this distance is ~18 cm, although St. Jude Medical has released a lead (Riata® defibrillation lead) with differing interelectrode distances (17–21 cm) which should be considered in patients with extreme of anatomy. Although not commonly performed, separate single coil leads may be implanted in the RV as well as in the superior vena cava (SVC), coronary sinus (CS), or in combination (47). Although seen to reduce the shocking impedance of a system, an additional shocking coil in the low right atrium has been demonstrated to be of no value in the reduction of DFTs (48).

Configuration refers to the anode and cathode electrodes between which current flows. By convention, the RV lead is usually designated the cathode, and the configuration is anodal to cathodal. For example, initial transvenous, abdominal systems defibrillated between an electrode in the RV and a second electrode either in the SVC or in the CS ("SVC → RV" or "CS → RV" configuration). With the implant of devices in the pectoral region, and thus in close proximity to the heart, a patch was hidden behind the generator housing ("can") to act as a second electrode ("can → RV" configuration). Now, an "active-can" configuration refers to a generator housing that is in fact integral to the system as another electrode.

Regardless of the number of leads and the combination used, successful defibrillation is more likely if a large, even current density can be distributed across a significant portion of the myocardium. Thus, because the pulse generator has a large surface area and can provide more even current distribution, defibrillation using the generator as one of the electrodes can be achieved with lower energies than defibrillation with a combination of leads and/or patches. Lower DFTs have been shown with the "can → RV" configuration than with "CS → RV" or with "SVC → RV" configurations, partially explained by the anatomically larger current density encompassing the entirety of the LV (49).

The introduction of a third electrode (a second shocking coil) was in an attempt to further reduce DFTs. The most common electrodes used in practice are the distal (RV) coil, the proximal (SVC) coil, and the pulse generator housing. Two electrodes may be connected, with the current flowing between the two joined electrodes (anodes) and a third common electrode (cathode). The area of the myocardium between the anodes should be minimized because there is no current flow between the two joined anodes. The lowest DFTs are achieved by joining the proximal coil and the pulse generator, with the distal coil as the common electrode. This "can/SVC → RV" configuration provides the most optimal current density across the myocardium. Anecdotally, reversing the polarity of the configuration by designating RV as the anode and SVC/can as the cathode ("RV → can/SVC" configuration) may lower DFTs. However, there is currently no definitive evidence that the polarity of the configuration significantly affects the DFT (50).

Sensing in an endocardial system is achieved through a distal electrode at the tip of the lead, using a high-voltage conductor similar to a conventional pacing electrode. Bipolar leads consist of two conductors, one for shocking and the other for sensing. Sensing, in this case, occurs between the tip of

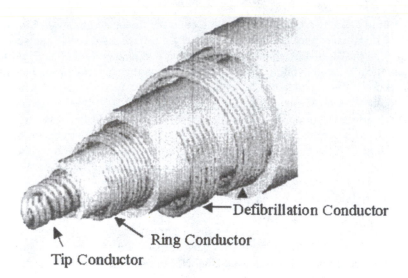

Tip Conductor

Ring Conductor

Defibrillation Conductor

Fig. 8.8 Coaxial (Gradaus R, Breithardt G, Bocker D. ICD leads: design and chronic dysfunctions. *Pacing Clin Electrophysiol* 2003;26:649–57.)

the lead and anywhere along the length of the shocking coil, and is termed "integrated bipolar sensing." Because of the distance between the tip and the coil, as well as the length of the coil, sensing in these leads is more susceptible to noise, far field artifacts, and postshock undersensing than true bipolar sensing (51). True bipolar sensing occurs between the distal tip of the lead and a ring located approximately 1 cm proximally from the tip. Newer lead technologies include a quadripolar lead, which consists of the two shocking coils, and true bipolar sensing with a distal tip and ring configuration (e.g., Medtronic Sprint Quattro™, St. Jude Medical Riata® ST).

The first available endocardial lead was the Endotak-C defibrillation lead (CPI and later Guidant, St. Paul, MN), with the first human implant in 1988. Original leads were coaxial in construction, with a layer of conducting material sheathed in insulation, wrapped again in conducting material, and again sheathed in insulation (Fig. 8.8) (52). Newer leads (e.g., Guidant Endotak Reliance®, Medtronic Quattro™, St. Jude Medical Riata®, Biotronik Kainox and SPS) all rely on multilumen lead construction in which each conductor is individually sheathed in insulation and then packaged in silicone housing. The advantage of multilumen design is its smaller size and increased resistance to compression.

The shocking coils are usually platinum based due to its resistance to corrosion in the body. New advances include coating with titanium nitride (TiN) and fractal iridium to increase the lead–myocardial interface and to reduce polarity without change in thresholds. Therefore, an alloy with iridium is usually used. The latest advance in ICD lead technology is assurance of isodiametry and reduction of tissue ingrowth.

As reviewed in the section on endocardial lead extraction, the irregularity of a shocking coil may promote tissue ingrowth and will increase risk of adhesion (53). In dual coil systems, the proximal coil has the potential to be placed with tissue tension along the SVC, a risk factor for adhesion. For this reason, the

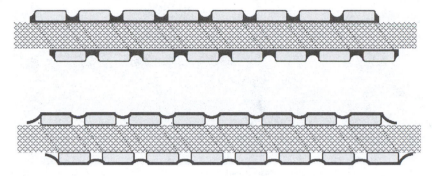

Fig. 8.9 Attempts at reduction of tissue ingrowth between defibrillator lead coils include either silicone backfilled coils as demonstrated on the top, compared to a coating of the entire coil as demonstrated on the bottom.

shocking coils are now treated to prevent this tissue ingrowth. As demonstrated in Fig. 8.9, the two most commonly used approaches include to backfill the coils with silicone to reduce irregularity in between the filars, or to coat the entire coil in ePTFE (Gore-Tex). Although animal models are promising (54), the leads have not been on the market long enough that definitive evidence of ease of extraction has been demonstrated in humans. Due to the potential of fibrosis and stenosis of the proximal coil, and the limited reduction in DFT, in many patients a single coil lead may be appropriate. This is especially true for young patients and children in whom multiple leads may be required over a lifetime.

Device Function

Tachyarrhythmia Detection

As previously described, R-waves are sensed when their amplitudes are detected above a set threshold. The time interval between two sensed events is the cycle length. Detection is the process of analyzing recent cycle lengths and R-wave morphologies to classify rhythms and determine appropriate programmed therapy. The ICD cannot distinguish between a macro-reentrant scar-related VT and chaotic VF. What it can do is distinguish arrhythmias based on rate. The labeling of fast rhythms as VT and even faster rhythms as VF is for operator convenience only. After initial detection, newer devices will distinguish based on morphology and A-V relationship for SVT discrimination, but the foundation is strictly rate-based.

Detection should be a rapid process so that therapy can be delivered before a patient develops symptoms or before an electrogram deteriorates, but not so rapid that self-limiting or nonsustained arrhythmias are aggressively treated. Because ventricular arrhythmias can be sustained or self-limiting, hemodynamically stable or unstable, ICDs should be able to respond to each episode by a sequence of detection, confirmation of arrhythmia prior to delivery of therapy, redetection if therapy is unsuccessful, and detection of nontachycardia rhythms after successful therapy to conclude the episode and to reset detection parameters.

The rate cutoff is defined as the heart rate above which the device will be triggered to deliver therapy. The original devices were not programmable,

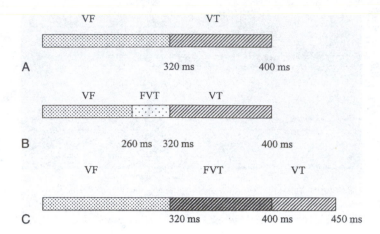

Fig. 8.10 Programmable detection zones. (**A**) Two zones, VF and VT, are programmed. (**B**) Fast VT (FVT) is programmed via the VF zone. (**C**) FVT is programmed via the VT zone. See text for details.

and the cutoff rate and sensitivity level were preset at the factory. Devices today have both programmable zones of detection, with different therapies possible for each zone (i.e., "tiered therapy"). Detection periods are zones of cycle lengths (CL) that are nonoverlapping and programmable. An average of the most recent cycle lengths of the sensed events is compared against various detection zones. For example, if the VF zone is programmed at 320 ms (~188 bpm), and the ventricular tachycardia (VT) zone is programmed at 400 ms (150 bpm), a detected CL will be classified into the VF zone if it is <320 ms (>188 bpm), and will be classified into the VT zone if it is between 320 and 400 ms (150–188 bpm). If a detected CL is >400 ms (<150 bpm), it is considered normal and therefore not classified as a tachycardia (Fig. 8.10).

For a tachyarrhythmia to be detected, a specified number of cycle lengths must be counted within a detection zone. Because VF CLs are often not regular, and VF EGMs may be intermittently below the set sensitivity, VF detection is usually programmed to occur when a specified percentage of the cycle lengths counted is within the VF detection zone. Although the proprietary names differ, the number of sensed events that occur within a detection zone to classify an event as VF is based on an average of the last several identified events (e.g., 12 of 16 sensed events in VF detection zone, or sustained classification for set time), and is programmable. Although some implanters use nominal settings, programming should be based on preimplant likelihood and suspected clinical response to an arrhythmic event. If an active patient with long QT syndrome has known nonsustained VF, and without immediate hemodynamic collapse during sustained episodes, one may prolong the number of sensed events required to initiate therapy (e.g., 18 of 24 events, or sustained classification for 2.5 s), if only to give the patient a chance to spontaneously terminate. Alternatively, if a patient is known to have high-risk substrate, with near-immediate hemodynamic collapse, a more sensitive setting may be desired, and possibly reduction of number of categorized events to initiate therapy is warranted (e.g., 8 of 12 sensed events, or sustained classification for 1 s). Increases in specificity of detection must be weighed against risk of syncope, degradation of rhythm to an under-sensed "fine VF", and the possibility of increased DFTs with ongoing metabolic derangement.

Because clinical VT is generally more stable than VF, and slower rhythms are generally more stable than faster rhythms, VT detection usually requires consecutive numbers of intervals that fall within the VT zone (i.e., 16 of 16 cycles), and the counter can be reset to zero by a single cycle length that falls outside the detection zone. In addition to VT and VF zones, newer devices have a third zone that can be programmed (fast VT "FVT" for Medtronic, "VT-1" for Guidant). When FVT is employed, it uses the detection algorithms assigned to either the VT or VF classifications, but therapy is tailored based on rate within the classification. When FVT detection is programmed via the VF counter, FVT is detected when the required number of cycle lengths falls between the FVT and VF detection zone. If only one cycle length falls below the VF detection zone, then VF is detected. Because it is programmed via the VF counter, consecutive intervals are not required, and therefore the detection is faster. In addition, more aggressive therapy is delivered because the default is the VF zone. This is ideal if a patient has a fast VT that is not well tolerated, but that may not require immediate high-energy defibrillation as in VF. If FVT is programmed via the VT counter, and the required number of cycle lengths falls between the FVT and VT zones, then slow VT will be detected. If one interval is less than the programmed FVT zone, then fast VT will be detected. This method may be associated with longer detection time, because detection of VT usually requires consecutive cycles. This programming is most often used in patients who have both a slow, hemodynamically stable VT, and a faster VT, which may require more aggressive therapy.

Although detection based on cycle lengths of sensed ventricular electrograms alone is highly reliable, inappropriate shocks can sometimes occur, accounting for 25–35% of therapies in conventional trials (55). This most commonly occurs with atrial fibrillation and sinus tachycardia, where the rates of these and other nonventricular arrhythmias fall within the detection zones (56). To decrease the risk of inappropriate shocks, newer devices offer additional detection parameters to increase the specificity of VT detection. Although limited to dual chamber systems, in 95% of all VTs, there are more ventricular than atrial events, and this should be a successful determinant of arrhythmia. However, the other 5%, most notably those with brisk V-A conduction, or double tachycardia with atrial fibrillation and VT, the risk of inappropriate therapy, or worse, withholding of therapy is too high. Medtronic's PR Logic attempts to utilize the A-V relationship by recognizing that within an R–R interval, sensed atrial activity that is nearly simultaneous with ventricular activity is likely to be of junctional origin, whereas sensed activity during the later half of the interval is more likely to be from an antegrade source, and finally, sensed atrial activity during the first half of the preceding R–R interval may be most consistent with retrograde conduction from a primary ventricular event. One problem with PR logic was that it was originally limited by 1°-AV block, whereby there would be shortening R–R intervals with exercise, and although the A-V relationship did not change, the sensed atrial activity relative to the R–R interval would be moved progressively closer to the first half, and eventually misclassified as retrograde activity and possibly of ventricular origin. Enhanced PR logic corrects this possible misclassification by allowing programmability of the zones in which SVT and VT are classified, most commonly with continued classification of SVT as those within 65% of RR, instead of 50% of R–R interval. For the faster zones (VF zones) discrimination parameters are generally not appropriate, with convention being early defibrillation for exceedingly fast ventricular rates offering the best chance of survival. These VT detection enhancements include sudden onset criterion, rate stability criterion, and morphology discrimination (57).

The *"sudden onset"* criterion is intended to distinguish sinus tachycardia with a gradual increase in rate from VT with a *"sudden onset."* With sudden onset turned on, the device inhibits therapy if the rate increase is gradual. The onset value can be programmed as a percentage of the last several cycle lengths or as an absolute value difference between intervals. The ICD locates and measures a pair of intervals where the cycle lengths decreased the most (onset). If the difference between this interval and previously measured intervals is above the programmed onset value, the ICD classifies the onset as sudden. If the difference is below the programmed onset value, it is classified as gradual, and therapy will be inhibited. Therapy is then delivered only if the rate accelerates to a higher tachycardia detection zone. This approach is highly specific for the exclusion of sinus tachycardia (58). The obvious shortcoming of this enhancement is ventricular tachycardia that begins during sinus tachycardia, such as onset of VT during exercise, which may be mistakenly classified as gradual onset and therefore not detected.

The *"rate stability"* criterion allows the ICD to withhold VT detection for rapid, supraventricular rhythms with irregular intervals, and can be used to differentiate VT with minor rate variability from atrial fibrillation with large variations in cycle lengths (58). The ICD begins to apply the criterion only after a certain number of events are already counted in a VT zone. Two commonly used methods include determination of variability from mean values and standard deviation, or a rate-adjusted determination of anticipated RR intervals. Sequential unstable intervals will reset the detected intervals that might otherwise be counted as VT. Some degree of variation, however, can be seen with monomorphic VT, particularly in the setting of antiarrhythmic drug therapy. If the VT stability intervals are programmed at a small value, for example, less than 30 ms, and if the differences in the R–R intervals of the VT exceed this value, the ICD will mark the intervals as unstable and fail to detect VT (59,60).

The concept of morphology discrimination is a fall back to the earliest arrhythmia detection algorithms incorporated in the AID-B device (Intec Systems, Pittsburgh, PA) known as probability density function, discussed earlier. Although deviation from isoelectric intervals was only short lived, the continued premise of alteration of depolarization identity continues. Although previous limited by complex calculations required to perform Guidant's VTC (vector and timing correlation), and St. Jude Medical's Morphology Discrimination, both are now regularly available, as are others. These algorithms evaluate the morphology of a QRS signal during known sinus rhythm, and use this as a template in which to compare later sensed events. The premise, much like a surface ECG, is that ventricular ectopy will have a different morphology than that as a result of normal His-Purkinje system depolarization both as a function of width and vector. In a single chamber system, an SVT or even a sinus tachycardia with rate dependent aberrancy may be misclassified as a VT, and generally morphology criteria are combined with additional criteria. More recent advances use time and frequency domain analysis with continued collection to determine features of normal depolarization specific for the patient, to include reclassification of aberrancy as SVT if appropriate.

The advantage of a dual-chamber ICD is the improvement in the detection and identification of arrhythmias to prevent inappropriate therapy, and availability of dual-chamber pacing capabilities. About 10–25% of patients receiving ICDs may require dual-chamber pacing at some point, and for the ICD recipient population, direct implantation of a dual-chamber device may be cost effective (61). Although there is controversy on the value of dual-chamber algorithms versus single-chamber rate and morphology criteria, there is little doubt that physician review of the event EGMs is greatly facilitated by determination of the A-V relationship (62,63). For an excellent review of current algorithms in depth, the reader is encouraged to review a 2004 article by Aliot et al (64). Rather than upgrade patients at a later date, our institution pursues dual-chamber ICD implantation if clinical circumstances or electrophysiology testing suggests the potential for significant disease in the sinoatrial or atrioventricular node. Newer atrial-based algorithms to minimize ventricular pacing (dynamic AAIR-DDIR mode switching) resolve the concern about inappropriate right ventricular pacing and deleterious remodeling (65,66).

Although the use of these detection enhancement parameters may increase specificity of VT detection, the concern exists that these parameters may mistakenly inhibit therapy, or delay time to detection, for true VT. To circumvent this, ICD programs allow therapy to be delivered when a tachycardia is sustained for a programmed period of time. If a therapy is withheld because of discriminators and the rate of the tachycardia remains in a detection zone, therapy will be delivered once the programmable duration period has expired. This feature ensures delivery of therapy if a tachycardia is sustained at a high rate for a period of time, regardless of whether the device categorizes it as SVT or VT.

The first ICDs were "committed" devices so that delivery of therapy could not be aborted once detection criteria for ventricular arrhythmias were met. Current devices can confirm a rhythm prior to discharge of energy, and therapy can be aborted if the tachycardia is nonsustained, thereby minimizing unnecessary and painful shocks. Confirmation does not occur prior to delivery of antitachycardia pacing (ATP), however, because ATP is meant to be delivered rapidly and painlessly. Indeed, one of the latest advances in Medtronic devices is the potential for the administration of ATP immediately upon detection, and during simultaneous charging of the capacitor for potential delivery of defibrillatory shock upon confirmation. Confirmation of a ventricular rhythm usually occurs during or after capacitor charging, and generally consists of checking a single cycle length to verify that it is still within a tachyarrhythmia detection zone. If the cycle length during confirmation falls within the VT or VF detection zone, therapy will be delivered. If VT had spontaneously terminated, then sinus rhythm would be detected during confirmation, and therapy would be aborted. Confirmation prevents delivery of therapy when the arrhythmia has terminated, which might actually initiate VF. Although rare, spontaneous termination of a rhythm to sinus, with intermittent premature ectopic beats may fall into the VT or VF zone leading to an inappropriate shock. Although confirmation of VT or VF prior to delivery of therapy is generally a very useful feature, a shock can be inappropriately diverted if there is variation in the arrhythmia cycle lengths so that one interval happens to fall outside a detection zone during confirmation. If therapy is either diverted inappropriately or if it is unsuccessful in restoring sinus rhythm, redetection of arrhythmia will begin. Most algorithms use a smaller number of intervals for meeting redetection criteria, and most devices will not allow confirmation in the redetection period after one diverted or unsuccessful therapy. In essence, therapy after redetection of VT/VF following a diverted or unsuccessful shock is committed, so that the overall duration of an episode is kept to a minimum. It is important to recognize that aborting a therapy does not mean the termination of a tachyarrhythmia detection episode. Termination of an episode requires that a specific number of CLs fall outside the detection zones, and results in the resetting of all detection counters to zero.

Therapy

Early devices were limited to a single form of therapy with a single high-energy shock. Today's devices offer a range of therapies, from programmable high-energy defibrillation shocks to low-energy synchronized cardioversion to antitachycardia pacing.

Defibrillation

The process of defibrillation involves halting ventricular fibrillation wavefronts within a critical mass of myocardium. Despite numerous studies, the exact mechanism of defibrillation remains controversial. The critical mass theory and the upper limit of vulnerability (ULV) theory are two widely recognized hypotheses, both seeking to explain failure of intermediate energy shocks to successfully defibrillate VF. The critical mass hypothesis states that shocks extinguish wavefronts near the electrode, but activation wavefronts continue in areas of low potential gradient far from the electrode. When these activation wavefronts continue in a region larger than the critical mass, VF is then propagated to the rest of the heart (67). The ULV hypothesis states that shocks extinguish *all* activities in the ventricle, and that VF is reinitiated when the shock falls on the vulnerable period of one or more myocardial regions. Because there will always be certain portions of the myocardium in the vulnerable period, the shock strength needed for successful defibrillation must not only depolarize a critical mass of the myocardium, but also be stronger than the ULV of all myocardial regions (68,69).

Defibrillation is a probabilistic function. Higher energy is more likely to defibrillate than lower energy, but the relationship is nonlinear and has significant covariables, to include autonomic or metabolic state. The DFT is usually taken to be the lowest energy at which defibrillation sometimes succeeds, and generally is lower than the minimum energy required for consistently successful defibrillation, which is not a clinically obtainable value (Fig. 8.11). In practice, the lowest energy that successfully converts VF to sinus rhythm during ICD testing is taken as the DFT, and the measured safety margin is the difference between the maximum output of a device and the DFT (70).

Many patients undergoing ICD implantations are also on antiarrhythmic drug (AAD) therapy, and the effects of AADs on DFTs should be taken into consideration. Class IC and IB agents, such as encainide, flecainide, lidocaine, and

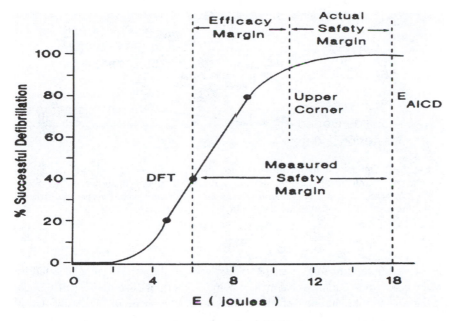

Fig. 8.11 Percent probability for successful defibrillation versus shock energy. The measured safety margin is the difference between the maximum output of the device and the measured DFT. The actual safety margin is the difference between the maximum output of the device and the energy required for consistent defibrillation success. ("upper corner," approximately the energy with 95% success rate.) (From Singer I, Lang D. Defibrillation threshold: clinical utility and therapeutic implications. *PACE* 1992;15:932–949, with permission.)

mexiletine, cause a reversible, dose-dependent increase in energy requirements for successful defibrillation (71–74). Amiodarone appears to have a bimodal effect on DFTs: acute administration may lower DFT in the animal model, but chronic use elevates DFTs (75,76). Type IA drugs, such as procainamide and quinidine, do not appear to affect DFTs significantly, whereas sotalol and *N*-acetyl-procainamide have been shown to lower DFTs (77).

Although higher energy strength is associated with increased defibrillation success, signs of cell damage can occur at higher stimulus strengths. A potential gradient of 60 V/cm can cause conduction block and inhibition of normal automaticity (78). Cell death occurs when the gradient of the shock is more than 100–200 V/cm (79). Therefore, it is desirable to obtain the lowest DFT possible in order to minimize myocardial injury. Initially, defibrillation was provided by an instrument developed by Zoll, which used 60-cycle alternating current (AC) for a duration of 150 ms, with available voltages from 180 to 750 V, applied with large electrodes across the closed chests of dogs (80). Lown compared the effects of AC on defibrillation with direct current (DC) discharged through a capacitor (81). He found that the use of capacitor discharge was associated with a higher success rate of defibrillation and a significantly lower incidence of ventricular and atrial arrhythmias, myocardial injury, and death. From that time, DC capacitor shocks became the standard energy form for defibrillation. Although recent capacitor technology has made miniaturization of generators possible, ongoing research has also

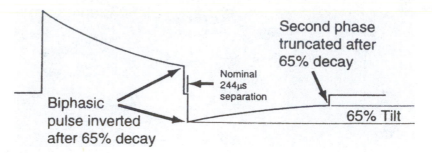

Fig. 8.12 Optimal biphasic tilt waveform. See text for details. (From Cohen SI, Schuger C. Implantable devices for the treatment of rhythm disturbances. In: Baim DS, Grossman W, eds. *Cardiac catheterization, angiography, and intervention*, 5th ed. Baltimore: Williams & Wilkins, 1996:508, with permission.)

focused on optimizing the shape and polarity of the waveforms generated by the capacitors to allow for delivery of lower energies. The number of phases, the tilt, and the duration of phases determine the shape of the defibrillation shock waveform.

Defibrillation waveforms can be delivered as a single monophasic pulse, sequential or simultaneous monophasic pulses, biphasic pulses with the two phases in opposite polarities, or triphasic pulses with the first and third pulses in the same polarity. Although previous work showed value to sequential delivery of monophasic pulses or simultaneous delivery through multiple leads, this vwork has been supplanted by the biphasic waveform (82,83). In one study comparing DFTs of monophasic and biphasic waveforms in 79 patients receiving nonthoracotomy leads, DFTs of less than 20 J are found in 91% of cases using biphasic waveforms, and in only 76% using monophasic pulses (84). An optimal biphasic waveform has an initial positive phase, followed by a negative terminal phase, with lower amplitude of the negative phase than of the positive phase, and the same duration and tilt for both phases (Fig. 8.12). Tilt is the difference between the voltage charge at the beginning of the phase and at the end of the phase, expressed as a percentage of the initial voltage, with original nominal values of 65%. Optimal values for maximizing defibrillation efficacy while minimizing refibrillatory phenomena are variable, and dependent on impedance of the system as a whole. While some studies have shown reduction of 15% in DFTs with a 50%/50% tilt, others have shown no benefit between 65%/65% and 42%/42% in DFTs (85–87). St. Jude Medical ICDs offer a variety of programming capability for changing tilt and duration that may allow for increased safety threshold in the patient with known high DFTs, although this circumstance should be rare (8). Triphasic waveforms continue to be investigated, but data so far suggests minimal incremental benefit (88,89).

Low-Energy Synchronized Cardioversions

Although VF often requires a relatively higher energy for termination, some ventricular tachycardias can be terminated with very low energies. Low-energy synchronized cardioversions have several advantages, including faster delivery of therapy, less patient discomfort, and conservation of battery energy.

Although each patient's pain threshold may vary, most patients tolerate a first shock of less than or equal to 1 J, although subsequent shocks are associated with increased perception of pain (90,91). There are unique differences identified when low-voltage shocks fail, with propagation of reentrant rhythms seen at very low shock values, and stimulation of automatic focus firing when low-voltage shocks fail that approximate the DFT of the myocardium (92). The risks of utilizing this therapy are acceleration of stable VT to VF and time delay to successful treatment if initial cardioversion is unsuccessful. Frequently, an initial 5 J defibrillatory shock will be delivered as the first of the defibrillations in the slower VT zones, mainly because of the speed with which the capacitor can be charged, although this low-voltage therapy should not be tried more than once, with subsequent defibrillations at or above the DFT.

Antitachycardia Pacing

The ability to terminate tachycardias with pacing was available prior to the advent of the ICD. However, because of the potential risk of accelerating VT to VF, the use of ATP was limited to the treatment of supraventricular tachycardias until the ability to defibrillate the heart was also available. Similar to low-energy cardioversions, the advantages of ATP include rapid delivery of therapy, less discomfort to the patient, and conservation of battery life (15,16,93). The concept of ATP in terminating VT is based on the fact that some VTs, such as those in patients with prior myocardial infarctions, are caused by reentrant circuits involving the border zones of prior myocardial infarctions (Fig. 8.13). In a reentrant circuit, the leading activation wavefront must encounter excitable tissue. The region of excitable tissue between the progressing activation wavefront and the "tail" of recovering tissue is known as the "excitable gap." Termination of VT occurs when a stimulus enters the

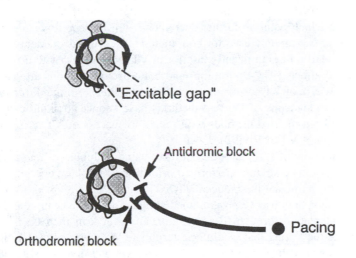

Fig. 8.13 (Top) Ventricular tachycardia is most commonly owing to a reentrant circuit at the border of injured (shaded islands) and normal tissue. The reentrant circuit is frequently characterized by an "excitable gap" of tissue. (Bottom) Rapid pacing can interact with the reentrant circuit by entering the "excitable gap." If pacing causes block in both the antidromic and orthodromic directions, the reentrant circuit is extinguished on cessation of pacing.

"excitable gap" and interacts with the reentrant circuit, resulting in a block in the forward direction (orthodromic) and backward direction (antidromic) (94,95).

The addition of multiple extrastimuli is used to increase the probability of a stimulus interacting with the tachycardia circuit, at a slightly increased risk of accelerating the VT. Almendral and associates showed that in 53 consecutive patients, interaction with the reentrant circuit (which is often called resetting by electrophysiologists) occurred in 55% with a single extrastimulus, 79% with double extrastimuli, and 85% with multiple stimuli (96). Increasing the number of extrastimuli increases the likelihood of tachycardia termination, because progressively earlier extrastimuli can "peel back" the refractoriness of intervening myocardial tissue, increasing the odds of one of the extrastimuli entering the excitable gap. Although increasing the number of pacing beats with burst pacing can increase the efficacy of tachycardia termination, longer pacing trains or more tightly coupled extrastimuli may be associated with acceleration of a stable VT to VF.

The two most commonly used methods of ATP are rate-adaptive burst pacing and autodecremental or ramp pacing. With rate-adaptive burst pacing, the device is programmed to deliver a set number of pulses at a constant coupling interval based on a percentage of the VT CL (Fig. 8.14). The sequence may be repeated in successive trains if VT is redetected. Each sequence is titrated by decrementing the coupling interval between pulses by a set amount per sequence, usually 10 ms. If the tachycardia accelerates during a pacing sequence, then the interval between pulses would be based on the percentage of the new tachycardia CL minus the decremental amount of the sequence, provided that the interval is not below the minimum set interval. In the autodecremental or ramp-pacing mode, the initial coupling interval within a sequence is also based on a percentage of the tachycardia CL. Within a sequence, each coupling interval is decremented by a set amount, usually 10 ms. Again, there is a minimum-coupling interval that acts as a safety device, at which point no further decrements will be seen. Pulse decrements of 10 ms are commonly used for both methods, because decrements less than 10 ms appear to be significantly inferior in VT termination, with no reduction in adverse effects (97). Both ramp- and burst-pacing methods are associated with a low risk of VT acceleration when drive trains are limited to nine beats or less. Comparisons of the two methods have shown no significant differences between the two methods with regard to success of VT termination or acceleration of VT to VF (98).

Programming of ATP can be performed using a number of methods. If an electrophysiologic study is performed prior to ICD implant, and burst pacing was able to terminate the induced VT, ATP can be programmed accordingly. Alternatively, noninvasive programmed stimulation (NIPS) can be performed after implantation through the generator, and ATP can then be tailored to determine the setting that would best terminate VT without accelerating it to VF. ATP can also be programmed empirically, which is a reasonable approach because the success of termination may be different between induced and spontaneous VT. A commonly used method is the "PainFREE" protocol (93), in which the ATP is assigned for rates from 240 to 320 ms as burst pacing at 88% of the tachycardia CL for two cycles, and then again at 88% minus 10 ms for two cycles, followed by defibrillation. This protocol has been demonstrated

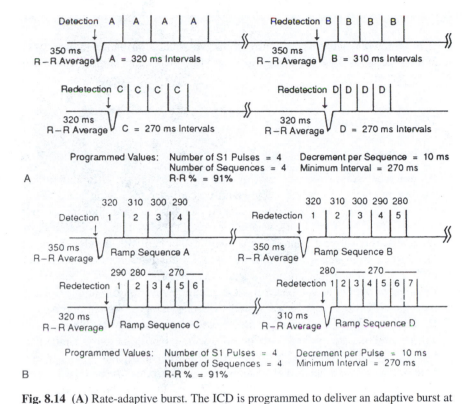

Fig. 8.14 (**A**) Rate-adaptive burst. The ICD is programmed to deliver an adaptive burst at 91% of the tachycardia cycle length on detection of VT. The number of pulses within the burst is programmed to four and the sequence will repeat itself four times on redetection of the tachycardia. The programmed decrement per sequence is 10 ms but the decrements may not go below a programmed minimum interval of 270 ms. In the example, a tachycardia at 350 ms is detected. The first burst sequence (A) should be 320 ms (350 ms × 91% = 320 ms). The first pulse is delivered accordingly at 320 ms from the R wave that fulfilled the programmed detection criteria. All subsequent pulses of this sequence are separated by 320 ms. Assuming that the VT is redetected and the RR interval remains at 350 ms, a second burst sequence (B) is decremented by 10 ms (320 ms − 10 ms = 310 ms). In the example, sequence (B) results in the acceleration of the tachycardia to 320 ms, which is again redetected. The calculated pulse interval (C) is now 270 ms (320 ms × 91% = 290 ms − 20 ms decrement = 270 ms). Assuming that the tachycardia is unaffected and redetected at 320 ms, the fourth and final burst sequence (D) will be 270 ms (the programmed minimum interval) despite the fact that the calculated pulse interval would have been 260 ms (320 ms × 91% = 280 ms − 30 ms decrement = 260 ms). (From Cohen SI, Schuger C. Implantable devices for the treatment of rhythm disturbances. In: Baim DS, Grossman W, eds. *Cardiac catheterization, angiography, and intervention*, 5th ed. Baltimore: Williams & Wilkins, 1996:513, with permission.) (**B**) Autodecremental ramp. The ICD is programmed in this case to deliver an autodecremental ramp of four pulses, starting at 91% of the average sensed RR, continuing on redetection for four sequences with a decrement per pulse of 10 ms, not to exceed a minimum interval of 270 ms. The first ramp sequence (A) should start at 320 ms (350 ms × 91% = 320 ms) with each interval thereafter shortened by 10 ms so that the fourth interval equals 290 ms. Assuming that the tachycardia is redetected (B), the initial ramp pulse will be 320 ms, with decrements of 10 ms with the ramp as above but with the addition of a fifth beat at 280 ms. Before the third ramp sequence (C), the average RR shortens to 320 ms. Accordingly, the initial pulse is 290 ms (320 ms × 91% = 290 ms). After a decrement of 10 ms for interval two, intervals three, four, and five and the additional sixth beat are all delivered at the programmed minimum of 270 ms. Acceleration of the tachycardia to 310 ms determines that the first pulse will be delivered at 280 ms, with intervals two to six and the additional seventh beat at the minimum programmed value of 270 ms. (From Cohen SI, Schuger C. Implantable devices for the treatment of rhythm disturbances. In: Baim DS, Grossman W, eds. *Cardiac catheterization, angiography, and intervention*, 5th ed. Baltimore: Williams & Wilkins, 1996:513, with permission.)

to be effective in termination of arrhythmia without defibrillation in over 89%. With the new "ATP during charging" offered by Medtronic, similar results can be expected.

ICD Implantation

Techniques

As previously discussed, the first available devices required a thoracotomy for placement of epicardial patches and epicardial rate-sensing leads. With the exception of cases involving congenital heart disease limiting access to the right side of the heart, venous obstruction or systemic bacteremia or fungemia, this surgical approach has been abandoned with the development of transvenous systems. Although the simultaneous intraoperative placement of 1 or 2 left ventricular epicardial leads may be prudent in select patients at the time of bypass or valve surgery, the routine extension of surgery for the placement of routine epicardial systems is unnecessary. Surgical approaches for implantation of epicardial patches include the anterolateral thoracotomy, subcostal thoracotomy, and subxiphoid and median sternotomy. Epicardial systems include two patch electrodes for delivering high-energy shocks and at least two unipolar epicardial sensing/pacing electrodes. In some cases, two additional epicardial electrodes are placed for backup use, because of a significant incidence of sensing lead failure. These are tunneled to the pocket and capped for future use. Patch electrodes can be placed either on the epicardium or on the pericardium. Care must be taken during surgical placement of the patches to avoid injury to the myocardium and to position the patches such that minimum DFTs are achieved. If the patch is to be outside the right atrium, it should be sewn to the outside of the pericardium to avoid perforation of the thin right atrial wall (42). The patches are positioned to adequately cover the myocardium, while keeping the borders apart to avoid shunting of current flow. In addition, the patches must be positioned such that the current flows across the septum and not near the coronary arteries. Postoperative complications include pericarditis, phrenic nerve damage, atrial arrhythmias, focal bleeding, patch displacement, and inflammation at the tissue–patch junction leading to sensing failures. Long-term complications include patch crumpling, lead fracture and dislodgment, infection, patch erosion, and constriction caused by the patches (41–45).

The first transvenous systems required abdominal implant because of the size of the pulse generator. Transvenous leads were tunneled subcutaneously to the abdomen. Additionally, subcutaneous patches or arrays were often required to achieve adequate DFTs because early devices used monophasic waveforms for defibrillation. Abdominal implants are now placed rarely, and usually only in patients (a) in whom a pectoral implant would carry significant risks of pocket erosion, (b) those with previous multiple pectoral pocket infections, or (c) those whose anatomy precludes pectoral implants. By the early 1990s, the size of the pulse generator had decreased sufficiently to allow for pectoral implantation. With the device in this location, the large surface area of the pulse generator could be used as an active electrode, which resulted in further lowering of DFTs to the range seen with epicardial implantation (99,100). Currently, left pectoral implantation using techniques similar to pacemaker implantations is the first choice for most institutions. Right pectoral locations, owing to the greater distance from the heart, are less effective but often adequate. Some patients desire subpectoral implants for cosmetic purposes. However, this location may be associated with increased peri-procedural complications and significant complication associated with generator changes (99). Subpectoral implants should be reserved for those in whom the risk of erosion is extremely high.

Initially, cardiothoracic surgeons in the operating room implanted ICDs, and this practice continues today in some hospitals. However, in most institutions with an active electrophysiology program, device implantation has become the responsibility of electrophysiologists. Implantation under local anesthesia combined with intravenous sedation, performed by electrophysiologists in a laboratory with air-filtering facilities similar to those used in the operating room, has been shown to have high success and low complication rates and short implantation and fluoroscopy time, and is associated with earlier discharge from the hospital (3,101). The perioperative mortality of pectoral device implant is very low (anticipated <1 in 500), and generally dependent on comorbidities such as renal and respiratory insufficiency, in addition to operator experience (102,103). Procedure-related complications are listed in Table 8.1. While a number of nonelectrophysiologist implanters have sought credentialing, physicians need to be aware of local market saturation, as studies have demonstrated that operators who perform >40 procedures per year have the lowest complication rate (102).

Implantation of transvenous ICD systems employs techniques similar to those used for permanent pacemaker implantations, and is discussed in detail in a separate chapter in this book. Connecting ICD leads to the device is slightly different than connecting pacemaker leads to pacemaker generators. All ICD pulse generators have at least three ports for single chamber devices (four ports for dual chamber devices, and five ports for CRT-D). One LV port is for the pace/sense IS-1 terminal pin, and two are for the defibrillation coil (usually DF+ and DF−). The second DF port may be capped if a single coil

Table 8.1 Procedure-related complications.

Associated with DFT testing
Inability to defibrillate
Hypotension
Associated with access using subclavian approach
Pneumothorax
Hemothorax
Subclavian artery puncture
Venous thromboembolism
Phrenic nerve stimulation
Right ventricular perforation
Pericardial effusion/tamponade
Generator pocket hematoma
CVA/TIA

lead is used, or is used to connect to subcutaneous patch if needed. The biggest difference between pacemaker and ICD implantation is not in placement of leads, but rather in testing and programming.

Intraoperative Testing

The ability to reliably sense and reproducibly defibrillate VF is fundamental to successful ICD implantation. Therefore, meticulous testing of leads and device function must be carried out at the time of implant. The ventricular lead must be tested for adequate sensing in sinus rhythm, with R wave amplitudes no less than 5 mV and preferably >10 mV. The slew rate is also obtained. The slew rate is the rate of rise of the signal voltage, and is large when the signal amplitude is large. The larger the slew rate, the more likely that R-waves, rather than T-waves, will be detected. Much like insertion of a pacemaker lead, care must be taken to obtain a stable position, to rule out diaphragmatic pacing and to rule out oversensing of myopotentials. Pacing threshold must also be acceptably low to ensure reliable backup pacing and successful capture during ATP. Repositioning of the lead must be carried out if any of the parameters are unsatisfactory.

An important part of ICD implantation that is not part of pacemaker implantation is testing of the device to determine DFTs. This is generally performed prior to closing the wound; after satisfactory lead positions and parameters are obtained, the leads are connected to the ICD, and the entire system is implanted into the subcutaneous pocket. To test the device, anesthesia with a short-acting agent such as propofol, or deep conscious sedation with a combination of narcotics and benzodiazepines is required. The testing is usually performed through the manufacturer's programmer, with a sterile interrogator head placed over the implanted pulse generator. Occasionally, testing may be performed through an emulator, which substitutes for the actual pulse generator and connects the defibrillation lead to the programmer. Although an emulator allows determination of DFTs prior to making a decision on ICD model, the emulator may not reflect the real-life response of the implanted ICD. An initial low-energy (1–2 J) synchronized shock may be considered to ensure that all connections are intact and to determine the high-voltage lead impedance before VF induction.

Today's devices offer a range of options for inducing VF. VF is commonly induced by critically timed T-wave shocks or high-frequency pacing. With T-wave shocks, paced beats are delivered at a fixed cycle length, followed by a low-voltage shock during the vulnerable period of the T wave to induce VF. Alternatively, rapid burst pacing at 50 Hz can be delivered, with the length of time of delivery at the discretion of the operator.

DFTs may be determined in several ways. The DFT testing protocol, or "step-down" approach, uses a series of inductions to determine the lowest energy that produces successful defibrillation. For example, with a device capable of a maximum energy output of 34 J, one may begin the test with a shock at 24 J (allowing for a 10 J safety-margin). If successful, then a shock at 12 J can be tested, decreasing to 6 J or even 3 J. The lowest energy that successfully defibrillates VF is reported as the DFT. Although this method more accurately determines DFTs, multiple VF inductions are needed. Alternatively, the margin-verification protocol requires testing of a selected energy that would allow for an adequate safety margin without determining the lowest energy that would successfully defibrillate. At least two shocks at the chosen energy must be successful to verify that a safety margin exists. For example, if two shocks at 12 J successfully defibrillate VF, a safety margin of at least 22 J would exist with a 34 J device, and testing can conclude at that point. Fewer numbers of VF inductions are needed with this latter method, and may be preferable in patients who may not tolerate repeated episodes of VF.

However, in most patients, we favor the "step-down" approach because having at least one shock that fails to defibrillate allows for redetection also to be tested. Owing to postshock lead polarization, autogain features (the gain may be dramatically decreased after shocks), and the potential for lead dislodgment postshock, failure to redetect VF after a failed shock is a genuine concern that should be addressed with testing during implantation. Redetection problems are encountered more frequently with integrated bipolar sensing leads than with true bipolar sensing leads. During testing, we choose to set the second shock at device maximum output. If the first shock fails, the device is allowed to redetect VF and deliver a second shock, and if this fails, we deliver a 360 J shock externally. Usually, 5 min intervals are allowed between each VF induction.

Although not routinely performed at our institution, data suggests a strong correlation between DFT and ULV (69,104–106). The ULV is that shock on a scanned T wave that induces VF. The hypothesis of the vulnerability theory of defibrillation is that a shock can both induce and terminate VF nearly simultaneously. If one delivers a T-wave shock (e.g., 1–2 J) and fails to defibrillate nearly simultaneously, this is within the limit of vulnerability and VF would be induced. If one performs a T-wave shock at 34 J, it would be anticipated that they would nearly simultaneously fibrillate and defibrillate the myocardium, and therefore be beyond the ULV, without ever having the hemodynamic consequence of VF. With successive lower output T-wave shocks, the ULV could be determined by stopping at that point in which VF was actually induced, or alternatively when a point at which a safety margin was identified. The advantage of this approach is that clinical VF is only induced on one occasion if at all. Studies have demonstrated that the ULV and DFT are within 5 J of another, and a safety margin of 15 J may therefore be equivalent to a 10 J DFT safety margin. With a 34 J device, one may consider performing ULV testing at 19 J, and if no VF is induced, feel comfortable with the safety margin of a 34 J defibrillation. This approach may be considered in a patient in whom brief deep sedation may not be advisable (e.g., significant respiratory or neurologic comorbidity) or in a patient in whom transient hemodynamic collapse may be considered high risk (e.g., fixed outlet obstruction, cerebrovascular disease, unrevascularized coronary distribution, recent surgical revascularization, or percutaneous revascularization). Studies of ULV testing have noted there may be inconsistent longitudinal results, but generally speaking, a low ULV (<10–11 J) or high ULV (>20 J) tends to correlate with low and high DFTs and success of first shock with programming based on ULV tends to be successful (69,105,106). Multiple tests relative to the T-wave peak (e.g., −40 ms, −20 ms, 0 ms) need to be performed to assure consistent results. One study found that those with no coronary artery disease may have a discrepancy in DFT-ULV correlation of >10 J, and DFT testing is preferred (104).

In addition to sensing, pacing, and determination of DFTs, other parameters, such as the impedance and charge time, must also be assessed during intraoperative testing to ensure that the device is performing adequately (39). Impedance must be measured for both the high-voltage electrodes and pacing electrodes. Impedance that is too high raises the concern of lead fracture or a poor connection between the lead and the ICD, and low impedance may signify an insulation break. If an unacceptable value is repeatedly obtained during testing, replacement of the lead may be necessary. Charge time is the time needed to charge the capacitor for energy delivery and may vary with generators, but should be short (less than 10 s) for new and normally functioning devices.

When adequate DFTs are not achievable with a single coil endocardial lead, reversing shocking polarity by designating the RV lead as the anode and the active pulse generator as the cathode may occasionally lower DFTs. Alternatively, using another electrode by changing to a dual coil lead or inserting a separate SVC or CS lead may be helpful. With today's devices, a subcutaneous patch or array, although effective, is rarely required (107,108). The entire system should be implanted and the wound closed only after satisfactory sensing of both sinus rhythm and VF, when pacing thresholds are low and lead impedances are acceptable. Because the DFT may increase over time because of fibrosis, migration, or the addition of antiarrhythmic drugs, a safety margin of 7–10 J above the DFT (of 15 J above the ULV) should be considered when programming therapies.

An important note should be mentioned regarding patients who have separate permanent pacemakers and ICDs. If the pacing spikes are large, ICDs may sense pacer stimulus artifacts and count them as R waves, which would lead to "double-counting" and may trigger inappropriate shocks. A more significant concern is that electrograms from VF are often small and may not be sensed by the pacemaker, thus triggering pacing. The large pacing spikes may reset the amplifier (decrease the gain) of the ICD, which may result in failure to sense VF. Unipolar leads are particularly problematic because they produce large pacing spikes. For this reason, implantation of a unipolar pacing lead is absolutely contraindicated in patients with preexisting ICDs. During intraoperative testing of a new ICD system in the setting of an existing pacemaker, the pacemaker should be programmed to full output (maximum amplitude and pulse width), pacing at either DOO or VOO mode in order to maximize pacer stimulus artifact size. If the pacemaker lead is not a committed bipolar lead, then it should be reprogrammed to unipolar during testing. The ICD is programmed at the least sensitive setting, to set up a worst-case scenario. Testing of the ICD must then include determination that these spikes do not interfere with VF sensing.

Immediate Postoperative Care

After implantation of an ICD, the ipsilateral arm is kept in a sling for at least 24 h. The wound is kept covered with a sterile dressing and checked frequently for evidence of oozing or hematoma formation. Infection remains a serious complication after device implantations. A recent meta-analysis of seven trials with more than 2,000 patients undergoing pacemaker implantation suggests a protective effect of antibiotics when given within 2 h of incision (109). No data are available regarding the length of antibiotic administration after implantation, but prophylactic antibiotics for 48 h after implantation are generally accepted. Portable chest radiographs should be obtained to rule out pneumothorax after implantations when the subclavian vein is accessed. Anticoagulation, if indicated, should be withheld for several hours after implantation to prevent bleeding complications. On postoperative day 1, anteroposterior and lateral chest radiographs should be obtained to check lead position, and the device should be interrogated to recheck sensing and pacing parameters prior to discharge. Occasionally, leads may migrate in 24 h after implantation, resulting in loss of capture or poor sensing, requiring revision of the lead. Lead revisions should be carried out as soon as possible, before significant scar tissue can form around the lead, which would make manipulation or extraction of the lead more difficult.

Controversy exists as to whether routine noninvasive programmed stimulations (NIPS) are necessary prior to discharge, to test for acute changes in DFTs or lead problems, and to set up ATP therapy. One study noted that in 97 patients undergoing routine predischarge testing, three had ineffective shocks at maximum device energy, despite an adequate safety margin during implant. No change in lead positions was detected on chest radiographs or under fluoroscopy in those patients (110). However, the devices implanted in that study were abdominal units, and these problems may be less likely with implantations of pectoral devices. At our institution, we do not routinely perform predischarge testing if lead positions are verified by chest radiographs and interrogation of the device is satisfactory.

References

1. Mirowski M, Mower MM, Reid PR. The automatic implantable defibrillator. *Am Heart J* 1980;100:1089–92.
2. Mirowski M, Reid PR, Mower MM, Watkins L, Gott VL, Schauble JF, Langer A, Heilman MS, Kolenik SA, Fischell RE, Weisfeldt ML. Termination of malignant ventricular arrhythmias with an implanted automatic defibrillator in human beings. *N Engl J Med* 1980;303:322–4.
3. Fitzpatrick AP, Lesh MD, Epstein LM, Lee RJ, Siu A, Merrick S, Griffin JC, Scheinman MM. Electrophysiological laboratory, electrophysiologist-implanted, nonthoracotomy-implantable cardioverter/defibrillators. *Circulation* 1994;89:2503–8.
4. Natale A, Kearney MM, Brandon MJ, Kent V, Wase A, Newby KH, Pisano E, Geiger MJ. Safety of nurse-administered deep sedation for defibrillator implantation in the electrophysiology laboratory. *J Cardiovasc Electrophysiol* 1996;7:301–6.
5. Buxton AE, Lee KL, Fisher JD, Josephson ME, Prystowsky EN, Hafley G. A randomized study of the prevention of sudden death in patients with coronary artery disease. Multicenter Unsustained Tachycardia Trial Investigators. *N Engl J Med* 1999;341:1882–90.
6. Moss AJ, Hall WJ, Cannom DS, Daubert JP, Higgins SL, Klein H, Levine JH, Saksena S, Waldo AL, Wilber D, Brown MW, Heo M. Improved survival with an implanted defibrillator in patients with coronary disease at high risk for ventricular arrhythmia. Multicenter Automatic Defibrillator Implantation Trial Investigators. *N Engl J Med* 1996;335:1933–40.
7. Moss AJ, Zareba W, Hall WJ, Klein H, Wilber DJ, Cannom DS, Daubert JP, Higgins SL, Brown MW, Andrews ML. Prophylactic implantation of a defibrillator in patients with myocardial infarction and reduced ejection fraction. *N Engl J Med* 2002;346:877–83.
8. Bardy GH, Lee KL, Mark DB, Poole JE, Packer DL, Boineau R, Domanski M, Troutman C, Anderson J, Johnson G, McNulty SE, Clapp-Channing N, Davidson-Ray LD, Fraulo ES, Fishbein DP, Luceri RM, Ip JH. Amiodarone or an implantable cardioverter-defibrillator for congestive heart failure. *N Engl J Med* 2005;352:225–37.
9. AVID. A comparison of antiarrhythmic-drug therapy with implantable defibrillators in patients resuscitated from near-fatal ventricular arrhythmias. The

Antiarrhythmics versus Implantable Defibrillators (AVID) Investigators. *N Engl J Med* 1997;337:1576–83.

10. Connolly SJ, Gent M, Roberts RS, Dorian P, Roy D, Sheldon RS, Mitchell LB, Green MS, Klein GJ, O'Brien B. Canadian implantable defibrillator study (CIDS): a randomized trial of the implantable cardioverter defibrillator against amiodarone. *Circulation* 2000;101:1297–302.

11. Kuck KH, Cappato R, Siebels J, Ruppel R. Randomized comparison of antiarrhythmic drug therapy with implantable defibrillators in patients resuscitated from cardiac arrest: the Cardiac Arrest Study Hamburg (CASH). *Circulation* 2000;102:748–54.

12. Gold MR, Shorofsky SR, Thompson JA, Kim J, Schwartz M, Bocek J, Lovett EG, Hsu W, Morris MM, Lang DJ. Advanced rhythm discrimination for implantable cardioverter defibrillators using electrogram vector timing and correlation. *J Cardiovasc Electrophysiol* 2002;13:1092–7.

13. Glikson M, Swerdlow CD, Gurevitz OT, Daoud E, Shivkumar K, Wilkoff B, Shipman T, Friedman PA. Optimal combination of discriminators for differentiating ventricular from supraventricular tachycardia by dual-chamber defibrillators. *J Cardiovasc Electrophysiol* 2005;16:732–9.

14. Compton SJ, Merrill JJ, Dorian P, Cao J, Zhou D, Gillberg JM. Continuous template collection and updating for electrogram morphology discrimination in implantable cardioverter defibrillators. *Pacing Clin Electrophysiol* 2006;29:244–54.

15. Sweeney MO, Wathen MS, Volosin K, Abdalla I, DeGroot PJ, Otterness MF, Stark AJ. Appropriate and inappropriate ventricular therapies, quality of life, and mortality among primary and secondary prevention implantable cardioverter defibrillator patients: results from the Pacing Fast VT REduces Shock ThErapies (PainFREE Rx II) trial. *Circulation* 2005;111:2898–905.

16. Wathen MS, DeGroot PJ, Sweeney MO, Stark AJ, Otterness MF, Adkisson WO, Canby RC, Khalighi K, Machado C, Rubenstein DS, Volosin KJ. Prospective randomized multicenter trial of empirical antitachycardia pacing versus shocks for spontaneous rapid ventricular tachycardia in patients with implantable cardioverter-defibrillators: Pacing Fast Ventricular Tachycardia Reduces Shock Therapies (PainFREE Rx II) trial results. *Circulation* 2004;110:2591–6.

17. Guidant. Factors that affect ICD longevity and replacement time Guidant Corporation Cardiac Rhythm Management – *Product Update*. St. Paul, MN, 2003.

18. Medtronic. CRM Product Performance Report. Minneapolis, MN, 2006.

19. SJM. CRM Product Performance Report. St. Paul, MN, 2006.

20. Guidant. CRM Product Performance Report. Guidant Corporation. St. Paul, MN, 2006.

21. Crespi A, Schmidt C, Norton J, Chen K, Skarstad P. Modeling and characterization of the resistance of lithium/SVO batteries for implantable cardioverter defibrillators. *J Electrochem Soc* 2001;148:A30–37.

22. Guidant. ERI Charge Time Limit Extended During Mid-Life in ICDs and CRT-Ds. Guidant Corporation Cardiac Rhythm Management – *Product Update*. St. Paul, MN, 2006.

23. Crespi A, Somdahl S, Hokanson K, Jain M, Skarstad P. Lithium-limited batteries for implantable cardioverter-defibrillators 202nd Meeting – The Electrochemical Society. Salt Lake City, UT, 2002.

24. Huffman FN, Migliore JJ, Robinson WJ, Norman JC. Radioisotope powered cardiac pacemakers. *Cardiovasc Dis* 1974;1:52–60.

25. Parsonnet V, Berstein AD, Perry GY. The nuclear pacemaker: is renewed interest warranted? *Am J Cardiol* 1990;66:837–42.

26. Mitcheson PD, Green TC, Yeatman EM, Holmes AS. Architectures for vibration-driven micropower generators. *J Microelectromech Syst* 2004;13:429–40.

27. Ozeki T, Chinzei T, Abe Y, Saito I, Isoyama T, Ono T, Kouno A, Ishimaru M, Takiura K, Baba A, Toyama T, Imachi K. A study on an energy supply method for a transcutaneous energy transmission system. *Artif Organs* 2003;27:68–72.

28. Tchin-Iou AV, Min BG. Design of the solar cell system for recharging the external battery of the totally-implantable artificial heart. *Int J Artif Organs* 1999;22:823–6.

29. Goto K, Nakagawa T, Nakamura O, Kawata S. An implantable power supply with an optically rechargeable lithium battery. *IEEE Trans Biomed Eng* 2001;48:830–3.

30. Langer A, Heilman MS, Mower MM, Mirowski M. Considerations in the development of the automatic implantable defibrillator. *Med Instrum* 1976;10:163–7.

31. Toivonen L, Viitasalo M, Jarvinen A. The performance of the probability density function in differentiating supraventricular from ventricular rhythms. *Pacing Clin Electrophysiol* 1992;15:726–30.

32. Aubert AE, Denys BG, Ector H, De Geest H. Detection of ventricular tachycardia and fibrillation using ECG processing and intramyocardial pressure gradients. *Pacing Clin Electrophysiol* 1986;9:1084–8.

33. Polikaitis A, Arzbaecher R, Bump T, Wilber D. Probability density function revisited: improved discrimination of VF using a cycle length corrected PDF. *Pacing Clin Electrophysiol* 1997;20:1947–51.

34. Winkle RA, Bach SM, Jr., Echt DS, Swerdlow CD, Imran M, Mason JW, Oyer PE, Stinson EB. The automatic implantable defibrillator: local ventricular bipolar sensing to detect ventricular tachycardia and fibrillation. *Am J Cardiol* 1983;52:265–70.

35. Dijkman B, Wellens HJ. Dual chamber arrhythmia detection in the implantable cardioverter defibrillator. *J Cardiovasc Electrophysiol* 2000;11:1105–15.

36. Olsen WH. Tachyarrhythmia sensing and detection. In: Singer I, ed. Implantable cardioverter defibrillator. Armonk, NY: Futura Publishing, 1994:777.

37. Berul CI, Callans DJ, Schwartzman DS, Preminger MW, Gottlieb CD, Marchlinski FE. Comparison of initial detection and redetection of ventricular fibrillation in a transvenous defibrillator system with automatic gain control. *J Am Coll Cardiol* 1995;25:431–6.

38. Niehaus M, Neuzner J, Vogt J, Korte T, Tebbenjohanns J. Adjustment of maximum automatic sensitivity (automatic gain control) reduces inappropriate therapies in patients with implantable cardioverter defibrillators. *Pacing Clin Electrophysiol* 2002;25:151–5.

39. Swerdlow CD, Friedman PA. Advanced ICD troubleshooting: Part I. *Pacing Clin Electrophysiol* 2005;28:1322–46.

40. Chugh A, Scharf C, Hall B, Cheung P, Good E, Horwood L, Oral H, Pelosi F, Jr., Morady F. Prevalence and management of inappropriate detection and therapies in patients with first-generation biventricular pacemaker-defibrillators. *Pacing Clin Electrophysiol* 2005;28:44–50.

41. Brodman R, Fisher JD, Furman S, Johnston DR, Kim SG, Matos JA, Waspe LE. Implantation of automatic cardioverter-defibrillators via median sternotomy. *Pacing Clin Electrophysiol* 1984;7:1363–9.

42. Ideker RE, Wolf PD, Alferness C, Krassowska W, Smith WM. Current concepts for selecting the location, size and shape of defibrillation electrodes. *Pacing Clin Electrophysiol* 1991;14:227–40.

43. Molina JE, Benditt DG, Adler S. Crinkling of epicardial defibrillator patches. A common and serious problem. *J Thorac Cardiovasc Surg* 1995;110:258–64.

44. Saksena S. Defibrillation thresholds and perioperative mortality associated with endocardial and epicardial defibrillation lead systems. The PCD investigators and participating institutions. *Pacing Clin Electrophysiol* 1993;16:202–7.

45. Chevalier P, Moncada E, Canu G, Claudel JP, Bellon C, Kirkorian G, Touboul P. Symptomatic pericardial disease associated with patch electrodes of the automatic implantable cardioverter defibrillator: an underestimated complication? *Pacing Clin Electrophysiol* 1996;19:2150–2.

46. Reid PR, Mirowski M, Mower MM, Platia EV, Griffith LS, Watkins L, Jr., Bach SM, Jr., Imran M, Thomas A. Clinical evaluation of the internal automatic

cardioverter-defibrillator in survivors of sudden cardiac death. *Am J Cardiol* 1983;51:1608–13.

47. BInner L, Stiller S, Brummer T, Stiller P, Grossmann G. Single coil ICD leads allow safe routine ICD implantation. [Abstract]. *Europace* 2005;7:93.

48. Rub N, Schweitzer O, Mewis C, Kettering K, Kuehlkamp V. Addition of a defibrillation electrode in the low right atrium to a right ventricular lead does not reduce ventricular defibrillation thresholds. *Pacing Clin Electrophysiol* 2004;27:346–51.

49. Bardy GH, Allen MD, Mehra R, Johnson G. An effective and adaptable transvenous defibrillation system using the coronary sinus in humans. *J Am Coll Cardiol* 1990;16:887–95.

50. Usui M, Walcott GP, Strickberger SA, Rollins DL, Smith WM, Ideker RE. Effects of polarity for monophasic and biphasic shocks on defibrillation efficacy with an endocardial system. *Pacing Clin Electrophysiol* 1996;19:65–71.

51. Sweeney MO, Ellison KE, Shea JB, Newell JB. Provoked and spontaneous high-frequency, low-amplitude, respirophasic noise transients in patients with implantable cardioverter defibrillators. *J Cardiovasc Electrophysiol* 2001;12:402–10.

52. Gradaus R, Breithardt G, Bocker D. ICD leads: design and chronic dysfunctions. *Pacing Clin Electrophysiol* 2003;26:649–57.

53. Epstein AE, Kay GN, Plumb VJ, Dailey SM, Anderson PG. Gross and microscopic pathological changes associated with nonthoracotomy implantable defibrillator leads. *Circulation* 1998;98:1517–24.

54. Wilkoff BL, Belott PH, Love CJ, Scheiner A, Westlund R, Rippy M, Krishnan M, Norlander BE, Steinhaus B, Emmanuel J, Zeller PJ. Improved extraction of ePTFE and medical adhesive modified defibrillation leads from the coronary sinus and great cardiac vein. *Pacing Clin Electrophysiol* 2005;28:205–11.

55. Germano JJ, Reynolds M, Essebag V, Josephson ME. Frequency and causes of implantable cardioverter-defibrillator therapies: is device therapy proarrhythmic? *Am J Cardiol* 2006;97:1255–61.

56. Grimm W, Flores BF, Marchlinski FE. Electrocardiographically documented unnecessary, spontaneous shocks in 241 patients with implantable cardioverter defibrillators. *Pacing Clin Electrophysiol* 1992;15:1667–73.

57. Gronefeld GC, Schulte B, Hohnloser SH, Trappe HJ, Korte T, Stellbrink C, Jung W, Meesmann M, Bocker D, Grosse-Meininghaus D, Vogt J. Morphology discrimination: a beat-to-beat algorithm for the discrimination of ventricular from supraventricular tachycardia by implantable cardioverter defibrillators. *Pacing Clin Electrophysiol* 2001;24:1519–24.

58. Swerdlow CD, Chen PS, Kass RM, Allard JR, Peter CT. Discrimination of ventricular tachycardia from sinus tachycardia and atrial fibrillation in a tiered-therapy cardioverter-defibrillator. *J Am Coll Cardiol* 1994;23:1342–55.

59. Swerdlow CD, Ahern T, Chen PS, Hwang C, Gang E, Mandel W, Kass RM, Peter CT. Underdetection of ventricular tachycardia by algorithms to enhance specificity in a tiered-therapy cardioverter-defibrillator. *J Am Coll Cardiol* 1994;24:416–24.

60. Le Franc P, Kus T, Vinet A, Rocque P, Molin F, Costi P. Underdetection of ventricular tachycardia using a 40 ms stability criterion: effect of antiarrhythmic therapy. *Pacing Clin Electrophysiol* 1997;20:2882–92.

61. Goldberger Z, Elbel B, McPherson CA, Paltiel AD, Lampert R. Cost advantage of dual-chamber versus single-chamber cardioverter-defibrillator implantation. *J Am Coll Cardiol* 2005;46:850–7.

62. Dorian P, Philippon F, Thibault B, Kimber S, Sterns L, Greene M, Newman D, Gelaznikas R, Barr A. Randomized controlled study of detection enhancements versus rate-only detection to prevent inappropriate therapy in a dual-chamber implantable cardioverter-defibrillator. *Heart Rhythm* 2004;1:540–7.

63. Theuns DA, Klootwijk AP, Goedhart DM, Jordaens LJ. Prevention of inappropriate therapy in implantable cardioverter-defibrillators: results of a prospective,

randomized study of tachyarrhythmia detection algorithms. *J Am Coll Cardiol* 2004;44:2362–7.

64. Aliot E, Nitzsche R, Ripart A. Arrhythmia detection by dual-chamber implantable cardioverter defibrillators. A review of current algorithms. *Europace* 2004;6: 273–86.

65. Sweeney MO, Ellenbogen KA, Casavant D, Betzold R, Sheldon T, Tang F, Mueller M, Lingle J. Multicenter, prospective, randomized safety and efficacy study of a new atrial-based managed ventricular pacing mode (MVP) in dual chamber ICDs. *J Cardiovasc Electrophysiol* 2005;16:811–7.

66. Wilkoff BL, Cook JR, Epstein AE, Greene HL, Hallstrom AP, Hsia H, Kutalek SP, Sharma A. Dual-chamber pacing or ventricular backup pacing in patients with an implantable defibrillator: the Dual Chamber and VVI Implantable Defibrillator (DAVID) Trial. *JAMA* 2002;288:3115–23.

67. Zhou X, Daubert JP, Wolf PD, Smith WM, Ideker RE. Epicardial mapping of ventricular defibrillation with monophasic and biphasic shocks in dogs. *Circ Res* 1993;72:145–60.

68. Chen PS, Shibata N, Dixon EG, Martin RO, Ideker RE. Comparison of the defibrillation threshold and the upper limit of ventricular vulnerability. *Circulation* 1986;73:1022–8.

69. Glikson M, Gurevitz OT, Trusty JM, Sharma V, Luria DM, Eldar M, Shen WK, Rea RF, Hammill SC, Friedman PA. Upper limit of vulnerability determination during implantable cardioverter-defibrillator placement to minimize ventricular fibrillation inductions. *Am J Cardiol* 2004;94:1445–9.

70. Singer I, Lang D. Defibrillation threshold: clinical utility and therapeutic implications. *Pacing Clin Electrophysiol* 1992;15:932–49.

71. Fain ES, Dorian P, Davy JM, Kates RE, Winkle RA. Effects of encainide and its metabolites on energy requirements for defibrillation. *Circulation* 1986;73:1334–41.

72. Reiffel JA, Coromilas J, Zimmerman JM, Spotnitz HM. Drug-device interactions: clinical considerations. *Pacing Clin Electrophysiol* 1985;8:369–73.

73. Dorian P, Fain ES, Davy JM, Winkle RA. Lidocaine causes a reversible, concentration-dependent increase in defibrillation energy requirements. *J Am Coll Cardiol* 1986;8:327–32.

74. Marinchak RA, Friehling TD, Kline RA, Stohler J, Kowey PR. Effect of antiarrhythmic drugs on defibrillation threshold: case report of an adverse effect of mexiletine and review of the literature. *Pacing Clin Electrophysiol* 1988;11: 7–12.

75. Huang J, Skinner JL, Rogers JM, Smith WM, Holman WL, Ideker RE. The effects of acute and chronic amiodarone on activation patterns and defibrillation threshold during ventricular fibrillation in dogs. *J Am Coll Cardiol* 2002;40:375–83.

76. Guarnieri T, Levine JH, Veltri EP, Griffith LS, Watkins L, Jr., Juanteguy J, Mower MM, Mirowski M. Success of chronic defibrillation and the role of antiarrhythmic drugs with the automatic implantable cardioverter/defibrillator. *Am J Cardiol* 1987;60:1061–4.

77. Movsowitz C, Marchlinski FE. Interactions between implantable cardioverter-defibrillators and class III agents. *Am J Cardiol* 1998;82:41I–8I.

78. Yabe S, Smith WM, Daubert JP, Wolf PD, Rollins DL, Ideker RE. Conduction disturbances caused by high current density electric fields. *Circ Res* 1990;66: 1190–203.

79. Jones JL, Jones RE, Balasky G. Microlesion formation in myocardial cells by high-intensity electric field stimulation. *Am J Physiol* 1987;253:H480–6.

80. Zoll PM, Paul MH, Linenthal AJ, Norman LR, Gibson W. The effect of external electric currents on the heart; control of cardiac rhythm and induction and termination of cardiac arrhythmias. *Circulation* 1956;14:745–56.

81. Lown B, Neuman J, Amarasingham R, Berkovits BV. Comparison of alternating current with direct electroshock across the closed chest. *Am J Cardiol* 1962;10:223–33.

82. Jones DL, Sohla A, Bourland JD, Tacker WA, Kallok MJ, Klein GJ. Internal ventricular defibrillation with sequential pulse countershock in pigs: comparison with single pulses and effects of pulse separation. *Pacing Clin Electrophysiol* 1987;10:497–502.

83. Jones DL, Klein GJ, Rattes MF, Sohla A, Sharma AD. Internal cardiac defibrillation: single and sequential pulses and a variety of lead orientations. *Pacing Clin Electrophysiol* 1988;11:583–91.

84. Block M, Hammel D, Bocker D, Borggrefe M, Budde T, Isbruch F, Wietholt D, Scheld HH, Breithardt G. A prospective randomized cross-over comparison of mono- and biphasic defibrillation using nonthoracotomy lead configurations in humans. *J Cardiovasc Electrophysiol* 1994;5:581–90.

85. Irnich W. How to program pulse duration or tilt in implantable cardioverter defibrillators. *Pacing Clin Electrophysiol* 2003;26:453–6.

86. Shepard RK, DeGroot PJ, Pacifico A, Wood MA, Ellenbogen KA. Prospective randomized comparison of 65%/65% versus 42%/42% tilt biphasic waveform on defibrillation thresholds in humans. *J Interv Card Electrophysiol* 2003;8:221–5.

87. Sweeney MO, Natale A, Volosin KJ, Swerdlow CD, Baker JH, Degroot P. Prospective randomized comparison of 50%/50% versus 65%/65% tilt biphasic waveform on defibrillation in humans. *Pacing Clin Electrophysiol* 2001;24:60–5.

88. Huang J, KenKnight BH, Rollins DL, Smith WM, Ideker RE. Ventricular vdefibrillation with triphasic waveforms. *Circulation* 2000;101:1324–8.

89. Zhang Y, Boddicker KA, Davies LR, Jones JL, Kerber RE. Surgical open-chest ventricular defibrillation: triphasic waveforms are superior to biphasic waveforms. *Pacing Clin Electrophysiol* 2004;27:941–8.

90. Lok NS, Lau CP, Tse HF, Ayers GM. Clinical shock tolerability and effect of different right atrial electrode locations on efficacy of low energy human transvenous atrial defibrillation using an implantable lead system. *J Am Coll Cardiol* 1997;30:1324–30.

91. Jung J, Hahn SJ, Heisel A, Buob A, Schubert BD, Siaplaouras S. Defibrillation efficacy and pain perception of two biphasic waveforms for internal cardioversion of atrial fibrillation. *J Cardiovasc Electrophysiol* 2003;14:837–40.

92. Chattipakorn N, Banville I, Gray RA, Ideker RE. Effects of shock strengths on ventricular defibrillation failure. *Cardiovasc Res* 2004;61:39–44.

93. Wathen MS, Sweeney MO, DeGroot PJ, Stark AJ, Koehler JL, Chisner MB, Machado C, Adkisson WO. Shock reduction using antitachycardia pacing for spontaneous rapid ventricular tachycardia in patients with coronary artery disease. *Circulation* 2001;104:796–801.

94. Stevenson WG, Friedman PL, Sager PT, Saxon LA, Kocovic D, Harada T, Wiener I, Khan H. Exploring postinfarction reentrant ventricular tachycardia with entrainment mapping. *J Am Coll Cardiol* 1997;29:1180–9.

95. Stevenson WG, Khan H, Sager P, Saxon LA, Middlekauff HR, Natterson PD, Wiener I. Identification of reentry circuit sites during catheter mapping and radiofrequency ablation of ventricular tachycardia late after myocardial infarction. *Circulation* 1993;88:1647–70.

96. Almendral JM, Rosenthal ME, Stamato NJ, Marchlinski FE, Buxton AE, Frame LH, Miller JM, Josephson ME. Analysis of the resetting phenomenon in sustained uniform ventricular tachycardia: incidence and relation to termination. *J Am Coll Cardiol* 1986;8:294–300.

97. Cook JR, Kirchhoffer JB, Fitzgerald TF, Lajzer DA. Comparison of decremental and burst overdrive pacing as treatment for ventricular tachycardia associated with coronary artery disease. *Am J Cardiol* 1992;70:311–5.

98. Newman D, Dorian P, Hardy J. Randomized controlled comparison of antitachycardia pacing algorithms for termination of ventricular tachycardia. *J Am Coll Cardiol* 1993;21:1413–8.

99. Gold MR, Peters RW, Johnson JW, Shorofsky SR. Complications associated with pectoral cardioverter-defibrillator implantation: comparison of subcutaneous and submuscular approaches. Worldwide Jewel Investigators. *J Am Coll Cardiol* 1996;28:1278–82.

100. Pacifico A, Wheelan KR, Nasir N, Jr., Wells PJ, Doyle TK, Johnson SA, Henry PD. Long-term follow-up of cardioverter-defibrillator implanted under conscious sedation in prepectoral subfascial position. *Circulation* 1997;95: 946–50.

101. van Rugge FP, Savalle LH, Schalij MJ. Subcutaneous single-incision implantation of cardioverter-defibrillators under local anesthesia by electrophysiologists in the electrophysiology laboratory. *Am J Cardiol* 1998;81:302–5.

102. Tobin K, Stewart J, Westveer D, Frumin H. Acute complications of permanent pacemaker implantation: their financial implication and relation to volume and operator experience. *Am J Cardiol* 2000;85:774–6, A9.

103. Pavia S, Wilkoff B. The management of surgical complications of pacemaker and implantable cardioverter-defibrillators. *Curr Opin Cardiol* 2001;16:66–71.

104. Gurevitz OT, Friedman PA, Glikson M, Trusty JM, Ballman KV, Rosales AG, Hayes DL, Hammill SC, Swerdlow CD. Discrepancies between the upper limit of vulnerability and defibrillation threshold: prevalence and clinical predictors. *J Cardiovasc Electrophysiol* 2003;14:728–32.

105. Green UB, Garg A, Al-Kandari F, Ungab G, Tone L, Feld GK. Successful implantation of cardiac defibrillators without induction of ventricular fibrillation using upper limit of vulnerability testing. *J Interv Card Electrophysiol* 2003;8:71–5.

106. Swerdlow CD, Peter CT, Kass RM, Gang ES, Mandel WJ, Hwang C, Martin DJ, Chen PS. Programming of implantable cardioverter-defibrillators on the basis of the upper limit of vulnerability. *Circulation* 1997;95:1497–504.

107. Gradaus R, Block M, Seidl K, Brunn J, Isgro F, Hammel D, Hauer B, Breithardt G, Bocker D. Defibrillation efficacy comparing a subcutaneous array electrode versus an "active can" implantable cardioverter defibrillator and a subcutaneous array electrode in addition to an "active can" implantable cardioverter defibrillator: results from active can versus array trials I and II. *J Cardiovasc Electrophysiol* 2001;12:921–7.

108. Kuhlkamp V, Dornberger V, Mewis C, Seipel L. Comparison of the efficacy of a subcutaneous array electrode with a subcutaneous patch electrode, a prospective randomized study. *Int J Cardiol* 2001;78:247–56.

109. Da Costa A, Kirkorian G, Cucherat M, Delahaye F, Chevalier P, Cerisier A, Isaaz K, Touboul P. Antibiotic prophylaxis for permanent pacemaker implantation: a meta-analysis. *Circulation* 1998;97:1796–801.

110. Goldberger JJ, Horvath G, Inbar S, Kadish AH. Utility of predischarge and one-month transvenous implantable defibrillator tests. *Am J Cardiol* 1997;79:822–6.

Section III

Pacing and Implantable Device Therapy for Specific Clinical Conditions

9

Sinus Node Dysfunction

Irene H. Stevenson, Paul B. Sparks, and Jonathan M. Kalman

Sinus node dysfunction was initially described in the early 1900s, and is the primary indication for pacemaker implantation in industrialized countries. The only effective treatment for symptomatic sinus node dysfunction is cardiac pacing. However, despite the widespread use of pacing therapy for this group of patients, the optimal pacing mode, pacing system and site of ventricular stimulation for sinus node dysfunction remains controversial. The available data for the diagnosis and treatment of sinus node dysfunction are reviewed in this chapter.

Sinus Node Anatomy and Physiology

Since Keith and Flack's original description in 1907 (1), the unique anatomic and functional characteristics of the sinus node have been extensively studied by numerous investigators (2–6). The sinus P wave arises from a "pacemaker complex" that is distributed over a large area, from the junction of the superior vena cava and right atrial appendage, extending inferiorly along the sulcus terminalis almost to the inferior vena cava. A close correspondence between the change in heart rate and the change in sites of impulse origin within this complex in response to certain autonomic influences was first observed by Lewis et al. and Meek and Eyster early in the century (7,8). More recently, Boineau and associates, using a computerized epicardial mapping system, have shown that, over a physiological range of spontaneous heart rates, the dominant pacemaker may occur over a wide distribution approximately 3 cm long, as far cranially as the right atrial-superior vena cava junction and as far caudally as the right atrial-inferior vena cava junction (9). These sites of origin were centered about the long axis of the sulcus terminalis and produced a P-wave axis on the surface electrocardiogram within the normal sinus spectrum. In addition, in response to autonomic manipulations, a close correspondence existed between the heart rate and the site of impulse origin within the sulcus terminalis, consistent with a graduated site-specific differential sensitivity to autonomic inputs (9–11). Vagal stimulation produced a decreased heart rate associated with change in location of the dominant pacemaker to a lower atrial site; conversely, isoproterenol infusion resulted in dominance of a more cranial and anterior pacemaker with an associated increase in heart rate.

This widely distributed physiologic pacemaker complex contrasts with the more localized and constant anatomic location of the histologically defined sinus node. The human sinus node lies immediately subepicardially within the sulcus terminalis of the right atrium at the junction of the anterior trabeculated appendage with the posterior smooth-walled venous component (2,5). The endocardial aspect of the sulcus terminalis is marked by the crista terminalis. In the majority of cases the node lies lateral to the crest of the atrial appendage, and specialized cells extend inferiorly in the sulcus terminalis for approximately 10 mm. In up to 10% of cases, the node extends across the crest of the appendage anterior to the superior vena cava (12).

The archetypal sinus node "P" cell, found in the centre of the sinoatrial node, is characterized by minimal organelles and contractile machinery in its cytoplasm. From the centre to the periphery there is then a gradation of many features of the sinus node cells until they resemble atrial contractile cells. These gradations occur in cell size, myofilament and mitochondrial content, and all aspects influencing sinus node function including conduction (gap junction density and type and cell orientation), action potential shape (ion channel expression), and pacemaking (ion channel expression/ionic currents and Ca handling) (13). This cellular diversity within the SA node is integral to its normal functioning.

Of primary importance is the presence of a pacemaker potential. Because the membrane depolarizes continuously during the diastolic phase, there is no well-defined resting potential in the nodal cell and the maximal negative potential lies between −50 and −70 mV. In addition, there is a markedly slower maximum rate of rise of the action potential compared with atrial muscle fibers leading to considerably slower impulse conduction (2–5 cm/s). The action potential of sinus pacemaker cells also exhibits a shorter duration than atrial and ventricular cells with the absence of a plateau phase. The conduction in the SA node is also very slow because of the paucity of connexins compared to atrial tissue. This poor electrical coupling is important for insulating the node from the suppressive influence of the atrial muscle. These characteristics however change gradually from the cells in the centre of the sinus node to the periphery and it is this complex structure which is essential for normal functioning of the node as a whole. Normally, the leading pacemaker site is in the centre with the periphery functioning to conduct the impulse to the surrounding atrial muscle. Only 1% of the SA node acts as the leading pacemaker site (14). Perhaps counterintuitively, the cells in the centre of the SA node have slower pacemaking ability with a *less* steep pacemaker potential than cells at the periphery. In fact, if central tissue is isolated, it shows *slower* pacemaking than isolated peripheral sinus node cells. Although the periphery of the SA node has the fastest pacemaking activity, it is not normally the leading pacemaker site because its activity is suppressed by surrounding atrial tissue. If however the surrounding atrial tissue is cut away, the pacemaking site shifts to the periphery and the pacemaker activity speeds up (13). This complexity of the SA node makes it a very robust structure with multiple pacemaker mechanisms allowing shift of the pacemaking site in response to various conditions. Certainly ablation of the SA node is notoriously difficult and generally of little clinical benefit.

A number of ionic currents have been described in single pacemaker cells from the sinus node region (15). In contrast to atrial and ventricular cells, the major time-dependent inward current in sinoatrial cells is not carried by sodium (I_{Na}), but rather by calcium (I_{Ca}). Two types of calcium current have been identified in sinus node cells, T- and L-types, which have different activation and inactivation thresholds and time courses. Calcium is the major ion responsible for the upstroke slope of the sinus node action potential but has also been demonstrated to play an important role in the genesis of the pacemaker potential. The delayed rectifier K-current (I_K) is the major outward current of the sinus node and is responsible for repolarization. However, the mechanism of spontaneous diastolic depolarization (the pacemaker potential) of the sinus node has not been entirely elucidated (15). In most studies, the most negative potential of the sinus node cell pacemaker potential ranges from −50 to −70 mV, and the rapid spike potential is initiated in the region of −40 mV (15). Therefore, the pacemaker potential ranges between −70 and −40 mV and only a very small current is necessary for depolarization. A number of currents have been postulated as being operative. Since the membrane depolarizes during the diastolic phase, the current responsible may be owing to a decay in the delayed rectifier outward potassium current (I_{Kr} and I_{Ks}) (16,17). However, since the net current to depolarize the membrane is inward, a decaying outward current is not sufficient to explain diastolic depolarization. Other currents that have been suggested include an increase in inward calcium ($I_{Ca,L}$ and $I_{Ca,T}$), an increase of inward background current (e.g., the Na^+/Ca^{2+} exchange current), a decrease of outward background current (e.g., a Na^+/K^+ pump current), Ca released from the sarcoplasmic reticulum (18,19), 4-aminopyridine-sensitive K+ currents (20), or an increase of I_f (15). The latter is an inward current activated on hyperpolarization (−40 to −60 mV) (15,21). It is carried by Na^+ and K^+. Because I_f is the inward current activated when the cell membrane hyperpolarizes, it tends to depolarize the cell membrane and maintain the low resting potential of the sinus node cell. This current is frequently called the pacemaker current in the nodal cell, but it is likely that no single ionic current is responsible for the pacemaker potential.

Modulation of the cardiac rate by the autonomic nervous system is mediated by both specific K-channels ($I_{K,Ach}$) as well as the I_f channel. The sinus node is densely innervated by vagal nerve endings and acetylcholine activates $I_{K,Ach}$ (22,23) as well as inhibits the I_f channel (24). It appears that the effect of acetylcholine on I_f rather than on $I_{K,Ach}$ is the primary cause of vagally mediated slowing of heart rate (25). The chronotropic action of β agonists is mediated by activation of the I_f current, causing a depolarizing shift in the activation curve rather than an increase in the current amplitude (21,26). The influence of β agonists causing Ca sarcolemmal transients has also been postulated as a mechanism for the rate increase with sympathetic activation (19,27).

Sinus Node Dysfunction

The sick sinus syndrome is a term that is commonly used to describe a wide variety of disturbances of sinus node function (28,29). More recently, the term sick sinus syndrome has been replaced by the phrase sinus node dysfunction, which will be used in this chapter. The spectrum of sinus node dysfunction includes sinus bradycardia, sinus pauses or sinus arrest, and sinoatrial exit block, which are frequently associated with atrial disease and disturbances

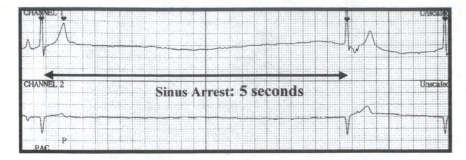

Fig. 9.1 After a premature atrial contraction (PAC), there is sinus node arrest for at least 5 s. After a long asystolic period, the first escape beat is a junctional beat with retrograde atrial activation.

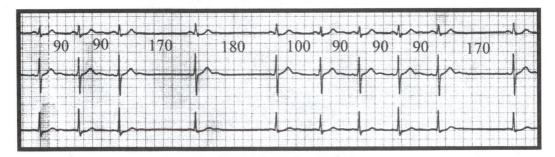

Fig. 9.2 An example of sinus node exit block (Wenckebach type). Progressive slowing of conduction within the sinus node leads to progressive reduction in the atrial rate until there is a long pause owing to blocked conduction.

of atrioventricular conduction (Figs. 9.1 and 9.2) (30). In particular, atrial tachyarrhythmias such as atrial fibrillation and atrial flutter frequently coexist and can produce symptoms either during the arrhythmia or at the time of termination when a prolonged sinus pause might induce syncope (tachycardia–bradycardia syndrome) (Fig. 9.3). The length of the pause may be compounded by coexistent failure of subsidiary pacemakers or distal conduction block (Fig. 9.1). The major symptoms of sinus node dysfunction include dizziness, presyncope, syncope, dyspnea, fatigue, and lethargy. The recognition that exertional symptoms may be owing to inadequate sinoatrial rate responsiveness (chronotropic incompetence) adds another dimension to the clinical spectrum (31). A precise definition of chronotropic incompetence is not well defined, although failure to increase the heart rate greater than 120 bpm (or 70% of the age-predicted maximum) is probably appropriate (32).

Pathophysiology of Sinus Node Dysfunction

Sinus node dysfunction has traditionally been considered in terms of intrinsic and extrinsic abnormalities (Table 9.1).

Intrinsic sinus node disease has been associated with a number of pathologic processes. For example, coronary artery disease is frequently associated with sinus node dysfunction, although a direct causal link has not been established.

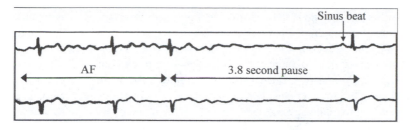

Fig. 9.3 A patient with the bradycardia–tachycardia form of sinus node dysfunction. On conversion from atrial fibrillation to sinus rhythm there is a 3.8 s pause.

Table 9.1 Etiologies of sinus node dysfunction.

Categories	Specific etiologies
Intrinsic	
Rheumatologic diseases	Rheumatic fever, scleroderma, ankylosing spondylitis, Reiter's syndrome, tuberous sclerosis
Congenital diseases	Correction of congenital heart defects, autosomal dominant sinus node dysfunction
Tumors	Lymphoma, granular cell tumor
SA nodal ischemia	Myocardial infarction, embolism
Infections	Chagas' disease
Trauma	After cardiac surgery, penetrating cardiac trauma
Infiltrative diseases	Sarcoidosis, amyloid, radiation therapy
Extrinsic	
Autonomic responses	Normal response, exaggerated vagal tone (carotid sinus hypersensitivity)
Electrolytes, hypoxia, and hormones	Thyroid disease, hyperkalemia, hypothermia, anorexia nervosa, hypoxia, sleep apnea
Medications	β-blockers, calcium channel blockers, antiarrhythmics, chemotherapy, lithium, phenothiazines, cimetidine, tricyclic antidepressants

In fact, a number of investigators have demonstrated that the sinus node artery is frequently patent in patients with sinus node dysfunction; one series found >50% stenosis of the artery in less than one-third of patients who died with sick sinus syndrome (33,34). Sinus node dysfunction also may be observed in cardiomyopathy, following cardiac surgery, and in a variety of inflammatory conditions of viral or connective tissue origin; however, the precise pathophysiology remains unknown in all of these conditions. Occasionally, sinus node dysfunction may have a familial basis (35). However, the specific cause is not apparent in the majority of cases of sinus node dysfunction. Degenerative loss of sinus node pacemaker cells and their replacement with fibrous tissue is frequently observed on pathologic examination of specimens from patients with sinus node dysfunction (36). This is a nonspecific finding, occurring in a wide variety of pathologic processes, and may be difficult to distinguish from the normal increase in fibrous tissue that occurs with aging (37).

Although sinus node dysfunction has previously been thought to be a localized condition there is growing evidence to suggest that in most instances, it is a disorder affecting the whole right atrial myocardium. Diffuse structural changes have been demonstrated in patients with sinus node dysfunction in the right atrium using electroanatomic mapping (38). Interestingly, in patients with heart failure who have similar structural abnormalities seen with electroanatomical mapping, a prolongation of sinus node recovery time (SNRT) was also observed (39). This suggests a diffuse process inclusive of the sinus node in these patients suffering from heart failure. Similar abnormalities of sinus node function have been demonstrated in people with atrial septal defects, another condition causing generalized right atrial structural remodeling (40). Pauses on reversion to sinus rhythm from atrial fibrillation are common and particularly prevalent in those suffering from the "tachy-brady" syndrome and a common indication for pacemaker insertion. Ablation of both atrial fibrillation (41) and atrial flutter (42) as well as following cardioversion of atrial flutter (43) have been demonstrated to result in "reverse remodeling" with normalization of the prolonged post reversion sinus pauses and sinus node depression.

Extrinsic causes of sinus node dysfunction are usually owing to autonomic inputs or drugs that affect sinus node function (Table 9.1). Excessive vagal tone, either alone or in the presence of coexistent structural disease, can produce many of the manifestations of sinus node dysfunction including sinus bradycardia, sinus pauses or sinus arrest, and sinoatrial exit block. It has been suggested that the clinical manifestations of neurally mediated syncope might be viewed as an expression of sinus node dysfunction produced by an exaggerated vagal response in conjunction with peripheral vasodepressor effects.

Indications for Pacing in Patients with Sinus Node Dysfunction

The only effective treatment for symptomatic sinus node dysfunction due to an intrinsic cause is pacing. Treatment of the condition is directed at symptoms. However, as every clinician knows, correlation of symptoms with a specific arrhythmia is not always possible in a condition with an episodic nature.

The indications for permanent pacing in sinus node dysfunction are published in the *ACC/AHA Guidelines for Implantation of Pacemakers and Arrhythmia Devices 1998* (44) together with the more recent update in 2002 (45). The standard format for indications was used: Class I (existence of evidence or general agreement), Class II (conflicting evidence and divergence of opinion exists), and Class III (evidence and general agreement that pacemaker implantation is not indicated). Class II was further divided into category IIa (weight of evidence or opinion is in favor of pacemaker implantation) and IIb (utility/efficacy less well established). Indications for pacing in sinus node dysfunction are summarized in Table 9.2. For sinus node dysfunction, the presence of symptoms in association with documented sinus bradycardia or sinus pauses is considered a Class I indication. If sinus bradycardia (<40 bpm) occurs in symptomatic patients but symptoms have not been clearly correlated with the bradycardia, this situation is considered a Class IIa indication for permanent pacing. In minimally symptomatic patients the presence of

Table 9.2 Indications for permanent pacing in patients with sinus node disease.

Class	Indications
I	Any type of sinus node dysfunction (including sinus bradycardia) clearly associated with symptoms
IIa	Symptomatic patients in whom symptoms have not been correlated directly with sinus node dysfunction
IIb	Minimally symptomatic patients with a heart rate <40 bpm while awake
III	Asymptomatic patients

documented (waking) bradycardia of <40 bpm is considered a Class IIb indication. Finally, in asymptomatic patients, even the presence of significant sinus bradycardia (<40 bpm) is considered a class III indication. Obviously in elderly patients with profound sinus bradycardia, one must take care not to overlook significant symptoms that may not necessarily be volunteered, such as fatigue and gradual impairment of exercise tolerance.

Investigation of Sinus Node Dysfunction

Although the ACC/AHA guidelines are relatively straightforward, all clinicians realize that it is frequently difficult to correlate symptoms of cerebral hypoperfusion with bradycardia. The 12-lead electrocardiogram may be diagnostic in a small proportion of patients, but is most often entirely normal. A variety of diagnostic strategies have been utilized for the evaluation of sinus node dysfunction and include heart rate monitoring for an extended period (Holter monitors and event recorders), tests of autonomic influence, and electrophysiologic testing.

Twenty-four-hour ambulatory (Holter) monitoring increases the rate of successful diagnosis and allows correlation between symptoms and recorded events. A positive result usually obviates the need for further invasive investigation (46). However, in view of the intermittent and sporadic nature of symptoms, the diagnostic yield of the Holter monitor is low (<2% in patients with syncope) (47). Although extended monitoring periods (48–72 h) may increase the diagnostic yield, the incremental increase in sensitivity is very low. For these patients, the use of an event recorder may provide useful information. Event recorders with the ability to loop back continuously may be helpful for patients who have infrequent events and who are unable to activate the recording during an episode. Recently, the diagnostic yield in syncope of unknown origin has been increased using an implantable loop recorder, especially in the elderly population. Brignole and associates reported on 103 patients, 78 over 65 years of age with recurrent unexplained syncope who underwent implantation of an implantable loop recorder (48). Fifty percent of the patients had a documented rhythm during a recurrent syncopal event over a mean follow up of 14 ± 10 months. No arrhythmias were seen in 25% of the episodes of recurrent syncope. In the remaining 75%, syncope was secondary to AV block

in 40%, gradual and progressive sinus bradycardia in 25%, atrial fibrillation/
tachycardia in 6%, and ventricular arrhythmias in 4%. The diagnostic value
of the implantable loop recorder was found to be significantly more useful in
patients over the age of 65 years with a diagnosis made for every 1.7 patients
selected for loop recorder insertion. A therapy could be started in 42% of
patients who would have been otherwise untreated.

Autonomic influences, either alone or in combination with structural sinus
node disease, can produce sinus node dysfunction. A number of tests have
been devised to assess the importance of autonomic influences, including
pharmacologic autonomic blockade for assessment of intrinsic heart rate and
evaluation of reflex reactions to upright tilt-testing. The clinical utility of these
tests in patients suspected of sinus node dysfunction is poorly understood.

A number of invasive diagnostic electro-physiological tests have been
developed in view of the difficulty frequently encountered in making the diagnosis of sinus node dysfunction in elderly patients with suggestive symptoms
(Table 9.3). These tests have been aimed at evaluating the various aspects of
sinus node function, including automaticity, sinoatrial conduction, and sinus
node refractoriness. Unfortunately, each test has significant drawbacks. The
sensitivity and negative predictive value for the SNRT and the sinoatrial
conduction time (SACT) are low. Although direct recording of the sinus node
electrogram can potentially provide very detailed information, recording the
sinus node electrogram is a time-consuming and painstaking procedure. The
clinical utility of all of these tests for confirmation of the diagnosis of sinus
node dysfunction, and for determining which patients will require permanent
pacing, remains limited (Fig. 9.4) (49).

To summarize, at the present time there is no definitive invasive diagnostic
method for evaluating the patient suspected of sinus node dysfunction. Most
commonly, the clinician will have to depend on extended ECG monitoring via
standard or implanted event recorders to correlate symptoms with sinus node
dysfunction. In many cases, the clinician must rely on clinical history and
indirect signs of sinus node dysfunction, and empiric pacing therapy may be
required in specific clinical situations.

Pacing Mode Choice in Patients with Sinus Node Dysfunction

The only effective treatment for symptomatic sinus node dysfunction is cardiac pacing. Despite two decades of clinical investigation, the optimal pacing
mode, pacing system and site of ventricular stimulation for bradycardia support for sinus node dysfunction remain uncertain. Selection of pacing mode
may be important for the clinical outcomes of quality of life, pacemaker
syndrome, atrial fibrillation, heart failure, thromboembolism, and mortality in
patients with sinus node dysfunction.

Patients with sinus node dysfunction may have single or dual-chamber
pacemakers programmed in one of four modes including DDD, AAI, VVI,
and DDI. Dual-chamber atrioventricular sequential pacing (DDD) refers to the
mode of cardiac pacing that incorporates atrial sensing or atrial pacing with subsequent ventricular pacing or ventricular sensing. Atrial and ventricular events
are separated by an interval that approximates the normal atrioventricular
conduction delay. In single-chamber atrial pacing (AAI), atrial pacing is

Table 9.3 Invasive tests for the evaluation of sinus node function.

Test	Technique	Comment
Sinus node recovery time (SNRT)	The atrium is paced for 30 s at a variety of rapid rates (80–180 bpm). Pacing is stopped, and the longest time required for the first sinus node activation at any of the paced rates is measured	Simple to perform
		In most patients, the SNRT has a maximal value at paced rates of 120–130 bpm.
		Large range for "abnormal" values: >1.2–1.5 s
		Clinical value is uncertain: Sensitivity: 25–70% Specificity: 45–100%
Sinoatrial conduction time (SACT)	Premature atrial contractions are introduced during sinus rhythm, and the interval between the premature beat and the subsequent sinus beat is measured. This interval will be the sum of conduction time "into" and "out of" the sinus node	Large range for "abnormal" values: >200–300 ms
		Clinical value is uncertain: Sensitivity: 54–63% Specificity: 57–88%
Sinus node electrogram	Direct measurement of the local sinus node electrogram using highly amplified signals	Potentially useful test, but at the present time clinical applicability is unknown
		Can be measured in only 50–80% of cases

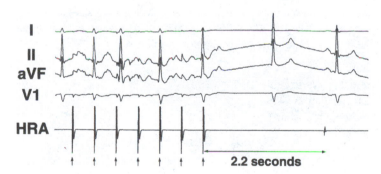

Fig. 9.4 Abnormal sinus node recovery time (SNRT). The atria are paced (arrows) at 150 bpm for 30 s. Notice that the patient has AV node block during pacing. With cessation of pacing, a junctional beat occurs, but it takes 2.2 s for spontaneous sinus node activity to return.

not followed by ventricular pacing. In patients with intact atrioventricular conduction, the AAI pacing mode maintains the normal atrioventricular relationship. In contrast, in single-chamber ventricular pacing (VVI), ventricular stimulation occurs without reference to the timing of atrial activity. During VVI pacing, the temporal relationship between atrial and ventricular contractions is not fixed and loss of the normal atrioventricular sequence results. In DDI pacing, atrial sensing inhibits both chambers, thus allowing native conduction to the ventricle but atrial pacing is followed by a paced ventricular beat unless a native ventricular beat is sensed. This nontracking mode may reduce ventricular stimulation in some cases.

The DDD and AAI pacing modes were often grouped together in study designs as "physiologic pacing," because both modes preserve the normal AV relationship. The expectation was that DDD pacing when compared to ventricular-based pacing, would improve quality of life, cardiac mortality and heart failure. Two large randomized trials, involving over 4,500 patients predominantly with sinus node dysfunction, have compared dual-chamber pacing with single-chamber ventricular pacing (50,51). No difference in total mortality or mortality from cardiovascular causes or stroke was demonstrated and only modest benefits seen for the progression of heart failure and development of atrial fibrillation which only emerge after years of follow-up. Recent evidence demonstrates that dual-chamber pacing, which confers the theoretical benefit of atrioventricular synchrony, has "unphysiologic," detrimental consequences, with forced right ventricular apical pacing producing ventricular dyssynchrony and left ventricular dysfunction (52). In the case of DDD pacing, there was usually significant amounts of ventricular pacing even in the group in which the pacing indication was sinus node dysfunction. In contrast, the study comparing the AAI to VVI modes (in which both AV and interventricular synchrony are maintained in the AAI group) did demonstrate benefits in all parameters including mortality after a longer follow-up of 5 years (53).

The Effect of Pacing Mode on Specific Outcomes in Patients with Sinus Node Dysfunction

The DDD, AAI, and VVI pacing modes are equally effective in preventing syncope owing to bradycardia in patients with sinus node dysfunction (54). However, as outlined in the following section, different pacing modes are associated with unique clinical outcomes (Table 9.4).

1. Quality of life
2. Pacemaker syndrome
3. Atrial fibrillation
4. Thromboembolic stroke
5. Heart failure
6. Mortality

Quality of Life

Although improved survival has not been demonstrated with dual chamber or pacing over ventricular pacing, available evidence suggests that patients with sinus node dysfunction experience an improvement in quality of life. The first randomized trial comparing AAI pacing to VVI pacing in 225 patients demonstrated a deterioration in quality of life with worsening heart failure in those patients assigned to VVI pacing (53). This benefit appears to be attenuated when VVI pacing is compared to DDD rather than AAI pacing (55,56). The Canadian Trial of Physiologic Pacing (CTOPP) was the first large-scale randomized study of pacing mode selection and compared

Table 9.4 Studies on effects of pacing mode on patients with sinus node dysfunction.

Study	Size	Pacing modes	Endpoints	Summary of results
Andersen 1997	225: All SND	VVI vs. AAI	*Mortality* – AAI relative risk: 0.66 (0.44–0.99); $p = 0.045$ *Cardiovascular mortality* – AAI relative risk: 0.47 (0.27–0.82); $p = 0.0065$ *Thromboembolism* – AAI relative risk: 0.47 (0.24–0.92); $p = 0.023$ *Atrial fibrillation* – AAI relative risk: 0.54 (0.33–0.89); $p = 0.012$	AAI pacing better than VVI in all clinical endpoints at long-term follow–up
PASE 1998	Total: 407 SND: 175	VVIR vs. DDDR	*Mortality* – DDDR 12%; VVIR 20%; $p = 0.9$ *Stroke or death* – DDDR 13%; VVIR 22%; $p = 0.11$ *Atrial fibrillation* – DDDR 19%; VVIR 28%; $p = 0.06$ *Stroke, death, or heart failure hospitalization* – DDDR 20%; VVIR 31%; $p = 0.07$ *QoL* – $p = 0.02$	Overall, no significant differences in any endpoints between DDDR and VVIR. In SND subgroup, a trend towards a reduction in atrial fibrillation and modest improvement in QoL with DDDR vs. VVIR. Table data are for SND group
CTOPP 2000	Total: 2,568, one-third SND alone	VVIR vs. AAIR (5.2%), DDDR (94.8%)	*Cardiovascular stroke or death* – AAIR/DDDR: 4.9%; VVIR: 5.5%; $p = 0.33$ *Atrial fibrillation* – AAIR, DDDR 5.3%; VVIR 6.6%; $p = 0.05$ *Heart failure* – AAIR/DDDR 3.1%; VVIR 3.1%; $p = NS$ *Stroke* – AAIR, DDDR 1.0%; VVIR 1.1%; $p = NS$	Data specifically for patients with SND are not available. Overall, only significant benefit of "physiological" pacing was reduction in atrial fibrillation which was not evident until after 2 years

(continued)

Table 9.4 (continued)

Study	Size	Pacing modes	Endpoints	Summary of results
MOST 2002	2010: All SND	VVIR vs. DDDR	*Total mortality and stroke* – DDDR 21.5%; VVIR 23%; *p* = 0.48	No differences in death or stroke. Atrial fibrillation, heart failure and pacemaker syndrome slightly less and quality of life slightly better with DDDR vs. VVIR
			Atrial fibrillation – DDDR hazard ratio 0.79 (0.66–0.94); *p* = 0.008	
			Heart failure hospitalization – DDDR hazard ratio 0.82 (0.63–1.06); *p* = 0.13 adjusted analyses 0.73 (0.56–0.95); *p* = 0.02	
			Pacemaker syndrome – 18.3% ventricular paced patients	
			QoL – Small incremental benefit of DDDR over VVIR some but not all questionnaires	
Nielsen 2003	177: All SND	AAI vs. DDDR-short AV vs. DDDR-long AV	*Atrial fibrillation* – AAIR 7.4%, DDDR-short AV 23.3%, DDDR-long AV 17.5%; *p* = 0.03	(1) Endpoints echocardiographic: all in favor of AAI pacing. (2) Endpoints clinical: Atrial fibrillation more common in DDD. No differences in thromboembolism, congestive heart failure or death
MOST substudy 2003	2010: All SND	VVIR vs. DDDR	*Cumulative % ventricular pacing* – DDDR (90%) vs. VVIR (58%); *p* = 0.001	An increased risk of both heart failure and atrial fibrillation with increased percentage ventricular pacing
			Heart failure – DDDR: Cum%VP >40% vs. ≤40%, hazard ratio 2.60 (1.05–6.47); *p* = 0.04	
			VVIR: Cum%VP >80% vs. ≤80%, hazard ratio 2.5 (1.44–4.36); *p* = 0.0012	
			Atrial fibrillation – DDDR: 1% ↑ risk of AF for every 1% ↑ in Cum%VP	
			VVIR: 0.7% ↑ risk of AF for every 1% ↑ in Cum%VP	

| ADEPT study | 872: 53% SND | DDD vs. DDDR & mode switch on vs. mode switch off | *Death* – DDD vs. DDDR & MS on vs. MS off; p = NS

Nonfatal MI – DDD vs. DDDR & MS on vs. MS off; p = NS

Stroke – DDD vs. DDDR & MS on vs. MS off; p = NS

Heart failure – DDD vs. DDDR; p = NS. MS on 9.4% vs. MS off 15.4%; $p < 0.01$

Atrial fibrillation – DDD vs. DDDR; p = NS. MS on 29% vs. MS off 21.1%; $p < 0.01$ | No advantage of rate-response function with respect to death, nonfatal MI, stroke, heart failure, or atrial fibrillation. In MS on vs. MS off patients, a statistically significant difference seen in incidence of AF (favoring MS off) & CHF hospitalizations (favoring MS on)

Lack of benefit of DDDR + MS calls into question the current clinical practice of routinely programming all features "on" |

SND = sinus node dysfunction.

"physiologic" pacing modes (AAIR-5%/DDDR-95%) and the VVIR pacing mode in patients undergoing pacemaker implantation for usual indications (51). Sick sinus syndrome was the indication for pacing in 34% of the 2,568 enrolled and randomized to receive either dual-or single-chamber ventricular pacemakers. Pacing mode choice did not influence quality of life although pacing-induced restoration of chronotropic competence did have a positive effect in the sinus node disease patients (57). There was also a lack of improvement in functional capacity detected. The MOST trial (The Mode Selection Trial in Sinus-Node Dysfunction), included 2,010 patients with sick sinus syndrome, 21% of whom also had AV block (50). A recently reported analysis of the MOST patients describes a small but significant improvement in several but not all measures of quality of life in those programmed to the DDD-mode compared to VVI-mode (58). Observations from the PASE Study, a prospective, randomized, and blinded-trial comparing DDDR and VVIR pacing in elderly patients (average age, 76) with standard indications for pacing (49% AV node disease, 43% sinus node dysfunction, 8% other), also suggest improved quality of life as well as significant improvement in cardiovascular functional status in patients who were assigned DDDR in contrast to VVIR pacing (56). In the patients with sinus node dysfunction, higher scores in the physical-role subscale, social-function subscale, and emotional-role subscale were observed with the DDDR pacing mode.

Overall it appears that maintenance of AV synchrony results in a slightly improved quality of life with DDD as opposed to VVI pacing.

Pacemaker Syndrome

The pacemaker syndrome refers to a constellation of symptoms that are associated with VVI pacing and loss of atrioventricular synchrony. Such symptoms include dizziness, presyncope, syncope, generalized weakness, headache, and features of cardiac failure (59). The prevalence of pacemaker syndrome varies markedly between published studies (0.1–83%), which probably reflects great variability in its definition as well as the ease or otherwise of crossover in the randomized studies (59,60). In the PASE study, 26% of patients assigned to ventricular pacing were crossed over to dual-chamber pacing during a 30 month follow-up because of symptoms relating to pacemaker syndrome (61). The patients who crossed over from ventricular pacing to dual-chamber pacing experienced significant improve-ments in quality of life. In the MOST trial, a total of 313 patients (31%) of those designated to the VVIR mode crossed over to DDDR with half of these crossovers attributed to the pacemaker syndrome (50). In contrast, the CTOPP trial (51) as well as the Danish study (62), found a much smaller incidence of pacemaker syndrome with crossover rates of only 5 and 1.8%, respectively. This is perhaps not unexpected as these trials were "hardware randomized" and thus necessitated a second procedure to achieve AV synchrony. The true incidence of pacemaker syndrome likely lies between these values. A reduction in pacemaker syndrome may be responsible for the improved quality of life reported by patients with pacing modes that preserve AV synchrony.

Atrial Fibrillation

Clinical trials have been uniformly positive in finding a reduction of atrial fibrillation with atrial-based pacing when compared to ventricular-based pacing (50,51,53,56,63,64). The early observational studies strongly suggested that the VVI pacing mode is associated with a two- to threefold increase in the incidence of atrial fibrillation compared with "physiologic" pacing modes (65–67). These findings have been corroborated in the larger prospective randomized trials although the benefit was not of the same magnitude. Andersen and associates demonstrated an increased risk of developing atrial fibrillation with VVI pacing compared with AAI pacing (53). However, this did not become evident until after 3 years of follow-up indicating a delay after pacemaker implantation of the benefit of atrial pacing or the deleterious effect of ventricular pacing. In the PASE trial in an elderly population, Lamas and associates demonstrated a 28% incidence of atrial fibrillation with VVIR pacing compared with a 19% incidence with DDDR pacing over 30 months in the subgroup of 175 patients with sick sinus syndrome ($p=0.06$) (56). This study was not specifically designed to address the effect of pacing mode on the development of atrial fibrillation and was not sufficiently powered to detect significant differences in the incidence of atrial fibrillation between the two pacing modes. Interpretation of outcome data from the PASE study is also complicated by a 26% crossover rate from VVIR to DDDR pacing because of pacemaker syndrome, which may have contributed to a smaller benefit of DDDR pacing over VVIR pacing. A subsequent multivariate analysis did demonstrate a benefit of DDDR pacing in incidence of atrial fibrillation (68). In a study of 210 patients, 110 of whom had "sick sinus syndrome" and no prior history of atrial fibrillation, patients were randomized to either a ventricular pacemaker or a "physiologic" pacemaker (63,64). An increased incidence of chronic atrial fibrillation was seen in the "sick sinus syndrome" subgroup who received ventricular pacing. The first large-scale trial of pacing mode selection was the CTOPP trial, in which 42% of the 2,568 patients had "sick sinus syndrome." There was a significant reduction in the incidence of atrial fibrillation with DDDR/AAIR pacing modes (5.3% per year) compared with the VVI pacing mode (6.6% per year) amounting to an 18.5% risk reduction (51). Again however, the Kaplan Meier curves did not separate until after 2 years of follow-up. After an extended follow-up of 6 years, the difference in atrial fibrillation between the two groups had increased slightly. In the MOST trial, the yearly incidence of atrial fibrillation was higher than in CTOPP, possibly because all patients had sinus node dysfunction (50). Nonetheless, the overall relative reduction in atrial fibrillation of 21% in MOST was similar to the 18.5% in CTOPP. An interesting observation in MOST is that in the DDDR arm, those patients who had no prior history of atrial fibrillation had a much greater reduction in atrial fibrillation risk of 50% compared to only a nonsignificant 14% reduction in those with a past history of atrial fibrillation. This suggests that perhaps patients with substrate which can already support atrial fibrillation are less responsive to the effect of pacing modalities to prevent or treat atrial fibrillation. A further benefit of AAI over DDD pacing in decreasing atrial fibrillation incidence in patients with sinus node dysfunction is supported by three studies (52,69,70). Although both AAI and DDD modes preserve AV synchrony, the ventricular desynchronization from right ventricular pacing in the DDD mode increases the likelihood of atrial fibrillation.

The likely mechanisms of increased atrial fibrillation with pacing are likely to be both AV and ventricular dyssynchrony. Although basic hemodynamic studies have convincingly demonstrated the benefits of maintaining AV synchrony, clinical trials, as described above, have failed to show the same impressive results expected from the physiological data. Changes in the relative timing of atrial and ventricular systole can result in marked changes in atrial pressure and volume (71–73). Acute VVI pacing is associated with an increase in right atrial and pulmonary capillary wedge pressures compared to DDD and AAI pacing. Two studies have demonstrated that peak and mean right atrial pressures were greater during dual-chamber pacing at an AV interval of 0 ms compared with pacing at an AV interval of 120–160 ms (73,74). Acute pacing studies comparing echocardiographic atrial dimensions have also been performed; Paxinos and associates demonstrated a 52% decrease in left atrial fractional shortening during acute VVI pacing compared with sinus rhythm (75).

Nielsen and colleagues have demonstrated that both VVI (76) and DDD (69) pacing when compared to AAI pacing in patients with sinus node dysfunction results in an increased left atrial size. These changes further translated into a significantly higher incidence of atrial fibrillation in the DDD pacing group. In addition to detrimental effects on left atrial size, VVI pacing has significant effects on left atrial mechanical function. In a prospective crossover study, Sparks and associates compared left atrial appendage function in 21 patients paced chronically in the VVI mode with a control group of 11 patients paced chronically in DDD mode for 3 months (77). Left atrial appendage function and the presence of spontaneous echo contrast (SEC) were determined with serial transesophageal echocardiography (TEE) performed within 24 h of pacemaker implantation, and after 3 months of follow-up. At 3 months, the VVI group was programmed to DDD and underwent a third TEE after DDD pacing for 3 months. Following chronic VVI pacing, there was a highly significant reduction in all parameters of left atrial appendage function, and four patients (19%) developed left atrial SEC, a known marker of thrombus formation. With the reestablishment of chronic AV synchrony with DDD pacing, parameters of left atrial appendage function returned to baseline values and SEC resolved in all patients. In the 11 patients undergoing chronic DDD pacing, no significant changes in left atrial appendage function were observed and SEC did not develop. The authors concluded that chronic loss of AV synchrony induced by VVI pacing is associated with mechanical global remodeling of the left atrium and reduced left atrial appendage function. Electrical remodeling of the atria with the loss of AV synchrony with decreased effective refractory period, increased SNRTs and increased P-wave durations has also been demonstrated with the loss of AV synchrony with VVI pacing (78). Importantly, these data also suggest that both the mechanical and electrical changes may reverse following the reestablishment of AV synchrony with DDD pacing.

Sophisticated pacing algorithms to prevent and treat atrial fibrillation have been developed over the past few years. However, trials to date have demonstrated minimal or even no efficacy (79,80–85).

Multisite atrial pacing techniques have been shown to prevent atrial dilatation, decrease total atrial contraction time, and decrease the conduction slowing which occurs with atrial premature beats which can trigger atrial fibrillation (86–88). Consequently, there has been significant interest in the potential of dual/multisite atrial pacing to decrease the rates of atrial fibrillation with early studies showing promise (89,90). However, the largest clinical trial in 118 patients only demonstrated a small incremental benefit in patients already on antiarrhythmic drugs in the rate of atrial fibrillation development with dual site as opposed to single site atrial pacing (91).

In summary, the lowest risk of atrial fibrillation is achieved with maintenance of both AV and interventricular synchrony where possible. However, the benefits appear to be relatively small and only become evident years after pacemaker implant. Multisite and alternate site pacing as well as pacing algorithms have not yet proven to be of significant benefit in atrial fibrillation prevention.

Thromboembolic Stroke

Reduction in the incidence of atrial fibrillation consequent to atrial pacing could plausibly decrease the incidence of thromboembolic stroke. However, as discussed above, the reduction in atrial fibrillation is relatively small and in the elderly pacemaker population, atrial fibrillation is only one of several causes of stroke. Additionally, the high use of anticoagulation in pacemaker patients (72% in the MOST study (50)) may substantially reduce the magnitude of benefit of prevention of atrial fibrillation with atrial-based pacing.

Despite this, in the only study using solely AAI pacing as the "physiologic" arm, Andersen and associates did demonstrate a twofold increase in thromboembolic events with chronic VVI pacing compared with AAI pacing over a follow-up period of 3.3 years (62), which was maintained out to 8 years (53). On multivariate analysis, atrial pacing was associated with a significant reduction in thromboembolic events (relative risk 0.47). At the time of randomization, VVI pacing and a history of bradycardia–tachycardia syndrome were independent predictors for the subsequent occurrence of thromboembolic events during follow-up. However, the large randomized controlled trials have not managed to demonstrate a reduction in stroke risk in those with atrial-based pacing when compared to ventricular-based pacing. In the CTOPP study, although there was a small reduction in the primary composite endpoint of cardiovascular death or stroke of 12% (from 5.3% per year in VVIR group to 4.8% per year in DDDR/AAIR group), this did not reach clinical significance (51). Specific data for the patients with sinus node dysfunction have not been published. The MOST study found an annualized incidence of stroke of 2.2% with no clear difference based on pacing mode (50). Thus, currently, dual-chamber pacing should not be selected for the prevention of stroke.

Heart Failure

The intuitive benefits of maintaining AV synchrony have not been fulfilled by the large randomized controlled pacing trials. Pacing mode choice, when comparing DDD pacing with ventricular-based pacing, has demonstrated an inconsistent benefit of "physiologic" DDD pacing with respect to the incidence of heart failure. This is likely to be explained by the dysynchronization imposed by forced right ventricular apical pacing in the DDD mode which negates any benefits conferred by maintenance of AV synchrony. Pacing from virtually any ventricular site disturbs the natural activation pattern and ventricular contraction because the impulse travels slowly through the myocardium rather than through the rapidly conducting His-Purkinje system. Ironically, of all ventricular sites, the right ventricular apex seems to be hemodynamically the least favorable (92,93). In humans, chronic RV apical pacing has been shown to result in asymmetric septal hypertrophy (94–96), ventricular dilatation 94, myocardial fiber disarray (97), increased catecholamine concentrations 98, and myocardial perfusion defects (99).

These physiological effects also translate into the clinical arena. Sweeney and colleagues, in a careful retrospective analysis of the MOST study data, demonstrated that an increase in the amount of ventricular pacing, in patients with a normal baseline QRS, is associated with an increased likelihood of congestive heart failure (52). This finding is augmented in patients with heart failure and no bradycardic pacing indication. The DAVID study, in patients with dual-chamber implantable cardioverter defibrillators, prospectively compares backup ventricular pacing (VVI, 40 bpm) to dual-chamber pacing (DDD/R, lower rate 70 bpm) (100). The study was terminated prematurely because of an excess of heart failure and deaths in the DDD/R arm. An increased frequency of ventricular pacing was associated with a 1.6-fold rise in the composite endpoint of congestive heart failure, hospitalization, and death (101). Analysis of the MADIT II trial showed similar negative consequences with an increase in cumulative percentage of right ventricular pacing regardless of pacing mode (102). Thus, it appears that dual-chamber pacing is a double-edged sword with the potential benefits of atrioventricular synchrony offset by the detrimental effect of inducing ventricular dysfunction. Of note, the smaller randomized controlled studies which compared AAI pacing to DDD pacing in SND with normal AV conduction, revealed an increase in heart failure hospitalizations in those with DDD/R pacing (53,69) supporting the theory of ventricular pacing induced dysfunction.

Nonetheless, the majority of patients who receive pacemakers for sinus node dysfunction do not experience heart failure that can be attributed to right ventricular apical pacing, even if paced a high percentage of the time. In randomized controlled trials of patients mostly with normal ventricular function it took 3–5 years before heart failure became manifest and then only occurred in <10% of patients. This is in contrast to the trials in patients with preexisting systolic heart failure and no bradycardic indications (DAVID and MADIT II) in which the effect was evident in less than a year. A recently published analysis of the MOST data has found that differences in heart failure risk relates to (1) atrioventricular synchrony (pacing mode); (2) ventricular synchrony (measured by ventricular "pacing burden"; and (3) underlying patient clinical and physiological variables ("substrate") (103,104). The "pacing burden" is the paced QRS duration (a measure of the "potency per dose"), together with cumulative percentage ventricular pacing (which is the frequency with which the dose is delivered). The "substrate" includes the underlying ventricular function, ventricular conduction, atrial rhythm, symptomatic heart failure, and myocardial infarction. The risk of heart failure hospitalization was found to be doubled in the DDDR mode with percentage pacing >40% versus cumulative percentage ventricular pacing ≤40%. However, in patients with a low-risk "substrate" (e.g., normal ejection fraction, no history of heart failure or myocardial infarction and normal baseline QRS), the risk might only increase from <1 to 2% as opposed to high risk patients (e.g., low baseline ejection fraction, history of symptomatic heart failure, baseline prolonged QRS duration, and myocardial infarction) where the risk of heart failure hospitalization rises from 20 to 40%. Thus, in these patients, the absolute increase in risk is much greater. A multicentered Danish study exploring the benefit of minimizing unnecessary ventricular pacing, comparing AAI pacing to DDD pacing (DANPACE), is ongoing. Another industry-sponsored trial is investigating the effect of an extendable AV delay in reducing ventricular pacing (SAVE-PACE).

The recognition of the adverse effects of right ventricular apical pacing has stimulated investigation not only of manipulation of pacing modes and timing cycles to minimize ventricular pacing, but also possible alternate ventricular site/s to attenuate the effects of ventricular dyssynchrony when ventricular pacing cannot be avoided. The studies looking at right ventricular outflow tract pacing have conflicting results possibly as there has not been any consistency in lead positioning (105,106). Newer atrial-based dual-chamber detection modes have been developed to overcome the limitations of the AAI/R and DDD/R modes in reducing undesirable ventricular pacing (107,108). Managed ventricular pacing, so called "MVP" (Medtronic) or "AAIsafeR2" (ELA) is a functional AAIR pacing mode that converts to DDDR pacing should there be loss of AV conduction or pauses. In sinus node dysfunction patients, this mode has been shown to reduce ventricular pacing by over 90% compared to the DDD/R mode (109). A study addressing the efficacy of MVP in ICD patients has just completed enrollment and is in the follow-up phase (110). It should be noted that these novel approaches to optimizing ventricular pacing have not been fully validated in randomized controlled trials. There are several ongoing studies running to test the hypothesis that minimizing right ventricular pacing and thus preserving ventricular synchrony will reduce the likelihood of atrial fibrillation, heart failure, and death.

Mortality

No trial comparing DDD to VVI pacing, has demonstrated a significant mortality benefit in patients paced for sinus node dysfunction based on mode selection. The MOST trial is the only trial to report cardiovascular mortality and showed no difference between the ventricular (8.9%) and DDD (9.2%) modes after a median follow-up of 33.1 months (50). In CTOPP (51) as well as in the PASE trial (56), a composite outcome of stroke or death due to cardiovascular cause also showed no difference after 5 years of follow-up in the group with sinus node disease according to pacing mode. In contrast, the smaller Danish trial, which compared AAI to VVI pacing, reported a decrease in both cardiovascular and all cause mortality in those with AAI pacing which only became evident at the long-term 8 year follow-up (53). This possibly reflects the detrimental effects of right ventricular pacing and dyssynchrony which have been shown to take 3–5 years to become manifest.

Other Issues Relating to Mode Selection and Pacemaker Programming

Risk of AV Block

A number of retrospective studies have suggested that patients with sinus node dysfunction have an increased risk of developing concomitant conduction disturbances and AV block in particular (111,112). Haywood and associates followed 24 patients with sinus node disease without evidence of conduction disturbance who were paced in AAI or AAIR modes. During a mean follow-up time of 10.7 ± 5 months, four patients required revision of pacing system as a result of development of AV block and one other patient manifested intermittent second-degree AV block (111). Vallins and Edhag demonstrated associated conduction disturbances at electrophysiologic study in 24 of 30 (80%) patients with symptomatic sinus node disease; however, only one of these 30 patients developed complete AV block during a 5-year follow-up period (113). In a literature survey of data from 28 different studies on atrial pacing with a median follow-up of 36 months there was a median annual incidence of second and third degree AV block of 0.6%, with a range of 0–4.5% (114). More recently, the Danish study compared AAI to VVI pacing in 225 patients with sinus node dysfunction and intact AV conduction (115). During a mean follow-up of 5.5 ± 2.4 years, as a group, atrioventricular conduction remained stable. However, 4 of 110 patients in the AAI group developed AV block that required upgrading of the pacemaker (0.6% per year). Two of these four patients had right bundle-branch block at pacemaker implantation. The authors concluded that treatment with single-chamber atrial pacing is safe and can be recommended to patients with sick sinus syndrome without bundle-branch block (115). Of note, a number of studies have demonstrated that when bundle branch block is present at implant there is a higher incidence of progression to AV block and implantation of a dual-chamber system is warranted (115–117).

Rate-Responsive Pacing

Increases in heart rate may be responsible for up to 75% of the increased cardiac output associated with exercise (118). Even in the healthy older population, heart rate increases to the same degree with exertion as in younger people (119). The advent of rate-responsive pacemakers in the mid-1970s represented a major advance in pacemaker technology. However, despite the convincing theoretical and physiological data (120), supporting the use of rate-responsive function, studies have failed to show a consistent benefit in clinical terms. Intuitively, significant symptomatic improvement would be greatest in patients with chronotropic incompetence, a hallmark of sinus node dysfunction. Although several small studies do support the concept that rate-responsive pacing improves quality of life (121,122), a larger randomized controlled trial (ADEPT study) does not support a global instigation of rate-responsive pacing in all patients in sinus rhythm with sinus node dysfunction (123). This trial randomized 874 patients with chronotropic incompetence to DDDR or DDD pacing and found no appreciable improvement in exercise capacity or quality of life. Indeed, a compelling concern in light of recent evidence is that more aggressive rate response programming may result in a greater percentage of ventricular pacing and resultant dyssynchrony.

Mode-Switching

The association of sinus node dysfunction with paroxysmal atrial arrhythmias has long been recognized and presents some specific issues with respect to pacing (32). Until relatively recently, patients with sinus node dysfunction and paroxysmal atrial arrhythmias were usually required to be paced in the VVIR or DDIR modes. Otherwise, inappropriate tracking of rapid atrial activity in atrial tachyarrhythmias leads to pacing at the upper rate limit. In recent years a wide range of pacemaker algorithms has been developed to ensure that the pacemaker does not inappropriately track unphysiologic high-rate atrial activity; the most commonly utilized algorithm is mode switching (124–126). If rapid atrial activity is detected by the pacemaker, the pacing mode is switched usually from the DDDR mode to either the VVIR or DDIR pacing modes. However, the benefits seen in patients with AV block and paroxysmal atrial fibrillation do not seem to extend to most patients with sinus node dysfunction and intact AV conduction. A subset of the MOST study examining the clinical benefits of mode switching in patients with sinus node dysfunction found no improvements in quality of life or cardiovascular symptoms (127). This is somewhat concerning given mode switching (and rate response) are nominally programmed on in virtually all patients without regard to clinical need. Restricted delays imposed by mode-switching algorithms can result in increased right ventricular pacing with its attendant possible adverse consequences. The recent ADEPT trial looked at both rate-response function and mode switching with respect to quality of life, death, stroke, heart failure, and atrial fibrillation (123). A statistically significant difference was noted in the incidence of atrial fibrillation (favoring mode switching off) and congestive heart failure hospitalizations (favoring mode switching on). The possible negative effects of both atrial pacing and ventricular pacing may explain the higher incidence of atrial fibrillation in the group with mode switching "on." These results emphasize the need for careful programming of cardiac rhythm devices to suit patients needs. One size does NOT fit all when it comes to pacemaker programming. It is not beneficial to have all programming options "on," "just in case" because of the potential negative consequences particularly relating to increased unnecessary ventricular pacing.

Summary of Pacing Mode Choice for Sinus Node Dysfunction

Goal 1. Prevent symptomatic bradycardia
Goal 2. Maintain AV synchrony
Goal 3. Maintain VV synchrony (minimize ventricular pacing) – especially in patients with baseline left ventricular dysfunction
Goal 4. Provide chronotropic support and mode-switching algorithms as required.

Various options are available which perform some if not all of these goals.

1. AAI/R: Single-chamber atrial pacing will potentially address all of these goals although there remains the risk of AV block. In sinus node dysfunction patients this annualized risk is reported to be as high as 4.5% although if patients are carefully selected, the risk is in the vicinity of 0.6% per year.
2. VVI/R: Does not maintain VV or AV synchrony but is still an option in certain clinical circumstances of minimal intervention or in the very elderly.
3. DDD/R: Dual-chamber pacing with a long atrioventricular delay is commonly used giving ventricular backup pacing should the AV node fail.

Nonetheless, even the longest programmable AV delays are sometimes not adequate at preventing ventricular pacing especially if the rate-responsive function is activated.

4. DDI/R: A nontracking mode which allows programming of long AV delays and protection from high-paced ventricular rates in those patients with sinus node dysfunction but intact AV conduction and normal QRS duration. This minimizes ventricular dyssynchrony due to ventricular pacing.

5. Novel minimal ventricular pacing modes: MVP or AAIsafeR2 which alternate between functional AAI/R to DDD/R pacing have theoretical advantages of reduction of unnecessary ventricular pacing. Trials assessing efficacy are ongoing.

Conclusion

Sinus node dysfunction remains the commonest indication for pacemaker insertion in the industrialized world. Cardiac pacing is one of the greatest medical achievements of the twentieth century. Although tremendous advances have been achieved in knowledge and technology, the ideal pacing mode and pacing site are still not totally defined. Large-scale randomized studies have induced a rethink regarding what was once thought of as the pinnacle of "physiologic" pacing, the DDDR mode. Future randomized trials will further refine our understanding of the ideal pacing system, mode, and site for patients with sinus node dysfunction.

References

1. Keith A, Flack M. The form and nature of the muscular connections between the primary divisions of the vertebrate heart. *J Anat Physiol.* 1907;41:172–189.
2. James TN. Anatomy of the human sinus node. *Anat Rec.* 1961;141:109–139.
3. James TN, Sherf L, Fine G, Morales AR. Comparative ultrastructure of the sinus node in man and dog. *Circulation.* 1966;34:139–163.
4. James TN. The sinus node. *Am J Cardiol.* 1977;40:965–986.
5. Anderson RH, Ho SY. The architecture of the sinus node, the atrioventricular conduction axis, and the internodal atrial myocardium. *J Cardiovasc Electrophysiol.* 1998;9:1233–1248.
6. Schuessler RB, Boineau JP, Bromberg BI. Origin of the sinus impulse. *J Cardiovasc Electrophysiol.* 1996;7:263–274.
7. Lewis T, Oppenheimer BS, Oppenheimer A. The site of origin of the mammalian heart beat: the pacemaker in the dog. *Heart.* 1911;2:147–169.
8. Meek WJ, Eyster JAE. Experiments on the origin and propagation of the mammalian heart beat: IV. The effect of vagal stimulation and of cooling on the location of the pacemaker within the sino-auricular node. *Am J Physiol.* 1914;34:368–383.
9. Boineau JP, Canavan TE, Schuessler RB, Cain ME, Corr PB, Cox JL. Demonstration of a widely distributed atrial pacemaker complex in the human heart. *Circulation.* 1988;77:1221–1237.
10. Kalman JM, Lee RJ, Fisher WG, Chin MC, Ursell P, Stillson CA, Lesh MD, Scheinman MM. Radiofrequency catheter modification of sinus pacemaker function guided by intracardiac echocardiography. *Circulation.* 1995;92:3070–3081.
11. Boineau JP, Schuessler RB, Roeske WR, Autry LJ, Miller CB, Wylds AC. Quantitative relation between sites of atrial impulse origin and cycle length. *Am J Physiol.* 1983;245:H781–H789.

12. Anderson KR, Ho SY, Anderson RH. Location and vascular supply of sinus node in human heart. *Br Heart J.* 1979;41:28–32.

13. Boyett MR, Honjo H, Kodama I. The sinoatrial node, a heterogeneous pacemaker structure. *Cardiovasc Res.* 2000;47:658–687.

14. Boyett MR, Dobrzynski H, Lancaster MK, Jones SA, Honjo H, Kodama I. Sophisticated architecture is required for the sinoatrial node to perform its normal pacemaker function. *J Cardiovasc Electrophysiol.* 2003;14:104–106.

15. Irisawa H, Brown HF, Giles W. Cardiac pacemaking in the sinoatrial node. *Physiol Rev.* 1993;73:197–227.

16. Ono K, Shibata S, Iijima T. Properties of the delayed rectifier potassium current in porcine sino-atrial node cells. *J Physiol.* 2000;524 Pt 1:51–62.

17. Matsuura H, Ehara T, Ding WG, Omatsu-Kanbe M, Isono T. Rapidly and slowly activating components of delayed rectifier K(+) current in guinea-pig sino-atrial node pacemaker cells. *J Physiol.* 2002;540:815–830.

18. Lipsius SL, Huser J, Blatter LA. Intracellular Ca2 + release sparks atrial pacemaker activity. *News Physiol Sci.* 2001;16:101–106.

19. Bogdanov KY, Vinogradova TM, Lakatta EG. Sinoatrial nodal cell ryanodine receptor and Na(+)-Ca(2+) exchanger: molecular partners in pacemaker regulation. *Circ Res.* 2001;88:1254–1258.

20. Lei M, Honjo H, Kodama I, Boyett MR. Characterisation of the transient outward K+ current in rabbit sinoatrial node cells. *Cardiovasc Res.* 2000;46:433–441.

21. DiFrancesco D. Pacemaker mechanisms in cardiac tissue. *Annu Rev Physiol.* 1993;55:455–472.

22. Sakmann B, Noma A, Trautwein W. Acetylcholine activation of single muscarinic K+ channels in isolated pacemaker cells of the mammalian heart. *Nature.* 1983;303:250–253.

23. Soejima M, Noma A. Mode of regulation of the ACh-sensitive K-channel by the muscarinic receptor in rabbit atrial cells. *Pflugers Arch.* 1984;400:424–431.

24. DiFrancesco D, Tromba C. Muscarinic control of the hyperpolarization-activated current (if) in rabbit sino-atrial node myocytes. *J Physiol.* 1988;405:493–510.

25. DiFrancesco D, Ducouret P, Robinson RB. Muscarinic modulation of cardiac rate at low acetylcholine concentrations. *Science.* 1989;243:669–671.

26. Brown HF, DiFrancesco D, Noble SJ. How does adrenaline accelerate the heart? *Nature.* 1979;280:235–236.

27. Huser J, Blatter LA, Lipsius SL. Intracellular Ca2 + release contributes to automaticity in cat atrial pacemaker cells. *J Physiol.* 2000;524(Pt 2):415–422.

28. Bernstein AD, Parsonnet V. Survey of cardiac pacing and defibrillation in the United States in 1993. *Am J Cardiol.* 1996;78:187–196.

29. Ferrer MI. The sick sinus syndrome in atrial disease. *JAMA.* 1968;206:645–646.

30. Strauss HC, Prystowsky EN, Scheinman MM. Sino-atrial and atrial electrogenesis. *Prog Cardiovasc Dis.* 1977;19:385–404.

31. Wiens RD, Lafia P, Marder CM, Evans RG, Kennedy HL. Chronotropic incompetence in clinical exercise testing. *Am J Cardiol.* 1984;54:74–78.

32. Kusumoto FM, Goldschlager N. Cardiac pacing. *N Engl J Med.* 1996;334:89–97.

33. Demoulin JC, Kulbertus HE. Histopathological correlates of sinoatrial disease. *Br Heart J.* 1978;40:1384–1389.

34. Shaw DB. Chronic sinus node disease and coronary artery disease. *Lancet.* 1988;1:1277.

35. Surawicz B, Hariman RJ. Follow-up of the family with congenital absence of sinus rhythm. *Am J Cardiol.* 1988;61:467–469.

36. Kaplan BM, Langendorf R, Lev M, Pick A. Tachycardia-bradycardia syndrome (so-called "sick sinus syndrome"). Pathology, mechanisms and treatment. *Am J Cardiol.* 1973;31:497–508.

37. Lev M. Aging changes in the human sinoatrial node. *J Gerontol.* 1954;9:1–9.

38. Sanders P, Morton JB, Kistler PM, Spence SJ, Davidson NC, Hussin A, Vohra JK, Sparks PB, Kalman JM. Electrophysiological and electroanatomic characterization of the atria in sinus node disease: evidence of diffuse atrial remodeling. *Circulation*. 2004;109:1514–1522.

39. Sanders P, Kistler PM, Morton JB, Spence SJ, Kalman JM. Remodeling of sinus node function in patients with congestive heart failure: reduction in sinus node reserve. *Circulation*. 2004;110:897–903.

40. Morton JB, Sanders P, Vohra JK, Sparks PB, Morgan JG, Spence SJ, Grigg LE, Kalman JM. Effect of chronic right atrial stretch on atrial electrical remodeling in patients with an atrial septal defect. *Circulation*. 2003;107:1775–1782.

41. Hocini M, Sanders P, Deisenhofer I, Jais P, Hsu LF, Scavee C, Weerasoriya R, Raybaud F, Macle L, Shah DC, Garrigue S, Le Metayer P, Clementy J, Haissaguerre M. Reverse remodeling of sinus node function after catheter ablation of atrial fibrillation in patients with prolonged sinus pauses. *Circulation*. 2003;108:1172–1175.

42. Daoud EG, Weiss R, Augostini RS, Kalbfleisch SJ, Schroeder J, Polsinelli G, Hummel JD. Remodeling of sinus node function after catheter ablation of right atrial flutter. *J Cardiovasc Electrophysiol*. 2002;13:20–24.

43. Sparks PB, Jayaprakash S, Vohra JK, Kalman JM. Electrical remodeling of the atria associated with paroxysmal and chronic atrial flutter. *Circulation*. 2000;102:1807–1813.

44. Gregoratos G, Cheitlin MD, Conill A, Epstein AE, Fellows C, Ferguson TB, Jr., Freedman RA, Hlatky MA, Naccarelli GV, Saksena S, Schlant RC, Silka MJ. ACC/AHA Guidelines for Implantation of Cardiac Pacemakers and Antiarrhythmia Devices: Executive Summary – a report of the American College of Cardiology/American Heart Association Task Force on Practice Guidelines (Committee on Pacemaker Implantation). *Circulation*. 1998;97:1325–1335.

45. Gregoratos G, Abrams J, Epstein AE, Freedman RA, Hayes DL, Hlatky MA, Kerber RE, Naccarelli GV, Schoenfeld MH, Silka MJ, Winters SL, Gibbons RJ, Antman EM, Alpert JS, Gregoratos G, Hiratzka LF, Faxon DP, Jacobs AK, Fuster V, Smith SC, Jr. ACC/AHA/NASPE 2002 guideline update for implantation of cardiac pacemakers and antiarrhythmia devices: summary article: a report of the American College of Cardiology/American Heart Association Task Force on Practice Guidelines (ACC/AHA/NASPE Committee to Update the 1998 Pacemaker Guidelines). *Circulation*. 2002;106:2145–2161.

46. Reiffel JA, Bigger JT, Jr., Cramer M, Reid DS. Ability of Holter electrocardiographic recording and atrial stimulation to detect sinus nodal dysfunction in symptomatic and asymptomatic patients with sinus bradycardia. *Am J Cardiol*. 1977;40:189–194.

47. Crook BR, Cashman PM, Stott FD, Raftery EB. Tape monitoring of the electrocardiogram in ambulant patients with sinoatrial disease. *Br Heart J*. 1973;35:1009–1013.

48. Brignole M, Menozzi C, Maggi R, Solano A, Donateo P, Bottoni N, Lolli G, Quartieri F, Croci F, Oddone D, Puggioni E. The usage and diagnostic yield of the implantable loop-recorder in detection of the mechanism of syncope and in guiding effective antiarrhythmic therapy in older people. *Europace*. 2005;7:273–279.

49. Reiffel JA, Kuehnert MJ. Electrophysiological testing of sinus node function: diagnostic and prognostic application-including updated information from sinus node electrograms. *Pacing Clin Electrophysiol*. 1994;17:349–365.

50. Lamas GA, Lee KL, Sweeney MO, Silverman R, Leon A, Yee R, Marinchak RA, Flaker G, Schron E, Orav EJ, Hellkamp AS, Greer S, McAnulty J, Ellenbogen K, Ehlert F, Freedman RA, Estes NA, III, Greenspon A, Goldman L. Ventricular pacing or dual-chamber pacing for sinus-node dysfunction. *N Engl J Med*. 2002;346:1854–1862.

51. Connolly SJ, Kerr CR, Gent M, Roberts RS, Yusuf S, Gillis AM, Sami MH, Talajic M, Tang AS, Klein GJ, Lau C, Newman DM. Effects of physiologic pacing versus ventricular pacing on the risk of stroke and death due to cardiovascular causes. Canadian Trial of Physiologic Pacing Investigators. *N Engl J Med*. 2000;342:1385–1391.

52. Sweeney MO, Hellkamp AS, Ellenbogen KA, Greenspon AJ, Freedman RA, Lee KL, Lamas GA. Adverse effect of ventricular pacing on heart failure and atrial fibrillation among patients with normal baseline QRS duration in a clinical trial of pacemaker therapy for sinus node dysfunction. *Circulation*. 2003;107:2932–2937.

53. Andersen HR, Nielsen JC, Thomsen PE, Thuesen L, Mortensen PT, Vesterlund T, Pedersen AK. Long-term follow-up of patients from a randomised trial of atrial versus ventricular pacing for sick-sinus syndrome. *Lancet*. 1997;350:1210–1216.

54. Grimm W, Langenfeld H, Maisch B, Kochsiek K. Symptoms, cardiovascular risk profile and spontaneous ECG in paced patients: a five-year follow-up study. *Pacing Clin Electrophysiol*. 1990;13:2086–2090.

55. Lamas GA, Lee KL, Sweeney MO, Silverman R, Leon A, Yee R, Marinchak RA, Flaker G, Schron E, Orav EJ, Hellkamp AS, Greer S, McAnulty J, Ellenbogen K, Ehlert F, Freedman RA, Estes NA, III, Greenspon A, Goldman L. Ventricular pacing or dual-chamber pacing for sinus-node dysfunction. *N Engl J Med*. 2002;346:1854–1862.

56. Lamas GA, Orav EJ, Stambler BS, Ellenbogen KA, Sgarbossa EB, Huang SK, Marinchak RA, Estes NA, III, Mitchell GF, Lieberman EH, Mangione CM, Goldman L. Quality of life and clinical outcomes in elderly patients treated with ventricular pacing as compared with dual-chamber pacing. Pacemaker Selection in the Elderly Investigators. *N Engl J Med*. 1998;338:1097–1104.

57. Newman D, Lau C, Tang AS, Irvine J, Paquette M, Woodend K, Dorian P, Gent M, Kerr C, Connolly SJ. Effect of pacing mode on health-related quality of life in the Canadian Trial of Physiologic Pacing. *Am Heart J*. 2003;145:430–437.

58. Fleischmann KE, Orav EJ, Lamas GA, Mangione CM, Schron E, Lee KL, Goldman L. Pacemaker implantation and quality of life in the Mode Selection Trial (MOST). *Heart Rhythm*. 2006;3:653–659.

59. Ausubel K, Furman S. The pacemaker syndrome. *Ann Intern Med*. 1985;103:420–429.

60. Heldman D, Mulvihill D, Nguyen H, Messenger JC, Rylaarsdam A, Evans K, Castellanet MJ. True incidence of pacemaker syndrome. *Pacing Clin Electrophysiol*. 1990;13:1742–1750.

61. Ellenbogen KA, Stambler BS, Orav EJ, Sgarbossa EB, Tullo NG, Love CA, Wood MA, Goldman L, Lamas GA. Clinical characteristics of patients intolerant to VVIR pacing. *Am J Cardiol*. 2000;86:59–63.

62. Andersen HR, Thuesen L, Bagger JP, Vesterlund T, Thomsen PE. Prospective randomised trial of atrial versus ventricular pacing in sick-sinus syndrome. *Lancet*. 1994;344:1523–1528.

63. Mattioli AV, Vivoli D, Mattioli G. Influence of pacing modalities on the incidence of atrial fibrillation in patients without prior atrial fibrillation. A prospective study. *Eur Heart J*. 1998;19:282–286.

64. Mattioli AV, Castellani ET, Vivoli D, Sgura FA, Mattioli G. Prevalence of atrial fibrillation and stroke in paced patients without prior atrial fibrillation: a prospective study. *Clin Cardiol*. 1998;21:117–122.

65. Hesselson AB, Parsonnet V, Bernstein AD, Bonavita GJ. Deleterious effects of long-term single-chamber ventricular pacing in patients with sick sinus syndrome: the hidden benefits of dual-chamber pacing. *J Am Coll Cardiol*. 1992;19:1542–1549.

66. Santini M, Alexidou G, Ansalone G, Cacciatore G, Cini R, Turitto G. Relation of prognosis in sick sinus syndrome to age, conduction defects and modes of permanent cardiac pacing. *Am J Cardiol*. 1990;65:729–735.

67. Stangl K, Seitz K, Wirtzfeld A, Alt E, Blomer H. Differences between atrial single chamber pacing (AAI) and ventricular single chamber pacing (VVI) with respect to prognosis and antiarrhythmic effect in patients with sick sinus syndrome. *Pacing Clin Electrophysiol*. 1990;13:2080–2085.

68. Stambler BS, Ellenbogen KA, Orav EJ, Sgarbossa EB, Estes NA, Rizo-Patron C, Kirchhoffer JB, Hadjis TA, Goldman L, Lamas GA. Predictors and clinical impact of atrial fibrillation after pacemaker implantation in elderly patients treated with dual chamber versus ventricular pacing. *Pacing Clin Electrophysiol*. 2003;26:2000–2007.

69. Nielsen JC, Kristensen L, Andersen HR, Mortensen PT, Pedersen OL, Pedersen AK. A randomized comparison of atrial and dual-chamber pacing in 177 consecutive patients with sick sinus syndrome: echocardiographic and clinical outcome. *J Am Coll Cardiol*. 2003;42:614–623.

70. Kristensen L, Nielsen JC, Mortensen PT, Pedersen OL, Pedersen AK, Andersen HR. Incidence of atrial fibrillation and thromboembolism in a randomised trial of atrial versus dual chamber pacing in 177 patients with sick sinus syndrome. *Heart*. 2004;90:661–666.

71. Ishikawa T, Kimura K, Yoshimura H, Kobayashi K, Usui T, Kashiwagi M, Ishii M. Acute changes in left atrial and left ventricular diameters after physiological pacing. *Pacing Clin Electrophysiol*. 1996;19:143–149.

72. Leclercq C, Gras D, Le Helloco A, Nicol L, Mabo P, Daubert C. Hemodynamic importance of preserving the normal sequence of ventricular activation in permanent cardiac pacing. *Am Heart J*. 1995;129:1133–1141.

73. Klein LS, Miles WM, Zipes DP. Effect of atrioventricular interval during pacing or reciprocating tachycardia on atrial size, pressure, and refractory period. Contraction-excitation feedback in human atrium. *Circulation*. 1990;82:60–68.

74. Calkins H, el Atassi R, Leon A, Kalbfleisch S, Borganelli M, Langberg J, Morady F. Effect of the atrioventricular relationship on atrial refractoriness in humans. *Pacing Clin Electrophysiol*. 1992;15:771–778.

75. Paxinos G, Katritsis D, Kakouros S, Toutouzas P, Camm AJ. Long-term effect of VVI pacing on atrial and ventricular function in patients with sick sinus syndrome. *Pacing Clin Electrophysiol*. 1998;21:728–734.

76. Nielsen JC, Andersen HR, Thomsen PE, Thuesen L, Mortensen PT, Vesterlund T, Pedersen AK. Heart failure and echocardiographic changes during long-term follow-up of patients with sick sinus syndrome randomized to single-chamber atrial or ventricular pacing. *Circulation*. 1998;97:987–995.

77. Sparks PB, Mond HG, Vohra JK, Yapanis AG, Grigg LE, Kalman JM. Mechanical remodeling of the left atrium after loss of atrioventricular synchrony. A long-term study in humans. *Circulation*. 1999;100:1714–1721.

78. Sparks PB, Mond HG, Vohra JK, Jayaprakash S, Kalman JM. Electrical remodeling of the atria following loss of atrioventricular synchrony: a long-term study in humans. *Circulation*. 1999;100:1894–1900.

79. Gillis AM, Unterberg-Buchwald C, Schmidinger H, Massimo S, Wolfe K, Kavaney DJ, Otterness MF, Hohnloser SH. Safety and efficacy of advanced atrial pacing therapies for atrial tachyarrhythmias in patients with a new implantable dual chamber cardioverter-defibrillator. *J Am Coll Cardiol*. 2002;40:1653–1659.

80. Carlson MD, Ip J, Messenger J, Beau S, Kalbfleisch S, Gervais P, Cameron DA, Duran A, Val-Mejias J, Mackall J, Gold M. A new pacemaker algorithm for the treatment of atrial fibrillation: results of the Atrial Dynamic Overdrive Pacing Trial (ADOPT). *J Am Coll Cardiol*. 2003;42:627–633.

81. Lee MA, Weachter R, Pollak S, Kremers MS, Naik AM, Silverman R, Tuzi J, Wang W, Johnson LJ, Euler DE. The effect of atrial pacing therapies on

atrial tachyarrhythmia burden and frequency: results of a randomized trial in patients with bradycardia and atrial tachyarrhythmias. *J Am Coll Cardiol.* 2003;41:1926–1932.

82. Blanc JJ, De Roy L, Mansourati J, Poezevara Y, Marcon JL, Schoels W, Hidden-Lucet F, Barnay C. Atrial pacing for prevention of atrial fibrillation: assessment of simultaneously implemented algorithms. *Europace.* 2004;6:371–379.

83. Padeletti L, Purerfellner H, Adler SW, Waller TJ, Harvey M, Horvitz L, Holbrook R, Kempen K, Mugglin A, Hettrick DA. Combined efficacy of atrial septal lead placement and atrial pacing algorithms for prevention of paroxysmal atrial tachyarrhythmia. *J Cardiovasc Electrophysiol.* 2003;14:1189–1195.

84. Israel CW, Barold SS. Can implantable devices detect and pace-terminate atrial fibrillation? *Pacing Clin Electrophysiol.* 2003;26:1923–1925.

85. Gillis AM. Clinical trials of pacing for maintenance of sinus rhythm. *J Interv Card Electrophysiol.* 2004;10(Suppl 1):55–62.

86. Prakash A, Delfaut P, Krol RB, Saksena S. Regional right and left atrial activation patterns during single- and dual-site atrial pacing in patients with atrial fibrillation. *Am J Cardiol.* 1998;82:1197–1204.

87. Prakash A, Saksena S, Hill M, Krol RB, Munsif AN, Giorgberidze I, Mathew P, Mehra R. Acute effects of dual-site right atrial pacing in patients with spontaneous and inducible atrial flutter and fibrillation. *J Am Coll Cardiol.* 1997;29:1007–1014.

88. Prakash A, Saksena S, Ziegler PD, Lokhandwala T, Hettrick DA, Delfaut P, Nanda NC, Wyse DG. Dual site right atrial pacing can improve the impact of standard dual chamber pacing on atrial and ventricular mechanical function in patients with symptomatic atrial fibrillation: further observations from the dual site atrial pacing for prevention of atrial fibrillation trial. *J Interv Card Electrophysiol.* 2005;12:177–187.

89. Saksena S, Prakash A, Hill M, Krol RB, Munsif AN, Mathew PP, Mehra R. Prevention of recurrent atrial fibrillation with chronic dual-site right atrial pacing. *J Am Coll Cardiol.* 1996;28:687–694.

90. Daubert C, Gras D, Berder V, Leclercq C, Mabo P. Permanent atrial resynchronization by synchronous bi-atrial pacing in the preventive treatment of atrial flutter associated with high degree interatrial block. *Arch Mal Coeur Vaiss.* 1994;87:1535–1546.

91. Saksena S, Prakash A, Ziegler P, Hummel JD, Friedman P, Plumb VJ, Wyse DG, Johnson E, Fitts S, Mehra R. Improved suppression of recurrent atrial fibrillation with dual-site right atrial pacing and antiarrhythmic drug therapy. *J Am Coll Cardiol.* 2002;40:1140–1150.

92. Prinzen FW, Peschar M. Relation between the pacing induced sequence of activation and left ventricular pump function in animals. *Pacing Clin Electrophysiol.* 2002;25:484–498.

93. Nahlawi M, Waligora M, Spies SM, Bonow RO, Kadish AH, Goldberger JJ. Left ventricular function during and after right ventricular pacing. *J Am Coll Cardiol.* 2004;44:1883–1888.

94. van Oosterhout MF, Prinzen FW, Arts T, Schreuder JJ, Vanagt WY, Cleutjens JP, Reneman RS. Asynchronous electrical activation induces asymmetrical hypertrophy of the left ventricular wall. *Circulation.* 1998;98:588–595.

95. Prinzen FW, Cheriex EC, Delhaas T, van Oosterhout MF, Arts T, Wellens HJ, Reneman RS. Asymmetric thickness of the left ventricular wall resulting from asynchronous electric activation: a study in dogs with ventricular pacing and in patients with left bundle branch block. *Am Heart J.* 1995;130:1045–1053.

96. Thambo JB, Bordachar P, Garrigue S, Lafitte S, Sanders P, Reuter S, Girardot R, Crepin D, Reant P, Roudaut R, Jais P, Haissaguerre M, Clementy J, Jimenez M. Detrimental ventricular remodeling in patients with congenital complete heart block and chronic right ventricular apical pacing. *Circulation.* 2004;110:3766–3772.

97. Adomian GE, Beazell J. Myofibrillar disarray produced in normal hearts by chronic electrical pacing. *Am Heart J.* 1986;112:79–83.

98. Lee MA, Dae MW, Langberg JJ, Griffin JC, Chin MC, Finkbeiner WE, O'Connell JW, Botvinick E, Scheinman MM, Rosenqvist M. Effects of long-term right ventricular apical pacing on left ventricular perfusion, innervation, function and histology. *J Am Coll Cardiol.* 1994;24:225–232.

99. Tse HF, Lau CP. Long-term effect of right ventricular pacing on myocardial perfusion and function. *J Am Coll Cardiol.* 1997;29:744–749.

100. Wilkoff BL, Cook JR, Epstein AE, Greene HL, Hallstrom AP, Hsia H, Kutalek SP, Sharma A. Dual-chamber pacing or ventricular backup pacing in patients with an implantable defibrillator: the Dual Chamber and VVI Implantable Defibrillator (DAVID) Trial. *JAMA.* 2002;288:3115–3123.

101. Sharma AD, Rizo-Patron C, Hallstrom AP, O'Neill GP, Rothbart S, Martins JB, Roelke M, Steinberg JS, Greene HL. Percent right ventricular pacing predicts outcomes in the DAVID trial. *Heart Rhythm.* 2005;2:830–834.

102. Steinberg JS, Fischer A, Wang P, Schuger C, Daubert J, McNitt S, Andrews M, Brown M, Hall WJ, Zareba W, Moss AJ. The clinical implications of cumulative right ventricular pacing in the multicenter automatic defibrillator trial II. *J Cardiovasc Electrophysiol.* 2005;16:359–365.

103. Shukla HH, Hellkamp AS, James EA, Flaker GC, Lee KL, Sweeney MO, Lamas GA. Heart failure hospitalization is more common in pacemaker patients with sinus node dysfunction and a prolonged paced QRS duration. *Heart Rhythm.* 2005;2:245–251.

104. Sweeney MO, Hellkamp AS. Heart failure during cardiac pacing. *Circulation.* 2006;113:2082–2088.

105. McGavigan AD, Roberts-Thomson KC, Hillock RJ, Stevenson IH, Mond HG. Right ventricular outflow tract pacing: radiographic and electrocardiographic correlates of lead position. *Pacing Clin Electrophysiol.* 2006;29:1063–1068.

106. McGavigan AD, Mond HG. Selective site ventricular pacing. *Curr Opin Cardiol.* 2006;21:7–14.

107. Sweeney MO, Shea JB, Fox V, Adler S, Nelson L, Mullen TJ, Belk P, Casavant D, Sheldon T. Randomized pilot study of a new atrial-based minimal ventricular pacing mode in dual-chamber implantable cardioverter-defibrillators. *Heart Rhythm.* 2004;1:160–167.

108. Frohlig G, Gras D, Victor J, Mabo P, Galley D, Savoure A, Jauvert G, Defaye P, Ducloux P, Amblard A. Use of a new cardiac pacing mode designed to eliminate unnecessary ventricular pacing. *Europace.* 2006;8:96–101.

109. Gillis AM, Purerfellner H, Israel CW, Sunthorn H, Kacet S, Anelli-Monti M, Tang F, Young M, Boriani G. Reducing unnecessary right ventricular pacing with the managed ventricular pacing mode in patients with sinus node disease and AV block. *Pacing Clin Electrophysiol.* 2006;29:697–705.

110. Sweeney MO, Ellenbogen KA, Miller EH, Sherfesee L, Sheldon T, Whellan D. The Managed Ventricular Pacingtrade mark Versus VVI 40 Pacing (MVP) Trial: clinical background, rationale, design, and implementation. *J Cardiovasc Electrophysiol.* 2006.

111. Haywood GA, Ward J, Ward DE, Camm AJ. Atrioventricular Wenckebach point and progression to atrioventricular block in sinoatrial disease. *Pacing Clin Electrophysiol.* 1990;13:2054–2058.

112. Bergfeldt L, Edvardsson N, Rosenqvist M, Vallin H, Edhag O. Atrioventricular block progression in patients with bifascicular block assessed by repeated electrocardiography and a bradycardia-detecting pacemaker. *Am J Cardiol.* 1994;74:1129–1132.

113. Vallin H, Edhag O. Associated conduction disturbances in patients with symptomatic sinus node disease. *Acta Med Scand.* 1981;210:263–270.

114. Rosenqvist M, Obel IW. Atrial pacing and the risk for AV block: is there a time for change in attitude? *Pacing Clin Electrophysiol*. 1989;12:97–101.

115. Andersen HR, Nielsen JC, Thomsen PE, Thuesen L, Vesterlund T, Pedersen AK, Mortensen PT. Atrioventricular conduction during long-term follow-up of patients with sick sinus syndrome. *Circulation*. 1998;98:1315–1321.

116. Brandt J, Anderson H, Fahraeus T, Schuller H. Natural history of sinus node disease treated with atrial pacing in 213 patients: implications for selection of stimulation mode. *J Am Coll Cardiol*. 1992;20:633–639.

117. Breivik K, Ohm OJ, Segadal L. Sick sinus syndrome treated with permanent pacemaker in 109 patients. A follow-up study. *Acta Med Scand*. 1979;206:153–159.

118. Benditt DG, Milstein S, Buetikofer J, Gornick CC, Mianulli M, Fetter J. Sensor-triggered, rate-variable cardiac pacing. Current technologies and clinical implications. *Ann Intern Med*. 1987;107:714–724.

119. Bjerregaard P. Mean 24 hour heart rate, minimal heart rate and pauses in healthy subjects 40–79 years of age. *Eur Heart J*. 1983;4:44–51.

120. Rosenqvist M, Aren C, Kristensson BE, Nordlander R, Schuller H. Atrial rate-responsive pacing in sinus node disease. *Eur Heart J*. 1990;11:537–542.

121. Hedman A, Nordlander R. QT sensing rate responsive pacing compared to fixed rate ventricular inhibited pacing: a controlled clinical study. *Pacing Clin Electrophysiol*. 1989;12:374–385.

122. Sulke N, Chambers J, Dritsas A, Sowton E. A randomized double-blind crossover comparison of four rate-responsive pacing modes. *J Am Coll Cardiol*. 1991;17:696–706.

123. NASPE 24th Annual Scientific Sessions. Late-Breaking Clinical Trials, Advanced Elements of Pacing Trial (ADEPT) May 17 2003, Washington DC. 2007.

124. den Dulk K, Dijkman B, Pieterse M, Wellens H. Initial experience with mode switching in a dual sensor, dual chamber pacemaker in patients with paroxysmal atrial tachyarrhythmias. *Pacing Clin Electrophysiol*. 1994;17:1900–1907.

125. Kamalvand K, Tan K, Kotsakis A, Bucknall C, Sulke N. Is mode switching beneficial? A randomized study in patients with paroxysmal atrial tachyarrhythmias. *J Am Coll Cardiol*. 1997;30:496–504.

126. Lau CP, Tai YT, Fong PC, Li JP, Chung FL. Atrial arrhythmia management with sensor controlled atrial refractory period and automatic mode switching in patients with minute ventilation sensing dual chamber rate adaptive pacemakers. *Pacing Clin Electrophysiol*. 1992;15:1504–1514.

127. Sweeney MO, Hellkamp AS, Ellenbogen KA, Glotzer TV, Silverman R, Yee R, Lee KL, Lamas GA. Prospective randomized study of mode switching in a clinical trial of pacemaker therapy for sinus node dysfunction. *J Cardiovasc Electrophysiol*. 2004;15:153–160.

Acquired Atrioventricular Block

S. Serge Barold and Bengt Herweg

There are many causes of atrioventricular (AV) block but progressive idiopathic fibrosis of the conduction system related to an aging process of the cardiac skeleton is the most common cause of chronic acquired AV block. Barring congenital AV block, Lyme disease is the most common cause of reversible third-degree AV block in young individuals and it is usually AV nodal. Before implantation of a permanent pacemaker, reversible causes of AV block such as Lyme disease, hypervagotonia, athletic heart, sleep apnea, ischemia, and drug, metabolic, or electrolytic imbalance must be excluded. Table 10.1 outlines the format used in the 2002 American College of Cardiology/American Heart Association/North American Society of Pacing and Electrophysiology (ACC/AHA/NASPE) guidelines for pacemaker implantation (1). The indications for permanent pacing in second- or third- degree AV block unlikely to regress are often straightforward in *symptomatic* patients but they are more difficult in *asymptomatic* patients.

Anatomic and Electrophysiologic Considerations

The specialized conduction system below the AV node consists of the bundle of His proximally and the three intraventricular fascicles distally – the right bundle branch, the anterior (superior) division of the left bundle branch, and the posterior (inferior) division of the left bundle branch (Fig.10.1). Although the left bundle branch does not exist as two discrete anatomic divisions, the functional separation into two fascicles is a useful concept clinically and electrocardiographically. Left anterior hemiblock (LAH) causes left axis deviation (−45° or more superior) or an axis in the right superior quadrant, and left posterior hemiblock (LPH) causes right inferior axis deviation in the frontal plane. Disease in any one of the three fascicles is of little clinical significance. When the ECG shows evidence of block in two fascicles (bifascicular block), only one pathway remains for AV conduction but AV block does not occur. Bifascicular block can be identified on the ECG when there is right bundle branch block (RBBB) with LAH, RBBB with LPH or left bundle branch block (LBBB) regardless of the axis in the

Table 10.1 Standard ACC/AHA/NASPE format for device indications.

Class I:	Conditions for which there is evidence and/or general agreement that a given procedure or treatment is beneficial, useful, and effective.
Class II:	Conditions for which there is conflicting evidence and/or a divergence of opinion about the usefulness/efficacy of a procedure or treatment.
Class IIa:	Weight of evidence/opinion is in favor of usefulness/effcacy.
Class IIb	Usefulness/efficacy is less well established by evidence/opinion.
Class III	Conditions for which there is evidence and/or general agreement that a procedure/treatment is not useful/effective, and in some cases may be harmful.

Reproduced with permission from (1).

Table 10.2 Pitfalls in diagnosis and treatment of AV block.

- Type I AV block can be physiological in athletes resulting from heavy physical training
- Type I AV block can be physiological during sleep in individuals with high vagal tone
- Failure to suspect vagally induced AV block, i.e. vomiting
- Failure to recognize reversible causes of AV block

  1. Lyme disease
  2. Electrolyte abnormalities
  3. Inferior myocardial infarction
  4. Sleep apnea

    - Poor correlation between narrow QRS type I block and symptoms.
    - Beliefs that all type I blocks with a wide QRS complex are AV nodal
    - Nonconducted atrial premature beats masquerading as AV Block
    - What appears to be narrow QRS type II block may be a type I variant.
    - Atypical type I sequence mistaken for type II block.
    - Making the diagnosis of type II block without seeing a truly conducted post block P-wave (shortage of PR intervals)
    - A recording that appears to show both types I and II and a narrow QRS complex may in fact represent only type I block.
    - Concealed extrasystoles causing pseudo-AV block. (Look for associated unexpected sudden PR prolongation, combination of what appears to be type I and type II and isolated retrograde P-waves from retrograde conduction of the concealed extrasystole)
    - Relying solely on a computer-rendered ECG diagnosis: Computer interpretations are notoriously error-prone

frontal plane. In LBBB, the frontal plane axis carries little value for the diagnosis of hemiblock. Right axis deviation with LBBB is rare and usually indicates the presence of a severe end-stage dilated cardiomyopathy while patients with LBBB and left axis deviation generally have more advanced myocardial disease than those with LBBB and a normal axis. In bifascicular block without documented second- or third-degree AV block, the functional status of the third fascicle cannot be evaluated from the ECG. During 1:1 AV conduction the diagnosis of trifascicular block can only be made in rare situations involving alternating RBBB and LBBB or RBBB with alternating LAH and LPH (2).

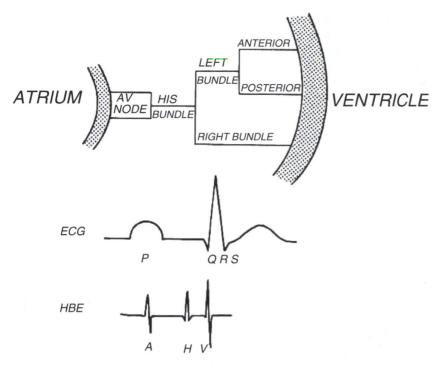

Fig. 10.1 Diagrammatic representation of the atrioventricular conduction system. The bundle branch system consists of a three-pronged system (two on the left side and one on the right side). At the bottom, the surface ECG is depicted simultaneously with a His bundle electrogram (HBE). The HBE is recorded near the septal leaflet of the tricuspid valve. A – reflects depolarization of the low atrium, H – depolarization of the His bundle, and V – depolarization of the upper ventricular septum. The AH interval reflects AV nodal conduction and the HV interval reflects conduction within the His-Purkinje system. The normal HV interval is 35–55 ms. A prolonged HV interval indicates delayed conduction in all three prongs of the conduction system and/or the His bundle. With His-Purkinje disease the HV interval (but not the surface QRS complex) remains normal as long as one of the three prongs conducts normally. (Barold SS. Pacemaker treatment of bradycardias, and selection of optimal pacing modes. In: Zipes DP (Ed.). *Contemporary Treatments in Cardiovascular Disease*, 1997;1:123, with permission.)

Intracardiac Recordings

The His bundle potential is easily recorded with an electrode catheter passed from the femoral vein to the level of the tricuspid valve. The "A" wave reflects depolarization of the low right atrium, the "V" deflection is produced by ventricular depolarization near the recording catheter and the "H" deflection is generated by rapid transmission of depolarization through the bundle of His and appears between the A- and V-waves (Fig. 10.1). The AH interval (normal is 60–140 ms) basically reflects AV nodal conduction (rarely intraatrial delay) and the HV interval (normal is 35–55 ms) reflects the conduction time from the His bundle to the beginning of ventricular activation – that is the His-Purkinje system. Bifascicular block is associated with a normal HV interval if conduction in the third fascicle remains intact. Consequently a prolonged HV interval strongly suggests delayed conduction in all three fascicles. However, HV delay may occasionally be within the His bundle itself or due to a combination of delay in the His bundle and the three fascicles. Prolongation of the PR interval in the ECG is an unreliable indicator of bifascicular or trifascicular disease because it may be due to prolongation of the AH and/or HV intervals. Consequently RBBB + LAH + first degree AV block should not be designated as trifascicular block unless invasive recordings demonstrate prolongation of the HV interval. Electrocardiographic documentation of true trifascicular block during 1:1 AV conduction is rare and involves either alternating or bilateral bundle branch block or fixed RBBB with alternating LAH and LPH. Finally asymptomatic patients with bundle branch block or bifascicular block do not require determination of the HV interval because the risk of developing complete AV block is very low at about 1–2% per year.

Complete AV Block

The 2002 ACC/AHA/NASPE guidelines designate *asymptomatic* complete AV block with ventricular escape rates > 40 bpm as a class II indication for pacing (1). The rate criterion of > 40 bpm is arbitrary and unnecessary. It is not the escape rate that is critical to stability, but rather the site of origin of the escape rhythm (junctional or ventricular). Rate instability may not be predictable or obvious. Irreversible acquired complete AV block should be a class I indication for pacing. In neuromuscular disease such as myotonic dystrophy, pacing should be considered much earlier in the course of the disease and offered to the asymptomatic patient once any conduction abnormality is noted and subsequent follow-up shows progression even when second-degree AV block has not yet developed. Waiting for the development of complete AV block may expose patients to a significant risk of syncope or even sudden death.

Second-Degree AV Block

Type I block and type II second-degree AV block are electrocardiographic patterns and as such should not be automatically equated with the anatomical site of block.

Type I Block (Wenckebach or Mobitz Type I)

Type I second-degree AV block is defined as the occurrence of a *single* nonconducted sinus P-wave associated with inconstant PR intervals before and after the blocked impulse provided there are at least two consecutive conducted P-waves (i.e., 3:2 AV block) to determine the behavior of the PR interval (3). The PR interval after the blocked impulse is always shorter if the P-wave is conducted to the ventricle (Fig. 10.2). The term "inconstant" PR or AV intervals is important because the majority of type I sequences are atypical and do not conform to the traditional teaching about the mathematical behavior of the PR intervals (4–6). The description of "progressive" prolongation of the PR interval is misleading because PR intervals may shorten or stabilize and show no discernible or measurable change anywhere in a type I sequence (Fig. 10.2). Indeed, atypical type I structures in their terminal portion can exhibit a number of consecutive PR intervals showing no discernible change before the single blocked beat (4). In such an arrangement the post-block PR interval is always shorter (Figs. 10.3A and 10.4A). A decrease or an increase of the sinus rate does not interfere with the diagnosis of type I block.

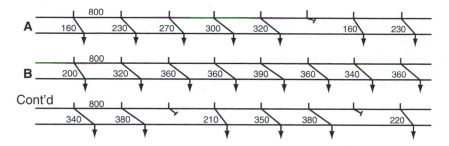

Fig. 10.2 Diagrammatic representation of AV block. The three levels represent activation of the atria, AV junction (PR intervals are shown between the lines), and ventricles, respectively. All values are in ms. (A) Classic type I AV block. (B) Relatively long and atypical type I sequence. Note the irregular fluctuations of the PR intervals before the dropped beat. Reproduced with permission from (11).

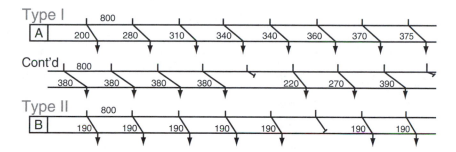

Fig. 10.3 Diagrammatic representation of various forms of second-degree AV block with the same format as in Fig. 10.2. (A) Relatively long and atypical type I sequence with several constant PR intervals before a dropped beat. Note the *shorter* PR interval after the blocked P-wave. This pattern should not be called type II AV block. It is essential to examine all the PR intervals in long rhythm strips and not merely several PR intervals preceding a blocked impulse. (B) True type II AV block. Every atrial impulse successfully traverses the AV node which is not afforded a long recovery time as occurring in type I AV block. Note that the PR interval *after* the blocked beat is unchanged. Reproduced with permission from (11).

Increments in AV Conduction

Increments in AV conduction (AV nodal – AH interval) in Type I AV nodal block are typically large. Type I infranodal block typically exhibits small increments in AV conduction (confined to the HV interval) and large increments in AV conduction (confined to the HV interval) occur uncommonly. The increments in AV nodal block may occasionally be so tiny that they superficially mimic type II second-degree AV block.

Site of Block: In *narrow QRS type I block*, the block is in the AV node in almost all the cases. Type I block can be physiological especially during sleep in normal individuals with high vagal tone and these people need no treatment. Asymptomatic type I second-degree AV block present throughout the day is generally considered benign. However, some workers in Britain recommend permanent pacing in this setting for prognostic reasons based on long-term mortality data from a single center (7–9). We believe that these observations need to be confirmed before recommending pacing for this situation.

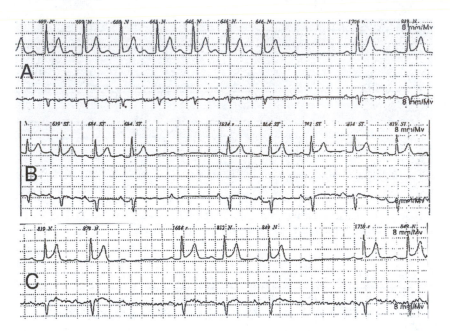

Fig. 10.4 Representative Holter recordings from an asymptomatic patient with a type I block variant that was misdiagnosed as type II block by several physicians. (A) Type I block with constant PR intervals before the blocked beat. Note that there is a slight increase in the sinus rate in the sequence before the blocked beat. However, the sinus rate then slows down and the blocked P-wave occurs in association with sinus slowing a combination consistent with a vagal phenomenon. The PR intervals after the blocked beat are inconstant. (B) Type I variant simulating type II block. The PR intervals are constant before and after the blocked beat. However, there is obvious sinus slowing simultaneously with the nonconducted P-wave. (C) Type I block. Note that in the presence of a narrow QRS complex, the occurrence of type I (with fairly large increments of the PR intervals) and what appears to be type II block basically rules out the presence of a true type II block.

IntraHisian narrow QRS type I block is rare. In practice, cases of narrow QRS intraHisian type I block due to chronic conduction system disease are not usually found because virtually all narrow QRS type I blocks are dismissed as being AV nodal. IntraHisian block although rare clinically, may be provoked by exercise in contrast to type I AV nodal block which generally improves with exercise. Improvement of AV block with exercise is highly suggestive of AV nodal second-degree AV block. His bundle recordings are unnecessary in an asymptomatic patient with narrow QRS type I block. However, if an electrophysiological study (performed for other reasons) in such a patient reveals infranodal block, a pacemaker should be recommended as a class I indication because diffuse His-Purkinje disease is likely to be present.

Type I second-degree AV block with bundle branch block (which is far less common than narrow QRS type I block) must not be automatically labeled as AV nodal. Outside of acute myocardial infarction, type I block and bundle branch block (QRS ≥ 0.12 s) occur in the His-Purkinje system in 60–70% of the cases (10) (Fig. 10.5). In such cases exercise is likely to aggravate the degree of AV block. Yet, many still believe that type I blocks are all AV nodal and therefore basically benign. It is believed that the prognosis of infranodal type I block is as serious as that of type II block and a permanent pacemaker

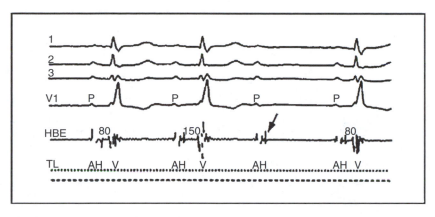

Fig. 10.5 Sinus rhythm with second-degree Type I 3:2 infranodal AV block, and RBBB. Note that the AH interval remains constant. The HV interval increases from 80 (following first P-wave) to 150 ms (following second P-wave). The third P-wave is followed by an H deflection but no QRS complex. AV block occurs in the His-Purkinje system below the site of recording of the His bundle potential (arrow). Note the shorter PR interval after the nonconducted P-wave, a feature typical of Type I second-degree AV block. HBE = His bundle electrogram, A = atrial deflection, H = His bundle deflection, V = ventricular deflection, P = P-wave. TL = time lines 50 ms. (Barold SS. Pacemaker treatment of bradycardias and selection of optimal pacing modes. In: Zipes DP (Ed.). *Contemporary Treatments in Cardiovascular Disease*, 1997;1:123, with permission.)

is generally recommended in both types regardless of symptoms. On this basis, patients with type I block and bundle branch block should undergo an invasive study to determine the level of second-degree block in the conduction system.

However, it is unknown whether underlying RBBB (unifascicular block) is prognostically different from underlying LBBB (bifascicular block) in the setting of asymptomatic type I second-degree infranodal block.

Type II Block (Mobitz Type II)

The definition of type II second-degree AV block continues to be problematic in clinical practice (3,11,12). Type II second-degree AV block is defined as the occurrence of a *single* non-conducted sinus P-wave associated with constant PR intervals before and *after* the blocked impulse, provided the sinus rate or the PP interval is constant and there are at least two consecutive conducted P-waves (i.e., 3:2 AV block) to determine the behavior of the PR interval (13,14). The pause encompassing the blocked P-wave should equal two (PP) cycles (Figs. 10.3B and 10.6). The PR interval is either normal or prolonged but remains constant. Type II block cannot be diagnosed whenever a single blocked impulse is followed by a shortened postblock PR interval or no P-wave at all. In this situation it is either a type I pattern or an unclassifiable sequence. Stability of the sinus rate is a very important criterion because a vagal surge can cause simultaneous sinus slowing and AV nodal block, generally a benign condition that can superficially resemble Type II second-degree AV block (3). In the presence of sinus arrhythmia, the diagnosis of type II block may not be possible if there is sinus slowing especially if the block occurs in one of the longer cycles. In contrast the diagnosis of type II block is possible with an increasing sinus rate.

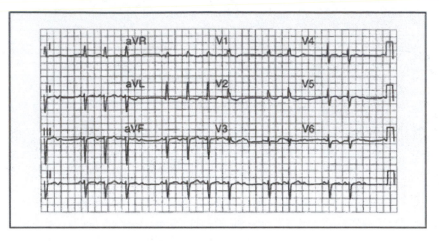

Fig. 10.6 Sinus rhythm with second-degree Type II AV block in the presence of right bundle branch block and LAH. There are tiny q-waves in V_2 and V_3 probably related to LAH rather than old anterior myocardial infarction. Note that the sinus rate is constant and the PR interval after the blocked beat remains unchanged. (Barold SS. Pacemaker treatment of bradycardias and selection of optimal pacing modes. In: Zipes DP (Ed.). *Contemporary Treatments in Cardiovascular Disease*, 1997;1:123, with permission.)

The 2002 ACC/AHA/NASPE guidelines introduced a new classification of type II second-degree AV block: wide QRS type II block (which makes up 65–80% of type II blocks) with a class I indication for pacing and narrow QRS type II block with a class II indication for permanent pacing (1). This differentiation is strange because there is no evidence that narrow QRS type II block is less serious than wide QRS type II block. The statement that "type II block is usually infranodal especially when the QRS is wide" may be the basis for this potentially misleading distinction. Type II block according to the strict definition is always infranodal and should be a class I indication regardless of QRS duration, symptoms or whether it is paroxysmal or chronic.

The literature on the diagnosis of type II block is replete with errors because the diagnostic importance of the rate criterion and need for an unchanged PR interval *after* a single blocked impulse are often ignored (3) (Fig. 10.7). A constant PR after the blocked beat is a sine qua non of Type II block. The diagnosis of Type II cannot be made if the P-wave after a blocked impulse is not conducted with the same PR interval as all the other conducted P-waves. The shorter PR interval after a single blocked P-wave may either be due to improved conduction (Type I block) or AV dissociation due to an escape AV junctional beat that bears no relationship to the preceding P-wave. In other words, Type II second-degree AV block cannot be diagnosed whenever a shortened AV interval occurs after the blocked P-wave. In such a situation the pattern is either Type I or unclassifiable. Type II block is sometimes described as having all the conducted PR intervals constant. There is an important loophole in this statement. It could be interpreted that the behavior of the first P-wave after the blocked impulse can be disregarded in the diagnosis (Figs. 10.3A and 10.8). If the P-wave is absent there is no opportunity to determine the behavior of the first PR interval after the blocked impulse and the diagnosis of type II block cannot be established.

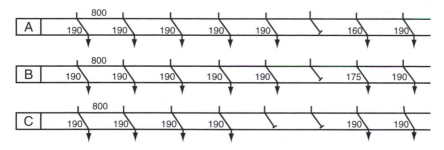

Fig. 10.7 Diagrammatic representation of various forms of second-degree AV block with the same format as in Fig. 10.2. (A) Dropped beat followed by a 30 ms shortening of the PR interval. This pattern should not be called type II AV block. It may be a type I AV block or unclassifiable if shortening of the PR interval is due to an AV junctional escape beat. (B) Type II AV block according to some of the old definitions. This is now labeled as type I with very small increments in conduction. Some workers still call this arrangement type II AV block. The diagnosis of type II block cannot be made if the PR interval *after* the blocked beat is not equal to all the other PR intervals. (C) Advanced second-degree AV block (failure of conduction of two consecutive P-waves without warning). All the PR intervals are constant including the first one after the block. This suggests infranodal AV block. Some workers cling to the original Mobitz definition and call this sequence type II block. Reproduced with permission from (11).

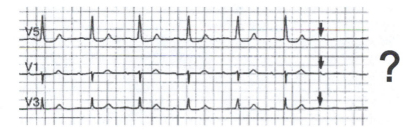

Fig. 10.8 Narrow QRS type I block registered in a 3-lead Holter recording. There is sinus arrhythmia. The last three PR intervals before the blocked beat (arrow) are constant. This pattern should not be classified as type II block when conduction of the postblock P-wave is not seen. Actually the P-wave after the block was conducted with a shorter PR interval consistent with type I block.

Site of Block

Type II according to the strict definition occurs in the His-Purkinje system and rarely above the site of recording of the His bundle potential in the proximal His bundle or nodo-Hisian junction. Type II block has not yet been convincingly demonstrated in the N zone of the AV node (3). Most if not all the purported exceptions involve reports where type I blocks (shorter PR interval after the blocked beat) are claimed to be type II blocks by using loopholes in the definitions of second-degree AV block. Because type II invariably occurs in the His-Purkinje system, it should be a class I indication for pacing.

Type II Second-Degree AV Block: True or False?

When confronted with a pattern that appears to be type II with a narrow QRS complex (especially in Holter recordings), one must consider the possibility of type I block without discernible or measurable increments in the PR intervals. Sinus slowing with AV block rules out type II block. Vagal AV block (discussed later) rarely involves more than block of two consecutive P-waves. Difficulty arises when the sinus rate is stable. When a type II-like pattern with a narrow QRS complex occurs in association with type I sequences, true type II block can be safely excluded because the coexistence of both types of block in the His bundle is almost unknown (Fig. 10.4). True narrow QRS type II block occurs without sinus slowing and is typically associated with sustained advanced second-degree AV block far more commonly than type I block. In other words, AV conduction ratios > 2:1 (3:1, 4:1) AV block are rare in vagal block (12).

Fixed-Ratio AV Block

2:1 AV block. 2:1 AV block can be AV nodal or in the His-Purkinje system. It cannot be classified as type I or type II block because there is only one PR interval to examine before the blocked P-wave (Fig. 10.9). 2:1 AV block is best labeled simply as 2:1 block (3,15). For the purpose of classification according to the World Health Organization and the ACC, it is considered as "advanced block" as are 3:1, 4:1 etc. AV block. Confusion arises when the term "advanced AV block" (defined in the ACC/AHA guidelines as a form of second-degree AV block of two or more P-waves) is used to describe both second- and third-degree AV blocks (1).

The site of the lesion in 2:1 AV block can often be determined by seeking the company 2:1 AV block keeps. An association with either type I or type II second-degree AV block helps localization of the lesion according to the correlations already discussed. Outside of acute myocardial infarction, sustained 2:1 and 3:1 AV block with a wide QRS complex occurs in the His-Purkinje system in 80% of cases and 20% in the AV node (3). It is inappropriate to label 2:1 or 3:1 AV nodal block as type I block and infranodal 2:1 or 3:1 AV block as type II block because the diagnosis of type I and type II blocks is based on electrocardiographic patterns and not on the anatomical site of block.

When stable sinus rhythm and 1:1 AV conduction are followed by sudden AV block of several impulses (> 1), and all the PR intervals before and after the block remain constant, such an arrangement strongly suggest infranodal block and the need for a pacemaker. This arrangement is sometimes called Type II block although it does not conform to the accepted contemporary definition of type II block. The purist will insist on calling this pattern (3:1, 4:1 AV block) type II AV block by citing the original description by Mobitz

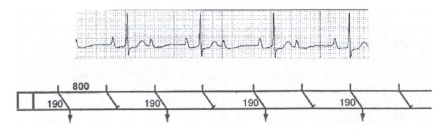

Fig. 10.9 Fixed 2:1 AV block. This cannot be classified as type I or type II block. Reproduced with permission from (11).

	75									
75	75	75	150	75	150	75	225		75	
	75	75	150	75	150	75	225		75	

Fig. 10.10 Diagrammatic representation of second-degree type II AV block from Mobitz's original article (16).

despite the accepted contemporary definitions that such patterns should not be labeled type II AV block (16) (Fig. 10.10). When the first PR interval after the blocked P-waves (in 3:1, 4:1 AV block) is not equal to previous PR intervals the block can be either in the AV node or the His-Purkinje system.

Paroxysmal AV block has been defined as the abrupt occurrence or repetitive block of the atrial impulses with a relatively long (approximately 2 s or more) ventricular asystole before the return of conduction or escape of a subsidiary ventricular pacemaker (17). We believe that this form of AV block does not represent a separate entity and is best considered simply as advanced or complete block.

First-Degree AV Block

It is now recognized that even an isolated markedly long PR interval can cause symptoms similar to the pacemaker syndrome especially in the presence of normal left ventricular (LV) function (18). During markedly prolonged anterograde AV conduction, the close proximity of atrial systole to the preceding ventricular systole produces the same hemodynamic consequences as continual retrograde ventriculoatrial conduction during VVI pacing (Figs. 10.11 and 10.12). This is why symptomatic marked first-degree AV block has been called "pacemaker syndrome without a pacemaker" but we believe that

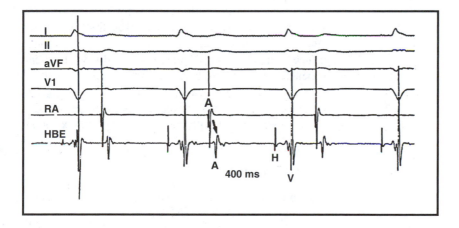

Fig. 10.11 Surface ECG and intracardiac recording from a patient with symptomatic marked first-degree AV block originally misdiagnosed as having as AV junctional rhythm with retrograde VA conduction. RA = high right atrial electrogram, HBE = Electrogram at site of His bundle recording. Note that the sequence of atrial activation (RA to HBE) is consistent with sinus rhythm and rules out retrograde atrial activation. The AH interval reflecting AV nodal conduction) is markedly prolonged. The patient had a normal left ventricular ejection fraction and complained of exertional dyspnea. (Barold SS. Acquired Atrioventricular Block. In: Kusumoto F, Goldschlager N (Eds), Cardiac Pacing for the Clinician, Philadelphia, PA: Lippincott, Williams & Wilkins, 2001 with permission).

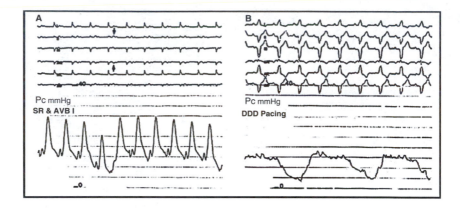

Fig. 10.12 (A) Same patient as Fig. 10.11. Pulmonary capillary wedge pressure shows large cannon waves. Scale 0–40 mm Hg. (B) Same patient after testing with a temporary dual chamber pacemaker with a physiologic AV delay. Note the normal pulmonary capillary wedge pressure. The patient was markedly improved after the implantation of a dual chamber pacemaker with AV delay optimization. (Barold SS. Acquired Atrioventricular Block. In: Kusumoto F, Goldschlager N (Eds), Cardiac Pacing for the Clinician, Philadelphia, PA: Lippincott, Williams & Wilkins, 2001 with permission).

the term "pacemaker-like syndrome" is more appropriate. An AV junctional rhythm with retrograde ventriculoatrial conduction may also produce the same pathophysiology. The 2002 ACC/AHA/NASPE guidelines for pacemaker implantation now advocate pacing in acquired marked first-degree AV block (>0.3s) as a Class IIa indication (1). Patients with a long PR interval may or may not be asymptomatic at rest. They are more likely to become symptomatic with mild or moderate exercise when the PR interval does not shorten appropriately and atrial systole shifts progressively closer toward ventricular systole. The class II recommendation does not really apply to patients with congestive heart failure, dilated cardiomyopathy, and marked first-degree AV block where biventricular pacing would be more beneficial than conventional dual chamber pacing. The clinician must decide in the individual patient whether there is a net benefit provided by two opposing factors: a positive effect from AV delay optimization and a negative effect impact of reduced LV function from aberrant pacemaker-controlled depolarization (Fig. 10.12). A recent study suggests that improvement with dual chamber pacing becomes evident with a PR interval > 0.28 s (19).

Intraventricular Conduction and Provocable AV Block

Although the meaning of bifascicular block is obvious, that of trifascicular block is not as simple. The term trifascicular block is often used rather loosely as previously emphasized. Bilateral bundle branch block, despite 1:1 AV conduction, carries a poor prognosis and should be a Class I indication for pacing, even in an asymptomatic patient.

Exercise

Permanent pacing is recommended as a class I indication in symptomatic or asymptomatic patients with exercise-induced AV block (absent at rest) because the vast majority are due to tachycardia-dependent block in the His-Purkinje system and carry a poor prognosis (20–22) (Fig. 10.13). This

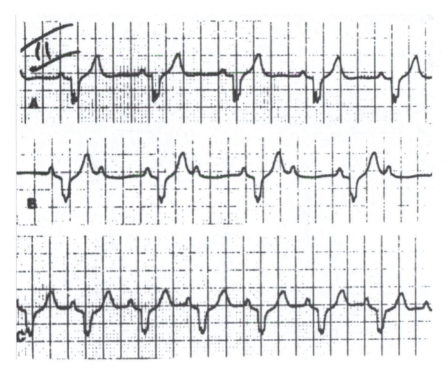

Fig. 10.13 (A) Lead II ECG in a patient with syncope intraventricular conduction block but no documented AV block at rest. (B) On exercise 2:1 AV block occurs and 1:1 AV conduction returns during the recovery period. A subsequent electrophysiological study revealed infranodal AV block at an atrial pacing rate of 110/min and a permanent pacemaker was implanted. No further syncope occurred.

form of AV block is often reproducible in the electrophysiology laboratory by rapid atrial pacing because it is tachycardia-dependent and rarely due to AV nodal disease. Exercise-induced AV block secondary to myocardial ischemia is rare and does not require pacing unless ischemia cannot be alleviated (23).

During an Electrophysiologic Study

When an electrophysiologic study is performed for the evaluation of syncope, many workers believe that AV block or delay in the following circumstances constitutes an indication for permanent pacing. (a) A markedly prolonged HV (from His bundle potential to earliest ventricular activation) interval ($\geq$100 ms: normal = 35–55 ms) identifies patients with a higher risk of developing complete AV block and need for a pacemaker (1) (Fig. 10.14). A study can define by a process of exclusion which patients might benefit from pacing in the presence of HV prolongation ($\geq$70 ms) and no other electrophysiological abnormality such as inducible ventricular tachycardia. (b) The development of second-or third-degree His-Purkinje block in an electrophysiological "stress test" performed by gradually increasing the atrial rate by pacing is an insensitive sign of conduction system disease but constitutes a class I indication for pacing because it correlates with a high incidence of third-degree AV block or sudden death (24). (c) Bradycardia-dependent (phase 4) block (not bradycardia-associated as in vagally induced AV block) is rare and always infranodal. It can be evaluated with His bundle recordings by producing bradycardia and pauses by the electrical induction of

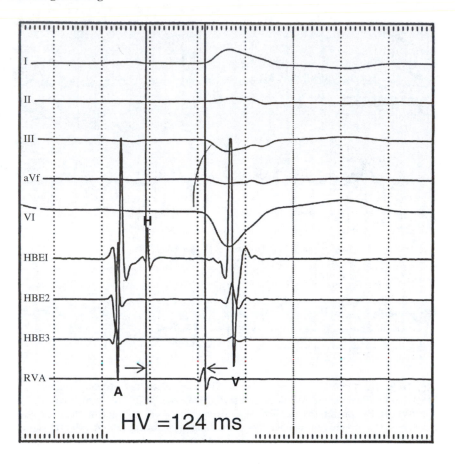

Fig. 10.14 Very long HV interval representing severe disease of the His-Purkinje system. His bundle recording in a patient with right bundle branch block and syncope. Left ventricular ejection fraction was normal. There was no documentation of second- or third-degree AV block before the electrophysiological study. Note the very long HV interval of 124 ms measured from the His bundle potential to the earliest ventricular activation either in the surface or intracardiac leads. (normal = 35–55 ms) responsible for the first-degree AV block. Time lines = 10 ms. A = low atrial depolarization, H = His bundle potential, V = Activation of high ventricular septum. Syncope disappeared after implantation of a permanent pacemaker.

atrial or ventricular premature beats. (d) A drug challenge with procainamide that depresses His-Purkinje conduction may be used to provoke HV interval prolongation or actual His-Purkinje block (according to published criteria) in susceptible patients and define the need for a pacemaker (25).

Permanent Pacing for AV Block after Acute Myocardial Infarction

The requirement for temporary pacing in acute myocardial infarction (MI) does not by itself constitute an indication for permanent pacing. Unlike many other indications, the need for permanent pacing after acute MI does not necessarily depend on the presence of symptoms.

Acute Inferior Myocardial Infarction

Permanent pacing is almost never needed in inferior MI and narrow QRS AV block. Pacemaker implantation should be considered only if second- or third-degree AV block persists for 14–16 days (26,27). The use of permanent pacing is required in only 1–2% of all the patients who develop acute second or third-degree AV block regardless of thrombolytic therapy. Narrow QRS type II second-degree AV block has not yet been reported in acute inferior MI (28–31).

Acute Anterior Myocardial Infarction

Patients who develop bundle branch block and transient second- and third-degree AV block during anterior MI have a high in-hospital mortality rate and are at a high risk of sudden death after hospital discharge. Sudden death usually is due to malignant ventricular tachyarrhythmias and less commonly related to the development of complete AV block with prolonged ventricular asystole. The use of permanent pacing in patients with transient trifascicular AV block or bilateral (alternating) bundle branch block is still controversial, but most workers recommend it with the aim of preventing sudden death from asystole despite the return of 1:1 AV conduction. Permanent pacing is not indicated in patients with acute anterior MI and residual bundle branch or bifascicular block without documented transient second- or third-degree AV block because there is no appreciable risk of late development of complete AV block. Measurement of the HV interval does not predict which patients will develop progressive conduction system disease.

Patients with an anterior MI who require permanent pacing often have a low LV ejection fraction that makes them potential candidates for a prophylactic implantable cardioverter-defibrillator. A recent study in patients who suffered an acute MI suggests waiting 3–6 months before implanting a defibrillator (32). Despite this recommendation, it makes sense to implant a cardioverter–defibrillator (which contains a pacemaker component) in patients who actually require only a permanent pacemaker at that juncture. Such patients are also at risk for sudden death from a ventricular tachyarrhythmia. It makes no sense to wait 3–6 months without protection for bradycardia until a cardioverter–defibrillator can be implanted on the basis of a poor LV ejection fraction according to the DINAMIT trial (32).

Vagally Mediated AV Block

Vagally mediated AV block is generally a benign condition considered a type I variant that can superficially resemble type II block (3,33). Vagally mediated AV block occurs in the AV node. Vagally induced AV block can occur in otherwise normal individuals and also in patients with coughing, swallowing, hiccups, micturition, etc. when vagal discharge is enhanced (Fig. 10.4). Electrophysiological studies in vagally mediated AV block are basically normal. Vagally mediated AV block is characteristically paroxysmal and often associated with sinus slowing. As a rule, AV nodal block is associated with obvious irregular and longer PP intervals and is bradycardia *associated* (not bradycardia dependent), i.e., both AV block and sinus slowing result from vagal effects. An acute increase in vagal tone may occasionally produce

AV block without preceding prolongation of the AH interval (constant PR), giving the superficial appearance of a Type II AV block mechanism, i.e., no PR prolongation before the blocked beat. In this situation, AH prolongation may occur during the initial several beats when AV conduction resumes. Vagally induced block is occasionally expressed in terms of constant PR intervals before and after the blocked impulse, an arrangement that may lead to an erroneous diagnosis of the more serious type II block if sinus slowing is ignored (Fig. 10.4). Sinus slowing can sometimes be subtle because the PP interval may increase by as little as 0.04 s.

AV Block in Athletes

Severe sinus bradycardia and third-degree AV block can occur at rest or after exercise in athletes and lead to symptoms such as lightheadedness, syncope, or even Stokes-Adams attacks. These changes are considered secondary to increased parasympathetic (hypervagotonia) and decreased sympathetic tone on the sinus and AV node related to physical training (34). Most patients become asymptomatic after physical deconditioning. If the latter produces no response or the patient refuses to decrease athletic activities, a permanent pacemaker becomes indicated. Some of the so-called "athletic patients" improved by pacing represent individuals who would otherwise benefit from pacing, i.e., subjects with sinus node disease rendered symptomatic by increased vagal tone related to training or athletes with spontaneous or exercise-induced infranodal block.

Atrioventricular block in athletes is most probably an expression of hypervagotonia. This form of AV block may or may not be associated with sinus bradycardia because the relative effects of sympathetic and parasympathetic systems on the AV and sinus node may differ. AV block in athletes responds to exercise or atropine. A number of authors have indicated that Mobitz Type II second-degree AV block (sometimes called Mobitz AV block as opposed to Wenckebach AV block) can occur in young athletes. The diagnosis of Type II AV block immediately raises the question of a permanent pacemaker, especially in symptomatic patients. We believe that Mobitz Type II second-degree AV block (always infranodal) does not occur in otherwise healthy athletes. The purported occurrence of Type II AV block in some reports appears related to failure of applying the correct definition of Type II second-degree AV block.

Selection of Optimal Pacing Mode for the Individual Patient

When selecting the type of pacemaker, the first question should be, "What is the status of the atrium and can it be paced and/or sensed?" The relatively unimportant contribution of AV synchrony to the cardiac output on *exercise* (as opposed to the increase in heart rate) should not detract from the well-established benefits of maintaining AV synchrony *at rest* for the prevention of hemodynamic (such as the pacemaker syndrome) and electrophysiological complications of atrial dysfunction (atrial fibrillation). One should be guided by the statement by the British Pacing and Electrophysiology Group that "the atrium should be paced/sensed unless contraindicated" (35). Therefore, the majority of patients with electrically responsive atria should be considered for dual-chamber pacing (VDD, DDD, or DDDR). Barring economic considerations, a DDDR device should be considered in all patients because the future risk of developing atrial chronotropic incompetence is largely unknown.

Alternative Right Ventricular Pacing Sites

Pooled data from many studies suggest that RV outflow (or septal) pacing provides somewhat better acute hemodynamic performance than RV apical pacing (36). An acute hemodynamic improvement does not necessarily translate into long-term improvement in LV function. So far, studies with longer follow-up, using RV pacing sites other than the RV apex have yielded mixed results in terms of LV function (37). These studies of alternative site RV pacing are difficult to interpret because of the small number of patients, wide range of starting LV function, spectrum of underlying heart disease, lack of standardization of the RV pacing sites, no quantification of the cumulative time of ventricular pacing as opposed to sensing, different endpoints, and varying durations of follow-up mostly too short for the continual duration of right ventricular outflow tract (RVOT) or right ventricular septal (RVS) especially in the crossover studies (37).

Two reports are favorable in terms of RVOT or RVS pacing. The study of Tse et al. (38) compared RVOT pacing (12 patients) versus right ventricular (RV) apical pacing (12 patients) all with dual chamber pacemakers, an optimized AV delay and > 95% ventricular pacing. The study revealed no change in left ventricular ejection fraction (LVEF) at 6 months but a significant drop in LVEF occurred after 18 months only in the patients with RV apical pacing. Victor et al. (39) followed 28 patients after ablation of the AV junction for permanent atrial fibrillation in whom a DDDR pacemaker was connected to two ventricular leads. One lead was screwed into the septum and another placed at the apex and the leads were connected to the atrial and ventricular ports, respectively. The septum or apex was paced by programming AAIR or VVIR modes, respectively. Patients were randomly assigned, 4 months later, to pacing at one site for 3 months, and crossed over to the other for 3 months. At 3 months, among patients with baseline LVEF ≤ 45%, LVEF was 42 ± 5% after septal pacing versus 37 ± 4% after apical pacing ($p < 0.001$). In patients with LVEF > 45%, no difference was found between the two pacing sites in LVEF.

Despite some encouraging data, the long-term benefit of alternative RV pacing sites (outflow tract, septum, and dual RV site) remains inconclusive and needs to be proven in much larger patient populations with normal LVEF for primary prevention of heart failure and patients with LV dysfunction being compared to biventricular and monochamber LV pacing. Nevertheless, there is a rapidly growing trend to pace the RV at the RVS or RVOT site especially in patients with abnormal LV function more on the basis of faith than solid data and the argument that no harmful effects of RVOT or RVS pacing has yet been reported.

VVI and VVIR Pacing

Atrial fibrillation/flutter with AV block or slow ventricular response (representing only 10–15% of patients requiring permanent pacing) constitutes the only indication for the VVI or VVIR pacing mode (35). Replacement of a depleted

VVI pacemaker with another VVI or VVIR unit is probably reasonable in truly asymptomatic patients. At the time of pacemaker replacement, such patients should be carefully evaluated to determine whether they might benefit from an upgrading procedure to a more physiologic pacing mode. Single-lead ventricular pacing may also be appropriate in patients who are incapacitated and inactive as well as those with other medical problems associated with short-life expectancy.

Single-Lead Dual-Chamber VDD Pacing

Satisfactory experience with single-lead VDD (or VDD/VVIR) pacing suggests that such dedicated VDD systems can provide an effective but less expensive pacing system than the DDD mode for patients with AV block and normal atrial chronotropic function. During sinus bradycardia, the VDD mode continues to pace effectively in the VVI or VVIR mode at the programmed lower rate with the risk of causing the pacemaker syndrome. The concern about implanting an appropriately programmed VDD device in patients with normal atrial chronotropic function and retrograde VA conduction is probably unwarranted, provided a Holter recording confirms the absence of significant sinus bradycardia, especially during waking hours. To guarantee absence of VVI pacing (with associated retrograde VA conduction), the lower rate of a VDD pulse generator should be programmed to a value less than the slowest sinus rate. Some sensor-driven pacemakers can automatically reset their lower rate during sleep to avoid loss of AV synchrony during relative bradycardia.

Cardiac Resynchronization for Primary Implantation in Patients with a Conventional Indication for Antibradycardia Pacing

The widespread acceptance that long-term RV apical pacing can impair LV function and precipitate heart failure raises the question as to whether biventricular pacing should be considered for the "primary prevention" of LV remodeling and development of heart failure (40,41). It can be hypothesized that patients requiring pacing for AV block, NYHA class III/IV and a LV ejection fraction (LVEF) ≤35% (regardless of the underlying conFiguration of the spontaneous QRS complex) might benefit from cardiac resynchronization therapy (CRT) at the time of the initial pacemaker implantation.

We believe that a CRT approach for initial pacemaker implantation might be worthwhile in selected patients with AV block. On the basis of little data (40–43), a number of workers now believe that it is reasonable to consider biventricular pacing if frequent or continuous RV pacing (i.e., when a large cumulative percentage of RV pacing as in complete AV block) is expected in the setting of a LVEF ≤35% (even without clinical heart failure) especially with associated mitral regurgitation. The cut-off point for LVEF is likely to change in the future with the emergence of more supportive data about the benefit of CRT in patients with less advanced forms of heart disease. The suggestion to consider biventricular pacing in selected patients requiring antibradycardia pacing is based on the concept derived from the Mode Selection trial (MOST) that it is the cumulative percentage of RV pacing time that ultimately determines the incidence of hospitalizations for congestive heart failure (44,45). The importance of minimizing RV pacing with special algorithms should be used in patients requiring intermittent RV pacing.

Conclusion

Second-degree AV block remains poorly understood despite the major advances in cardiac electrophysiology in the last 35 years. The literature abounds with varying definitions of second-degree AV block especially Mobitz Type II block. It should therefore not be surprising that during formal testing, physicians score more poorly with second-degree AV block ECGs than with those of other arrhythmias (46). Indeed it was stated a few years ago that "Mobitz II block is misunderstood more than any other abnormality of rhythm or conduction."(47). Much of the prevailing confusion surrounding second-degree AV block would disappear with the proper application of strict and uniform definitions. The understanding of second-degree AV block is basically an exercise in clinical logic that centers on appreciating the definitions of type I and type II blocks.

Portions of this chapter have been excerpted with permission from Barold SS, Herweg B. The spectrum of acquired AV block in clinical practice. Hospital Chronicles 2006.

References

1. Gregoratos G, Abrams J, Epstein AE, Freedman RA, Hayes DL, Hlatky MA, Kerber RE, Naccarelli GV, Schoenfeld MH, Silka MJ, Winters SL, Gibbons RI, Antman EM, Alpert JS, Hiratzka LF, Faxon DP, Jacobs AK, Fuster V, Smith SC Jr. American College of Cardiology/American Heart Association Task Force on Practice Guidelines American College of Cardiology/American Heart Association/North American Society for Pacing and Electrophysiology Committee. ACC/AHA/NASPE 2002 guideline update for implantation of cardiac pacemakers and antiarrhythmia devices: summary article. A report of the American College of Cardiology/American Heart Association Task Force on Practice Guidelines (ACC/AHA/NASPE Committee to Update the 1998 Pacemaker Guidelines). J Cardiovasc Electrophysiol 2002;13:1183–1199.
2. Rosenbaum MB, Elizari MV, Lazzari JO. Clinical evidence of hemiblock: syndrome of RBBB and intermittent LAH and LPH. Trifascicular block. In: Rosenbaum MB, Elizari MV, Lazzari JO, (Eds.). The Hemiblocks. Oldsmar, FL, Tampa Tracings 1970;55–69.
3. Barold SS, Hayes DL. Second-degree atrioventricular block: a reappraisal. Mayo Clin Proc 2001;76:44–57.
4. El-Sherif N, Aranda J, Befeler B, Lazzara R. Atypical Wenckebach periodicity simulating Mobitz type II AV block. Brit Heart J 1978;40:1376–1383.
5. Friedman HS, Gomes JAC, Haft JI. An analysis of Wenckebach periodicity. J Electrocardiol 1975;8:307–315.
6. Denes P, Levy L, Pick A, Rosen KM. The incidence of typical and atypical AV Wenckebach periodicity. Am Heart J 1975;89:26–31.
7. Connelly DT, Steinhaus DM. Mobitz type I atrioventricular block: an indication for permanent pacing? PACE 1996;19:261–264.
8. Shaw DB, Kekwick CA, Veale D, Gowers J, Whistance T. Survival in second-degree atrioventricular block. Br Heart J 1985;53:587–593.
9. Shaw DB, Gowers JI, Kekwick CA, New KH, Whistance AW. Is Mobitz type I atrioventricular block benign in adults? Heart 2004;90:169–174.
10. Barold SS. Lingering misconceptions about type I second-degree atrioventricular block. Am J Cardiol 2001;88:1018–1020.
11. Barold SS, Friedberg HD. Second degree atrioventricular block. A matter of definition. Am J Cardiol 1974;33:311–315.

12. Lange HW, Ameisen O, Mack R, Moses SW, Kligfield P. Prevalence and clinical correlates of non-Wenckebach narrow QRS complex second degree atrioventricular block detected by ambulatory ECG. Am Heart J 1988;115:114–120.
13. WHO/ISC Task Force. Definition of terms related to cardiac rhythm. Am Heart J 1978;95:796–806.
14. Surawicz B, Uhley H, Borun R, Laks M, Crevasse L, Rosen K, Nelson W, Mandel W, Lawrence P, Jackson L, Flowers N, Clifton J, Greenfield J Jr, De Medina EO. The quest for optimal electrocardiography. Task Force I: standardization of terminology and interpretation. Bethesda Conference co-sponsored by the American College of Cardiology and Health Resources Administration of the Department of Health, Education, and Welfare Task Force 1. Standardization of terminology and interpretation. Am J Cardiol 1978;41:130–144.
15. Barold SS. 2:1 atrioventricular block: order from chaos. Am J Emerg Med 2001;19:214–217.
16. Möbitz W. Uber die unvollstandige storung der erregungsuberleitung zwischen vorhof und kammer des menschlichen herzems. Z Ges Exp Med 1924;41:180–237.
17. Shohat-Zabarski R, Iakobishvili Z, Kusniec J, Mazur A, Strasberg B. Paroxysmal atrioventricular block: clinical experience with 20 patients. Int J Cardiol 2004;97:399–405.
18. Barold SS. Indications for permanent cardiac pacing in first-degree AV block: class I, II, or III? PACE 1996;19:747–751.
19. Iliev II, Yamachika S, Muta K, Hayano M, Ishimatsu T, Nakao K, Komiya N, Hirata T, Ueyama C, Yano K. Preserving normal ventricular activation versus atrioventricular delay optimization during pacing: the role of intrinsic atrioventricular conduction and pacing rate. PACE 2000;23:74–83.
20. Luscure M, Dechandol AM, Lagorge P, Marot M, Goutner C, Donzeau P. Blocs auriculo-ventriculaires d'effort. Ann Cardiol Angeiol 1995;44:486–492.
21. Sumiyoshi M, Nakata Y, Yasuda M, Tokano T, Ogura S, Nakazato Y, Yamaguchi H. Clinical and electrophysiologic features of exercise-induced atrioventricular block. Am Heart J 1996;2:1277–1281.
22. Barold SS, Jaïs P, Shah DC, Takahashi A, Haïssaguerre M, Clémenty J. Exercise-induced second-degree AV block: is it type I or type II? J Cardiovasc Electrophysiol 1997; 8:1084–1086.
23. Deaner A, Fluck D, Timmis AD. Exertional atrioventricular block presenting with recurrent syncope: successful treatment by coronary angioplasty. Heart 1996;75:640–641.
24. Petrac D, Radic B, Birtic K, Gjurovic J. Prospective evaluation of infrahisal second-degree AV block induced by atrial pacing in the presence of chronic bundle branch block and syncope. PACE 1996;19:784–792.
25. Englund A, Bergfeldt L, Rosenqvist M. Pharmacological stress testing of the His-Purkinje system in patients with bifascicular block. PACE 1998;21:1979–1987.
26. Harthorne JW, Barold SS. Atherosclerosis, the conduction system and cardiac pacing. In: Fuster V, Ross R, Topol EJ (Eds.): Atherosclerosis and Coronary Artery Disease. Philadelphia, Lippincott-Raven, 1996:1013–1030.
27. Barold SS. American College of Cardiology/American Heart Association guidelines for pacemaker implantation after acute myocardial infarction. What is persistent advanced block at the atrioventricular node? Am J Cardiol 1997;80:770–774.
28. Barold SS. Narrow QRS Mobitz type II second-degree atrioventricular block in acute myocardial infarction: true or false? Am J Cardiol 1991;67:1291–1294.
29. Scheinman MM, Gonzalez RP. Fascicular block and acute myocardial infarction. JAMA 1980;244:2646–2649.
30. Sclarovsky S, Strasberg B, Hirshberg A, Arditi A, Lewin RF, Agmon J. Advanced early and late atrioventricular block in acute inferior wall myocardial infarction. Am Heart J 1984;108:19–24.

31. Behar S, Zissman E, Zion M, Hod H, Goldbourt U, Reicher-Reiss H, Shalev Y, Kaplinsky E, Caspi A. Prognostic significance of second-degree atrioventricular block in inferior wall acute myocardial infarction. SPRINT Study Group. Am J Cardiol 1993;72:831–834.

32. Hohnloser SH, Kuck KH, Dorian P, Roberts RS, Hampton JR, Hatala R, Fain E, Gent M, Connolly SJ; DINAMIT Investigators. Prophylactic use of an implantable cardioverter-defibrillator after acute myocardial infarction. N Engl J Med 2004;351:2481–2488.

33. Massie B, Scheinman MM, Peters R, Desai J, Hirschfield D, O'Young J. Clinical and electrophysiologic findings in patients with paroxysmal slowing of the sinus rate and apparent Mobitz type II atrioventricular block. Circulation 1978;58:305–314.

34. Barold SS. Cardiac pacing in special and complex situations. Indications and modes of stimulation. Cardiol Clin 1992;10:573–591.

35. Clarke M, Sutton R, Ward D, et al. Recommendations for pacemaker prescription for symptomatic bradycardia. Report of a working party of the British Pacing and Electrophysiology Group. Br Heart J 1991;66:185–191.

36. de Cock CC, Giudici MC, Twisk JW. Comparison of the haemodynamic effects of right ventricular outflow-tract pacing with right ventricular apex pacing: a quantitative review. Europace 2003;5:275–278.

37. Barold SS, Herweg B. Right ventricular outflow tract pacing: not ready for prime-time. J Interv Card Electrophysiol 2005;13:39–46.

38. Tse HF, Yu C, Wong KK, Tsang V, Leung YL, Ho WY, Lau CP. Functional abnormalities in patients with permanent right ventricular pacing: the effect of sites of electrical stimulation. J Am Coll Cardiol 2002;40:1451–1458.

39. Victor F, Mabo P, Mansour H, Pavin D, Kabalu G, de Place C, Leclercq C, Daubert JC. A randomized comparison of permanent septal versus apical right ventricular pacing: short-term results. J Cardiovasc Electrophysiol 2006;17:238–242.

40. Barold SS, Lau CP. Primary prevention of heart failure in cardiac pacing. Pacing Clin Electrophysiol 2006;29:217–219.

41. Tse HF, Lau CP. Selection of permanent ventricular pacing site: how far should we go? J Am Coll Cardiol 2006;48:1649–1651.

42. Sweeney MO, Prinzen FW. A new paradigm for physiologic ventricular pacing. J Am Coll Cardiol 2006;47:282–288.

43. Doshi RN, Daoud EG, Fellows C, Turk K, Duran A, Hamdan MH, Pires LA. Left ventricular-based cardiac stimulation post AV nodal ablation evaluation (The PAVE Study). J Cardiovasc Electrophysiol 2005;16:1160–1165.

44. Sweeney MO, Hellkamp AS, Ellenbogen KA, Greenspon AJ, Freedman RA, Lee KL, Lamas GA, for the MOST Investigators. Adverse effect of ventricular pacing on heart failure and atrial fibrillation among patients with normal baseline QRS duration in a clinical trial of pacemaker therapy for sinus node dysfunction. Circulation 2003;107:2932–2937.

45. Sweeney MO, Hellkamp AS. Heart failure during cardiac pacing. Circulation 2006;113:2082–2088.

46. Gillespie ND, Brett CT, Morrison WG, Pringle SD. Interpretation of the emergency electrocardiogram in junior hospital doctors. J Accid Emerg Med 1996;13:395–397.

47. Phibbs BP. Diagnosis of complex forms of AV block: some tricks, some booby traps. In: Phibbs BP, Advanced ECG. Boards and Beyond, Boston MA, Little, Brown, 1997:110–124.

Cardiac Resynchronization Therapy for Congestive Heart Failure

Nitish Badhwar and Byron K. Lee

Introduction

Over the past 20 years there have been many groundbreaking advances in the pharmacologic treatment of congestive heart failure. However, there are still many end-stage patients, who despite optimal medical management, still have severe and refractory symptoms, along with an overall poor prognosis (1,2). Cardiac resynchronization therapy (CRT), which is also known as biventricular pacing has been shown to be an effective nonpharmacologic approach that can help many of these patients with advanced heart failure. Since the early pilot studies of CRT in the mid 1990s there has been extensive research in this area. Now we have several published large scale randomized controlled trials that prove CRT not only improves symptoms, but also decreases mortality. Based on these trials, CRT has become the standard of care for selected patients with moderate to severe heart failure.

Abnormal Electrical Conduction in Heart Failure

In advanced heart failure, it is common to see abnormal electrical conduction. Heart failure patients can have first-degree heart block and/or intraventricular conduction delay. The intraventricular conduction delay is usually manifest as left bundle branch block. It has been estimated that one-third of patients with systolic heart failure have a QRS duration greater than 120 ms (3).

These conduction disturbances typically worsen overall cardiac function. The AV delay seen with first degree heart block can lead to suboptimal contribution of atrial systole, less filling time for the LV, and worsened mitral regurgitation (4,5). The intraventricular conduction abnormality can lead to regional LV wall motion delay, which is termed LV dyssynchrony. In LBBB, the LV lateral wall typically depolarizes late and therefore, contracts late. This delayed contraction of the LV lateral wall occurs when the septum is already in its relaxation phase. On echo, it can be seen that the relaxed septum moves paradoxically away from the lateral wall late in systole. This is inefficient contraction since the septum and lateral walls are not moving in unison to squeeze blood forward. It has been shown that this LV dyssynchrony is associated with increased mortality among heart failure patients (6–8).

Mechanism

CRT typically involves placing pacing leads in the right atrium, right ventricle, and a lateral branch of the coronary sinus. The lead in the coronary sinus is also known as the LV lead since it activates the lateral wall of the LV. Chapter 5 describes in detail the techniques for implantation of LV leads.

With leads in the RA, RV, and coronary sinus, the electrical disturbances that exacerbate heart failure can be minimized. The AV interval is adjustable and can be shortened by programming the device to pace the ventricles with less delay following atrial activation (paced or intrinsic). The timing of RV pacing and LV pacing can also be adjusted to coordinate the contraction of the septum and the LV lateral wall, thereby reducing LV dyssynchrony. In the older CRT devices, the RV and LV pacing could only be programmed to pace simultaneously. However in newer devices, the timing of RV and LV pacing can be offset to further optimize cardiac output. It has been shown that in 85% patients, offsetting the timing of RV and LV pacing is better than simultaneous pacing of the RV and LV leads (9) (Fig. 11.1).

By shortening AV delay and reducing LV dyssynchrony, CRT can increase LV filling time, increase stroke volume, and reduce mitral regurgitation (5,10,11). These are the underlying mechanism of acute improvement with CRT. In fact, patients frequently feel better almost immediately after implantation. Occasionally, we see patients with end-stage heart failure who cannot be weaned off inotropic support be successfully weaned 1–2 days after CRT implantation.

CRT also appears to confer long-term benefits on cardiac function. Several studies support a positive effect of CRT on cardiac remodeling. Yu et al. assessed CRT patients serially over 3 months. They found that there was progressive improvement in EF, LV end systolic volume, and LV end diastolic volumes (12). The MIRACLE trial similarly found progressive improvement of these parameters over 6 months of CRT patients (11). We frequently see patients continue to have symptomatic improvement several months after the procedure.

Clinical Trials

To date, there is extensive evidence supporting the benefits of CRT for the treatment of heart failure. More than 4000 patients now have been randomized in single or double blinded controlled trials (Fig.11.2). Although the inclusion criteria of these trials were slightly different, the results of these trials have consistently shown that CRT improves symptoms. More recently, trials have shown that CRT also decreases mortality. A few of the seminal trials are highlighted below and in Table 11.1.

MIRACLE Study

The MIRACLE (Multicenter InSync Randomized Clinical Evaluation) trial was the first large scale, prospective, randomized, double-blind trial of CRT (11). It was started in October 1998 and was eventually published in June

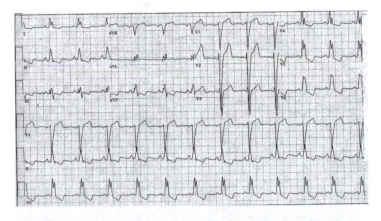

Panel A

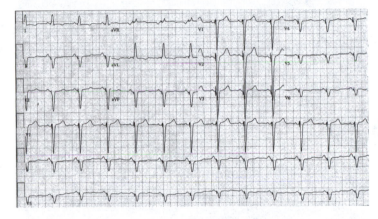

Panel B

Fig. 11.1 ECG of a patient before CRT (Panel A) and after CRT (Panel B). Note the QRS is clearly narrowed with CRT pacing.

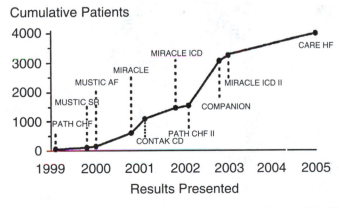

Fig. 11.2 Cumulative enrollment of patients into randomized controlled CRT trials. (Reproduced with permission from Abraham WT. Prog Cardiovasc Dis 2006;48(4): 232–38.)

Table 11.1 Randomized clinical trials of Cardiac Resynchronization Therapy.

Study	Design	No. of patients	Mean follow-up (months)	Results	p value
MUSTIC (NEJM 2001)	Crossover CRT *vs* no CRT in patients with CHF NYHA III, EF < 35%, QRS > 150 ms, LVEDD > 60 mm, NSR	58	6	Improved 6MWT	<0.001
				QOL	<0.001
				Hospitalization	<0.05
				Peak V_{O2}	<0.03
MIRACLE (NEJM 2002)	Parallel arms CRT *vs* no CRT in patients with CHF NYHA III, EF < 35%, QRS > 130 ms, LVEDD > 55 mm, 6MWT < 450 m, NSR	453	6	Improved 6MWT	=0.005
				NYHA class	<0.001
				QOL	=0.001
				LVEF	<0.001
				Peak V_{O2}	=0.009
PATH-CHF (JACC 2002)	Crossover CRT (LV or BiV) *vs* no CRT in patients with CHF NYHA III-IV, EF < 35%, QRS > 120 ms, PR > 150 ms, NSR	41	12	Improved 6MWT	=0.03
				Peak V_{O2}	=0.002
				QOL	=0.062
				NYHA class	<0.001
				LV and BiV had similar improvement	
MIRACLE ICD (JAMA 2003)	Parallel arms CRT + ICD *vs* CRT in patients with CHF NYHA III, EF < 35%, QRS > 130 ms, LVEDD > 55 mm, cardiac arrest due to VT/VF, spontaneous VT or inducible VT/VF, NSR	369	6	Improved NYHA class	=0.007
				QOL	=0.02
				No change	
				6MWT	=0.36

CONTAK CD (JACC 2003)	Crossover, parallel controlled CRT vs no CRT in patients undergoing ICD implantation with CHF NYHA II-IV, EF < 35%, QRS > 120 ms, NSR, indications for ICD implantation	490	6	Improved 6MWT	= 0.043
				Peak V_{O_2}	= 0.030
				LVEF	< 0.001
				LV volumes	= 0.02
				No significant change	
				NYHA class	= 0.10
				QOL	= 0.40
				HF progression	= 0.35
PATH-CHF II (JACC 2003)	Crossover CRT (LV only) vs no CRT in patients with CHF NYHA II-IV, EF < 30%, QRS > 120 ms, NSR, Peak V_{O_2} < 18 ml/min/kg	86	6	Improved 6MWT	= 0.021
				QOL	= 0.015
				Peak V_{O_2}	< 0.001
				No benefit in QRS 120–150 ms	
COMPANION (NEJM 2004)	Parallel arms Optimal pharmacological therapy (OPT) vs CRT vs CRT + ICD (CRT-D) in patients with CHF NYHA III-IV, EF ≤ 35%, QRS > 120 ms	1520	16	Death or hospitalization for CHF reduced by 34% in CRT, 40% in CRT-D	< 0.002
				As compared to OPT	< 0.001
				All cause mortality reduced by 36% in CRT-D	= 0.003
			Stopped early by DSMB	24% in CRT	= 0.05

(continued)

Table 11.1 (continued)

Study	Design	No. of patients	Mean follow-up (months)	Results	p value
CARE-HF (NEJM 2005)	Open label, randomized Medical therapy vs Medical therapy + CRT in patients with CHF NYHA III-IV, EF ≤ 35%, QRS > 120 ms with dyssynchrony (aortic preejection > 140 ms, interventricular mechanical delay > 40 ms, delayed activation of postlateral LV) QRS > 150 ms (no dyssynchrony evidence needed)	814	29.4	All cause mortality/ hospitalization reduction by 37% in CRT	<0.001
				All cause mortality reduced by 36% in CRT	<0.002
				Improvement in QOL	<0.01
				LVEF	
				LVESV	
				NYHA class	

6MWT, 6-min walk test; *AF*, atrial fibrillation; *CARE-HF*, Cardiac Resynchronization- Heart Failure study group; *CHF*, congestive heart failure; *CONTAK-CD*, CONTAK-cardiac defibrillator; *COMPANION*, Comparison of Medical Therapy, Resynchronization, and Defibrillation Therapies in Heart Failure study group; *CRT*, cardiac resynchronization therapy; *DSMB*, data safety monitoring board; *EF*, ejection fraction; *ICD*, implantable cardioverter-defibrillator; *JACC*, Journal of American College of Cardiology; *JAMA*, Journal of American Medical Association; *LVEDD*, LV end diastolic diameter; *LVESV*, LV end systolic volume; *MIRACLE*, Multicenter Insync Randomized Clinical Evaluation trial; *MUSTIC*, Multisite Stimulation in Cardiomyopathies study group; *NEJM*, New England Journal of Medicine; *NSR*, normal sinus rhythm; *NYHA*, New York Heart Association; *QOL*, quality of life; *PACE*, pacing and clinical electrophysiology; *PATH-CHF*, Pacing Therapies in Heart Failure study group; *VT*, ventricular tachycardia; *VF*, ventricular fibrillation.

2002. In this study, 453 patients with NYHA class III or IV heart failure, EF≤35%, and QRS duration ≥130 ms were all implanted with a CRT device. Patients were randomized to have the CRT feature turned *on* or *off*. At 6 months, patients randomized to CRT *on* had significant improvement in quality of life, 6 min walk distance (39 vs. 10 m, $p = 0.005$), NYHA functional class, exercise treadmill time, EF ($+4.6$ vs. -0.2%, $p < 0.001$), and peak VO_2 consumption. Furthermore, patients in the CRT on group had significantly fewer hospitalizations and fewer intravenous medications for the treatment of worsening heart failure. This study was instrumental in securing FDA approval for CRT devices in August 2001.

COMPANION Study

The Comparison of Medical Therapy, Pacing, and Defibrillation in Heart Failure (COMPANION) Study was the first large scale, randomized CRT trial to suggest that in addition to symptomatic improvement, CRT may confer mortality benefit (13). COMPANION was started in early 2000 and was eventually published in May 2004. In this trial, 1,520 patients with NYHA class III and IV heart failure and QRS duration ≥120 ms were randomized to optimal medical therapy, implantation of CRT device, or implantation of a CRT device with defibrillator capability. Mean follow-up was over 11 months. Like MIRACLE, COMPANION showed that CRT improved heart failure symptoms based on exercise tolerance testing and quality of life surveys. COMPANION additionally showed that in the patients who got either type of CRT device, there was a significant 20% reduction in the primary endpoint that was a composite of all-cause mortality and all-cause hospitalization. COMPANION's most impressive finding was in terms of all-cause mortality, which was one of their secondary endpoints. In the patients who got CRT without defibrillator capability, there was a trend toward decreased overall mortality when compared to optimal medical therapy (24% risk reduction, $p = 0.059$). In the patients who got CRT with defibrillator capability, there was a significant 36% ($p = 0.03$) risk reduction of overall mortality when compared to optimal medical therapy.

CARE-HF Study

The CARE-HF (Cardiac Resynchronization-Heart Failure) study was designed specifically to evaluate the effects of CRT on morbidity and mortality (1). This trial was started in January 2001 and was published in April 2005. Eight hundred nineteen patients with EF ≤35% and evidence dyssynchrony were randomized to optimal medical therapy or CRT. Dyssynchrony was defined as either a QRS duration ≥150 ms or a QRS duration of 120–149 ms with echocardiographic evidence of dyssynchrony. In the CRT group, there was a 37% risk reduction ($p < 0.001$) in the primary endpoint, which was a composite of death from any cause or unplanned hospitalization for a major cardiac event (Fig. 11.3). In terms of all-cause mortality (secondary endpoint), there was a 36% risk reduction ($p < 0.002$) in the CRT group compared to optimal medical therapy. This study went beyond COMPANION by showing that CRT alone, even without the defibrillator, could improve survival.

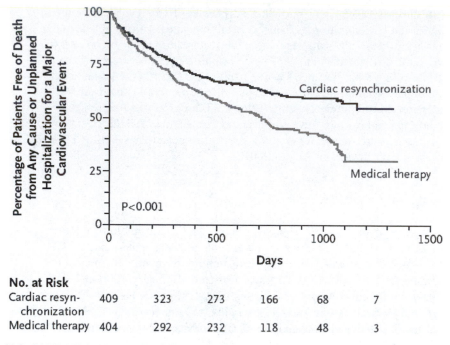

Fig. 11.3 CARE-HF Study: Kaplan-Meier curve for all cause mortality or an unplanned hospitalization for a major cardiovascular event, which was the primary endpoint. CRT group had a 37% risk reduction as compared to medical therapy group. (Reproduced with permission from Cleland JGF, Daubert J-C, Erdmann E, et al. N Engl J Med 2005;352: 1539–49.)

Patient Selection

In 2005, the ACC/AHA published guidelines for the treatment of chronic heart failure which included a description of our current target population for CRT based on the many published clinical trials: patients with LVEF ≤35%, sinus rhythm, and NYHA functional class III or ambulatory class IV symptoms despite recommended, optimal medical therapy and who have cardiac dyssynchrony, which is currently defined as a QRS duration greater than 120 ms (14). This guideline defined cardiac dyssynchrony specifically as a wide QRS since most of the CRT trials used only this criterion as an indicator of dyssynchrony. However, several studies have since shown that echocardiography, MRI, and nuclear imaging may be better at measuring dyssynchrony than QRS duration (15) and ongoing prospective studies are evaluating their utility in predicting response (clinical improvement and LV reverse remodeling) to CRT (16). Beyond the target population described by the ACC/AHA guidelines, there are other patient populations that may also derive benefit from CRT. There is a high prevalence of atrial fibrillation (AF) in patients with end-stage heart failure. Preliminary data from the MUSTIC trial and a few small studies suggest functional and acute hemodynamic improvement in patients with AF and complete AV block with CRT when compared with right ventricular (RV) pacing

(17–19). Furthermore, Gasparini et al. (20) showed better long-term clinical outcomes in heart failure patients with permanent AF after CRT. Patients with QRS prolongation due to pacing device may also benefit from CRT. Data from the DAVID trial (21) has shown the negative impact of RV pacing in patients with cardiomyopathy undergoing ICD implantation, suggesting that a wide QRS complex from RV pacing is also deleterious. Leon et al. (18) upgraded traditional RV pacing devices to CRT devices in patients with chronic AF and heart failure and showed fewer hospitalizations and improvement in EF. These data suggest that we should expand the indications for CRT to patients with heart failure and AF (with prolonged QRS duration) as well as those with heart failure and RV pacing induced prolonged QRS duration.

In the near future, we may find out that CRT also benefits patients with early heart failure by preventing progression of disease. The MIRACLE-ICD II trial was a pilot study that showed LV reverse remodeling in patients with NYHA functional class II (22). This is undergoing further evaluation in the ongoing REVERSE and MADIT-CRT trials which are prospectively looking at clinical events and mortality in patients with mild heart failure (NYHA I-II) and wide QRS at baseline (23,24).

Use of Echocardiography and Other Imaging Modalities in CRT

Electrical dyssynchrony (wide QRS complex) is a surrogate marker of mechanical dyssynchrony, which is used to select patients for CRT. Mechanical dyssynchrony can occur between the atrium and the ventricle, between the RV and the LV (interventricular), and between the walls of a single ventricle (intraventricular). The baseline QRS duration is a good marker of *interventricular* (RV–LV) dyssynchrony; however subsequent studies have shown that *intraventricular* (LV) dyssynchrony is a more accurate predictor of response to CRT (15) and this does not correlate with the baseline QRS duration (25). Hence, there can be patients with wide QRS who do not have LV dyssynchrony and hence will not respond to CRT. At the same time there can be patients with advanced heart failure and narrow QRS complex who have LV dyssynchrony and will benefit from CRT (25–29).

This emphasizes the need for an imaging modality that can accurately assess LV dyssynchrony to select appropriate patients for CRT. In this section, we will present some promising approaches for assessing dyssynchrony. At present, it is not clear which imaging approach is superior in identifying the patients that are most likely to benefit from CRT.

Echocardiography

Echocardiography is a cost-effective imaging modality that is portable, easily accessible at most medical centers, and has a high temporal resolution. It has been used as a screening tool to assess EF in patients with advanced heart failure. Most of the CRT clinical trials have used 2D echo to assess the EF. Echo has also been used to assess mechanical dyssynchrony and to program optimal atrioventricular (AV) timing and interventricular (VV) timing after CRT implantation to achieve maximal hemodynamic benefit with biventricular

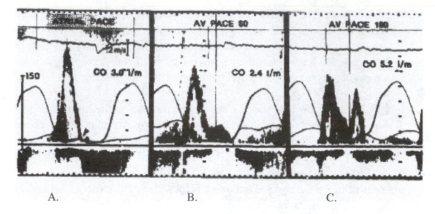

Fig. 11.4 Mitral flow velocity curve and simultaneous left atrial and left ventricular pressure curves in a 76-year old man with long PR interval and severe left ventricular dysfunction (ejection fraction 25%) due to severe coronary artery disease. He has New York Heart Association functional class IV symptoms. (A) Atrial pacing with antegrade native conduction and a long atrioventricular (AV) delay. There is an increase in left ventricular pressure above left atrial pressure during atrial relaxation in mid-diastole (arrowhead), culminating in a shortening of the diastolic filling time and the onset of diastolic regurgitation. The baseline cardiac output (CO) is 3.0 l/min. (B) Atrioventricular pacing at a short AV interval of 60 ms. Diastolic filling occurs through all of diastole. Atrial contraction now occurs simultaneously with left ventricular contraction, resulting in a lower cardiac output than that in panel A. Note that the mean left atrial pressure increased from 31 mm Hg in the left panel to 42 mm Hg in the center panel. (C) Atrioventricular pacing at the optimal AV interval of 180 ms. The relationship of atrial contraction to the onset of ventricular contraction is now optimal, resulting in diastolic filling throughout the entire diastolic filling period. An appropriate relation now exists between mechanical left atrial and left ventricular contraction, so that the mean left atrial pressure is maintained at a low level (34 mm Hg), with left atrial contraction occurring just before left ventricular contraction. This causes an increase in left ventricular end-diastolic pressure to 43 mm Hg, and the cardiac output has increased to 5.2 l/min. (Reproduced with permission from Nishimura RA, Hayes DL, Homes DR. J Am Coll Cardiol 1995;25:281–8.)

pacing. Echo evaluation also can assess the long-term effects of CRT on the heart (reverse remodeling) that include changes in EF, LV end diastolic volume, LV end systolic volume and mitral regurgitation (11,12,30).

Echo has been used to assess all levels of mechanical dyssynchrony: dyssynchrony between the atrium and the ventricle, *interventricular* dyssynchrony, and *intraventricular* dyssynchrony. Echo Doppler imaging at the level of the mitral valve inflow shows the effects of a long AV interval (fused E and A waves with diastolic mitral regurgitation), short AV interval (truncation of A wave with loss of atrial kick), and optimal AV interval (aortic systolic flow starts at the end of A wave) (5,31). This is illustrated in Fig. 11.4. Pulsed-wave Doppler echocardiography has been used to evaluate interventricular dyssynchrony that is defined as the time difference between right and left ventricular pre-ejection intervals. This is usually measured from the onset of the QRS complex on the EKG (that correlates with the end of diastole) to the onset of the aortic and pulmonary ejection. Delayed aortic ejection time (>40–50 ms) has been used as a marker of interventricular dyssynchrony that improves with CRT (32–34).

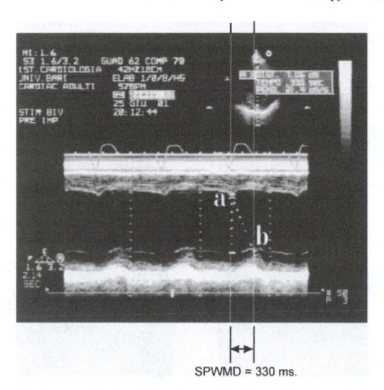

SPWMD = 330 ms.

Fig. 11.5 M-mode short-axis view of the echocardiographic image taken at the level of the papillary muscles. Calculation of septal-to-posterior wall motion delay (SPWMD) obtained by measuring the shortest interval between the maximal posterior displacement of the septum (a) and the posterior wall (b). (Reproduced with permission from Pitzalis MV, Iacoviello M, Romito R, et al. J Am Coll Cardiol 2002;40:1615–22.)

Recent studies have shown that intraventricular dyssynchrony (in the LV) is a better predictor of response to CRT (35,36). Pitzalis et al. have shown that M-mode echocardiography derived septal to posterior wall motion delay (SPWMD) >130 ms is a marker of intraventricular dyssynchrony that predicts a favorable response to CRT (37,38) (Fig. 11.5). However, this technique has limited utility in patients with ischemic cardiomyopathy who have an akinetic septum. A recent retrospective analysis of the CONTAK-CD database showed that SPWMD did not correlate with LV reverse remodeling (39). A 2D echo (apical four-chamber view) derived regional wall motion curves have also been used to quantify LV dyssynchrony (septal–lateral wall phase angle difference). These curves were compared by a mathematical phase analysis, based on Fourier transformation. Patients showing lateral wall phase angle delay >25° showed the best acute hemodynamic benefit with CRT (40,41).

Tissue Doppler imaging (TDI) which is a feature in some of the newer echo machines is a promising approach to assess dyssynchrony. It measures the time to peak systolic velocity (from the onset of QRS complex) in different segments of the LV and the delay between them is used as a marker of LV dyssynchrony (Fig. 11.6). These measurements can be obtained by pulsed-wave TDI or color-coded TDI that requires postprocessing. Initial studies used

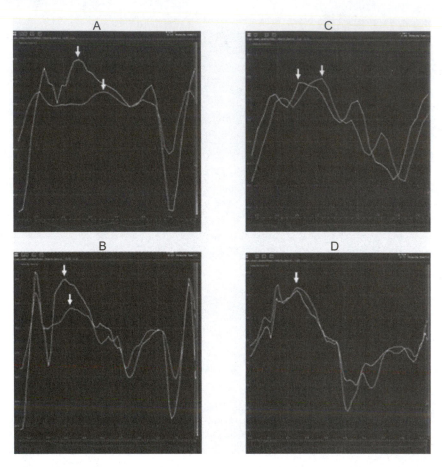

Fig. 11.6 Regional myocardial velocity curves obtained by tissue Doppler imaging at the basal septal (yellow) and basal lateral (green) segments. (A) In a patient with left bundle branch block with QRS duration of 180 ms, there was delay in peak systolic contraction (arrows) of 95 ms in the lateral wall compared to the septal wall. (B) After biventricular pacing, there was improvement in synchronicity as reflected by the near overlapping of myocardial velocity curves with a difference of only 20 ms. (C) Another patient with mildly prolonged QRS duration of 135 ms with intraventricular conduction delay. There was delay in peak systolic conduction of 125 ms in the lateral wall compared to the septal wall (arrow). (D) After biventricular pacing, systolic synchronicity was achieved as reflected by the perfect overlapping of the myocardial velocity curves. In both cases, there was significant left ventricular reverse remodeling with reduction of LV end-systolic volume of 37% and 40%, respectively. (Reproduced with permission from Yu CM, Fung JW, Chan CK, et al. J Cardiovasc Electrophysiol 2004;15:1058–65.)

a four-segment model (septal, lateral, inferior, and anterior) and showed that a delay >65 ms predicted response to CRT (35). Yu et al. used a 12-segment model (6 basal and 6 mid segment) and derived a LV dyssynchrony index from the standard deviation of all 12 intervals (12,36). LV dyssynchrony index >31 ms yielded a sensitivity and specificity of 96% and 78% to predict LV reverse modeling (36). Based on this technique they showed that dyssynchrony was present in 64% of heart failure patients with wide QRS complex and 43% of the patients with narrow QRS complex (42). Penicka et al. used pulsed-wave TDI to show that sum asynchrony (sum of interventricular and intraventricular) >102 ms was a good predictor of response to CRT (43).

Table 11.2 Echocardiographic parameters of intraventricular dyssynchrony.

- M-mode: Septal to posterior wall motion delay (>130 ms)
- 2D echo:
  - a. Aortic Pre-ejection interval >140 ms
  - b. Wall motion phase analysis (lateral delay >25°)
  - c. Contrast enhanced systolic regional fractional area
- TDI:
  - a. Difference in time to peak systolic velocity (4 segment >65 ms)
  - b. 12 segment LV dyssynchrony index >31 ms
  - c. Tissue tracking, strain and strain-rate imaging
  - d. TSI
- 3D echo

TDI is limited by its inability to differentiate between myocardial velocity due to systolic contraction and passive motion. Strain and strain rate analysis allows direct assessment of the extent and timing of myocardial deformation during systole and can overcome this limitation. Breithardt et al. showed reversal of septal–lateral wall strain pattern after CRT (44). However, Yu et al. compared TDI and strain rate imaging and showed that TDI was superior in prediction of reverse remodeling (36). Tissue synchronization imaging (TSI) is the latest addition to TDI that automatically detects peak velocity and color codes the time to peak velocities (green for normal timing, orange for moderate delay and red for severe delay). LV dyssynchrony is defined as the difference in time to peak velocity of opposing walls, a cut off value of >65 ms predicted acute response to CRT (45,46).

Three-dimensional echocardiography is another new approach to assess dyssynchrony. It shows real time and accurate measurement of LV volumes and EF. This method examines regional LV contraction at approximately 3,000 points over the endocardial surface and can be used to measure LV dyssynchrony based on the degree of dispersion in the timing of the point of minimum volume for each segment (47). This technique is very promising and needs correlation with response to CRT.

Currently, TDI is the most validated measure of LV dyssynchrony out of all the echo-derived parameters summarized in Table 11.2. The limitations of all the echo-derived parameters include operator dependence, inability to get good acoustic windows in some patients, signal to noise ratio, increased time consumption and lack of reproducibility of some parameters. Nevertheless, echo remains a very attractive approach to assess dyssynchrony mainly because it is so readily accessible at most hospitals.

Magnetic Resonance Imaging (MRI)

Cine MRI is an excellent imaging modality for dyssynchrony that provides reproducible, high-resolution three-dimensional assessment of global and regional myocardial function (48). MRI tagging measures myocardial deformation during systole and early diastole and gives quantitative analysis of regional LV function. A 3D regional myocardial motion or strain (relative shortening) can be computed in circumferential, longitudinal, and radial manner using different techniques (49). Comprehensive 3-D strain maps of the entire LV can be constructed and the magnitude of strain at different times can be displayed using a color-coded map. LV dyssynchrony can be calculated based on the regional temporal variance of strain (similar to TDI), regional variance vector of principal strain, and temporal uniformity of strain (49). Animal and human studies have shown that the variance of circumferential strain (and not longitudinal strain) is a better predictor of response to CRT (50,51).

Although MRI provides 3-D assessment of LV dyssynchrony, it is more expensive and has a lower temporal resolution than echocardiography. It is contraindicated in patients with pacemakers and defibrillators, which means MRI is not an option for device optimization after implant. However, a recent study has shown that it may be safe to do MRI in patients with modern devices (52).

Equilibrium Radionuclide Angiography (ERNA)

ERNA is a nuclear medicine based imaging modality that is also referred to as multiple gated blood pool scintigraphy (MUGA). It has been used as an objective, accurate, and reproducible assessment of cardiac wall motion and EF for many years. This imaging modality is not contraindicated in patients with implanted devices. ERNA derived phase method has been used to monitor and characterize abnormalities of both contraction and related electrical conduction (53). ERNA derived phase image analysis, a functional method based on the first Fourier harmonic fit of the gated blood pool vs. radioactivity curve, generates the parameters of amplitude (A) and phase angle ($\emptyset$). Amplitude (A) measures the magnitude of regional contraction and phase angle ($\emptyset$) represents the timing of regional contraction. Standard deviation of phase (SD $\emptyset$) has been shown to measure baseline interventricular dyssynchrony that predicts changes in EF after CRT (54). Recently two new scintigraphic parameters to assess intraventricular (LV) dyssynchrony called synchrony (S) and entropy (E) have been described that are highly reproducible and well differentiated among model ventricles with normal motion, ventricles with aneurysm, ventricles with diffuse dysfunction, and ventricles with severe regional dysfunction (55). S and E have shown the best correlation with clinical response in heart failure patients requiring CRT in preliminary studies (56). The limitations of ERNA include cost, exposure to radiation, and temporal resolution. However, it is a promising approach that deserves more investigation.

Pacing Modes and Programming Features

In the initial CRT trials, the device was programmed in a VDD mode (atrial sensed and ventricular paced) to achieve atrial synchronous biventricular pacing with no or minimal atrial pacing. The PV delay was programmed short and the upper tracking rate was programmed relatively high to ensure maximal biventricular pacing. In clinical practice, devices are typically programmed to DDDR mode with rate response *on,* which usually leads to atrial pacing. This rate-adaptive mode has been shown to increase exercise capacity in CRT patients with chronotropic incompetence (57). PEGASUS CRT is an ongoing multicenter trial that will further examine rate-adaptive mode in CRT. It will randomize CRT patients to DDD (lower rate of 40 bpm), DDD (lower rate of 70 bpm) or DDDR (lower rate of 40 bpm) to evaluate the effect of atrial support pacing on clinical outcomes in these patients (58).

The AV delay is empirically programmed to a short AV interval to ensure biventricular pacing. Echo can be used to optimize the AV delay in CRT patients as outlined in the previous section. The goal of AV optimization is to have LV systolic contraction after optimal LV filling. Strohmer et al. used echocardiographic and hemodynamic data and showed that optimal AV delay was achieved by programming a delay of 100 ms from the end of the P wave to the nadir/peak of the QRS complex on the surface ECG in patients with AV block (59). The various echocardiographic parameters to achieve optimal AV delay include mitral Doppler inflow pattern (optimal E and A waves), diastolic mitral regurgitation, LV dp/dt, and aortic velocity time integral (VTI) (4,60–62). Kerlan et al. showed that AV optimization guided by aortic VTI yields a higher systolic improvement in a prospective study comparing different echo methods (62).

As mentioned previously, RV and LV pacing can be offset in the newer generation CRT devices. Various studies have used different echocardiographic methods like aortic VTI, LV dp/dt and TDI to achieve an optimal VV interval that leads to maximal systolic function (9,63–65). Patients with ischemic cardiomyopathy may require longer VV intervals due to the presence of scar that causes slower conduction (66). Another study showed that optimal AV delay was significantly shorter during RV preactivation than LV preactivation emphasizing the need for optimizing the AV interval for different VV intervals (65). Data from the Insync III trial showed significant improvement in exercise tolerance in patients with optimization of the VV interval (67). A device based method to optimize AV and VV timings based on the intracardiac electrograms was recently validated with echo data and has been incorporated into some devices (68).

Approach to Nonresponders

Analysis of patients in many CRT studies has shown that 30–40% of the patients failed to respond to CRT as measured by clinical improvement (NYHA class, hospitalization from heart failure, improved exercise capacity) or more objective echocardiographic parameters (LV ejection fraction, LV volumes, mitral regurgitation) (1,11,13,36). The response to CRT cannot be reliably predicted by currently accepted EKG criteria for implantation (QRS width greater than 120 ms). In fact, many patients with widened QRS complexes do not respond while many who do respond do not show changes in their QRS complex (25). Figure 11.7 shows the lack of correlation between the QRS duration on EKG and mechanical dyssynchrony evaluated with TDI.

The presence of LV dyssynchrony and the site of placement of the LV lead are two important determinants of response to CRT. The role of imaging modalities like echocardiography, MRI, and ERNA in measuring LV dyssynchrony and predicting response to CRT has been discussed in detail in the previous section. The site of LV lead placement is also important; better outcomes have been noted with lateral LV pacing as compared to anterior LV

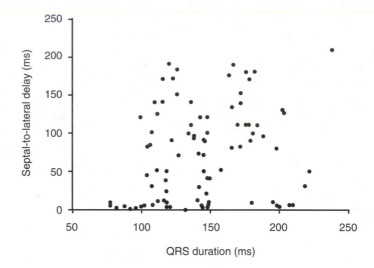

Fig. 11.7 Lack of correlation between QRS duration and LV dyssynchrony measured as septal to lateral wall delay using echocardiographic tissue Doppler imaging. (Reproduced with permission from Bleeker GB, Schalij MJ, Molhoek SG, et al. J Cardiovasc Electrophysiol 2004;15:544–9.)

pacing (69). Echocardiogram with TDI has been used to select regions of latest activation in the LV that will be ideal sites for placement of the LV lead (70). Surgical LV lead placement should be considered when the area of latest activation does not have a suitable coronary sinus branch vein that allows transvenous lead placement (71–73). Radiographic LV–RV interlead distance has been shown to predict acute hemodynamic response to CRT as measured by a rise in dp/dt; this can be used to improve the success rate at the time of lead implantation (74).

Imaging with PET or contrast enhanced cardiovascular magnetic resonance can identify areas of LV scar. The placement of the LV lead at areas of LV scarring will show no response to CRT and can lead to worsening of heart failure due to unopposed RV pacing (75) or worsening of ventricular tachycardia (76). Bleeker et al. showed that patients with transmural scar in the posterolateral LV (as assessed by MRI) did not show clinical or echocardiographic response with CRT (77).

Narrowing of the baseline QRS complex was the only independent parameter that significantly correlated with clinical response to CRT in a recent retrospective study (78); this highlights the role of the post-CRT EKG in predicting response. Molhoek et al. also showed that reduction in QRS duration >50 ms was highly specific (88%) but not very sensitive (18%) to predict response to CRT (79).

In managing nonresponders after CRT, the first step is to evaluate device related causes like ineffective biventricular pacing and also suboptimal atrioventricular (AV) and interventricular (VV) timing. More biventricular pacing can often be achieved by adding AV nodal blocking agents that prevent native AV conduction, shortening the programmed AV delay, or AV nodal ablation in patients with AF and rapid ventricular conduction. A recent study on CRT in patients with AF showed the additive value of AV nodal ablation in

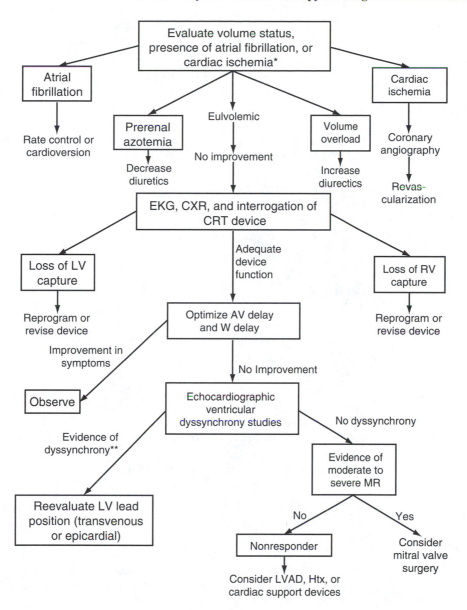

Fig. 11.8 Stepwise algorithm for management of heart failure patients who are nonresponders to CRT. AV = atrioventricular; CXR = chest X-ray; EKG = electrocardiogram; Htx = heart transplant; LV = left ventricular; LVAD = left ventricular assist device; MR = mitral regurgitation; RV = right ventricular; VV = interventricular. *Cardiac ischemia is evaluated in patients with ischemic cardiomyopathy. **Evidence of dyssynchrony includes septal to posterior wall motion delay ≥ 130 ms, intraventricular mechanical delay ≥40 ms, and tissue Doppler imaging ≥ 65 ms. (Reproduced with permission from Aranda JM, Woo GW, Schofield RS, et al. J Am Coll Cardiol 2005;46:2193–8.)

ensuring maximal biventricular pacing and better clinical outcomes (20). The EKG and chest X-ray should also be assessed to verify LV lead capture and to rule out lead dislodgement.

The next step in device evaluation for CRT optimization is programming an optimal AV and VV delay with the help of 2D echocardiogram using the mitral Doppler inflow pattern, LV dp/dt, and aortic VTI (9,60,61,64). These studies have shown incremental response to CRT in selected patients (67). Anodal stimulation should be evaluated in patients with unipolar LV pacing who are programmed to LV early (VV interval) as it can lead to noncapture of the RV lead (80). Although algorithms for MRI or ERNA are still being developed, these are other imaging modalities that may also guide CRT optimization in the future.

Finally, one needs to address the medical reasons for lack of response to CRT. These include suboptimal drug therapy for heart failure, significant mitral regurgitation, other comorbidities (obesity, anemia, severe COPD), and end-stage heart failure (restrictive pattern on echo, RV enlargement). Due consideration should be given to surgical correction of mitral regurgitation and coronary revascularization in patients with ischemic cardiomyopathy.

Aranda et al. (81) have proposed an algorithm for a step-by-step approach to CRT nonresponders as shown in Fig.11. 8.

Conclusion

Cardiac resynchronization therapy refers to biventricular pacing that improves mechanical dyssynchrony in patients with advanced heart failure, decreased EF, and wide QRS complex at baseline. It has now been shown to improve symptoms and survival based on randomized trials of over 4,000 patients. About 30% of the patients who receive CRT do not respond to this therapy. Imaging modalities like echocardiography, MRI and ERNA can improve the response to CRT by guiding both patient selection (based on LV dyssynchrony) and placement of the LV lead at the site of latest mechanical activation. Optimal programming of the AV and the VV intervals in CRT devices can improve effectiveness. Ongoing prospective randomized studies are evaluating the role of CRT in patients with mild heart failure (NYHA Class I and II) to prevent disease progression.

References

1. Cleland JG, Daubert JC, Erdmann E, Freemantle N, Gras D, Kappenberger L, Tavazzi L. The effect of cardiac resynchronization on morbidity and mortality in heart failure. N Engl J Med 2005;352:1539–49.
2. Khand A, Gemmel I, Clark AL, Cleland JG. Is the prognosis of heart failure improving? J Am Coll Cardiol 2000;36:2284–6.
3. Farwell D, Patel NR, Hall A, Ralph S, Sulke AN. How many people with heart failure are appropriate for biventricular resynchronization? Eur Heart J 2000;21:1246–50.
4. Auricchio A, Stellbrink C, Block M, Sack S, Vogt J, Bakker P, Klein H, Kramer A, Ding J, Salo R, Tockman B, Pochet T, Spinelli J. Effect of pacing chamber and atrioventricular delay on acute systolic function of paced patients with congestive heart failure. The Pacing Therapies for Congestive Heart Failure Study Group. The Guidant Congestive Heart Failure Research Group. Circulation 1999;99:2993–3001.
5. Nishimura RA, Hayes DL, Holmes DR, Jr., Tajik AJ. Mechanism of hemodynamic improvement by dual-chamber pacing for severe left ventricular dysfunction: an acute Doppler and catheterization hemodynamic study. J Am Coll Cardiol 1995;25:281–8.
6. Xiao HB, Roy C, Fujimoto S, Gibson DG. Natural history of abnormal conduction and its relation to prognosis in patients with dilated cardiomyopathy. Int J Cardiol 1996;53:163–70.

7. Unverferth DV, Magorien RD, Moeschberger ML, Baker PB, Fetters JK, Leier CV. Factors influencing the one-year mortality of dilated cardiomyopathy. Am J Cardiol 1984;54:147–52.

8. Shamim W, Francis DP, Yousufuddin M, Varney S, Pieopli MF, Anker SD, Coats AJ. Intraventricular conduction delay: a prognostic marker in chronic heart failure. Int J Cardiol 1999;70:171–8.

9. Bordachar P, Lafitte S, Reuter S, Sanders P, Jais P, Haissaguerre M, Roudaut R, Garrigue S, Clementy J. Echocardiographic parameters of ventricular dyssynchrony validation in patients with heart failure using sequential biventricular pacing. J Am Coll Cardiol 2004;44:2157–65.

10. Auricchio A, Klein H, Spinelli J. Pacing for heart failure: selection of patients, techniques and benefits. Eur J Heart Fail 1999;1:275–9.

11. Abraham WT, Fisher WG, Smith AL, Delurgio DB, Leon AR, Loh E, Kocovic DZ, Packer M, Clavell AL, Hayes DL, Ellestad M, Trupp RJ, Underwood J, Pickering F, Truex C, McAtee P, Messenger J. Cardiac resynchronization in chronic heart failure. N Engl J Med 2002;346:1845–53.

12. Yu CM, Chau E, Sanderson JE, Fan K, Tang MO, Fung WH, Lin H, Kong SL, Lam YM, Hill MR, Lau CP. Tissue Doppler echocardiographic evidence of reverse remodeling and improved synchronicity by simultaneously delaying regional contraction after biventricular pacing therapy in heart failure. Circulation 2002;105:438–45.

13. Bristow MR, Saxon LA, Boehmer J, Krueger S, Kass DA, De Marco T, Carson P, DiCarlo L, DeMets D, White BG, DeVries DW, Feldman AM. Cardiac-resynchronization therapy with or without an implantable defibrillator in advanced chronic heart failure. N Engl J Med 2004;350:2140–50.

14. Hunt SA, Abraham WT, Chin MH, Feldman AM, Francis GS, Ganiats TG, Jessup M, Konstam MA, Mancini DM, Michl K, Oates JA, Rahko PS, Silver MA, Stevenson LW, Yancy CW, Antman EM, Smith SC, Jr., Adams CD, Anderson JL, Faxon DP, Fuster V, Halperin JL, Hiratzka LF, Jacobs AK, Nishimura R, Ornato JP, Page RL, Riegel B. ACC/AHA 2005 Guideline Update for the Diagnosis and Management of Chronic Heart Failure in the Adult: a report of the American College of Cardiology/American Heart Association Task Force on Practice Guidelines (Writing Committee to Update the 2001 Guidelines for the Evaluation and Management of Heart Failure): developed in collaboration with the American College of Chest Physicians and the International Society for Heart and Lung Transplantation: endorsed by the Heart Rhythm Society. Circulation 2005;112:e154–235.

15. Bax JJ, Abraham T, Barold SS, Breithardt OA, Fung JW, Garrigue S, Gorcsan J, 3rd, Hayes DL, Kass DA, Knuuti J, Leclercq C, Linde C, Mark DB, Monaghan MJ, Nihoyannopoulos P, Schalij MJ, Stellbrink C, Yu CM. Cardiac resynchronization therapy: Part 1–issues before device implantation. J Am Coll Cardiol 2005;46:2153–67.

16. Yu CM, Abraham WT, Bax J, Chung E, Fedewa M, Ghio S, Leclercq C, Leon AR, Merlino J, Nihoyannopoulos P, Notabartolo D, Sun JP, Tavazzi L. Predictors of response to cardiac resynchronization therapy (PROSPECT) –study design. Am Heart J 2005;149:600–5.

17. Leclercq C, Walker S, Linde C, Clementy J, Marshall AJ, Ritter P, Djiane P, Mabo P, Levy T, Gadler F, Bailleul C, Daubert JC. Comparative effects of permanent biventricular and right-univentricular pacing in heart failure patients with chronic atrial fibrillation. Eur Heart J 2002;23:1780–7.

18. Leon AR, Greenberg JM, Kanuru N, Baker CM, Mera FV, Smith AL, Langberg JJ, DeLurgio DB. Cardiac resynchronization in patients with congestive heart failure and chronic atrial fibrillation: effect of upgrading to biventricular pacing after chronic right ventricular pacing. J Am Coll Cardiol 2002;39:1258–63.

19. Doshi RN, Daoud EG, Fellows C, Turk K, Duran A, Hamdan MH, Pires LA. Left ventricular-based cardiac stimulation post AV nodal ablation evaluation (the PAVE study). J Cardiovasc Electrophysiol 2005;16:1160–5.

20. Gasparini M, Auricchio A, Regoli F, Fantoni C, Kawabata M, Galimberti P, Pini D, Ceriotti C, Gronda E, Klersy C, Fratini S, Klein HH. Four-year efficacy of cardiac resynchronization therapy on exercise tolerance and disease progression: the importance of performing atrioventricular junction ablation in patients with atrial fibrillation. J Am Coll Cardiol 2006;48:734–43.

21. Wilkoff BL, Cook JR, Epstein AE, Greene HL, Hallstrom AP, Hsia H, Kutalek SP, Sharma A. Dual-chamber pacing or ventricular backup pacing in patients with an implantable defibrillator: the Dual Chamber and VVI Implantable Defibrillator (DAVID) Trial. Jama 2002;288:3115–23.

22. Abraham WT, Young JB, Leon AR, Adler S, Bank AJ, Hall SA, Lieberman R, Liem LB, O'Connell JB, Schroeder JS, Wheelan KR. Effects of cardiac resynchronization on disease progression in patients with left ventricular systolic dysfunction, an indication for an implantable cardioverter-defibrillator, and mildly symptomatic chronic heart failure. Circulation 2004;110:2864–8.

23. Linde C, Gold M, Abraham WT, Daubert JC. Rationale and design of a randomized controlled trial to assess the safety and efficacy of cardiac resynchronization therapy in patients with asymptomatic left ventricular dysfunction with previous symptoms or mild heart failure–the REsynchronization reVErses Remodeling in Systolic left vEntricular dysfunction (REVERSE) study. Am Heart J 2006;151:288–94.

24. Moss AJ, Brown MW, Cannom DS, Daubert JP, Estes M, Foster E, Greenberg HM, Hall WJ, Higgins SL, Klein H, Pfeffer M, Wilber D, Zareba W. Multicenter automatic defibrillator implantation trial-cardiac resynchronization therapy (MADIT-CRT): design and clinical protocol. Ann Noninvasive Electrocardiol 2005;10:34–43.

25. Bleeker GB, Schalij MJ, Molhoek SG, Verwey HF, Holman ER, Boersma E, Steendijk P, Van Der Wall EE, Bax JJ. Relationship between QRS duration and left ventricular dyssynchrony in patients with end-stage heart failure. J Cardiovasc Electrophysiol 2004;15:544–9.

26. Ghio S, Constantin C, Klersy C, Serio A, Fontana A, Campana C, Tavazzi L. Interventricular and intraventricular dyssynchrony are common in heart failure patients, regardless of QRS duration. Eur Heart J 2004;25:571–8.

27. Achilli A, Sassara M, Ficili S, Pontillo D, Achilli P, Alessi C, De Spirito S, Guerra R, Patruno N, Serra F. Long-term effectiveness of cardiac resynchronization therapy in patients with refractory heart failure and "narrow" QRS. J Am Coll Cardiol 2003;42:2117–24.

28. Bleeker GB, Holman ER, Steendijk P, Boersma E, van der Wall EE, Schalij MJ, Bax JJ. Cardiac resynchronization therapy in patients with a narrow QRS complex. J Am Coll Cardiol 2006;48:2243–50.

29. Turner MS, Bleasdale RA, Vinereanu D, Mumford CE, Paul V, Fraser AG, Frenneaux MP. Electrical and mechanical components of dyssynchrony in heart failure patients with normal QRS duration and left bundle-branch block: impact of left and biventricular pacing. Circulation 2004;109:2544–9.

30. St John Sutton MG, Plappert T, Abraham WT, Smith AL, DeLurgio DB, Leon AR, Loh E, Kocovic DZ, Fisher WG, Ellestad M, Messenger J, Kruger K, Hilpisch KE, Hill MR. Effect of cardiac resynchronization therapy on left ventricular size and function in chronic heart failure. Circulation 2003;107:1985–90.

31. Bax JJ, Abraham T, Barold SS, Breithardt OA, Fung JW, Garrigue S, Gorcsan J, 3rd, Hayes DL, Kass DA, Knuuti J, Leclercq C, Linde C, Mark DB, Monaghan MJ, Nihoyannopoulos P, Schalij MJ, Stellbrink C, Yu CM. Cardiac resynchronization therapy: Part 2–issues during and after device implantation and unresolved questions. J Am Coll Cardiol 2005;46:2168–82.

32. Bax JJ, Ansalone G, Breithardt OA, Derumeaux G, Leclercq C, Schalij MJ, Sogaard P, St John Sutton M, Nihoyannopoulos P. Echocardiographic evaluation of cardiac resynchronization therapy: ready for routine clinical use? A critical appraisal. J Am Coll Cardiol 2004;44:1–9.

33. Rouleau F, Merheb M, Geffroy S, Berthelot J, Chaleil D, Dupuis JM, Victor J, Geslin P. Echocardiographic assessment of the interventricular delay of activation and correlation to the QRS width in dilated cardiomyopathy. Pacing Clin Electrophysiol 2001;24:1500–6.

34. Bordachar P, Garrigue S, Lafitte S, Reuter S, Jais P, Haissaguerre M, Clementy J. Interventricular and intra-left ventricular electromechanical delays in right ventricular paced patients with heart failure: implications for upgrading to biventricular stimulation. Heart 2003;89:1401–5.

35. Bax JJ, Bleeker GB, Marwick TH, Molhoek SG, Boersma E, Steendijk P, van der Wall EE, Schalij MJ. Left ventricular dyssynchrony predicts response and prognosis after cardiac resynchronization therapy. J Am Coll Cardiol 2004;44:1834–40.

36. Yu CM, Fung JW, Zhang Q, Chan CK, Chan YS, Lin H, Kum LC, Kong SL, Zhang Y, Sanderson JE. Tissue Doppler imaging is superior to strain rate imaging and postsystolic shortening on the prediction of reverse remodeling in both ischemic and nonischemic heart failure after cardiac resynchronization therapy. Circulation 2004;110:66–73.

37. Pitzalis MV, Iacoviello M, Romito R, Guida P, De Tommasi E, Luzzi G, Anaclerio M, Forleo C, Rizzon P. Ventricular asynchrony predicts a better outcome in patients with chronic heart failure receiving cardiac resynchronization therapy. J Am Coll Cardiol 2005;45:65–9.

38. Pitzalis MV, Iacoviello M, Romito R, Massari F, Rizzon B, Luzzi G, Guida P, Andriani A, Mastropasqua F, Rizzon P. Cardiac resynchronization therapy tailored by echocardiographic evaluation of ventricular asynchrony. J Am Coll Cardiol 2002;40:1615–22.

39. Marcus GM, Rose E, Viloria EM, Schafer J, De Marco T, Saxon LA, Foster E. Septal to posterior wall motion delay fails to predict reverse remodeling or clinical improvement in patients undergoing cardiac resynchronization therapy. J Am Coll Cardiol 2005;46:2208–14.

40. Breithardt OA, Stellbrink C, Kramer AP, Sinha AM, Franke A, Salo R, Schiffgens B, Huvelle E, Auricchio A. Echocardiographic quantification of left ventricular asynchrony predicts an acute hemodynamic benefit of cardiac resynchronization therapy. J Am Coll Cardiol 2002;40:536–45.

41. Kawaguchi M, Murabayashi T, Fetics BJ, Nelson GS, Samejima H, Nevo E, Kass DA. Quantitation of basal dyssynchrony and acute resynchronization from left or biventricular pacing by novel echo-contrast variability imaging. J Am Coll Cardiol 2002;39:2052–8.

42. Yu CM, Fung JW, Chan CK, Chan YS, Zhang Q, Lin H, Yip GW, Kum LC, Kong SL, Zhang Y, Sanderson JE. Comparison of efficacy of reverse remodeling and clinical improvement for relatively narrow and wide QRS complexes after cardiac resynchronization therapy for heart failure. J Cardiovasc Electrophysiol 2004;15:1058–65.

43. Penicka M, Bartunek J, De Bruyne B, Vanderheyden M, Goethals M, De Zutter M, Brugada P, Geelen P. Improvement of left ventricular function after cardiac resynchronization therapy is predicted by tissue Doppler imaging echocardiography. Circulation 2004;109:978–83.

44. Breithardt OA, Stellbrink C, Herbots L, Claus P, Sinha AM, Bijnens B, Hanrath P, Sutherland GR. Cardiac resynchronization therapy can reverse abnormal myocardial strain distribution in patients with heart failure and left bundle branch block. J Am Coll Cardiol 2003;42:486–94.

45. Gorcsan J, 3rd, Kanzaki H, Bazaz R, Dohi K, Schwartzman D. Usefulness of echocardiographic tissue synchronization imaging to predict acute response to cardiac resynchronization therapy. Am J Cardiol 2004;93:1178–81.

46. Yu CM, Zhang Q, Fung JW, Chan HC, Chan YS, Yip GW, Kong SL, Lin H, Zhang Y, Sanderson JE. A novel tool to assess systolic asynchrony and identify responders

of cardiac resynchronization therapy by tissue synchronization imaging. J Am Coll Cardiol 2005;45:677–84.

47. Kapetanakis S, Kearney MT, Siva A, Gall N, Cooklin M, Monaghan MJ. Real-time three-dimensional echocardiography: a novel technique to quantify global left ventricular mechanical dyssynchrony. Circulation 2005;112:992–1000.

48. Doherty NE, 3rd, Seelos KC, Suzuki J, Caputo GR, O'Sullivan M, Sobol SM, Cavero P, Chatterjee K, Parmley WW, Higgins CB. Application of cine nuclear magnetic resonance imaging for sequential evaluation of response to angiotensin-converting enzyme inhibitor therapy in dilated cardiomyopathy. J Am Coll Cardiol 1992;19:1294–302.

49. Lardo AC, Abraham TP, Kass DA. Magnetic resonance imaging assessment of ventricular dyssynchrony: current and emerging concepts. J Am Coll Cardiol 2005;46:2223–8.

50. Nelson GS, Curry CW, Wyman BT, Kramer A, Declerck J, Talbot M, Douglas MR, Berger RD, McVeigh ER, Kass DA. Predictors of systolic augmentation from left ventricular preexcitation in patients with dilated cardiomyopathy and intraventricular conduction delay. Circulation 2000;101:2703–9.

51. Helm RH, Leclercq C, Faris OP, Ozturk C, McVeigh E, Lardo AC, Kass DA. Cardiac dyssynchrony analysis using circumferential versus longitudinal strain: implications for assessing cardiac resynchronization. Circulation 2005;111:2760–7.

52. Roguin A, Zviman MM, Meininger GR, Rodrigues ER, Dickfeld TM, Bluemke DA, Lardo A, Berger RD, Calkins H, Halperin HR. Modern pacemaker and implantable cardioverter/defibrillator systems can be magnetic resonance imaging safe: in vitro and in vivo assessment of safety and function at 1.5 T. Circulation 2004;110:475–82.

53. Botvinick E, Dunn R, Frais M, O'Connell W, Shosa D, Herfkens R, Scheinman M. The phase image: its relationship to patterns of contraction and conduction. Circulation 1982;65:551–60.

54. Kerwin WF, Botvinick EH, O'Connell JW, Merrick SH, DeMarco T, Chatterjee K, Scheibly K, Saxon LA. Ventricular contraction abnormalities in dilated cardiomyopathy: effect of biventricular pacing to correct interventricular dyssynchrony. J Am Coll Cardiol 2000;35:1221–7.

55. O'Connell JW, Schreck C, Moles M, Badwar N, DeMarco T, Olgin J, Lee B, Tseng Z, Kumar U, Botvinick EH. A unique method by which to quantitate synchrony with equilibrium radionuclide angiography. J Nucl Cardiol 2005;12:441–50.

56. Badhwar N, Viswanathan M, O'Connell JW, De Marco T, Schreck C, Lee BK, Tseng ZH, Lee RL, Olgin JE, Botvinick EH. Novel scintigraphic parameters to assess left ventricular dyssynchrony predict clinical response in heart failure patients requiring cardiac resynchronization therapy (abstract). J Nuc Med. 2006;47 (Supplement 1):1P.

57. Tse HF, Siu CW, Lee KL, Fan K, Chan HW, Tang MO, Tsang V, Lee SW, Lau CP. The incremental benefit of rate-adaptive pacing on exercise performance during cardiac resynchronization therapy. J Am Coll Cardiol 2005;46:2292–7.

58. Martin DO, Stolen KQ, Brown S, Yu Y, Christie C, Doshi SK, Smith JM, Gold MR, Day JD. Pacing Evaluation-Atrial SUpport Study in Cardiac Resynchronization Therapy (PEGASUS CRT): design and rationale. Am Heart J 2007;153:7–13.

59. Strohmer B, Pichler M, Froemmel M, Migschitz M, Hintringer F. Evaluation of atrial conduction time at various sites of right atrial pacing and influence on atrioventricular delay optimization by surface electrocardiography. Pacing Clin Electrophysiol 2004;27:468–74.

60. Kindermann M, Frohlig G, Doerr T, Schieffer H. Optimizing the AV delay in DDD pacemaker patients with high degree AV block: mitral valve Doppler versus impedance cardiography. Pacing Clin Electrophysiol 1997;20:2453–62.

61. Meluzin J, Novak M, Mullerova J, Krejci J, Hude P, Eisenberger M, Dusek L, Dvorak I, Spinarova L. A fast and simple echocardiographic method of determina-

tion of the optimal atrioventricular delay in patients after biventricular stimulation. Pacing Clin Electrophysiol 2004;27:58–64.

62. Kerlan JE, Sawhney NS, Waggoner AD, Chawla MK, Garhwal S, Osborn JL, Faddis MN. Prospective comparison of echocardiographic atrioventricular delay optimization methods for cardiac resynchronization therapy. Heart Rhythm 2006;3:148–54.

63. van Gelder BM, Bracke FA, Meijer A, Lakerveld LJ, Pijls NH. Effect of optimizing the VV interval on left ventricular contractility in cardiac resynchronization therapy. Am J Cardiol 2004;93:1500–3.

64. Sogaard P, Egeblad H, Pedersen AK, Kim WY, Kristensen BO, Hansen PS, Mortensen PT. Sequential versus simultaneous biventricular resynchronization for severe heart failure: evaluation by tissue Doppler imaging. Circulation 2002;106:2078–84.

65. Porciani MC, Dondina C, Macioce R, Demarchi G, Pieragnoli P, Musilli N, Colella A, Ricciardi G, Michelucci A, Padeletti L. Echocardiographic examination of atrioventricular and interventricular delay optimization in cardiac resynchronization therapy. Am J Cardiol 2005;95:1108–10.

66. Rodriguez LM, Timmermans C, Nabar A, Beatty G, Wellens HJ. Variable patterns of septal activation in patients with left bundle branch block and heart failure. J Cardiovasc Electrophysiol 2003;14:135–41.

67. Leon AR, Abraham WT, Brozena S, Daubert JP, Fisher WG, Gurley JC, Liang CS, Wong G. Cardiac resynchronization with sequential biventricular pacing for the treatment of moderate-to-severe heart failure. J Am Coll Cardiol 2005;46:2298–304.

68. Porterfield. Device based intracardiac delay optimization vs. echo in ICD patients (acute IEGM AV/PV and VV study).(abstract). Europace 2006;8 (Supplement 1).

69. Butter C, Auricchio A, Stellbrink C, Fleck E, Ding J, Yu Y, Huvelle E, Spinelli J. Effect of resynchronization therapy stimulation site on the systolic function of heart failure patients. Circulation 2001;104:3026–9.

70. Ansalone G, Giannantoni P, Ricci R, Trambaiolo P, Fedele F, Santini M. Doppler myocardial imaging to evaluate the effectiveness of pacing sites in patients receiving biventricular pacing. J Am Coll Cardiol 2002;39:489–99.

71. Dekker AL, Phelps B, Dijkman B, van der Nagel T, van der Veen FH, Geskes GG, Maessen JG. Epicardial left ventricular lead placement for cardiac resynchronization therapy: optimal pace site selection with pressure-volume loops. J Thorac Cardiovasc Surg 2004;127:1641–7.

72. Koos R, Sinha AM, Markus K, Breithardt OA, Mischke K, Zarse M, Schmid M, Autschbach R, Hanrath P, Stellbrink C. Comparison of left ventricular lead placement via the coronary venous approach versus lateral thoracotomy in patients receiving cardiac resynchronization therapy. Am J Cardiol 2004;94:59–63.

73. Fernandez AL, Garcia-Bengochea JB, Ledo R, Vega M, Amaro A, Alvarez J, Rubio J, Sierra J, Sanchez D. Minimally invasive surgical implantation of left ventricular epicardial leads for ventricular resynchronization using video-assisted thoracoscopy. Rev Esp Cardiol 2004;57:313–9.

74. Heist EK, Fan D, Mela T, Arzola-Castaner D, Reddy VY, Mansour M, Picard MH, Ruskin JN, Singh JP. Radiographic left ventricular-right ventricular interlead distance predicts the acute hemodynamic response to cardiac resynchronization therapy. Am J Cardiol 2005;96:685–90.

75. Kanhai SM, Viergever EP, Bax JJ. Cardiogenic shock shortly after initial success of cardiac resynchronization therapy. Eur J Heart Fail 2004;6:477–81.

76. Guerra JM, Wu J, Miller JM, Groh WJ. Increase in ventricular tachycardia frequency after biventricular implantable cardioverter defibrillator upgrade. J Cardiovasc Electrophysiol 2003;14:1245–7.

77. Bleeker GB, Kaandorp TA, Lamb HJ, Boersma E, Steendijk P, de Roos A, van der Wall EE, Schalij MJ, Bax JJ. Effect of posterolateral scar tissue on clinical and echocardiographic improvement after cardiac resynchronization therapy. Circulation 2006;113:969–76.

78. Lecoq G, Leclercq C, Leray E, Crocq C, Alonso C, de Place C, Mabo P, Daubert C. Clinical and electrocardiographic predictors of a positive response to cardiac resynchronization therapy in advanced heart failure. Eur Heart J 2005;26:1094–100.

79. Molhoek SG, L VANE, Bootsma M, Steendijk P, Van Der Wall EE, Schalij MJ. QRS duration and shortening to predict clinical response to cardiac resynchronization therapy in patients with end-stage heart failure. Pacing Clin Electrophysiol 2004;27:308–13.

80. van Gelder BM, Bracke FA, van der Voort PH, Meijer A. Right ventricular anodal capture during left ventricular stimulation in CRT-implantable cardioverter defibrillators (ICD). Pacing Clin Electrophysiol 2006;29:337; author reply 337–8.

81. Aranda JM, Jr., Woo GW, Schofield RS, Handberg EM, Hill JA, Curtis AB, Sears SF, Goff JS, Pauly DF, Conti JB. Management of heart failure after cardiac resynchronization therapy: integrating advanced heart failure treatment with optimal device function. J Am Coll Cardiol 2005;46:2193–8.

Pacing Therapies for Atrial Fibrillation

Michael Platonov and Anne M. Gillis

Atrial fibrillation (AF) occurs frequently in the pacemaker population particularly in those with sinus node dysfunction as the primary indication for cardiac pacing (1–3). Clinical trials have demonstrated that atrial pacing prevents paroxysmal and persistent AF in the general pacemaker population and the greatest benefit is observed in patients with sinus node disease (1–4). Many dual chamber pacemakers now have specific algorithms designed to suppress AF (4,5). In addition, there has been considerable interest in selective atrial pacing sites and prevention of AF (4,5). The mechanisms by which atrial pacing might prevent AF include:

1. prevention of bradycardia-induced dispersion of atrial repolarization which may provide a substrate for AF;
2. overdrive suppression of atrial premature beats which may trigger AF;
3. selected atrial pacing sites may shorten total atrial conduction time (otherwise termed atrial resynchronization) thus minimizing areas of slow conduction and reducing atrial dispersion of repolarization that might contribute to re-entry;
4. maintenance of atrioventricular (AV) conduction may prevent valvular regurgitation and elevation of atrial pressures that may lead to adverse atrial electrical remodeling that begets AF.

The present chapter will review clinical trials of atrial pacing for prevention of AF, trials of specific atrial pacing algorithms for prevention of AF, studies of selected atrial pacing sites for prevention of AF and pacing modalities to be considered following AV node ablation.

Clinical Trials of Pacing for Prevention of AF

A number of clinical trials have compared single chamber ventricular pacing modes to either atrial or dual chamber pacing modes on clinical outcomes including AF (1–4,6–8). Single chamber ventricular pacing, although simple, may create clinically undesirable outcomes. Ventricular pacing disrupts AV synchrony, may cause pacemaker syndrome, and precipitates mitral and tricuspid regurgitation in some. Dual-chamber pacing, has been considered to be more physiologic but confers additional cost and complexity.

The Danish Study

The Danish Investigators randomized 225 consecutive patients with sinus node disease to atrial (AAI) or ventricular (VVI) pacing (1). Over 5.5 years of follow-up, the risk of developing AF was significantly lower in the AAI group (4.1% per year) compared to the VVI group (6.6% per year, $p = 0.012$). Thromboembolic events were also to lower in AAI group (2.1% per year) compared to the VVI group (4.1% per year, $p = 0.023$).

Pacemaker Selection in the Elderly

The pacemaker selection in the elderly (PASE) trial investigators followed 407 patients age 65 or older (6) who were randomized to dual chamber or ventricular pacing for 30 months. The primary study endpoint was quality of life determined by the SF-36. Although quality of life improved significantly after pacemaker implantation, there were no differences in quality of life between the two pacing groups. Patients with sinus node dysfunction had moderately better quality of life and functional status with DDD pacing compared to VVI pacing. Patients with sinus node disease randomized to DDD pacing tended to experience less AF (12.6% per year) compared to those treated with VVI pacing (18.6% per year, $p = 0.06$). In a subgroup analysis, the PASE investigators concluded that ventricular pacing compared to dual chamber pacing was an independent predictor of AF development in patients with sinus node disease (9).

Canadian Trial of Physiologic Pacing: CTOPP

The CTOPP investigators randomized 2,568 patients from a general pacemaker population to physiologic or ventricular pacing (2). Over 3.1 years of follow-up, the risk of developing AF was significantly lower in the physiologic group (5.3% per year) compared to the ventricular pacing group (6.3% per year, $p = 0.05$). This benefit of physiologic pacing persisted over extended surveillance (Fig. 12.1). Over 6.4 years of follow-up, the risk of developing AF remained significantly lower in the physiologic group (4.5% per year) compared to the ventricular pacing group (5.7% per year, $p = 0.009$) (10). The benefit of physiologic pacing for the prevention of AF did not materialize until two years of follow-up. This suggests a delayed biological effect of pacing on the emergence of AF.

Mode Selection Trial

The mode selection trial (MOST) investigators randomized 2,010 patients with sinus node disease to dual-chamber or ventricular pacing (3). Over 33 months of follow-up, the risk of developing AF was significantly lower in the physiologic group (7.9% per year) compared to the ventricular pacing group (10.0% per year, $p = 0.008$). The beneficial effect of dual chamber pacing for prevention of AF appeared within 6 months of pacemaker implantation. The major benefit of physiologic pacing for prevention of AF was observed in those patients without a prior history of AF (50% relative risk reduction). The MOST investigators also reported a 56% relative risk reduction in the development of permanent AF in patients randomized to physiologic pacing compared to ventricular pacing ($p < 0.001$). A MOST substudy reported that

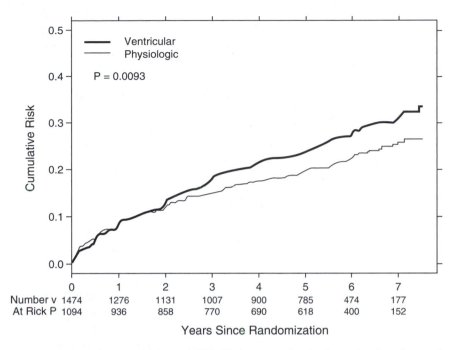

Fig. 12.1 The cumulative risk of developing atrial fibrillation according to the mode of cardiac pacing. Patients with an atrial or dual chamber pacemaker were significantly less likely to develop AF compared to patients receiving a ventricular pacemaker. Reprinted with permission from Kerr CR, Connolly SJ, Abdollah MB et al. Circulation 2004;109:357–62.

patients who were more frequently paced in the ventricle were more likely to develop AF. The risk of developing AF increased by 0.7% – 1% for each 1% increase in ventricular pacing in the dual chamber and ventricular pacing groups, respectively (11).

United Kingdom Pacing and Cardiovascular Events Trial: UKPACE

The UKPACE investigators randomized 2,021 patients aged 70 or older with AV block to dual chamber or ventricular pacing (7). Single chamber patients were sub-randomized to fixed or rate-adaptive pacing. Over 4.6 years of follow-up, the risk of developing AF was similar in the dual chamber pacing group (2.8% per year) compared to the ventricular pacing group (3.0% per year, p = NS).

Atrial Versus Dual Chamber Pacing in Sinus Node Disease

Neilsen et al. randomized 177 patients with sinus node disease to atrial rate adaptive pacing or dual chamber rate adaptive pacing with either a short (150 ms) or long (300 ms) (8) AV delay. Over 2.9 ± 1.1 years of follow-up, the risk of developing AF was lower in the atrial pacing group (7.3%) compared to the dual chamber pacing groups (23.3% and 17.5% for short and long AV delays, respectively, p = 0.03) The patients randomized to a short AV delay were paced in the ventricle 90% of the time whereas the patients randomized to the long AV delay were paced in the ventricle 17% of the time. These data suggest that even a modest amount of ventricular pacing increases risk of AF.

Meta Analysis of Trials

One meta-analysis reviewed individual patient data for five randomized controlled trials comparing atrial-based to ventricular pacing (12). This analysis included 35,000 patient-years of follow-up. No significant reduction in mortality or heart failure was seen with atrial-based pacing compared with ventricular pacing. A significant reduction in the occurrence of AF (Hazard Ratio 0.80, 95% CI 0.72–0.89, $p = 0.00003$), and stroke (Hazard Ratio 0.81, 95% CI 0.67–0.99, $p = 0.035$) were observed for atrial based pacing compared to ventricular pacing. The stroke reduction is consistent with prevention of AF, itself a risk factor for stroke.

Cost Benefit of Dual Chamber Pacing

The MOST investigators reported that the incremental cost per quality-adjusted year of life gained based over the first 4 years following pacemaker implantation was $53,000 (13). This cost decreased when the data were projected over the life of a pacemaker patient to $6,800 per quality-adjusted year of life gained. In contrast, the CTOPP investigators reported that the incremental cost-effectiveness of physiologic pacing was $297,600 Canadian per life-year gained and $74,000 per episode of AF avoided in the 1,058 patients who participated in a cost analysis substudy (14). In those deemed to be pacemaker dependent, the cost per life-year saved was reduced to $16,634 Canadian.

Clinical Implications

Dual chamber pacemakers are more expensive and are also associated with an almost two fold risk of implant-related complications compared to ventricular pacing (2,15). Most of these additional complications are related to the atrial lead (e.g. dislodgement, perforation). Ventricular pacing is more likely to cause pacemaker syndrome particularly in patients with sinus node dysfunction (1,16). For patients with sinus node disease, atrial pacing should be considered for those with intact AV conduction and dual chamber pacemakers should be considered for those with associated AV node conduction abnormalities (17). The dual chamber pacemakers should be programmed to minimize the amount of ventricular pacing.

There is little evidence to support the use of dual chamber pacing in those with permanent complete heart block (7,17). However, a number of patients with an AV block indication have intrinsic conduction much of the time (18). Given the concerns that a high burden of ventricular pacing increases the risk of heart failure and AF over time (11), such patients may benefit from newer algorithms in pacemakers designed to minimize ventricular pacing.

Selective Pacing Algorithms for Prevention of AF

AF Suppression Algorithms

A number of pacing algorithms have been developed specifically for the prevention of AF (4,5). These algorithms are summarized in Table 12.1. A number of clinical trials have evaluated the efficacy of one or more of these algorithms to prevent AF. While studies in small populations were promising, larger randomized clinical trials have not demonstrated substantial

Table 12.1 Atrial Pacing Algorithms to Prevent AF.

Algorithm	Biotronik	ELA	Guidant	Medtronic	St. Jude	Vitatron
Inhibit pauses following a PAC		Post-extrasystolic pause suppression (PEPS)		Atrial rate stabilization (ARS)		Post PAC response
Continuously pace atrium	DDD+	Sinus rhythm overdriving (SRO)	Atrial preference pacing (APP)	Atrial pacing preference (APP)	Dynamic atrial overdrive (DAO)	Pace conditioning
						Rate smoothing
Increase pacing rate following PACs		Acceleration on PAC (APAC)	Pro-act			PAC suppression
Transiently pace the atrium at high rate (following termination of AF)			Post atrial therapy pacing	Post modeswitch overdrive pacing (PMOP)		Post AF response
Prevent rapid heart rate response drop following exercise						Post exercise

AF, atrial fibrillation; PAC, premature atrial contraction.

benefits of these therapies for preventing AF (4,5). The Atrial Dynamic Overdrive Pacing Trial (ADOPT) Investigators randomized 399 patients with sinus node dysfunction and paroxysmal AF to DDDR pacing compared to DDDR pacing plus the dynamic atrial overdrive pacing algorithm (19). Patients were evaluated 1, 3, and 6 months following pacemaker insertion. The primary study outcome measure was symptomatic AF burden defined as percentage of days in symptomatic AF and documented using event recorders. Symptomatic AF burden decreased progressively in both groups but was lower in the treatment group at each follow-up visit. The atrial over-drive pacing algorithm was associated with a very modest but statistically significant reduction in symptomatic AF during follow-up (2.50% control versus 1.87% treatment, $p = 0.005$). However, the absolute risk reduction diminished over time, 1.25% at 1 month compared to 0.36% at 6 months. Furthermore, total AF burden estimated using the pacemaker stored data of the duration of automatic mode switching was similar in both groups. The reduction in symptomatic AF over time noted in both groups may reflect the elimination of bradycardia and the ability to reinitiate antiarrhythmic drug therapy.

The ASPECT (Atrial Septal Pacing Clinical Efficacy Trial) Investigators studied the role of septal pacing and three atrial pace prevention algorithms (Atrial Preference Pacing, Atrial Rate Stabilization and Post Mode Switch Overdrive Pacing) for prevention of AF (20). These investigators randomized 298 patients with symptomatic bradycardia and paroxysmal AF to septal or right atrial appendage (RAA) pacing. After a one-month stabilization period, patients were randomized in a crossover design to 3 months of the three AF pacing prevention algorithms ON or OFF. This was followed by 3 months of pacing in the alternate strategy. The primary outcome measure was AF burden recorded from the diagnostic counters in the pacemaker and reported as percent time in AF. The combined three-pacing prevention algorithms did not significantly reduce AF burden despite demonstration of a significant reduction in atrial premature beat frequency. Several other studies comparing these and other pacing algorithms have been conducted and published in abstract form (4,5). Together, these studies suggest that AF pace prevention algorithms have modest to minimal incremental benefit compared to standard atrial pacing for the prevention of AF.

Might there be subsets of patients who benefit from these therapies? Lewalter et al. classified patients with paroxysmal AF and pacemakers into a substrate or trigger group based on the frequency of atrial premature beats observed in the 5 min prior to AF onset (21). The trigger group had more frequent atrial premature beats prior to AF onset and were treated with pacing algorithms aimed at preventing premature beats. The substrate group was treated with continuous atrial overdrive pacing. For the trigger group, these investigators reported a statistically significant 28% reduction in AF burden (median AF burden: 2.06 h/day in the nontreatment phase compared to 1.49 h/day in the therapy phase; $p = 0.03$). In contrast, there was no reduction in AF burden in the substrate group (median AF burden: 1.82 h/day in the nontreatment phase compared to 2.38 h/day in the therapy phase; $p = 0.12$). In association with the reduction in AF burden, atrial premature beats were suppressed in the trigger group but not in the substrate group.

Purerfellner et al. randomized 50 patients to postmode switch overdrive pacing at 90 or 120 bpm for 10 min following termination of AF (22). They reported that this algorithm prevented early recurrence of AF but did not impact AF frequency or AF burden. This study also demonstrated some shortcomings of the existing post-mode switch overdrive pacing algorithm. These investigators reported that AF recurred frequently before initiation of the overdrive pacing algorithm due to delays in classifying termination of the previous episode of AF.

Atrial Antitachycardia Pacing (ATP) for Prevention/Termination of AF

Atrial tachycardia and atrial flutter occur commonly in patients with AF and these arrhythmias frequently transition during episodes of AF (23,24). An example of AF which organizes into atrial flutter and is then effectively terminated by atrial ATP therapy is shown in Fig. 12.2. Atrial ATP efficacy for termination of atrial tachycardia or atrial flutter has been reported to range from 30–50% (4,23,24). The hypothesis that pace termination of atrial tachycardia or atrial flutter would prevent the development of AF and therefore reduce overall AF burden was tested in the ATTEST (Atrial Therapy Efficacy and Safety Trial) (25). This was a parallel study design

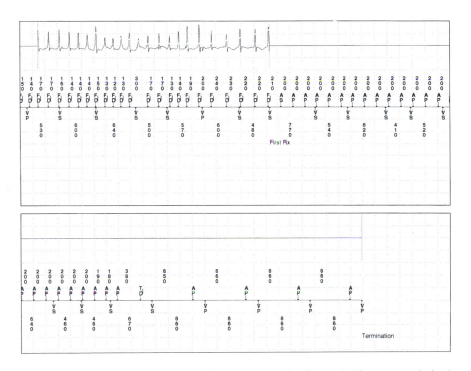

Fig. 12.2 An example of atrial fibrillation (AF) organizing into atrial flutter. A. The upper strip in the top panel demonstrates the atrial electrogram (EGM) and the lower strip demonstrates the annotated markers indicating how the pacemaker classifies each atrial and ventricular event as well as the cycle length (in ms) between each interval. The atrial electrogram shows the rapid irregular atrial rhythm which subsequently transitions into an organized atrial tachycardia. B. Atrial antitachycardia pacing (ATP) therapy – a burst train followed by two premature extrastimuli is delivered restoring atrial paced rhythm. The marker channel notations indicate how the device classifies each beat. Inter-beat intervals are also shown (in ms). AP – atrial paced event; VP – ventricular paced event; AR – atrial event sensed in atrial refractory period; FS – AF sensed event; TD – tachycardia detected; TS – tachycardia sensed event. Courtesy AM Gillis.

randomizing 370 patients to DDDR pacing or DDDR pacing with atrial pace prevention therapies and atrial ATP therapies programmed "ON". Patients were followed for 3 months following randomization. Although over 15,000 episodes of an atrial tachyarrhythmia were treated by atrial ATP therapies and device-classified efficacy was 41%, AF frequency and AF burden were not significantly reduced by the delivery of the AF pace prevention therapies or atrial ATP therapies. It is likely that ATP efficacy was exaggerated in the ATTEST study and other studies (4,23). Although ATP therapy was delivered frequently, many episodes likely terminated spontaneously and were unaffected by the delivered ATP therapy. The Medtronic AT500 used in the ATTEST study defined effective termination of AT/AF by ATP if sinus or atrial paced rhythm occurred before redetection of AT/AF. Although this redetection time is variable, it may take up to 3 min from the last therapy for redetection to occur. By shortening the redetection time, we have demonstrated that atrial ATP efficacy is lower than previously reported – atrial ATP terminated only 26% of all atrial tachyarrhythmias, and 32% of AT episodes (23).

The Low Energy in Atrial Fibrillation (LEAF) Study investigators randomized 243 patients to two periods, each 6 months in duration, to DDDR pacing or DDDR pacing plus atrial ATP and AF pace prevention therapies programmed on (26). No difference in AF burden was observed between the observation period (2.36 h/day) and the treatment period (2.14 h/day, $p = 0.25$).

Are there subsets likely to benefit from atrial ATP? We compared AT/AF burden in 261 patients who received a Medtronic AT500 pacemaker for treatment of AT/AF (27). Patients with frequent episodes of AT/AF before and after atrial ATP therapy initiation were identified from four clinical studies performed in 72 centers worldwide. Patients were divided into two groups based on device-classified atrial ATP efficacy <60% (low efficacy group) and 60% (high efficacy group). Total AT/AF burden increased slightly in the low ATP efficacy group following programming of atrial ATP therapy, (median 2.77 [25th–75th percentiles 0.84–5.86] h/day versus 2.92 [0.59–8.12] h/day, $p = 0.01$). Total AT/AF burden decreased significantly in the high efficacy group (median 2.46 [0.29–8.88] h/day versus 0.68 [0.13–2.97] h/day, $p < 0.001$). These data suggest that there is a subset of patients with AF who have coexisting pace terminatable atrial tachyarrhythmias that respond to atrial ATP therapy.

Clinical Implications

At present there is no overwhelming data to support the use of selective pacing algorithms for prevention or termination of AF. Some data suggest that individual patients may benefit from AF prevention algorithms and others may benefit from atrial ATP therapies. It is possible that some of these pacing therapies in conjunction with antiarrhythmic drug use may lead to suppression of AF in selected individuals. However, it is also possible that these algorithms may be proarrhythmic in some patients. Accordingly, therapy must be individualized and the impact of therapy re-evaluated over time. If therapies are ineffective they should be inactivated as some therapies, if used frequently, may consume considerable current and impact device longevity.

Alternative Atrial Pacing Sites

Experimental and clinical studies have demonstrated that atrial septal pacing, dual site right atrial pacing and biatrial pacing shorten total atrial activation time and reduce overall dispersion of atrial refractoriness, thus counteracting some of the consequences of AF induced electrical remodeling (4,28–30). It has been hypothesized that electrical resynchronization of atrial depolarization and repolarization achieved through site-specific pacing might prevent AF (4,28,30–32).

Atrial Septal Pacing

Electrical connections between the right and left atria are supplied primarily by Bachmann's bundle (BB) and the coronary sinus (CS) musculature (29,33,34). In Bachmann's original experiments, clamping these fibres produced significant delay in interatrial conduction (33,34). Conversely, pacing BB is associated with the shortest atrial activation times compared with other single atrial pacing sites. Yu et al. showed that BB pacing produced shorter atrial activation times and longer atrial refractory periods compared to RAA pacing (28). In addition, these investigators demonstrated that patients consistently had AF induced with early RAA extrastimulation coupled to RAA drive pacing, whereas AF could not be induced with RAA extrastimulation coupled to pacing at BB. Bailin et al. randomized 120 patients to pacing at Bachmann's bundle compared to pacing the RAA. After one year of follow-up, those with BB pacing were 75% free from chronic AF compared with 47% of patients undergoing RAA pacing ($p = 0.01$) (34).

The CS muscular sleeve has also been considered a preferential conduction route between the atria (29). Pacing at the CS os has been reported to shorten total atrial activation time compared to pacing at the RAA. Yu et al. reported that in patients in whom AF was consistently induced with early RAA extrastimulation coupled to RAA drive pacing, no patient had AF induced with RAA extrastimulation coupled to pacing at the distal CS (28). However, Duytschaever et al. reported that pacing at the CS os could prevent initiation of paroxysms of atrial tachyarrhythmia triggered by single, but not by multiple right atrial premature beats (35). Furthermore, in some subjects with AF, pacing at the CS os failed to shorten atrial conduction times. Farfield R wave oversensing is a distinct limitation of placing the pacing lead near the CS os.

Bennett et al. reported that atrial activation times were similar when pacing from the CS os, Bachmann's Bundle or the interatrial septum (30). Of these three options, septal lead placement may be preferable given its relative lack of technical complexity. Indeed, Hermida et al. showed no difference in feasibility and reliability comparing septal and RAA pacing sites, whereas septal pacing was associated with shorter interatrial activation times and reduced left atrial electromechanical delay (36).

Overall, clinical trials of septal pacing compared to RAA pacing have reported mixed results for the prevention of AF. Padeletti et al. compared RAA to septal lead placement in 46 patients with PAF and sinus bradycardia (32). AF burden was significantly lower in the septal pacing group compared to the RAA group (47 ± 84 min/d versus 140 ± 217, $p < 0.05$). However, in the larger ASPECT Trial, 298 patients were randomized to a septal or nonseptal lead location. No significant reduction in the burden of AF was observed between the two groups (31). Hermida et al. randomized 124 patients to septal or RAA pacing (37). Survival free from AF was similar in both groups. Since many patients enrolled in these studies did not experience AF following pacemaker implantation, these studies may have been underpowered to detect a benefit of septal pacing over RAA pacing.

Dual Site Right Atrial Pacing

Dual site right atrial pacing involving placement of one lead in the high right atrium and a second lead near the CS os has been studied for control of AF. Saksena et al. randomized 118 patients with paroxysmal drug refractory AF to a crossover design of three treatment periods (support pacing at a low rate, right atrial overdrive at 80 bpm or dual site overdrive at 80 bpm) (38). Each treatment period lasted 6 months in duration. Event free survival from AF tended to be prolonged with dual site right atrial pacing compared to right atrial pacing. The greatest benefit dual site pacing was observed in patients treated with Class I or III antiarrhythmic drug therapy. This therapy is more complex (requires a Y adaptor) and costly. To date the clinical data does not support this lead configuration compared to traditional RAA or septal lead locations.

Biatrial Pacing

Biatrial pacing (BAP) has also been explored for the prevention of AF (39–43). BAP shortens overall atrial activation times and it has been hypothesized that this would "resynchronize" atrial activation and repolarization rendering atrial tissue less susceptible to re-entry (28). However, not all studies have confirmed that biatrial pacing reduces dispersion of atrial repolarization (44). Biatrial pacing may also provide hemodynamic benefits which affect the electrical substrate for AF. Naito et al. reported that biatrial pacing reduced the incidence of AF following coronary artery bypass surgery compared to right atrial pacing and that effect was associated with improved cardiac output and lowered pulmonary artery wedge pressure compared to right atrial pacing (45). Other investigators have reported that these hemodynamic benefits were greatest in patients with marked interatrial conduction delay (46). Thus the hemodynamic improvements observed with biatrial pacing may have prevented AF through lower left atrial pressures, reduced atrial stretch and perhaps a reduction in atrial premature beats.

Several trials of biatrial pacing for prevention of AF have been undertaken in a small number of patients (total 149 subjects) with paroxysmal or persistent AF (39–43). D'Allonnes treated 86 patients with persistent AF in a prospective noncontrolled study (43). They reported that 55 patients (64%) remained in sinus rhythm, including 28 patients (33%) without documented recurrence of AF over a mean of 33 months. The greatest benefit was observed in patients with less marked interatrial conduction delays. However, other investigators have not been able to demonstrate a benefit of biatrial pacing compared to right atrial pacing for prevention of AF (39). The requirement for a second atrial lead to be placed in the CS increases the complexity and cost of therapy. Given the marginal therapeutic benefit of biatrial pacing compared to right atrial pacing sites, this technique has not been widely embraced for the pacemaker population with AF.

Atrial Pacing following Cardiac Surgery

The cardiac surgical population is a relevant target for therapeutic atrial pacing as up to 40% of patients will develop post-operative AF (47). A number of clinical trials of various atrial pacing sites for prevention of AF have been conducted in the post operative cardiac surgical population (45,48–53). Crystal et al. evaluated outcomes in 10 trials of temporary pacing using standard epicardial wires for prevention of postoperative AF (47). These trials were small with treatment groups ranging from 9 to 100 patients. The treatment protocols used different locations of pacing electrodes (right atrial, left atrial, and biatrial pacing) and also differed in the type of pacing algorithms employed – simple overdrive at a fixed heart rate versus more complex overdrive algorithms. All 3 pacing sites decreased AF occurrence: biatrial (744 patients enrolled) OR, 0.46 (95% CI, 0.30–0.71); right atrial (581 patients enrolled) OR, 0.68 (95% CI, 0.39–1.19); and left atrial (148 patients enrolled) OR, 0.57 (95% CI, 0.28–1.16) (Fig. 12.3). Concurrent β-blockade must be implemented to realize the benefits of atrial pacing for prevention of post operative AF. Some, but not all studies reported that BAP reduced the length of stay in the intensive care unit and total hospital stay (49,50). Debrunner also reported that fewer patients were discharged on antiarrhythmic medications (48).

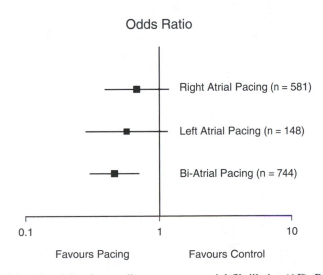

Fig. 12.3 Impact of atrial pacing following cardiac surgery on atrial fibrillation (AF). Biatrial pacing was more effective at preventing AF compared to left atrial pacing or right atrial pacing. Data from Crystal E, Connolly SJ, Sleik K et al. Circulation 2002;106:75–80.

Atrial pacing using the epicardial approach is not without the potential for complications. Undersensing may develop over time resulting in asynchronous atrial stimulation that may be proarrhythmic, i.e. initiate AF (52). Diaphragmatic stimulation has also been reported to be a significant complication (53). The rapid failure of epicardial leads due to elevation of pacing thresholds or undersensing mandates short courses of post-operative therapy. However, this usually overlaps the course of post operative AF development, which peaks at 48 h post-operatively. More recent studies have reported fewer technical limitations (48). Although promising, atrial pacing for prevention of post cardiac surgery AF has not yet been widely embraced.

Pacing following AV Junction Ablation

Permanent pacing and AV junction ablation may be undertaken for rate control of AF when drug therapy is ineffective or poorly tolerated (54–56). Overall, clinical studies have reported improvements in ventricular function, functional capacity, quality of life and general well being (54). The improvement in ventricular function has been attributed, in part, to reversal of tachycardia-induced cardiomyopathy and, in part, to regularization of the ventricular rate. Survival in patients undergoing AV junction ablation has been reported to be similar to survival in patients with AF who received drug therapy (57).

Optimal Pacing Mode Post AV Junction Ablation?

There are concerns in this patient population that continuous right ventricular apical pacing over the long term is deleterious and may increase the risk of developing heart failure (58–60). This fear has generated debate over the optimal pacing lead configuration(s) following AV junction ablation. Doshi et al. compared chronic biventricular pacing to right ventricular pacing in patients undergoing AV junction ablation for the management of AF with rapid ventricular rates (58). These investigators reported that at 6 months of follow-up patients treated with biventricular pacing had significant improvement in 6 min walk distance (31% above baseline) compared to patients treated with right ventricular pacing, (24% above baseline, $p = 0.04$). The left ventricular ejection fraction in the biventricular group (0.46 ± 0.13) was also significantly greater compared to patients in the right ventricular pacing group (0.41 ± 0.13, $p = 0.03$). However, there were no significant differences in the quality-of-life measures. Not surprisingly, the major benefit of biventricular pacing was observed in patients with depressed left ventricular function and symptomatic heart failure.

Tops et al. recently reported on the development of left ventricular dyssynchrony and heart failure symptoms during long term right ventricular pacing following AV junction ablation in 55 patients with preserved systolic function at the time of ablation (59). Patients were followed for 3.8 ± 1.7 years. During follow-up, 27 patients (49%) developed left ventricular dyssynchrony and worsened heart failure symptoms. The New York Heart Association functional class increased from 1.8 ± 0.6 to 2.2 ± 0.7, $p < 0.05$. The left ventricular ejection fraction decreased from $48 \pm 7\%$ to $43 \pm 7\%$, $p < 0.05$ and left ventricular end diastolic volumes increased. Patients without LV dyssynchrony did develop heart failure.

These studies raise questions about the optimal lead pacing site and pacing mode for patients undergoing AV junction ablation. Some data suggest that alternate right ventricular pacing sites may be associated with preserved ventricular function compared to right apical pacing (60,61). However, emerging data suggest that hemodynamic studies are required to identify the optimal right ventricular pacing site (62). Cardiac resynchronization therapy should be considered for patients with significant left ventricular dysfunction at the time of AV junction ablation. However, at present we have no systematic way of predicting which patients experience improvement in left ventricular dysfunction following AV junction ablation and which patients will experience a deterioration of left ventricular function over time. Future studies are required to determine if biventricular pacing is superior over the long term compared to alternate right ventricular pacing sites.

Dual or Single Chamber Pacing Post AV Junction Ablation?

Following AV junction ablation there is an increased risk of progression from paroxysmal to permanent AF (63–66). This may occur for two reasons: discontinuation of Class I/III antiarrhythmic drugs and the impact of continuous ventricular pacing causing mechanical and electrical remodeling that contribute to the substrate for permanent AF. The rate at which patients progress to develop permanent AF varies between studies reported and is likely dependent, in part, on the burden of AF at the time of ablation, the underlying systolic function and whether antiarrhythmic drugs are discontinued.

Brignole et al. reported that the burden of AF had increased to 30% six months following AV junction ablation in 63 patients (56). Gianfranchi et al. reported that the actuarial estimate of progression to permanent AF was 22%, 40% and 56%, respectively, 1, 2, and 3 years after AV junction ablation and implantation of a dual chamber pacemaker in 63 patients with antiarrhythmic drug refractory paroxysmal AF (63). In the second phase of the PA (3) (Atrial Pacing Peri-ablation for Prevention of Atrial Fibrillation) study, patients were randomized to dual chamber pacing versus atrial sensed ventricular pacing in a cross over study design (65). Of the 67 patients randomized, 42% developed permanent AF within one year following ablation. AF frequency and burden increases early following AV junction ablation suggesting that ventricular pacing even in an atrial synchronous mode promotes AF. Some data suggest that the rate of progression to permanent AF is higher with ventricular pacing compared to dual chamber pacing (64). The PA3 investigators performed a subgroup analysis on patients maintained on stable antiarrhythmic therapy pre and post AV junction ablation (66). The burden of AF increased threefold in the immediate 2-week period post-ablation, rising from 3.6 h/day to 10.4 on average, compared with a stable burden in the medical therapy group who had elected to defer ablation. Thus, this data suggests that continuous right ventricular pacing post AV junction ablation promotes the development of AF. Whether alternate right ventricular lead sites or biventricular pacing delays this progression is unknown. Given the high probability of permanent AF developing early following ablation, ventricular pacing appears to be the appropriate pacing mode for patients undergoing total AV junction ablation (17).

Clinical Implications

Following AV junction ablation ventricular function improves in many due to optimal rate control. However, ventricular function may deteriorate over time, in some, due to ventricular dyssynchrony secondary to right ventricular apical pacing. While patients with significant left ventricular dysfunction may benefit from cardiac resynchronization therapy, long-term studies demonstrating a significant impact on important clinical outcomes such as survival and/or hospitalization for heart failure do not exist at present. Since a significant number of patients progress fairly rapidly to develop permanent AF following AV junction ablation, AV synchronous pacing does not appear to be indicated.

References

1. Andersen HR, Nielsen JC, Thomsen FEB, et al. Long-term follow-up of patients from a randomized trial of atrial versus ventricular pacing for sick-sinus syndrome. Lancet 1997;350:1210–16.
2. Connolly SJ, Kerr CR, Gent M, et al. Effects of physiologic pacing versus ventricular pacing on the risk of stroke and death due to cardiovascular causes. N Eng J Med 2000;342:1385–91.
3. Lamas GA, Lee KL, Sweeney MO, et al. Ventricular pacing or dual-chamber pacing for sinus-node dysfunction. N Eng J Med 2002;346:1854–62.
4. Gillis AM. Clinical trials of pacing for maintenance of sinus rhythm. J Interv Card Electrophysiol 2004;10(Suppl 1):55–62.
5. Savelieva I, Camm AJ. The results of pacing trials for the prevention and termination of atrial tachyarrhythmias: is there any evidence of therapeutic breakthrough? J Interv Card Electrophysiol 2003;8:103–15.
6. Lamas GA, Orav EJ, Stambler BS, et al. Quality of life and clinical outcomes in elderly patients treated with ventricular pacing as compared with dual-chamber pacing. N Eng J Med 1998;338:1097–104.
7. Toff WD, Camm AJ, Skehan JD. Single-chamber versus dual-chamber pacing for high-grade atrioventricular block. N Eng J Med 2005;353:145–55.
8. Nielsen JC, Lene Kristensen, Henning R. Andersen, et al. A randomized comparison of atrial and dual-chamber pacing in177 consecutive patients with sick sinus syndrome: echocardiographic and clinical outcome. J Am Coll Cardiol 2003;42:614–23.
9. Stambler BS, Ellenbogen KA, Orav EJ, et al. Predictors and clinical impact of atrial fibrillation after pacemaker implantation in elderly patients treated with dual chamber versus ventricular pacing. PACE 2003;26:2000–7.
10. Kerr CR, Connolly SJ, Abdollah MB, et al. Canadian trial of physiological pacing: effects of physiological pacing during long-term follow-up. Circulation 2004;109:357–62.
11. Sweeney MO, Hellkamp AS, Ellenbogen KA, et al. Adverse effect of ventricular pacing on heart failure and atrial fibrillation among patients with normal baseline QRS duration in a clinical trial of pacemaker therapy for sinus node dysfunction. Circulation 2003;107:2932–7.

12. Healey JS, Toff WD, Lamas GA, et al. Cardiovascular outcomes with atrial-based pacing compared with ventricular pacing. Circulation 2006;114:11–17.

13. Fleischmann KE, Orav EJ, Lamas GA, et al. Pacemaker implantation and quality of life in the Mode Selection Trial (MOST). Heart Rhythm 2006;3:653–9.

14. O'Brien BJ, Blackhouse G, Goeree R, et al. Cost-effectiveness of physiologic pacing: results of the Canadian health economic assessment of physiologic pacing. Heart Rhythm 2005;2:270–5.

15. Ellenbogen KA, Hellkamp AS, Wilkoff BL, et al. Complications arising after implantation of DDD pacemakers: the MOST experience. Am J Cardiol 2003;92:740–9.

16. Gillis AM. Redefining physiologic pacing: lessons learned from recent clinical trials. Heart Rhythm 2006;3:1367–72.

17. Link MS, Hellkamp AS, Estes NAM, et al. High incidence of pacemaker syndrome in patients with sinus node dysfunction treated with ventricular-based pacing in the Mode Selection Trial. J Am Coll Cardiol 2004;43:2066–71.

18. Gillis AM, Purerfellner H, Israel CW, et al. Reducing unnecessary right ventricular pacing with the managed ventricular pacing mode in patients with sinus node disease and AV block. Pacing Clin Electrophysiol 2006;29:697–705.

19. Carlson MD, Ip J, Messenger J, Beau S, Kalbfleisch S, et al. A new pacemaker algorithm for the treatment of atrial fibrillation: results of the Atrial Dynamic Overdrive Pacing Trial (ADOPT). J Am Coll Cardiol. 2003;42:627–33.

20. Padeletti L, Purerfellner H, Adler SW, et al. Combined efficacy of atrial septal lead placement and atrial pacing algorithms for prevention of paroxysmal atrial tachyarrhythmia. J Cardiovasc Electrophysiol 2003;14:1189–95.

21. Lewalter T, Yang A, Pfeiffer D, et al. Individualized selection of pacing algorithms for the prevention of recurrent atrial fibrillation: Results from the VIP registry. Pacing Clin Electrophysiol 2006;29:124–34.

22. Purerfellner H, Ruiter JH, Widdershoven JW, et al. Reduction of atrial tachyarrhythmia episodes during the overdrive pacing period using the post-mode switch overdrive pacing (PMOP) algorithm. Heart Rhythm 2006;3:1164–71.

23. Gillis AM, Unterberg-Buchwald C, Schmidinger H, et al. Safety and efficacy of advanced atrial pacing therapies for atrial tachyarrhythmias in patients with a new implantable dual chamber cardioverter-defibrillator. J Am Coll Cardiol 2002;40:1653–9.

24. Israel CW, Ehrlich JR, Gronefeld G, et al. Prevalence, characteristics and clinical implications of regular atrial tachyarrhythmias in patients with atrial fibrillation: insights from a study using a new implantable device. J Am Coll Cardiol 2001;38:355–63.

25. Lee MA, Weachter R, Pollak S, et al. The effect of atrial pacing therapies on atrial tachyarrhythmia burden and frequency: results of a randomized trial in patients with bradycardia and atrial tachyarrhythmias. J Am Coll Cardiol 2003;41:1926–32.

26. Mabo P and the Leaf Study Group. The LEAF (Loe Energy in Atrial Fibrillation) study results: Evaluation of device based therapies for atrial tachyarrhythmia prevention and termination. Heart Rhythm 2005;2:S17.

27. Gillis AM, Koehler J, Morck M, et al. High atrial antitachycardia pacing therapy efficacy is associated with a reduction in atrial tachyarrhythmia burden in a subset of patients with sinus node dysfunction and paroxysmal atrial fibrillation. Heart Rhythm 2005;2:791–6.

28. Yu W, Tsai C, Hsieh M, et al. Prevention of the initiation of atrial fibrillation: mechanism and efficacy of differential atrial pacing modes. Pacing Clin Electrophysiol 2000;23:373–9.

29. Ants M, Otomo K, Arruda M, et al. Electrical conduction between the right atrium and the left atrium via the musculature of the coronary sinus. Circulation 1998; 98:1790–5.

30. Bennett DH. Comparison of the acute effects of pacing the atrial septum, right atrial appendage, coronary sinus os, and the latter two sites simultaneously on the duration of atrial activation. Heart 2000; 84:193–6.

31. Padeletti L, Pieragnoli P, Ciapetti C, et al. Randomized crossover comparison of right atrial appendage pacing versus interatrial septum pacing for prevention of paroxysmal atrial fibrillation in patients with sinus bradycardia. Am Heart J 2001;142:1045–55.

32. Padeletti L, Purerfellner H, Adler S, et al. Combined efficacy of atrial septal lead placement and atrial pacing algorithms for prevention of paroxysmal atrial tachyarrhythmia. J Cardiovasc Electrophysiol 2003;14:1189–95.

33. Khaja A, Flaker G. Bachmann's Bundle: does it play a role in atrial fibrillation? Pacing Clin Electrophysiol 2005;28:855–63.

34. Bailin SJ. Is Bachmann's Bundle the only right site for single-site pacing to prevent atrial fibrillation? Results of a multicenter randomized trial. Card Electrophysiol Rev 2003;7:325–8.

35. Duytschaever M, Firsovaite V, Colpaert R, et al. Limited benefit of septal pre-excitation in pace prevention of atrial fibrillation. J Cardiovasc Electrophysiol 2005;16:269–77.

36. Hermida J, Carpentier C, Kubala M, et al. Atrial septal versus atrial appendage pacing: feasibility and effects on atrial conduction, interatrial synchronization and atrioventricular sequence. Pacing Clin Electrophysiol 2003;26 [Pt. 1]:26–35.

37. Hermida JS, Kulbala M, Lescure FX, et al. Atrial septal pacing to prevent atrial fibrillation in patients with sinus node dysfunction: results of a randomized controlled study. Am Heart J 2004;148:312–7.

38. Saksena S, Prakash A, Hill M, et al. Prevention of recurrent atrial fibrillation with chronic dual-site right atrial pacing. J Am Coll Cardiol 1996;24:687–94.

39. Levy T, Walker S, Rochelle J, et al. Evaluation of biatrial pacing, right atrial pacing, and no pacing in patients with drug refractory atrial fibrillation. Am J Cardiol 1999;82:426–9.

40. Mirza I, James S, Holt P. Biatrial pacing for paroxysmal atrial fibrillation. J Am Coll Cardiol 2002;40:457–63.

41. Fragakis N, Shakespeare CF, Lloyd G, et al. Reversion and maintenance of sinus rhythm in patients with permanent atrial fibrillation by internal cardioversion followed by biatrial pacing. Pacing Clin Electrophysiol 2002;25:278–86.

42. Birnie D, Connors SP, Veinot JP, et al. Left atrial vein pacing: a technique of biatrial pacing for the prevention of atrial pacing. Pacing Clin Electrophysiol 2004;27:240–5.

43. D'Allones GR, Pavin D, Leclerq C, et al. Long-term effects of biatrial synchronous pacing to prevent drug-refractory atrial tachycarrhythmia: a nine-year experience. J Cardiovasc Electrophysiol 2000;11:1081–91.

44. Gilligan DM, Fuller IA, Clemo HF, et al. The acute effects of biatrial pacing on atrial depolarization and repolarization. Pacing Clin Electrophysiol 2000;23: 1113–20.

45. Naito S, Tada H, Kaneko T, et al. Biatrial epicardial pacing prevents atrial fibrillation and confers hemodynamic benefits after coronary artery bypass surgery. Pacing Clin Electrophysiol 2005;28:S146–S149.

46. Doi A, Takagi M, Toda I, et al. Acute haemodynamic benefits of biatrial atrioventricular sequential pacing: comparison with single atrial atrioventricular sequential pacing. Heart 2004;90:411–41.

47. Crystal E, Connolly SJ, Sleik K, et al. Interventions on prevention of postoperative atrial fibrillation in patients undergoing heart surgery. Circulation 2002;106:75–80.

48. Debrunner M, Naegeli B, Genoni M, et al. Prevention of atrial fibrillation after cardiac valvular surgery by epicardial, biatrial synchronous pacing. Eur J Cardio-thoracic Surg 2004;25:16–20.

49. Levy T, Fotopoulos G, Walker S, et al. Randomized, controlled study investigating the effect of biatrial pacing in prevention of atrial fibrillation after coronary artery bypass surgery. Circulation 2000;102:1382–7.

50. Greenberg MD, Katz NM, Iuliano S, et al. Atrial pacing for the prevention of atrial fibrillation after cardiovascular surgery. J Am Coll Cardiol 2000;35:1416–22.

51. Gerstenfeld EP, Khoo M, Martin RC, et al. Effectiveness of bi-atrial pacing for reducing atrial fibrillation after coronary artery bypass graft surgery. J Int Card Electrophys 2001;5:275–83.

52. Kurz DJ, Naegell B, Kunz M, et al. Epicardial, biatrial synchronous pacing for prevention of atrial fibrillation after cardiac surgery. Pacing Clin Electrophysiol 1999;22:721–6.

53. Gerstenfeld EP, Hill MRS, French SN, et al. Evaluation of right atrial and biatrial temporary pacing for the prevention of atrial fibrillation after coronary artery bypass surgery. J Am Coll Cardiol 1999;33:1981–7.

54. Wood MA, Brown-Mahoney C, Kay GN, et al. Clinical outcomes after ablation and pacing therapy for atrial fibrillation. Circulation 2000;101:1138–44.

55. Gillis AM, Wyse DG, Connolly SJ, et al. Atrial pacing periablation for prevention of paroxysmal atrial fibrillation. Circulation 1999;99:2553–8.

56. Brignole M, Gianfranchi L, Menozzi C, et al. Assessment of atrioventricular junction ablation and DDDR mode-switching pacemaker versus pharmacological treatment in patients with severely symptomatic paroxysmal atrial fibrillation. Circulation 1997;96:2617–24.

57. Ozcan C, Jahangir A, Friedman PA, et al. Long-term survival after ablation of the atrioventricular node and implantation of a permanent pacemaker in patients with atrial fibrillation. N Engl J Med. 2001;344:1043–51.

58. Doshi RN, Daoud EG, Fellows C, et al. Left ventricular-based cardiac stimulation post AV nodal ablation evaluation (the PAVE study). J Cardiovasc Electrophysiol 2005;16:1160–5.

59. Tops LF, Schalij MJ, Holman ER, et al. Right ventricular pacing can induce ventricular dyssynchrony in patients with atrial fibrillation after atrioventricular node ablation. J Am Coll Cardiol 2006;48:1642–8.

60. Gillis AM, Chung MK. Pacing the right ventricle: to pace or not to pace? Heart Rhythm 2005;2:201–6.

61. Victor F, Mabo P, Mansour H, et al. A randomized comparison of permanent septal versus apical right ventricular pacing: short-term results. J Cardiovasc Electrophysiol 2006;17:238–42.

62. Lieberman R, Padeletti L, Schreuder J, et al. Ventricular pacing lead location alters systemic hemodynamics and left ventricular function in patients with and without reduced ejection fraction. J Am Coll Cardiol 2006;48:1634–41.

63. Gianfranchi L, Brignole M, Menozzi C, et al. Progression of permanent atrial fibrillation after atrioventricular junction ablation and dual-chamber pacemaker implantation in patients with paroxysmal atrial tachycardias. Am J Cardiol 1998;81:351–4.

64. Gillis AM, Connolly SJ, Lacombe P, et al. Randomized crossover comparison of DDDR versus VDD pacing after atrioventricular junction ablation for prevention of atrial fibrillation. Circulation 2000;2102:736–41.

65. McComb JM, Gribbin GM. Chronic atrial fibrillation in patients with paroxysmal atrial fibrillation, atrioventricular node ablation and pacemakers. Europace 1999;1:30–34.

66. Willems R, Wyse DG, Gillis AM. Atrial Pacing Periablation for Paroxysmal Atrial Fibrillation (PA3) Study Investigators. Total atrioventricular nodal ablation increases atrial fibrillation burden in patients with paroxysmal atrial fibrillation despite continuation of antiarrhythmic drug therapy. J Cardiovasc Electrophysiol. 2003;14:1296–301.

Pacemakers and Syncope

Ehab A. Eltahawy and Blair P. Grubb

Pathophsiology/Epidemiology

Syncope is the abrupt and transient loss of consciousness due to a temporary reduction in cerebral blood flow. It is associated with an absence of postural tone and followed by a rapid and usually complete recovery. Syncope may be both benign or the only warning before an episode causing sudden death (1). Recurrent episodes of syncope may result from a variety of disorders, all of which cause a temporary reduction in cerebral blood flow sufficient to disturb the normal functions of the brain. Neurocardiogenic (vasovagal) syncope is the most common of a group of reflex (neurally mediated) syncopes, characterized by a sudden failure of the autonomic nervous system (ANS) to maintain blood pressure, and occasionally heart rate, at a level sufficient to maintain cerebral perfusion and consciousness (2–4). Syncope accounts for 3.5% of all emergency room visits and 1–6% of all hospital admissions annually in the USA (5).

The current opinion is that neurocardiogenic syncope (NCS) is only one component of a broad and varied group of disturbances in the normal functioning of the ANS. Any one of the disorders may result in orthostatic intolerance, hypotension and, ultimately, syncope.

Basic Physiology of Standing

The evolution of the upright posture has provided a unique challenge to a blood pressure control system that had principally evolved to meet the needs of animals that spent the majority of their time in a dorsal position (6–9). The ANS provides the principal means for both short- and long-term responses to changes in position (10). When standing, there is a gravity-mediated downward displacement of approximately 300–800 ml of blood to the vasculature of the abdomen and lower extremities (11). This represents a volume drop of between 25 and 30%, half of which occurs within the first few minutes of standing. This sudden redistribution of blood results in a fall in venous return to the heart. Because the heart can only pump the blood that it receives, this causes a fall in stroke volume of approximately 40% and a decline in arterial pressure.

In addition, standing produces a substantial increase in the transmural capillary pressure present in the dependent areas of the body, which causes a rise in fluid filtration into tissue spaces. This process reaches a steady state after approximately 30 min of upright posture and can produce a decline in plasma volume of up to 10% (6,10,11).

Successful maintenance of upright posture (and cerebral perfusion) requires the interplay of several cardiovascular regulatory systems and orthostatic stabilization usually occurs within 1 min. The exact response to postural change differs with standing (an active process) compared with responses seen during head-up tilt (a more passive process).

This fall in both arterial pressure and cardiac filling leads to the activation of two different groups of pressure receptors, consisting of the high-pressure receptors of the carotid sinus and aortic arch and the low-pressure receptors of the heart and lungs (2). Within the heart there are mechanoreceptors linked by unmyelinated vagal afferents in all four cardiac chambers. These mechanoreceptors produce a tonic inhibitory effect on the cardiovascular control centers of the medulla.

Reduced venous return and the fall in filling pressure that occur during upright posture reduce the stretch on these receptors. As their firing rates decrease, there is a change in medullary input, which triggers an increase in sympathetic outflow. This causes a constriction not only of the systemic resistance vessels, but also of the splanchnic capacitance vessels as well. In addition, there is a focal axon reflex (the venoarteriolar axon reflex) that can constrict flow to the skin, muscle, and adipose tissue. This may contribute up to 50% of the increase in limb vascular resistance seen during upright posture (4).

During head-up tilt, there is also activation of the high-pressure receptors in the carotid sinus. The afferent impulses generated by stretch on the arterial wall are then transmitted via the sensory fibers of the carotid sinus nerve and terminate in the nucleus tractus solitarii in the medulla (5). The initial increase in heart rate seen during tilt is thought to be modulated by a decline in carotid artery pressure. The slow rise in diastolic pressure seen during upright tilt is believed to be more closely related to a progressive increase in peripheral vascular resistance.

In summary, the early steady state adjustments to upright posture consist of an increase in heart rate of approximately 10–15 bpm, an increase in diastolic blood pressure of 10 mmHg and little or no change in systolic blood pressure (3).

Disturbances in Orthostatic Control

A growing number of autonomic disturbances of orthostatic regulation have been identified. The system in Fig. 13.1 follows that developed by the American Autonomic Society and attempts to represent current understanding of these disorders in a clinically useful framework (12).

Reflex Syncopes

NCS is a component of what is termed "reflex syncopes." These are a group of disorders that occur because of a sudden failure of the ANS to maintain adequate vascular tone during orthostatic stress, resulting in hypotension (frequently associated with bradycardia) and consequently cerebral hypoperfusion and loss of consciousness.

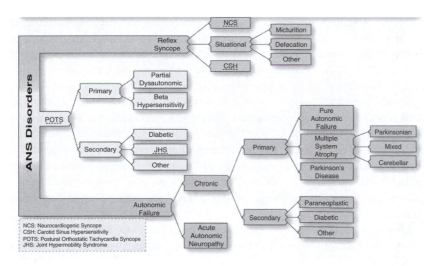

Fig. 13.1 Disorders of the autonomic nervous system associated with orthostatic intolerance.

The two most frequent types of reflex syncopes are NCS and carotid sinus syndrome. While both can represent the consequences of augmented vagal tone with similar resultant clinical manifestations, NCS occurs in a vdifferent patient population and is often associated with sympathetic inhibition as described below. NCS can be quite varied in presentation (1).

Clinical Picture: The syndrome tends to occur in younger patients and often exhibits three distinct phases that consist of a distinct prodrome (usually light-headedness, nausea, diaphoresis or visual changes) followed by a sudden loss of consciousness. The loss of consciousness is usually brief (30 s–5 min) but may be longer, particularly in older patients. Patients may occasionally have seizure-like movements during an episode (convulsive syncope). Recovery is usually quite rapid and postictal states are rare, although in older patients, confusion may occur for up to 10 min after the event. Afterward, the patient may appear pale and have an headache, weakness, or fatigue. However, nearly one-third of patients (most commonly older adults) will experience few, if any, prodromal symptoms and loss of consciousness occurs suddenly with little warning. For unclear reasons, episodes may occur in clusters, followed by a long event-free period (1,2).

Impact of Vasovagal Syncope: Almost 20% of the population experience at least one episode of neurally mediated syncope in their lifetime, and 9% faint recurrently (13). Several studies of vasovagal syncope reported that patients had medians of 5–15 syncopal spells and had been fainting for 2–10 years, and many patients fainted at least several times a year (14–21). Patients with frequent vasovagal syncope have a quality of life similar to that of patients with severe rheumatoid arthritis or chronic low back pain and to that of psychiatric inpatients (21). Their quality of life is inversely proportional to the frequency of syncopal spells (22). Vasovagal syncope is common, affects people of all ages, can occur frequently, and can be a chronic, persistent problem.

Etiology: Although the cause is still controversial (23), NCS is believed to occur in persons who have a predisposition to the condition as a result of excessive peripheral venous pooling that causes a sudden drop in peripheral venous return (24). There is growing evidence that serotonin plays a key role in CNS regulation of both heart rate and blood pressure (25). In the reflex syncopes, there is thought to be disturbances in the production of serotonin as well as postsynaptic receptor density centrally, which leads to a hypersensitive state, with excessive responses to fluctuations in sensory input on a peripheral level. This results in a cardiac hypercontractile state, which activates mechanoreceptors that normally only respond to stretch. The increase in afferent neural traffic to the brain mimics the conditions seen in hypertension and provokes an apparent paradoxical reflex bradycardia and a drop in peripheral vascular resistance (26).

Mechanoreceptors are present throughout the body (in the bladder, rectum, esophagus, and lungs) and it is thought that the sudden activation of a large number of these receptors (urination, defecation, swallowing or coughing) in susceptible individuals also sends afferent signals to the brain, which provokes a similar response (1). These result in what is frequently referred to as "situational syncope," since the syncopal episode occurs in the particular situations mentioned.

Evaluation

Diagnosis

A detailed history and physical examination are central to diagnosis (27), which requires ruling out cardiovascular or neurological disease. The recently published The Evaluation of Guidelines in Syncope Study (EGSYS)-2 demonstrated that clinical history had the highest yield in diagnosing vasovagal syncope (28). The patient should be asked about the frequency and circumstances of each event (including prodromal symptoms), as well as any precipitating factors, such as prolonged standing, fear or pain. Situational syncope is suggested if the event occurred with defecation, urination, coughing or swallowing. Patients should be asked about a family history of cardiovascular disorders or unexplained sudden death, which may direct the investigation to other more malignant etiologies. The accounts of bystanders are valuable in providing information about the duration of the loss of consciousness, changes in skin color and associated myoclonic or tonic–clonic activity. The presence of a cardiac or vascular murmur or focal neurological signs necessitates further investigation, such as echocardiography or brain magnetic resonance imaging. The European Society of Cardiology (ESC) Guidelines on syncope suggest that standard 12-lead electrocardiography should be performed routinely (with attention to rhythm, duration of the QT interval, bundle-branch morphology, and evidence of myocardial ischemia or hypertrophy) and that echocardiography be performed if there is any question regarding whether the heart is normal (29).

As mentioned previously, a detailed, careful history and a physical examination will have a much greater yield than the indiscriminate ordering of multiple laboratory examinations (28). In the absence of another identifiable cause, a compatible history is often sufficient to make the diagnosis of NCS (30). However, if the diagnosis remains uncertain, further testing is warranted.

Tilt-table testing is the only method for the diagnosis of NCS that has undergone rigorous evaluation (30). A positive test is one that provokes a hypotensive episode that reproduces the patient's symptoms. Tilt-table testing is based on the concept that an orthostatic stress, such as prolonged upright posture, could be used to cause venous pooling and thereby provoke the previously discussed responses in predisposed individuals (30). In contrast to standing, the patient is strapped to a table that is able to incline at an angle of 60–70° that serves to inhibit the skeletal muscle pump and thus force the autonomic system to function on its own. Deprived of a component of the compensatory mechanism that the person has come to depend on, abnormal hemodynamic and rate changes are more likely to be observed.

There have been numerous studies on the utility of tilt-table testing in the evaluation of neurocardiogenic syncope, that have made it a well-established component in the diagnostic work-up of this disorder (31–36).

The specificity of tilt-table testing (without pharmacological challenge) is close to 90%, but is less with pharmacological provocation. The false-positive rate is 10%. Short-term (days to weeks) reproducibility of results is approximately 80–90%, whereas long-term reproducibility (>1 year) is nearly 60% (37). As there is no true "gold standard" against which to compare it, the exact sensitivity of tilt-table testing is unknown (38). The stress induced during tilt-table testing is different from that which the patient experiences clinically. The recent International Study of Syncope of Uncertain Etiology (ISSUE) (39) compared tilt-induced syncopal episodes with spontaneously recorded episodes (with an implantable loop recorder) and demonstrated that spontaneous events were more likely to be associated with significant bradycardia (40).

Guidelines for tilt-table testing have been issued by the American College of Cardiology and the ESC, the latter being part of an updated 2004 statement on the overall management of syncope (29,41). Although useful for diagnosing NCS, tilt-table testing has not proved useful in determining the efficacy of therapy.

Abnormal responses to tilt-table testing can be grouped into five basic types. The first of these is the classic neurocardiogenic (or vasovagal) response, which is characterized by a rapid drop in blood pressure (with or without associated bradycardia). The second pattern, which the authors have termed "dysautonomic," demonstrates a gradual fall in blood pressure (with little change in heart rate) that ultimately results in the loss of consciousness (usually seen in the autonomic failure syndromes). The third pattern, a postural tachycardia response, consists of a more than 30-bpm increase in heart rate (or a heart rate of >120 bpm during the first 10 min of the baseline tilt). The fourth pattern is termed "cerebral syncope" (42); these individuals will experience syncope in the absence of systemic hypotension, associated with intense cerebral vasoconstriction (as measured by a transcranial Doppler) and cerebral hypoxia (as measured by an electroencephalogram). The last response is referred to as 'psychogenic'; in this pattern, syncope occurs during tilt in the absence of hypotension or of any identifiable change in transcranial Doppler or electroencephalogram (43).

Implantable Devices for Evaluation (Loop Recorders)

Introduction

While clinical assessment and abnormal lab tests help reach a diagnosis in most patients, elusive, infrequent arrhythmias are less easily detected. In such cases, prolonged monitoring with external and, more recently, implanted loop recorders (ILRs) has been of much benefit. This has allowed a correlation of symptoms with specific abnormal rhythms in the majority of patients suspected of having an arrhythmia.

The Implantable Loop Recorder

The only currently available loop recorder is the Reveal© Minneapolis, MN. With an operating life of about 14 months, it is implanted in the left pectoral region for optimal amplitude signal. The recorder bipolar electrocardiogram (ECG) signal is stored in the memory. This can hold 21 min of uncompressed signal or 42 min of compressed signal. The memory buffer is frozen using a hand-held activator given to the patient at the time of the implant. Interrogation with a standard Medtronic 9790 pacemaker programmer allows stored events to be downloaded.

The current version of the device (Reveal Plus©) has programmable automatic detection of high and low heart rates, and pauses. The memory configuration allows for division of multiple 1–2 min automatic rhythm strips in addition to 1–3 manual recordings. Thus, in patients unable to manually activate the device, automatic event acquisition can occur to detect extreme heart rates or pauses as preprogrammed.

Trials

The prototype of the ILR was implanted in patients with recurrent and unexplained syncope after extensive noninvasive and invasive testing was unrevealing (44). The device allowed a correlation between symptoms and rhythms with 85% success. In another trial (45) the ILR provided symptom–rhythm correlation in 7 (47%) of 15 patients who had unexplained syncope and a negative work-up. This included a negative tilt-table test and electrophysiological study.

The ILR also has a role in patients with syncope who have not undergone such extensive preimplant testing. (46–48) Studies by Krahn et al., and Nierop et al. have shown that the ILR in such circumstances lowers the likelihood of recurrent syncope by 30–70%. The utility of the ILR in establishing a symptom–rhythm correlation has been established in other populations also including pediatric and geriatric patients (46,49,50).

The ISSUE investigators (International Study on Syncope of Uncertain Etiology) have published several landmark trials on the utility of ILR in syncope. The first trial examined implantation of ILRs in three different groups of syncope patients to obtain ECG correlation with spontaneous syncope after conventional testing (51–53). The first study performed tilt tests in 111 patients with unexplained syncope suspected to be vasovagal, and implanted loop recorders after the tilt test regardless of results. Syncope recurred in 34% of patients in both the tilt-positive and tilt-negative groups, with marked bradycardia or asystole the most common recorded arrhythmia during follow-up (46% and 62%, respectively). The heart rate-response during tilt testing did not predict spontaneous heart rate during episodes, with a much higher incidence of asystole noted than expected based on the tilt response. The study highlighted the limitations of tilt testing, and suggested that bradycardia is more common than previously recognized.

The second part of the ISSUE study performed long-term monitoring in 52 patients with syncope and bundle-branch block with negative electrophysiological testing (52). Syncope recurred in 22 of the 52 patients. Long-term monitoring demonstrated marked bradycardia due to complete AV block in 17 patients. This study confirmed the previous view that negative EP testing does not exclude intermittent complete AV block, and that syncope may be a clue that conduction system disease is progressive.

The third part of the ISSUE study examined the spontaneous rhythm in 35 patients with syncope and structural heart disease who had negative electrophysiological testing (53). The underlying heart disease was predominantly ischemic heart disease or hypertrophic cardiomyopathy with moderate left ventricular dysfunction. Only two of the 35 patients had ejection fractions less than 30% which would have made them candidates for primary prevention of sudden death with AICD therapy in keeping with the MADIT-2 trial (54). Symptoms recurred in 19 of the 35 patients (54%), with bradycardia in four, supraventricular tachyarrhythmias in five, and ventricular tachycardia in only one patient. There were no sudden deaths during 16 ± 11 months of follow-up. The study supports a monitoring strategy in patients with moderate left ventricular dysfunction related to ischemic heart disease when electrophysiological testing is negative.

A single center, prospective, randomized trial compared primary use of the ILR for prolonged monitoring to traditional testing in patients with unexplained syncope (49,55). Sixty patients (aged 66 ± 14 years, 33 male) with unexplained syncope were randomized to "conventional" testing with an external loop recorder, tilt and electrophysiological testing, or immediate prolonged monitoring with an ILR for up to a year. Patients were offered crossover to the alternate strategy if they remained undiagnosed after their assigned strategy. They were excluded if they had a left ventricular ejection fraction less than 35%.

A diagnosis was obtained in 14 of 30 patients randomized to prolonged monitoring compared to 6 of 30 undergoing conventional testing (47 versus 20%, $p = 0.029$), Crossover was associated with diagnosis in of 6 patients undergoing initial monitoring, compared to 8 of 21 who began with conventional testing (17 versus 38%, $p = 0.44$). Bradycardia was detected in 14 patients undergoing monitoring, compared to 3 patients with conventional testing (40 versus 8%, $p = 0.005$). These data illustrate the limitations of conventional diagnostic techniques for detection of arrhythmia particularly bradycardia.

These data suggests that tilt testing has a modest yield at best when used as a screening test in all patients undergoing investigation for syncope, and confirms that electrophysiological testing has very limited utility in patients with preserved left ventricular function. Cost analysis showed that an initial monitoring strategy with the ILR had a higher initial cost, but was more cost-effective because the higher diagnostic yield reduced cost per diagnosis by 26% (55).

Following this, the ISSUE-2 trial (56) was a prospective multicenter observational study aiming to assess the efficacy of specific therapy based on ILR diagnostic observations in patients with recurrent suspected neurally mediated syncope (NMS).

Patients were enrolled if they had three or more clinically severe syncopal episodes in the last 2 years without significant electrocardiographic and cardiac abnormalities. Orthostatic hypotension and carotid sinus syncope were excluded. After ILR implantation, patients were followed until the first documented syncope (Phase I). The ILR documentation of this episode determined the subsequent therapy and commenced Phase II follow-up. Among 392 patients, the 1-year recurrence rate of syncope during Phase I was 33%. One hundred and three patients had a documented episode and entered Phase II: 53 patients received specific therapy (46) a pacemaker because of asystole of a median 11.5 s duration and six anti-tachyarrhythmia therapy (catheter ablation: four, implantable defibrillator: one, anti-arrhythmic drug: one)] and the remaining 50 patients did not receive specific therapy. The 1-year recurrence rate in 53 patients assigned to a specific therapy was 10% (burden 0.07 ± 0.2 episodes per patient/year) compared with 41% (burden 0.83 ± 1.57 episodes per patient/year) in the patients without specific therapy (80% relative risk reduction for patients, $p = 0.002$, and 92% for burden, $p = 0.002$). The 1-year recurrence rate in patients with pacemakers was 5% (burden 0.05 ± 0.15 episodes per patient/year). Severe trauma secondary to syncope relapse occurred in 2% and mild trauma in 4% of the patients.

The study showed that a strategy based on early diagnostic ILR application, with therapy delayed until documentation of syncope allows a safe, specific, and effective therapy in patients with NMS.

Loop Recorder Outcome

All reports using the ILR have suggested a low incidence of life-threatening arrhythmia or significant morbidity during follow-up. This verifies the general good prognosis of recurrent unexplained syncope in the absence of severe left ventricular dysfunction or when electrophysiological testing is negative, and supports the safety of a monitoring strategy. Syncope resolves in almost one-third of patients during long-term monitoring despite frequent episodes prior to implantation of the loop recorder. This suggests that syncope is frequently self-limited, or reflects a transient physiological abnormality.

The literature clearly supports the use of the ILR in patients with recurrent, unexplained syncope who have failed a noninvasive work-up and continue to have syncope. This represents a select group that has been referred for further testing, where ongoing symptoms are likely and a symptom–rhythm correlation is a feasible goal. Widespread use of the ILR is likely to reduce the diagnostic yield as the probability of recurrent syncope is less in "all-comers" (45,50). The optimal patient for prolonged monitoring with an external and implantable loop recorder has recurrent symptoms suspicious for arrhythmia; namely, abrupt onset with minimal prodrome, a typically brief loss of consciousness, and complete resolution of symptoms within seconds to minutes. Many use a left ventricular ejection fraction cut-off of 35% or less for performing electrophysiological testing prior to prolonged monitoring (54).

Loop Recorder Use

There may be a low-risk population where ILR is not warranted. This would include patients without heart disease and with relatively low burden of syncope. Testing in this group would have a low yield and the diagnosis is almost certainly benign.

Cost considerations are very relevant in decisions regarding ILRs. Cost modeling and recent cost analysis suggest that the device is cost-effective after non-invasive testing has been performed when a diagnosis is aggressively sought, comparing favorably with a conventional work-up (55).

Future Directions in Monitoring Devices

The ILR represents what is only the beginning in an emerging field of long-term physiological monitoring (57,58). Ideally, the device would include a measure of blood pressure, invaluable in the evaluation of bradycardia and possible vasovagal syncope. Sensor development will bring us commercial products capable of monitoring blood pressure, glucose, oxygen saturation, brain function, and many other physiological parameters (58). Such exciting tools for risk stratification will better enable us to manage a variety of chronic and often elusive conditions.

Therapeutic Modalities

In cases where syncope occurs only under exceptional circumstances, management primarily entails education of the patient and their family regarding the nature of the disorder and the predisposing factors to be avoided (such as extreme heat, dehydration and drugs that may precipitate syncope, for example, alcohol and vasodilators). Patients should be instructed to lie down at the onset of any prodromal symptoms.

Non-pharmacological treatments should be encouraged. Moderate aerobic and isometric exercise enhances peripheral muscle strength, thereby facilitating the ability of the skeletal muscle pump to augment venous return to the heart. Sleeping with the head of the bed upright (~6 in.) is useful in autonomic failure syndromes, as are elastic support hose that are at least waist high and provide a minimum of 30 mmHg of ankle counter pressure. Isometric counter maneuvers, such as leg and arm muscle tensing, are useful in preventing NCS if used at the earliest sign of symptoms (59,60). Biofeedback therapy has also been helpful in preventing NCS induced by various psychological stimuli (61,62).

Increasing fluid and salt intake may prevent further syncopal episodes. A reduced frequency of syncopal episodes was reported among adolescents with NCS who increased fluid intake (almost 2 L in the morning, followed by enough fluid to keep the urine clear) (63). In a small randomized trial of patients with NCS, daily supplementation with 120 mmol of sodium (~7 g of salt) for 8 weeks increased both blood pressure during tilt-table testing and plasma volume, compared with placebo, although effects on symptoms were not reported (64). Some practitioners have advocated tilt training (standing for 10–30 min each day against a wall) to desensitize patients to the effects of orthostatic stress (65); however, data on the use of this method are conflicting and long-term compliance appears poor (66).

Pharmacological Management

For patients who experience sudden, recurrent, and unpredictable episodes of syncope of neurocardiogenic origin, particularly those who have had recurrent injuries or whose occupations place them or others at severe risk for injury or

Table 13.1 Potential therapies for neurocardiogenic syncope.

Lifestyle changes	Treatment	Use and dosage	Problems
	Fluid intake	About 2 L/day	Poor compliance, frequent urination
	Salt intake[a]	120 mmol/day	Edema, gastrointestinal upset
	Physical maneuvers[a]	Isometric arm contraction; leg crossing	Unable to use in absence of prodrome
	Tilt training	10–30 min/day of standing	Poor compliance
Drugs and devices	Midodrine[a]	2.5–10 mg three times daily	Nausea, scalp pruritis, hypertension
	Fludrocortisone	0.1–0.2 mg daily	Bloating, hypokalemia, headache
	β-blockers[a]	Drugs such as metoprolol (50 mg one to two times daily)	Prosyncope, fatigue, bradycardia
	Selective serotonin-reuptake inhibitors[a]	Drugs such as paroxetine (20 mg daily) or escitalopram (10 mg daily)	Nausea, diarrhea, insomnia, agitation
	Permanent cardiac pacing[a,b]	DDD mode with rate-drop algorithm	Invasive, expensive, infection, bleeding thrombosis

[a] This treatment has been reported to be effective in at least one randomized clinical trial. For β-blockers, other randomized clinical trials showed no benefit.
[b] Recent well-controlled randomized trials showed no benefit. DDD denotes dual-chamber cardiac pacing.

death from syncope, prophylactic therapy is appropriate. The goal of therapy is to reduce both the frequency and the severity of syncopal events and to prevent fall-related injuries.

Although a variety of agents are used to prevent recurrent NCS (Table 13.1), there are limited data from randomized controlled trials to support their use and no drug has been approved by the US FDA for this indication (67).

β-blockers were among the first agents used to prevent NCS and are presumed to work owing to their negative inotropic actions that lessen the degree of cardiac mechanoreceptor activation during periods of reduced venous return. Although β-blockers were reported to be effective in several uncontrolled studies, they did not demonstrate any benefit in five out of seven controlled studies (68–74).

Fludrocortisone is a mineralocorticoid that expands fluid volume and increases peripheral α-receptor sensitivity, thus promoting vasoconstriction (75). Although very useful in treating orthostatic hypotension, its use in NCS is less well studied. In uncontrolled studies, the drug has appeared effective in reducing recurrent NCS. One randomized trial that compared fludrocortisone with atenolol in adolescents with NCS found similar results for the two drugs, although no placebo group was studied (76).

A variety of vasoconstrictive agents have been used in the treatment of autonomic disorders, including NCS. The 1-receptor agonist clonidine has been demonstrated to produce a paradoxic increase in blood pressure in autonomic failure patients who have profound postganglionic sympathetic disturbances (77). Midodrine hydrochloride, a direct 1-receptor agonist and vasoconstrictor approved in the USA for the treatment of symptomatic orthostatic hypotension, is also used for recurrent NCS (78–80). In a randomized, double-blind, crossover trial, patients receiving midodrine (5 mg three times daily) for 1 month had significantly more symptom-free days (mean difference: 7.3) and a better quality of life than the placebo group, and were significantly less likely to experience tilt-induced syncope (79).

Recently, investigators at the Mayo Clinic, MN, USA, reported that the acetylcholinesterase inhibitor pyridostigmine was effective in preventing orthostatic hypotension without exacerbating supine hypertension (81). Further randomized trials of this promising agent are now underway.

Because serotonin may have a role in regulating sympathetic nervous system activity (25,82,83), selective serotonin-reuptake inhibitors have been proposed as a potential therapy and open-label studies have found that these agents may reduce recurrent NCS (25,84). In a randomized placebo-controlled trial, 82% of patients who were randomly assigned to receive paroxetine were free of syncope for 25 months, compared with 53% of the placebo group ($p < 0.001$) (85).

It had long been noted that many patients with autonomic failure may also be anemic. Hoeldtke and Streeten published a landmark study demonstrating that erythropoietin given via subcutaneous injection could cause significant elevations in blood pressure and increasing blood counts (86). Subsequent studies have suggested that these effects are independent of each other and that erythropoietin possesses direct vasoconstrictive effects related to its effects on peripheral nitric oxide (87,88).

There is perhaps no other treatment modality that is more controversial than the role of permanent cardiac pacing. Some episodes of NCS, both spontaneous and tilt-induced, are associated with profound bradycardia or asystole which led to the impetus to test pacemakers as therapy. There have been numerous trials on pacing in syncope, the results of which have been mixed. This has led to a certain degree of uncertainty regarding the role pacemakers can play in syncope if any at all.

Pacemakers in Syncope

Trial Data for Pacing in Patients with Autonomic Dysfunction (Vasovagal/CSH)

The trials for pacing in neurocardiogenic syncope have gone through several phases. The initial results were based on observational studies. These were followed by historically controlled studies (17–19), randomized open-label controlled studies, and most recently placebo-controlled studies.

The first reports on the use of permanent pacing for neurocardiogenic syncope demonstrated that VVI mode pacing is almost always ineffective and may actually aggravate syncope because of retrograde ventriculoatrial conduction (89). In their original paper on tilt-table testing, Kenny et al. (90) also reported the successful use of dual-chamber cardiac pacing for neurocardiogenic syncope. Later, Fitzpatrick and Sutton (91) reported the results of pacing in 20 tilt-positive patients with induced symptomatic bradycardia(<60 bpm). Syncope was eliminated in about half of the patients, while the remainder experienced fewer syncopal episodes of a less severity. Fitzpatrick et al. (92) then investigated tilt-table testing performed with a temporary dual-chamber pacemaker in place. They found that temporary DVI pacing with hysteresis could abort about 85% of the cases of neurocardiogenic syncope induced by 60° head-up tilt. Both McGuinn et al. (93) and Samoil et al. (94) also found that in a small number of patients, temporary dual-chamber pacing could prevent tilt-induced syncope or at least prolong the time from onset of symptoms to syncope.

These findings are in contrast to those of Sra et al (95), who studied the effects of temporary pacing in 22 patients; 20 with sinus rhythm during AV sequential pacing and two with atrial fibrillation who had ventricular pacing alone. All 22 had an initial positive baseline tilt test. After repeating the tilt with pacing at a rate 20% higher than the supine resting heart rate, one patient remained asymptomatic, one had dizziness without hypotension, and 15 experienced presyncope rather than syncope. Only five patients had recurrent syncope during the following tilt. Afterward, all patients had repeated tilt table testing while on pharmacological therapy; metoprolol was effective in 10 of 22 patients, theophylline in 3 of 12 patients, and disopyramide in 6 of 9 patients. From this the authors concluded that pacing was of little benefit, although it could also be concluded that pacing offered a clear benefit for some patients.

Finally, Peterson et al. (18) presented data on the long-term effects of permanent pacing in patients with severe recurrent syncope and reproducible tilt-induced neurocardiogenic syncope with a pronounced bradycardic component. Dual-chamber permanent pacemakers were implanted in 37 patients who were then followed for 50 ± 24 months. Approximately 89% had a marked reduction in symptoms, while 27% had complete elimination of symptoms. There was a reduction in the overall frequency of syncopal episodes from 136 to 11 episodes/year. Interestingly, the clinical features that best predicted the usefulness of permanent pacing included a relatively younger age (56 compared to 76 years) and the absence of a prodrome (84).

The first randomized trial that appeared was the North American Vasovagal Pacemaker Study (VPS1) trial (20). Initially the study planned to recruit 280 patients randomized to pacemaker placement or previous therapy, but was stopped after recruitment of only 54 patients because of the dramatic difference between time to syncopal recurrence in the two groups. Shortly thereafter the VASIS trial reported similar results, despite the fact that there were a number of significant differences between the trials (35). Patients in the VASIS trial tended to be older and had fewer symptoms than those in the VPS study, and the follow-up was longer. The difference in syncope recurrence between the paced group and the no-therapy group was quite significant in terms of syncope recurrence.

The potential benefit of a rate-drop response pacemaker was evaluated by Ammirati et al. in the SYDIT trial (96). They studied a total of 20 patients over a 17 ± 4 month follow-up period and found that the rate drop pacing algorithm was better than rate hysteresis. Ammirati et al. (97) later reported the results of a multicenter, randomized trial of medical therapy with atenolol compared to dual-chamber cardiac pacing. The paced group had significantly lower syncope recurrence than did the atenolol group.

Two recent trials have cast some doubt on the efficacy of pacing in neurocardiogenic syncope. The VPS2 trial was a randomized, double blinded trial of 100 patients who all received dual-chamber pacemakers and were then randomized to being "ON" (DDD mode) or "OFF" (ODO; sensing without pacing) (98). Patients included had six or more episodes of syncope during their lifetime or had at least three episodes during the prior 2 years. They also had positive tilt-table tests; however, no standardized test protocol was employed and provocation was with either nitroglycerine or isoproterenol. Interestingly, only 15–23% of patients had recorded heart rates of less than 40 bpm. No significant difference was observed in time to first syncopal recurrence between the two groups over a 6-month follow-up period – the pacing "ON" group had a relative risk reduction of 30%. It is interesting to speculate if this trend may have become more significant had the study continued for a longer period of time; however, at 6 months the groups were then changed to rate drop response versus conventional rate hyteresis.

A similar study was the SYNPACE trial (99) which compared 29 patients with pacemakers turned "ON" versus those turned "OFF." While there was no significant difference in syncope recurrence between the two groups, those patients who had asystolic preimplant tilt table tests showed a significant increase in time to recurrence compared to those who only experienced bradycardia (91 days versus 11 days). Interestingly, in the VASIS trial 85% of patients had tilt-induced asystole, and in the SYNDIT trial 60% had asystole. This raises the possibility that asystole during tilt testing may be a predictor of response to permanent cardiac pacing. Also, patients in both the VASIS and SYDIT trials were older, raising the question as to whether age may be a predictor of pacing response.

Can Tilt Test Result Predict a Successful Response to Pacing?

Petersen et al. (18) found that the degree of cardio inhibition did not correlate with the degree of benefit from permanent pacing. More recently, the ISSUE investigators reported that asystole during tilt testing did not predict asystole during follow-up (39); indeed, some patients with tilt-induced asystole had syncope without bradycardia (vasodepressor syncope). An asystolic response during recurrent syncope was found even if the patient had a vasodepressor response during the tilt-table test. Finally, the authors followed 40 syncope patients with pacemakers for a median of 5 years. Syncope recurred in nearly 75%, and bradycardia during tilt testing did not predict a response to pacing at all (100). Together, these data suggest that the hemodynamic response during tilt-table testing (including trough heart rate) does not predict the hemodynamic responses during spontaneous syncope, and does not predict the response to permanent pacemaker insertion.

Indications for Permanent Pacing in Patients with Autonomic Dysfunction

In an attempt to organize the available trial data into practical recommendations, the AHA/ACC have established guidelines for the use of permanent pacemakers in carotid hypersensitivity and neurally mediated syncope (Table 13.2). (101)

Table 13.2 Indications for permanent pacing in hypersensitive carotid sinus syndrome and neurally mediated syncope.

Class I

1. Recurrent syncope caused by carotid sinus stimulation; minimal carotid sinus pressure induces ventricular asystole of >3-s duration in the absence of any medication that depresses the sinus node or AV conduction. (Level of evidence: C)

Class IIa

1. Recurrent syncope without clear, provocative events and with a hypersensitive cardioinhibitory response. (Level of evidence: C)

2. Syncope of unexplained origin when major abnormalities of sinus node function or AV conduction are discovered or provoked in electrophysiological studies. (Level of evidence: C)

Class IIb

1. Neurally mediated syncope with significant bradycardia reproduced by a head-up tilt with or without isoproterenol or other provocative maneuvers. (Level of evidence: B)

Class III

1. A hyperactive cardio inhibitory response to carotid sinus stimulation in the absence of symptoms.

2. A hyperactive cardio inhibitory response to carotid sinus stimulation in the presence of vague symptoms such as dizziness, light-headedness, or both.

3. Recurrent syncope, light-headedness, or dizziness in the absence of a hyperactive cardio inhibitory response.

4. Situational vasovagal syncope in which avoidance behavior is effective.

Gabriel Gregoratos, Melvin D. Cheitlin, Alicia Conill, Andrew E. Epstein, Christopher Fellows, T. Bruce Ferguson, Jr, Roger A. Freedman, Mark A. Hlatky, Gerald V. Naccarelli, Sanjeev Saksena, Robert C. Schlant, and Michael J. Silka. ACC/AHA Guidelines for Implantation of Cardiac Pacemakers and Antiarrhythmia Devices: Executive Summary: A Report of the American College of Cardiology/American Heart Association Task Force on Practice Guidelines (Committee on Pacemaker Implantation). *Circulation* 97:1325–1335.

Optimal Mode for Sensing in Vasovagal Syncope

Early detection of impending vasovagal syncope is a key factor in the development of an effective pacing strategy. Unlike other conditions requiring pacing, the fall in heart rate during vasovagal syncope is often insidious rather than abrupt. Pacemakers with a rate drop response algorithm are therefore considered particularly appropriate as they take account of the rate of fall, as opposed to the more conventional rate hysteresis systems that pace when a particular heart rate is reached.

In a randomized trial, Ammirati et al. compared rate drop responsiveness and rate hysteresis in 20 patients with recurrent syncope (96). This study demonstrated a benefit for those with rate drop responsiveness (0 of 12 fainted) compared with rate hysteresis (3 of 8 fainted). The second phase of VPS II (97) hopes to establish whether dual-chamber pacing with rate drop sensing is superior to dual-chamber pacing at an escape rate of 50 bpm.

Optimal Mode for Pacing in Vasovagal Syncope

Early studies showed single-chamber ventricular demand pacing (VVI) to be ineffective in preventing vasovagal syncope (89,94).The absence of atrioventricular synchrony appears to aggravate the peripheral vasodilatation, perhaps by retrograde activation of atria and release of natriuretic peptides. Invasive hemodynamic studies have demonstrated that dual-chamber pacing achieves a reduction in the rate of fall of arterial pressure as heart rate drops, which in the clinical setting may sufficiently prolong consciousness to allow injury to be avoided.

McLeod et al. (102) assessed the relative usefulness of single-chamber pacing (VVI) and dual-chamber pacing (DDD) in the prevention of vasovagal syncope in 12 highly symptomatic young children (19). In a three way, double blind randomized crossover design, the pacemakers were programmed to no pacing, ventricular pacing with rate hysteresis, or dual-chamber pacing with rate drop responsiveness. Each treatment exposure lasted 4 months. Both pacing modes were equivalent, and more effective than no pacing, in preventing syncope. DDD pacing was superior to VVI pacing in preventing presyncope. Dual-chamber pacing has now been clinically assessed in randomized trials of pacing in vasovagal syncope, and is generally considered to be the pacing mode of choice (20,35,84).

However, the optimal pacemaker intervention rate is still the subject of debate. It has been suggested that high rate intervention (>120 bpm) may be better than standard rate pacing (80–90 bpm) in improving symptoms and/or aborting syncope (20).

Selecting Patients for Pacing

The crucial issue is to identify individuals who could benefit from pacing. Pacemakers should be considered for patients with frequent and medically refractory vasovagal syncope in whom there is evidence for bradycardia. Patients with specific drug intolerances or contraindications may be considered earlier. The VASIS group proposed a classification of the hemodynamic collapse patterns seen on tilt testing for the purpose of identifying potential candidates for drug or pacemaker trials (35).

Patients with predominant bradycardia (cardio inhibition) are the target for pacing. Within this group there is further subdivision into more severe or less severe forms. The expectation is that those with the more severe form will derive the greatest benefit from pacing. However, there is concern with pacing this group as it appears that more severe cardio inhibition is more prevalent in the younger population. Pacing young people has a considerable long-term burden, not least of which is the need for periodic system replacement. The other groups that may benefit from pacing are those with chronotropic incompetence. This usually affects a much older population, so there is less reluctance to pace these patients.

Limitations of Cardiac Pacing

Cardiac pacing cannot address the profound vasodilatation that occurs together with cardio inhibition in vasovagal syncope. Therefore, pacing should not be seen in isolation or always as an alternative to pharmacological intervention. Recently, there has been interest in a combined approach, using pharmacological support for the vasodepressor component and pacing for the cardio inhibitory component – for example, fludrocortisone to minimize intravascular volume depletion and pacing to modify the heart rate response.

Conclusion

As Sutton noted (103), pacing appears to be a very effective means of symptom control, and there is no doubt that it does work in some patients. Based on the physiological processes at play in neurocardiogenic syncope, it should be remembered that a fall in blood pressure usually precedes the fall in heart rate. Thus, pacing determined by rate criteria alone may represent "too little too late." The development of newer sensor technology that allows for the direct or indirect measurement of blood pressure would permit the onset of pacing at the earliest point in the syncopal episode.

Sra (104) has noted that evaluation of any therapy in neurocardiogenic syncope has been undermined by a number of factors. Amongst these he cites "difficulty in demonstrating efficacy of therapy under controlled conditions, unrealistic end-points (i.e. a goal of eliminating all symptoms) and inadequate understanding of the natural history of the problem."

At present pacing should not be employed as first-line therapy for a number of reasons. Many patients will respond to conservative measures, or a number of potential pharmacotherapeutic agents. Also, as the VPS2 and SYNPACE trial seem to indicate, pacing differs little from standard therapy. However, for patients who demonstrate a significant bradycardic or asystolic component of their syncope, cardiac pacing may significantly prolong the time from the onset of symptoms to loss of consciousness. For patients who experience little or no warning prior to syncope, pacing may cause a more gradual fall in blood pressure that can be perceived as a prodrome, thereby allowing them to take appropriate evasive actions such as lying or sitting down.

Treatment of Specific Unusual Conditions (Autonomic Dysfunction)

While there has been several trials investigating the use of pacemakers in neurocardiogenic syncope, there is less data available on the use of pacing in orthostatic intolerance and autonomic dysfunction. Moss et. al (105) and Weismann et. al (106) initially reported that cardiac tachypacing could be beneficial and improves symptoms in selected patients with severe orthostatic hypotension. Abe et al (107) reported on two patients with severe refractory orthostatic hypotension, in whom tachypacing at 100 bpm improved the blood pressure drop in the upright position and prevented syncope.

Two further small case series by Sahul et al. (108), and Fortrat et al. (109) showed no improvement in either symptoms or hemodynamic variables in patients with severe orthostatic hypotension. In fact the report by Fortrat actually suggested a worsening in upright blood pressure response. Both studies would seem to indicate that tachycardia alone cannot compensate for an upright fall in blood pressure, and that there are other mechanisms at play. Further studies on the role of pacemakers are certainly warranted in these conditions.

Conclusions/Summary Recommendations

Future Perspective

Over the next few years, it is anticipated that major advances will be made in understanding the pathogenetic etiology of the autonomic disorders, including NCS. Similar to the technological advances that have permitted the identification and analysis of the genes responsible for almost all patients with a congenital long QT syndrome, it is highly likely that by elucidating the genotypic and molecular basis for the autonomic disorders, we may be able to individualize the management of the various phenotypic presentations.

Such fundamental knowledge has already been gained with a relatively new subgroup of disorders currently referred to as the postural tachycardia syndrome (Fig. 13.1). This appears to be a milder, less severe form of autonomic insufficiency that is characterized by excessive increases in heart rate while in the upright position. Recent investigations have suggested a genetic basis for this group of disorders. A landmark study by Shannon and colleagues has identified the exact genes responsible for this subgroup in one family with a number of severely affected members (110). The defect was in the genetic code for a protein responsible for recycling norepinephrine in the intrasynaptic cleft, which allowed for excessively high levels of serum norepinephrine. There may be multiple genetic forms of this and other autonomic disorders and studies are underway to determine this.

In addition, it is very likely that other molecular or pathophysiological etiologies will be unraveled, leading to unique approaches to treatment. In a recent paper by Schroeder and colleagues, antibodies against the ganglionic acetylcholine receptors were detected in the serum of a patient with long-standing severe autonomic failure (111). Removal of the antibodies by means of plasma exchange resulted in a dramatic clinical improvement. The authors suggest that patients with autonomic failure that is not otherwise explained should be tested for the presence of antiganglionic acetylcholine receptor antibodies. This may be one of many such auto antibodies, knowledge of which will pave the way for a more individualized approach to both the diagnosis and the therapy of autonomic disorders in general.

With regards to pacemakers and device therapy in syncope, further refinement in the ability to detect incipient syncope may arise from the recognition of other sensing strategies, such as changes in the QT interval, right ventricular pressure, central venous temperature or changes in respiratory pattern. Minute ventricular sensing together with heart rate change may offer earlier detection of impending vasovagal syncope than can heart rate alone (112) Pacemakers with varying capabilities are now available, and could prove to be a significant adjunct to current sensing modes.

Conclusion

NCS can be a challenging and potentially frustrating syndrome for both the patient and the physician. Even if the cause is benign, recurrent episodes of syncope do not only result in injury, but may provoke substantial anxiety among patients and their families, producing a degree of functional impairment similar to that seen in many chronic debilitating disorders. There are a few data available on the natural history of this disorder and the results of a few large, randomized trials guide decision-making regarding the optimal therapy. Further investigations will aid in our understanding of this disorder, at the same time identify better diagnostic and therapeutic modalities, and clarify the role device recorders and pacemakers can play in management.

References

1. Grubb BP: Neurocardiogenic syncope. In: Syncope: mechanisms and management. Grubb B, Olshansky B (Eds.) Malden, Mass, Blackwell/Futura Publishing 47–71 (2005).
2. Grubb BP, Karas B: Clinical disorders of the autonomic nervous system associated with orthostatic intolerance: an overview of classification, clinical evaluation, and management. Pacing Clin. Electrophysiol. 22(5), 798–810 (1999).
3. Wieling W, van Lieshout J: Maintenance of postural normotension in humans. In: Clinical Autonomic Disorders: Evaluation and Management, 2nd Edition. Low PA (Ed.), Philadelphia, Lippincott-Raven, PA, USA 73–82 (1997).
4. Shepherd RFJ, Shepherd JT: Control of the blood pressure and the circulation in man. In: Autonomic Failure: A Textbook of Clinical Disorders of the Autonomic Nervous System, 4th Edition. Mathias CJ, Bannister R (Eds.), Oxford University Press, Oxford, England, 72–75 (1999).
5. Goldschlager N, Epstein AE, Grubb BP et al.: Etiologic considerations in the patient with syncope and an apparently normal heart. Arch. Intern. Med. 163, 151–162 (2003).
6. Bannister R, Mathias CJ: Introduction and classification of autonomic disorders. In: Autonomic Failure: A Textbook of Clinical Disorders of the Autonomic Nervous System. Mathias C, Bannister R (Eds.) Oxford Press, Oxford, UK, xvii–xxii (1999).
7. Calabrese R, Gordon T, Hawkins R, Qian N: Essentials of Neural Science and Behaviour. Appleton & Lange, Norwalk, CT (1995).
8. Bennaroch E: The Central Autonomic Network: Functional Organization and Clinical Correlations. Futura Press, Armonk, NY, USA (1997).
9. Appenzeller O, Oribe E: The Autonomic Nervous System: An Introduction to Basic and Clinical Concepts. Elsevier Science, Amsterdam, The Netherlands (1997).
10. Joyner M, Sheppard T: Autonomic regulation of the circulation. In: Clinical Autonomic Disorders, 2nd Edition. Low P (Ed.), Lippincott-Raven, Philadelphia, PA 61–71 (1997).
11. Thompson WO, Thompson PK, Dailey ME: The effect of upright posture on the composition and volume of the blood in man. J. Clin. Invest. 5, 573–609 (1988).
12. Consensus Committee of the American Autonomic Society and the American Academy of Neurology on the definition of orthostatic hypotension, pure autonomic failure and multiple system atrophy. Neurology 46, 1470–1471 (1996).
13. Chen LY, Shen WK, Mahoney DW, et al.: Prevalence of self-reported syncope: an epidemiologic study from Olmsted County, MN [abstract]. J. Am. Coll. Cardiol. 39, 114A–115A (2002).
14. Sheldon R, Rose S, Flanagan P, et al.: Risk factors for syncope recurrence after a positive tilt-table test in patients with syncope. Circulation 93, 973–981 (1996).
15. Grimm W, Degenhardt M, Hoffman J, et al.: Syncope recurrence can better be predicted by history than by head-up tilt testing in untreated patients with suspected neurally mediated syncope. Eur. Heart. J. 18, 1465–1469 (1997).
16. Natale A, Geiger MJ, Maglio C, et al.: Recurrence of neurocardiogenic syncope without pharmacologic interventions. Am. J. Cardiol. RF77, 1001–1003 (1996).
17. Benditt DG, Sutton R, Gammage MD, et al.: Clinical experience with Thera DR rate-drop response pacing algorithm in carotid sinus syndrome and vasovagal syncope. The International Rate-Drop Investigators Group. Pacing. Clin. Electrophysiol. 20, 832–839 (1997).

18. Petersen ME, Chamberlain-Webber R, Fitzpatrick AP, et al.: Permanent pacing for cardioinhibitory malignant vasovagal syndrome. Br. Heart. J. 71, 274–281 (1994).

19. Sheldon R, Koshman ML, Wilson W, et al.: Effect of dual-chamber pacing with automatic rate-drop sensing on recurrent neurally mediated syncope. Am. J. Cardiol. 81, 158–162 (1998).

20. Connolly SJ, Sheldon R, Roberts RS, Gent M. The North American vasovagal pacemaker study (VPS): a randomized trial of permanent cardiac pacing for the prevention of vasovagal syncope. J. Am. Coll. Cardiol. 33, 16–20 (1999).

21. Linzer M, Pontinen M, Gold DT, et al.: Impairment of physical and psychosocial function in recurrent syncope. J. Clin. Epidemiol. 44, 1037–1043 (1991).

22. Rose MS, Koshman ML, Spreng S, et al.: The relation between health-related quality of life and frequency of spells in patients with syncope. J. Clin. Epidemiol. 53, 1209–1216 (2000).

23. Mosqueda-Garcia R, Furlan R, Tank J, Fernandez-Violante R: The elusive pathophysiology of neurally mediated syncope. Circulation 102, 2898–2906 (2000).

24. Kosinski D, Grubb BP, Temesy-Armos P: Pathophysiological aspects of neurocardiogenic syncope: current concepts and new perspectives. Pacing Clin. Electrophysiol. 18, 716–724 (1995).

25. Grubb BP, Karas BJ: The potential role of serotonin in the pathogenesis of neurocardiogenic syncope and related autonomic disturbances. J. Intervent. Cardiac Electrophysiol. 2, 325–332 (1998).

26. Lurie KG, Benditt D: Syncope and the autonomic nervous system. J. Cardiovasc. Electrophysiol. 7, 760–776 (1996).

27. Linzer M, Yang EH, Estes NA III et al.: Diagnosing syncope. 1. Value of history, physical examination, and electrocardiography: Clinical Efficacy Assessment Project of the American College of Physicians. Ann. Intern. Med. 126, 989–996 (1997).

28. Brignole M, Menozzi C, Bartoletti A et al.: For the Evaluation of Guidelines in Syncope Study 2 (EGSYS-2) group: a new management of syncope: prospective systematic guideline-based evaluation of patients referred urgently to general hospitals. Eur. Heart J. 27(1), 76–82 (2006).

29. Brignole M, Alboni P, Benditt D et al.: Task force on syncope, European Society of Cardiology. Guidelines on management (diagnosis and treatment) of syncope – Update 2004. Executive summary. Europace 6, 467–537 (2004).

30. Grubb BP, Kosinski D: Tilt table testing: concepts and limitations. Pacing Clin. Electrophysiol. 20, 781–787 (1997).

31. Grubb BP: Tilt table testing. In: Syncope: mechanisms and management. Grubb B, Olshansky B (Eds.) Blackwell/Futura Publishing, Malden, MA (2005).

32. Garcia-Civera R, Ruiz-Granell R, Morell-Cabedo S et al.: Significance of tilt table testing in patients with suspected arrhythmic syncope and negative alectrophysiologic study. J. Cardiovasc. Electrophysiol. 16(9), 938–942 (2005).

33. Sagristà-Sauleda J, Romero B, Permanyer-Miralda G, Moya A, Soler-Soler J: Reproducibility of sequential head-up tilt testing in patients with recent syncope, normal ECG and no structural heart disease. Eur. Heart J. 23, 1706–1713 (2002).

34. Kenny RA, O'Shea D, Parry SW: The Newcastle protocols for head-up tilt table testing in the diagnosis of vasovagal syncope, carotid sinus hypersensitivity, and related disorders. Heart 83, 564–569 (2000).

35. Sutton R, Brignole M, Menozzi C et al. for the Vasovagal Syncope International Study (VASIS) Investigators: Dual-chamber pacing in the treatment of neurally mediated tilt-positive cardioinhibitory syncope: pacemaker versus no therapy: a multicenter randomized study. Circulation 102(3), 294–299 (2000).

36. Hermosillo AG, Jordan JL, Vallejo M, Kostine A, Marquez MF, Cardenas M: Cerebrovascular blood flow during the near syncopal phase of head-up tilt test: a comparative study in different types of neurally mediated syncope. Europace 8(3), 199–203 (2006).

37. Sutton R, Benditt D: The basic autonomic assessment. In: The Evaluation and Management of Syncope. Benditt D, Blanc JJ, Brignole M, Sutton R (Eds.). Blackwell-Futura, Malden, MA 71–79 (2003).

38. Krahn A, Klein GJ, Yee R, Skanes AC: Randomized assessment of syncope trial: conventional diagnostic testing versus a prolonged monitoring strategy. Circulation 104, 46–51 (2001).

39. Menozzi C, Brignole M, Garcia-Civera R et al.: International Study on Syncope of Uncertain Etiology (ISSUE): mechanism of syncope in patients with heart disease and negative electrophysiologictest. Investig. Circulation 105(23), 2741–2745 (2002).

40. Benditt D, Ferguson D, Grubb BP, Kapoor WN, Kugler J, Lerman BB: Tilt table testing for accessing syncope and its treatment: an American College of Cardiology Consensus document. J. Am. Coll. Cardiol. 28, 263–267 (1996).

41. Brignole M, Alboni P, Benditt L et al.: Guidelines on the management, diagnosis and treatment of syncope. Euro. Heart J. 22, 1256–1306 (2001).

42. Grubb BP, Samoil D, Kosinski D et al.: Cerebral syncope: loss of consciousness associated with cerebral vasoconstriction in the absence of systemic hypotension. Pacing Clin. Electrophysiol. 21, 652–658 (1988).

43. Grubb BP, Gerard G, Wolfe DA, Samoil D, Davenport CW, Homan RW: Syncope and seizure of psychogenic origin: identification with head upright tilt table testing. Clin. Cardiol. 15, 839–842 (1992).

44. Krahn AD, Klein GJ, Norris C, Yee R. The etiology of Syncope in patients with negative tilt table and electrophysiological testing. Circulation 92, 1819–1824 (1995).

45. Garcia-Civera R, Ruiz-Granell R, Morell-Cabedo S, et al. Selective use of diagnostic tests in patients with syncope of unknown cause. JACC 41, 787–790 (2003).

46. Krahn AD, Klein GJ, Yee R, Takle-Newhouse T, Norris C. Use of an extended monitoring strategy in patients with problematic syncope. Reveal Investigators. Circulation 99, 406–410 (1999).

47. Nierop PR, van Mechelen R, van Elsacker A, Luijten RH, Elhendy A. Heart rhythm during syncope and presyncope: results of implantable loop recorders. Pacing Clin. Electrophysiol. 23, 1532–1538 (2000).

48. Krahn AD, Klein GJ, Yee R, Norris C. Final results from a pilot study with an implantable loop recorder to determine the etiology of syncope in patients with negative non-invasive and invasive testing. Am. J Cardiol. 82, 117–119 (1998).

49. Ermis C, Zhu AX, Pham S, et al. Comparison of automatic and patient-activated arrhythmia recordings by implantable loop recorders in the evaluation of syncope. Am J Cardiol 92, 815–819 (2003).

50. Krahn AD, Klein GJ, Yee R, Skanes AC. Randomized assessment of syncope trial: conventional diagnostic testing versus a prolonged monitoring strategy. Circulation 104, 46–51 (2001).

51. Moya A, Brignole M, Menozzi C, et al. Mechanism of syncope in patients with isolated syncope and in patients with tilt-positive syncope. Circulation 104, 1261–1267 (2001).

52. Brignole M, Menozzi C, Moya A et al. Mechanism of syncope in patients with bundle branch block and negative electrophysiological test. Circulation 104, 2045–2050 (2001).

53. Menozzi C, Brignole M, Garcia-Civera R, et al. Mechanism of syncope in patients with heart disease and negative electrophysiological test. Circualtion 105, 2741–2745 (2002).

54. Moss AJ, Zareba W, Hall WJ, et al. Prophylactic implantation of a defibrillator in patients with myocardial infacrtion and reduced ejection fraction. N Engl J Med 346, 877–883 (2002).

55. Krahn AD, Klein GJ, Yee R, Hoch JS, Skanes AC. Cost implications of testing strategy in patients with syncope: randomized assessment of syncope trial. J Am Coll Cardiol 42, 495–501 (2003).

56. Michele Brignole, Richard Sutton, Carlo Menozzi, Roberto Garcia-Civera, Angel Moya, Wouter Wieling, Dietrich Andresen, David G. Benditt, Panos Vardas, and for the International Study on Syncope of Uncertain Etiology 2 (ISSUE 2) Group. Early application of an implantable loop recorder allows effective specific therapy in patients with recurrent suspected neurally mediated syncope. Eur Heart J 27(9): 1085–1092 (2006). Ebub 2006 Mar 28.

57. Farwell D, Freemantle N, Sulke N. Use of implantable loop recorders in the diagnosis and management of syncope. Eur Heart J 25, 1257–1263 (2004).

58. Kapoor W. Is there an effective treatment for neurally-mediated syncope? JAMA 289, 2272–2275 (2003).

59. Brignole M, Croci F, Menozzi C et al.: Isometric arm counter-pressure maneuvers to abort impending vasovagal syncope. J. Am. Coll. Cardiol. 40, 2054–2060 (2002).

60. Krediet P, van Dijk N, Linzer M, Lieshout J, Wieling W: Management of vasovagal syncope: controlling or aborting faints by leg crossing and muscle tensing. Circulation 106, 1684–1689 (2002).

61. McGrady AV, Bush EG, Grubb BP: Outcome of biofeedback-assisted relaxation for neurocardiogenic syncope and headache: a clinical replication series. Appl. Psychophysiol. Biofeedback 22 (1), 63–72 (1997).

62. McGrady AV, Kern-Buell C, Bush E, Devonshire R, Claggett AL, Grubb BP: Biofeedback-assisted relaxation therapy in neurocardiogenic syncope: a pilot study. Appl. Psychophysiol. Biofeedback 28(3), 183–192 (2003).

63. Younoszai AK, Franklin WH, Chan DP, Cassidy SC, Allen HD: Oral fluid therapy: a promising treatment for vasodepressor syncope. Arch. Pediatr. Adolesc. Med. 152, 165–168 (1998).

64. El-Sayed H, Hainsworth R: Salt supplement increases plasma volume and orthostatic tolerance in patients with unexplained syncope. Heart 75, 134–140 (1996).

65. Ector H, Reybrouck T, Heidbuchel H, Gewillig M, Van de Werf F: Tilt training: a new treatment for recurrent neurocardiogenic syncope or severe orthostatic intolerance. Pacing Clin. Electrophysiol. 21, 193–196 (1998).

66. Foglia Manzillo G, Giada F, Gaggioli G et al.: Efficacy of tilt training in the treatment of neurally mediated syncope: a randomized study. Europace 6, 199–204 (2004).

67. Brignole M: Randomized clinical trials of neurally mediated syncope. J. Cardiovasc. Electrophysiol. 14, S64–S69 (2003).

68. Brignole M, Menozzi C, Gianfranchi L, Lolli G, Bottoni N, Oddone D: A controlled trial of acute and long-term medical therapy in tilt-induced neurally mediated syncope. Am. J. Cardiol. 70, 339–342 (1992).

69. Sheldon R, Rose S, Flanagan P, Koshman ML, Killam S: Effect of β blockers on the time to first syncope recurrence in patients after a positive isoproterenol tilt table test. Am. J. Cardiol. 78, 536–539 (1996).

70. Di Girolamo E, Di Iorio C, Sabatini P et al.: Evaluation of the effects of diverse therapeutic treatments versus no treatment of patients with neurocardiogenic syncope. Cardiologia 43, 833–837 (1998).

71. Madrid AH, Ortega J, Rebollo JG et al.: Lack of efficacy of atenolol for the prevention of neurally mediated syncope in a highly symptomatic population: a prospective, double-blind, randomized and placebo-controlled study. J. Am. Coll. Cardiol. 37, 554–559 (2001).

72. Ventura R, Maas R, Zeidler D et al.: A randomized and controlled pilot trial of β-blockers for the treatment of recurrent syncope in patients with a positive or negative response to head-up tilt test. Pacing Clin. Electrophysiol. 25, 816–821 (2002).

73. Flevari P, Livanis EG, Theodorakis GN, Zarvalis E, Mesiskli T, Kremastinos DT: Vasovagal syncope: a prospective, randomized, cross-over evaluation of the effects of propranolol, nadolol and placebo on syncope recurrence and patients' well-being. J. Am. Coll. Cardiol. 40, 499–504 (2002).

74. Sheldon R, Connolly S, Rose S et al. and the POST Investigators: Prevention Of Syncope Trial (POST): a randomized pacebo-controlled study of metoprolol in the prevention of vasovagal syncope. Circulation 113(9), 1164–1170 (2006).

75. Hickler RB, Thompson GR, Fox LM, Hamlin JT: Successful treatment of orthostatic hypotension with 9-X-fluohydrocortisone. N. Engl. J. Med. 261, 788–791 (1959).

76. Scott WA, Pongiglione G, Bromberg BI et al.: Randomized comparison of atenolol and fludrocortisone acetate in the treatment of pediatric neurally mediated syncope. Am. J. Cardiol. 76, 400–402 (1995).

77. Grubb BP, Kosinski D: Orthostatic hypotension: causes, classification and treatment. Pacing Clin. Electrophysiol. 26, 892–901 (2003).

78. Parry SW, Kenny RA: The management of vasovagal syncope. QJM 92, 697–705 (1999).

79. Low PA, Gilden JL, Freeman R et al.: Efficacy of midodrine vs placebo in neurogenic orthostatic hypotension: a randomized, double-blind multicenter study. JAMA 278, 388 (1997).

80. Ward CR, Gray JC, Gilroy JJ, Kenny RA: Midodrine: a role in the management of neurocardiogenic syncope. Heart 79, 45–49 (1998).

81. Singer W, Opfen-Gehrking, McPhee BR, Hiltz MJ, Bharucha AE, Low P: Acetylcholinesterase inhibition: a novel approach in the treatment of orthostatic hypotension. J. Neurol. Neurosurg. Psychiatry 74, 1294–1298 (2003).

82. Kuhn DM, Wolfe WA, Lovenberg W: Review of the central serotonergic neuronal system in blood pressure regulation. Hypertension 2, 243–255 (1980).

83. Grubb BP, Wolfe DA, Samoil D, Temesy-Armos P, Hahn H, Elliott L: Usefulness of fluoxetine hydrochloride for prevention of resistant upright tilt-induced syncope. Pacing Clin. Electrophysiol. 16, 458–464 (1993).

84. Benditt D, Peterson ME, Lurie K, et al. Cardiac pacing for prevention of recurrent vasovagal syncope. Ann Intern Med 122, 204–209 (1995).

85. Di Girolamo E, Di Iorio C, Sabatini P, Leonzio L, Barbone C, Barsotti A: Effects of paroxetine hydrochloride, a selective serotonin reuptake inhibitor, on refractory vasovagal syncope: a randomized, double-blind, placebo-controlled study. J. Am. Coll. Cardiol. 33, 1227–1230 (1999).

86. Hoeldkte RD, Streeten DH: Treatment of orthostatic hypotension with erythropoietin. N. Engl. J. Med. 329, 611–615 (1993).

87. Biaggioni S, Robertson D, Krantz S, Jones M, Hale V: The anemia of primary autonomic failure and its reversal with recombinant erythropoietin. Ann. Intern. Med. 121, 181–186 (1994).

88. Grubb BP, Lachant N, Kosinski D: Erythropoietin as a therapy for severe refractory orthostatic hypotension. Clin. Auton. Res. 4, 212 (1994) (Abstract).

89. Fitzpatrick AP, Travill CM, YardasPE, et al. Recurrent symptoms after ventricular pacing in unexplained syncope. Pacing Clin Electrophysiol. 1990;13:619–624.

90. Kenny RA, Ingram A, Baylor J, Sutton R. Head up tilt: a useful test for explaining unexplained syncope. Lancet 1, 1352–1355 (1989).

91. Fitzpatrick A, Sutton R. Tilting toward a diagnosis in recurrent unexplained syncope. Lancet 1, 658–660 (1989).

92. Fitzpatrick A, Theodorakis G, Ahmed R. Dual Chamber pacing aborts vasovagal syncope induced by head up 60 degree tilt. Pacing Clin Electrophysiol 14, 13–19 (1991).

93. McGuinn P, Moore S, Edel T, et al. Temporary dual chamber pacing during tilt table testing for vasovagal syncope: predictor of therapeutic success (Abstract). Pacing Clin Electrophysiol 14, 734 (1991).

94. Samoil D, Grubb BP, Brewster P, et al. Comparison of single and dual chamber pacing techniques in the prevention of upright tilt-induced vasovagal syncope. Eur J Card Pacing Electrophysiol 3, 36–41 (1993).

95. Sra J, Jazayeri M, Avitall B et al. Comparison of cardiac pacing with drug therapy in the treatment of neurocardiogenic (vasovagal) syncope with bradycardia or asystole. N Engl J Med 328, 1085–1090 (1993).

96. Ammirati F, Colivicchi F, Toscano S et al. DDD pacing with rate-drop function versus DDI with rate hysteresis pacing for cardioinhibitory vasovagal sncope. PACE 21, 2178–2181 (1998).

97. Ammirati F, Colivicchi F, Santini M. Permanent cardiac pacing versus medical treatment for the prevention of recurrent vasovagal syncope: a multicenter, randomized controlled trial. Circulation 104, 52–57 (2001).

98. Connolly S, Sheldon R, Thorpe K, et al. Pacemaker therapy for prevention of syncope in patients with recurrent severe vasovagal syncope. Second vasovagal pacemaker study (VPSII): a randomized trial. JAMA 289, 2224–2229 (2003).

99. Giada F, Raviele A, Menozzi C, et al. The vasovagal syncope and pacing trial (SYNPACE): a randomized placebo controlled study of permanent cardiac pacing for treatment of recurrent vasovagal syncope. PACE 26, 1016 (2003).

100. Raj SR, Koshman ML, Sheldon RS: Five-year follow-up of patients with dual chamber pacemakers for vasovagal syncope [abstract]. Can J Cardiol 18, xxx (2002).

101. Gabriel Gregoratos, Melvin D. Cheitlin, Alicia Conill, Andrew E. Epstein, Christopher Fellows, T. Bruce Ferguson, Jr, Roger A. Freedman, Mark A. Hlatky, Gerald V. Naccarelli, Sanjeev Saksena, Robert C. Schlant, and Michael J. Silka. ACC/AHA Guidelines for Implantation of Cardiac Pacemakers and Antiarrhythmia Devices: Executive Summary: A Report of the American College of Cardiology/American Heart Association Task Force on Practice Guidelines (Committee on Pacemaker Implantation). Circulation 98, 1325–1335 (1998).

102. McLeod K, Wilson N, Hewitt J et al. Cardiac pacing for severe childhood neurally mediated syncope with reflex anoxic seizures. Heart 82, 721–725 (1999).

103. Sutton R. Has cardiac pacing a role in vasovagal syncope? J Interv Card Electrophysiol 9, 145–149 (2003).

104. Sra JS. Can we assess the efficacy of therapy in neurocardiogenic syncope? J Am Coll Cardiol 37, 560–561 (2001).

105. Moss AJ, Glaser W, Topal E. Atrial tachypacing in the treatment of a patient with primary orthostatic hypotension. N Engl J Med 302, 1456–1457 (1980).

106. Weismann P, Chin M, Moss AJ. Cardiac tachypacing for severe refractory idiopathic orthostatic hypotension. Ann Intern Med 116, 650–651 (1992).

107. Abe H, Numata T, Hanada H, Kohshi K, Nakashima Y. Successful treatment of severe orthostatic hypotension with cardiac tachypacing in dual chamber pacemakers. Pacing Clin Electrophysiol 23, 137–139 (2000).

108. Sahul ZH, Trusty JM, Erickson M, Low PA, Shen WK. Pacing does not improve hypotension in patients with severe orthostatic hypotension – a prospective randomized cross-over pilot study. Clin Auton Res 14(4), 255–258 (2004).

109. Fortrat JO, Lemarie C, Bellard E, Victor J. Do we need a reflex tachycardia to stand up? PACE 28, 962–967 (2005).

110. Shannon J, Flatten NL, Jordan T et al.: Orthostatic intolerance and tachycardia associated with norepinephrine-transporter deficiency. N Engl J Med 342, 541–549 (2000).

111. Schroeder C, Vernino S, Birkenfeld AL et al.: Plasma exchange for primary autoimmune autonomic failure. N Engl J Med 353(15), 1585–1590 (2005).

112. Kurbaan A, Erickson M, Peterson M et al. Respiratory changes in vasovagal syncope. J Cardiovasc Electrophysiol 11, 607–611 (2000).

14

Indications for Implantable Cardioverter Defibrillators

Salam Sbaity and Brian Olshansky

Sudden death caused by cardiac arrest due to ventricular tachycardia or ventricular fibrillation remains a serious health problem worldwide. In the United States alone, cardiovascular disease accounts for over 900,000 deaths annually (1). Of these deaths, 350,000 are due to out-of-hospital cardiac arrest (2), two-thirds of which occur without prior recognition of cardiac disease (1). In the United States, 15–20% of all fatalities and 50% of all cardiac fatalities are sudden. Although sudden death caused by asystole or pulseless electrical activity is not preventable, sudden death caused by a ventricular arrhythmia can be. Prompt treatment to stop the ventricular arrhythmia before it causes death is possible.

Most individuals who die suddenly from a cardiac cause have no warning and are not even diagnosed with a cardiac condition (1). The challenge is to identify the high-risk individuals for whom sudden death due to ventricular fibrillation is likely and for whom a defibrillation shock could be life saving. Although ventricular tachycardia and ventricular fibrillation can also simply represent the last cardiac rhythm in a cascade of comorbid events, a large body of data now suggests that life can be restored, meaningful life can be extended, and the risk for sudden death can be reduced by use of implantable cardioverter defibrillators (ICDs) to correct ventricular tachyarrhythmias.

This chapter addresses the role of and indications for ICD therapy to treat patients with cardiovascular disease at risk for sudden cardiac death (SCD) caused by ventricular arrhythmias. Important clinical trials are reviewed that contrast medical therapies with the ICD in specific high-risk patient populations. The benefits, technological advances, and emerging areas in ICD therapy are considered in light of practical patient applications and recent clinical guidelines.

Sudden Cardiac Death

Causes

Although fatal and poorly tolerated ventricular tachyarrhythmias are initiated and perpetuated by one of three fundamental mechanisms (reentry, triggered automaticity, and abnormal automaticity), clinically, they arise from a broad range of pathologic conditions that are difficult, if not impossible, to quantify, characterize, and predict (3). The underlying trigger may be structural (e.g., prior myocardial infarction), metabolic (e.g., electrolyte abnormality), ischemic, functional (e.g., depression (4)), autonomic (5) (e.g., sympathetic excess), or electrical (e.g., primary ion channel abnormality in the congenital long QT interval syndrome).

Initiating factors, often multifactorial, include ectopic beats, ischemia, alteration in conduction or refractoriness, electrolyte disturbances, drugs, and autonomic perturbations. Factors that result in sudden death because of a ventricular arrhythmia are complex and understood poorly. Any simplistic medical approach that alters the arrhythmic "substrate" (such as drug therapy or even catheter ablation) may fail to reduce risk and may make things worse. Alternatively, a defibrillation shock, timed properly, can stop ventricular fibrillation.

Conditions that Increase the Risk for Sudden Cardiac Death

Sudden cardiac death, by definition, occurs unexpectedly. Without obvious clues of an impending catastrophe or without a catastrophe actually occurring, only identification of specific risk factors can provide adequate evidence that therapies, such as an ICD, should be initiated. The annual risk of SCD due to a cardiac arrest is 0.1–0.2% in the general population (1). This risk is not considered high enough to implant ICDs in the entire population.

Specific demographic factors associated with SCD that identify high-risk individuals in the general population include: male gender (6–9), age >45 years (10–12), smoking (13), sympathomimetic drugs, hypertension (14,15), hypercholesterolemia (5), metabolic syndrome (16), intraventricular conduction delay (17,18), rapid sinus rate (19,20), and atrial fibrillation (21,22). However, no single factor is specific or sensitive enough to target any specific medical intervention. At this time, no prophylactic therapy or specific intervention for prevention of SCD can be recommended. Instead, general preventive approaches, such as smoking cessation, exercise, appropriate diet, and lowering of elevated cholesterol levels, may offset the risk of SCD.

At higher risk are patients with myocardial ischemia, valvular heart disease, congenital heart disease, myocardial infarction, congestive heart failure, and primary myocardial disease, especially when concomitant ventricular dysfunction is present. Myocardial infarction, even if old, adds substantial, and continued, risk. Less common conditions associated with sudden death include hypertrophic cardiomyopathy, the long QT interval syndrome, Brugada syndrome, infiltrative diseases, peripartum cardiomyopathy, sarcoidosis, right ventricular dysplasia, among others (Table 14.1) (23–26). Currently, the presence of any of these conditions is not reason enough to warrant impromptu evaluation for an antiarrhythmic therapy even though risk for SCD exists. These patients, and patients with idiopathic ventricular fibrillation or other uncommon causes for sudden death, at highest risk, may ultimately become better identified with genetic mapping and genetic screening (27–34).

Patients identified as being at highest risk include those with a history of aborted cardiac arrest due to ventricular fibrillation, or sustained, poorly tolerated, ventricular tachycardia not related to a reversible cause and syncope associated with inducible ventricular tachycardia at electrophysiology testing. Patients with these conditions have up to a 30% risk of death in the first year after their index event (23–26) and many of these deaths are SCDs.

Table 14.1 Cardiac conditions associated with continued risk for sudden death due to ventricular arrhythmias.

Common

   Ischemic cardiomyopathy

   Dilated cardiomyopathy

   Valvular cardiomyopathy (aortic/mitral)

Unusual

   Long (and short) QT interval syndrome

   Right ventricular dysplasia

   Hypertrophic cardiomyopathy

   Idiopathic ventricular fibrillation

   Infiltrative heart disease

      Amyloidosis

      Sarcoidosis

      Hemochromatosis

   Congenital heart diseases (cyanotic and acyanotic)

   Congenital complete heart block

   Peripartum cardiomyopathy

   Myocarditis

   Coronary anomalies

   Brugada syndrome

   Wolff-Parkinson-White syndrome

Catecholaminergic polymorphic ventricular tachycardia

Other conditions of possible but unclear relation: myotonic dystrophy, epilepsy, various drugs/supplements, schizophrenia and sleep apnea

Methods to Identify Risk

Patients with cardiac disease can be further risk stratified. New York Heart Association Functional Class, ventricular function, as measured by the ejection fraction and age, remain the best predictors of sudden death and total cardiac mortality for patients with dilated cardiomyopathy and coronary artery disease (35–37). In the future, genetic profiling and inflammatory markers may allow better assessment of individual risks for SCD (35,37–39).

Other indicators of risk include ongoing myocardial ischemia and ventricular arrhythmias but even these are nonspecific. Methods to better target the highest-risk individual for aggressive antiarrhythmic therapy (drugs or ICDs) have included clinical assessment, treadmill testing, Holter monitoring, cardiac catheterization, electrophysiologic testing, and various non-invasive tests. Unfortunately, the clinical utility of noninvasive and invasive tests is limited. No failsafe method to predict survival is available. The level of risk that raises concern is not well defined.

Noninvasive Assessment

Noninvasive markers have been evaluated to help identify high-risk patients. Ventricular ectopy is associated with an increased risk for cardiac arrest. Premature ventricular contractions (PVCs) and nonsustained ventricular tachycardia identify increased risk for death, even in patients with no obvious heart disease (40–43). PVCs and nonsustained ventricular tachycardia provide prognostic information in patients with coronary artery disease. In the GISSI trial, >10 PVCs/h was associated with tripling in mortality in patients with myocardial infarction (44). In some conditions, such as dilated cardiomyopathy, PVCs and nonsustained ventricular tachycardia have little prognostic value because they are so ubiquitous. The sensitivity and specificity of ventricular ectopy to predict mortality in any cardiac condition, however, is low.

Other noninvasive techniques to identify risk, such as baroreflex sensitivity, spectral turbulence (45–47), heart rate variability, T-wave alternans (48–51), QT interval prolongation, QT dispersion (52,53), and late potentials (by the signal averaged ECG) (54–56), have been considered in select patient populations (Table 14.2). All have failed to live up to initial promises.

The most novel of the noninvasive techniques involves evaluation of microvolt T-wave alternans (MTWA). This noninvasive diagnostic approach detects minute changes in electrical activity in the T-wave as it alternates in shape, amplitude, and timing beat by beat. A positive MTWA test has been linked to inducible (48–51) and spontaneous (57,58) malignant ventricular arrhythmias.

MTWA abnormalities occur at lower thresholds but at higher heart rates in patients at high risk for SCD (51). It is critical to measure MTWA at heart rates within a fixed range to maximize the predictive value with an optimal rate of 110 beats/minute. Exercise and pacing have been used for this but it can be difficult to maintain a fixed rate in the proper range especially in patients with atrial fibrillation. A recent meta-analysis estimated a negative predictive value of 97% but a positive predictive value of only 19%. The risk of an indeterminate test is high.

Recent data highlight weaknesses of measuring MTWA. The ABCD trial, a trial of 566 patients followed for 1.9 years, showed that electrophysiology testing and MTWA had comparable 1-year positive predictive values of 11% and 9%, respectively (59). They also had comparable negative predictive values of 96% and 95%, respectively. The event rates were low for both groups; many patients had indeterminate tests. In this study, there was no pure MTWA group. The noninvasive testing group included electrophysiological testing and MTWA. There was no specific analysis of MTWA by itself. Sixty-seven percent who had negative or indeterminate MTWA and electrophysiology testing group received an ICD. Since 33% of these patients received an ICD shock, sudden death was eliminated in this population. It therefore becomes difficult to determine the value of MTWA alone.

In an SCD-HeFT (Sudden Cardiac Death Heart Failure Trial) substudy of MTWA, 490 patients were enrolled at 37 sites and followed for a mean of 35 months prospectively with a composite of primary endpoint of SCD, sustained ventricular arrhythmias, or an appropriate ICD discharge. This was a sick population of heart failure patients. MTWA was positive in 37%, negative in 22%, and indeterminate in 41%. There is no significant difference in survival between the MTWA positive and negative patients in the ICD and placebo arms. Mortality did not differ significantly between groups. These data indicate that MTWA results are frequently indeterminate and their ability to predict outcomes is limited.

Electrophysiology Testing

Invasive electrophysiology testing has been a time honored "gold standard" to assess long-term risk of SCD in various patient populations (60–63). Despite

Table 14.2 Noninvasive tests.

Noninvasive test	What it measures	Some possibly useful parameters	How measured
Heart rate	Spectral analysis of beat-to-beat to changes in RR interval assessing patterns that may correlate with changes in sympathetic/parasympathetic tone	Normal values given SDNN[a] 141 ms r-MSSD 27 ms pNN50[d] ULF power[f]	Measures changes beat-to-beat from prolonged recordings (e.g., Holter) LF power[b] 54nn (1170ms[c]) HF power[e] LF:HF ratio[g] 1.5–2.0
Signal averaged ECG	Conduction through the ventricles. Late potentials or delayed contraction have been associated with slow conduction and potential for reentry arrhythmias	QRS duration > 115–120 ms Low amplitude signal voltage < 20 μV Duration of low amplitude > 40 ms	Signal averaging of multiple QRS complexes to increase signal/noise ratio. *Specially filtered*
QT dispersion	Difference between the maximal and minimal QT on the surface ECG. May predict dispersion of repolarization and mortality	QTd > 100 ms likely abnormal	From surface 12-lead EKG
T-wave alternans	Microvolt beat-to-beat T-wave charges that may occur in patients at risk for sudden death	Beat-to-beat alternans (1.9 μV)	Special equipment to filter T wave. Bicycle exercise to keep HR at 100
Baroflex sensitivity (BRS)	Systolic BP and heart rate during phase IV of Valsalva maneuver or after phenylephrine	BRS < 3 ms/mmHg is abnormal	Phenylephrine infusion of Valsalva maneuver increases heart rate and blood pressure

[a] Standard deviation of all normal RR intervals in the entire 24-hour ECG recording.
[d] Percentage of differences between adjacent normal RR intervals that are greater than 50ms computed over the entire 24-hour ECG recording.
[f] Ultralow frequency.
[b] The energy in the heart period power spectrum between 0.04 and 0.15 Hz.
[c] Root mean square successive difference, the square root of the mean of the squared differences between adjacent normal RR intervals over the entire 24-hour ECG recording.
[e] The energy in the heart period power spectrum between 0.15 and 0.40 Hz.
[g] The ratio of low to high frequency power.

extensive investigation, even after definition of a "proper" protocol (three extrastimuli from two right ventricular sites and at two cycle lengths), the overall predictive value of electrophysiology testing in any population remains questionable and may be no better than MTWA even though electrophysiology testing is still considered to identify high-risk individuals in select populations.

In patients after myocardial infarction, Richards showed that induction of sustained ventricular tachycardia at electrophysiologic testing was associated with a 10.4-fold higher risk of dying (64). In a follow-up of > 3,000 survivors of acute myocardial infarction, Bourke found that benefit is obtained by restricting electrophysiologic testing to infarct survivors whose left ventricular ejection fraction is < 0.40 (65). In other studies induction of sustained monomorphic ventricular tachycardia at electrophysiologic testing allowed accurate identification of patients who may profit by prophylactic antiarrhythmic therapy (66).

The results of electrophysiology testing are patient-, symptom-, and disease-specific. Even under the best of circumstances, the predictive value is relatively poor. In hypertrophic cardiomyopathy, for example, electrophysiology testing has no predictive value (67,68). In several primary prevention trials electrophysiology testing, even in patients with coronary artery disease, was not a robust predictor of outcomes (69).

The benefits of electrophysiology testing are even less clear when the prognosis is known to be poor. A patient who survives a cardiac arrest from ventricular fibrillation, when no reversible cause is apparent, will derive little benefit from electrophysiology testing, because the risk of recurrent arrhythmia and cardiac arrest remains high no matter the results of the test. The test will be unlikely to reproduce the clinical arrhythmia in a patient who sustained a cardiac arrest even if the patient remains at continued risk. The chance of inducing sustained monomorphic ventricular tachycardia in a patient who survives a cardiac arrest caused by a ventricular arrhythmia is only about 50%, even if the underlying condition is coronary artery disease, a condition for which the electrophysiology test has the greatest sensitivity to detect a clinically apparent arrhythmia (70).

The electrophysiology test has been used to guide antiarrhythmic drug therapy but its predictive value is poor. High-risk patients had similar survival with empiric use of β-adrenergic blockers alone compared with a serial-guided drug approach (63). The ESVEM (Electrophysiologic Study Versus Electrocardiographic Monitoring) trial showed that the recurrence rate of ventricular tachycardia for patients with ventricular tachycardia or ventricular fibrillation was high even if the electrophysiology test showed apparent complete suppression of inducibility of ventricular tachycardia (71). Indeed, in ESVEM, the electrophysiology test was only as good a predictor as the Holter monitor. Serial drug evaluation guided by electrophysiology testing was abandoned because this and several other studies showed lack of efficacy of antiarrhythmic drugs that were considered effective by electrophysiology testing. The test has limited predictive value in conditions such as dilated cardiomyopathy, hypertrophic cardiomyopathy, valvular cardiomyopathy, long QT syndrome, right ventricular dysplasia, or most congenital anomalies that place individuals at risk of SCD.

MUSTT (Multicenter UnSustained Tachycardia Trial), a large randomized trial of patients with nonsustained ventricular tachycardia, coronary artery disease, and impaired left ventricular function indicated that electrophysiology testing in this "high-risk" population provided only slight predictive benefit (69). Other reports confirm lack of such a benefit. Based on its low predictive value, several randomized, multicenter, controlled trials, including the MADIT II (Multicenter Automatic Defibrillator Implant Trial II) and the AVID (Antiarrhythmics Versus Implantable Defibrillators) trial, a secondary prevention trial, abandoned electrophysiology testing to predict outcome or the need for therapy (72,73).

Long-term follow-up of survivors of acute myocardial infarction indicates that electrophysiology testing has low positive predictive value for the induction of sustained ventricular tachycardia (21%) and ventricular fibrillation (12%) (74). Electrophysiology testing has a low specificity and low positive predictive accuracy even in this setting (65,75).

The electrophysiology test may be useful for specific clinical situations. The electrophysiology test may be useful for patients with wide complex tachycardia of unclear mechanism (76) and for patients with syncope and impaired left ventricular function or structural heart disease (76). Examples include a patient with left ventricular dysfunction and a recent non-Q-wave myocardial infarction who has suffered a sustained arrhythmia near the time of the acute myocardial infarction and a patient who has a cardiac arrest after cardiac surgery, in the throes of acute congestive heart failure, or during infusion of an inotropic drug.

It makes little sense to consider electrophysiology testing if the endpoint is going to be the same: an ICD implant.

Therapy to Reduce the Risk of Sudden Cardiac Death

General Therapies

Several standard drug therapies can markedly improve survival from cardiovascular disease in select patient populations. These include β-blockers (77–79), aspirin (80,81), angiotensin converting enzyme (ACE) inhibitors (82,83), angiotensin receptor blockers (ARBs) (84–86), anticoagulants (including warfarin and aspirin) (87–90), aldosterone antagonists (91), and HMG-CoA reductase inhibitors (78–80,83,86,92–98).

Myocardial revascularization, when obstructive coronary artery disease is causing active ischemia, or valve replacement, for aortic stenosis, can reduce risk in these select patient subgroups (80,99–107). Unfortunately, these therapies, although effective, do not eliminate the risk of death. The risk can remain high in patients with underlying cardiovascular disease who have congestive heart failure or ventricular dysfunction.

The congestive heart population is a large (5 million), high-risk group (1), with an incidence approaching 10 per 1,000 population among persons > 65 years of age (108) and a 10% 1-year and a 50% 5-year mortality. Those with New York Heart Association Functional Class II and III congestive heart failure often die of an SCD (109). ACE inhibitor use has been consistently associated with improved survival in heart failure patients, but risk of death remains high (27–35% at 2.5 years), with a large percentage of sudden cardiac arrhythmia (23–52%) (109–111).

In randomized trials, β-blockers such as carvedilol, bisoprolol, and metoprolol have been associated with a reduction in total mortality and sudden death in congestive heart failure patients (78,79,93,94). Nevertheless, even with carvedilol, the mortality approaches 20% at 1 year (93). In the CIBIS II trial, the majority of deaths were sudden, even with β-blocker therapy (112). Ironically, drug therapy that improves left ventricular function can have a neutral effect (digoxin) or worsen survival (Milrinone) in patients with congestive heart failure (113,114).

Statins may lower mortality in heart failure patients independent of any effects on coronary artery disease. This has been shown through SCD-HeFT data. Statins can also reduce appropriate ICD discharge in few studies including MADIT II post hoc subanalysis (92,115). To date, no randomized controlled trial has evaluated the influence of statins on malignant ventricular arrhythmias or cardiac death independent of the effect on coronary artery disease.

Specific Antiarrhythmic Drug Approaches

Specific antiarrhythmic drug therapy has been advocated for patients who are at high risk for arrhythmic death, SCD, and total mortality, as standard therapies mentioned are limited in their ability to reduce total mortality in high-risk populations. Several randomized, multicenter antiarrhythmic drug trials have been completed (116–124). Antiarrhythmic drugs used in the post myocardial infarction period or in association with congestive heart failure have not been shown to provide benefit. They may also cause harm.

Class I Drugs
Prophylactic antiarrhythmic drug use does not improve total survival. The Cardiac Arrhythmia Suppression Trial (CAST) (125), based on the supposition that frequent PVCs after myocardial infarction are associated with increased risk of sudden death, evaluated the long-term benefits of antiarrhythmic drug therapy for those patients with ≥ 10 PVCs/h after myocardial infarction. After PVC suppression was shown to occur on the antiarrhythmic drug, patients were randomized to the antiarrhythmic drug showing apparent benefit (Class I antiarrhythmic drugs: moricizine, encainide, or flecainide) or a placebo (126–129). The mortality at 10 months was substantially higher (almost triple) in the drug-treated group, despite evidence for PVC suppression.

CAST-II compared moricizine with placebo. The protocol for the CAST-II was modified in an attempt to enroll patients more likely to experience serious arrhythmias and to observe for early risk of antiarrhythmic drugs. The qualifying ejection fraction was lowered to ≤ 0.40, a higher dose of moricizine could be used, and the definition of disqualifying ventricular tachycardia was changed to allow patients with more serious arrhythmias to be entered into the trial. CAST II was subsequently terminated prematurely because patients treated with moricizine had an increased cardiac mortality rate during the first 2 weeks of exposure to the drug, a time point not assessed in CAST. There was no evidence of long-term benefit with moricizine (129).

Similarly, the IMPACT (International Mexiletine and Placebo Antiarrhythmic Coronary Trial) using mexiletine showed the same increased mortality after myocardial infarction despite early data suggesting benefit (130).

Sotalol
Similar to CAST, the SWORD (Survival With Oral d-Sotalol) trial investigated whether an antiarrhythmic drug affected mortality. SWORD used d-sotalol, a class III antiarrhythmic drug without substantial beta blocking

effects reduced all-cause mortality in patient post myocardial infarction who have left ventricular dysfunction. Patients who have a left ventricular ejection fraction ≤ 0.40 and a recent (6–42 days) myocardial infarction or symptomatic heart failure with a remote (>42 days) myocardial infarction were randomly assigned d-sotalol or placebo. The study was stopped prematurely as there was an increase in mortality in the sotalol arm due to arrhythmic deaths (116).

The ESVEM trial, a randomized, NIH-sponsored multicenter trial, was designed to determine the best method to guide drug therapy for patients who had malignant ventricular arrhythmias: Holter monitoring versus electrophysiology testing (71). Patients needed to have sustained ventricular tachycardia, ventricular fibrillation, or syncope (and inducible sustained ventricular tachycardia at electrophysiology testing), in addition to ≥10 PVCs/h on Holter monitoring. It was difficult to find a drug therapy that was effective based on criteria developed in this prospective study. Death and arrhythmia recurrence were the same, based on antiarrhythmic therapy guided by Holter monitoring or electrophysiology testing. Sotalol (racemic d, l sotalol, a Class II/III antiarrhythmic drug) was associated with the highest efficacy rate; however, it still had an unacceptably high arrhythmia recurrence rate (131). Arrhythmia recurrence was high (60%), even though patients were placed on a drug considered successful based on the results of electrophysiology testing or Holter monitoring.

In ESVEM, amiodarone, ICDs, and placebo were not included and the data applied only to a highly select population. Most ESVEM patients ultimately did receive an ICD when antiarrhythmic drugs failed (as they generally did). The high costs of finding a therapy(132), and, even then, an ineffective therapy, made the ESVEM approach unfeasible and impractical.

Amiodarone

EMIAT (European Myocardial Infarction Amiodarone Trial), CAMIAT (Canadian Amiodarone/Arrhythmia Myocardial Infarction Trial), and BASIS (Basel Antiarrhythmic Study of Infarct Survival) evaluated the use of empiric amiodarone after myocardial infarction (122,123,133). These studies did not show that amiodarone had a survival advantage; however, a small but statistically significant reduction of sudden death (CAMIAT) and arrhythmic events (EMIAT) was observed.

The use of amiodarone in patients with congestive heart failure has been evaluated by several large trials, including, CHF-STAT (Congestive Heart Failure Survival Trial of Antiarrhythmia Therapy) and GESICA (Grupo de Estuldo de la Sobrevida en la Insoficiencia Cardiac en Argentina) (110,134). CHF-STAT, a study of 674 American veterans who had left ventricular ejection fractions ≤0.40 and frequent PVCs (≥10/h), showed no survival benefit of amiodarone over placebo. GESICA showed survival benefit with amiodarone. In GESICA, 516 patients were randomized from 26 hospitals. Amiodarone reduced mortality from 41 to 34% at 2 years, but mortality remained high even for patients taking amiodarone. The disparate results may result from the patient populations in the two studies. CHF-STAT included more patients with ischemic heart disease. When considering only nonischemic patients in CHF-STAT, amiodarone showed a trend toward benefit. In both studies, the total mortality and arrhythmic death mortality were high, whether or not amiodarone was used. In these multi-center randomized trials, patients were requested to stop amiodarone for real or perceived side effects; the discontinuation rate was approximately 20–40%.

Amiodarone was not associated with worsening in prognosis often associated with Class I antiarrhythmic drugs in high-risk populations. Amiodarone, the only antiarrhythmic shown to be at least as safe as placebo in high-risk patients with structural heart disease, has not been (and cannot be) tested against placebo in the highest-risk population, those with a history of cardiac arrest (135). Although data conflict, there is ongoing concern about the use of antiarrhythmic drug therapy as the primary means to improve survival in high-risk patients. It appears, for the population tested, that empiric use of almost any antiarrhythmic drug appears to be of little long-term survival benefit.

SCD-HeFT was a prospective, randomized trial that enrolled patients with left ventricular ejection fraction ≤ 0.35 and New York Heart Association Functional Class II–III congestive heart failure to evaluate whether amiodarone or an ICD improved survival compared to a placebo pill. The primary end point of the trial was death from any cause. Amiodarone therapy did not affect outcomes compared to placebo (54). A few studies and one meta-analysis of several large studies have shown reduction in SCD using amiodarone for LV dysfunction due to prior myocardial infarction and nonischemic dilated cardiomyopathy (117,136). Any long-term survival benefit from amiodarone is doubtful.

Azimilide

The AzimiLide post-Infarct surVival Evaluation (ALIVE) trial (137), a double-blind, placebo-controlled, multinational trial, assessed the effect of azimilide on survival in high-risk post myocardial infarction (within 6–21 days) and patients with left ventricular ejection fractions between 0.15 and 0.35. There was no survival advantage from azimilide but no harm caused by the drug.

Summary of Antiarrhythmic Drug Therapy

No antiarrhythmic drug has been shown to improve survival. Antiarrhythmic drugs may suppress ventricular arrhythmias and therefore have some use particularly in patients with ICDs. However, there are no potential advantages seen with any antiarrhythmic drug to reduce the risk of mortality in patients who are at risk for cardiovascular events. Antiarrhythmic drugs can have proarrhythmic effects and, with the complexity of the substrate responsible for SCD, it is not surprising that affecting a single ion channel would not have benefit.

Radiofrequency Catheter Ablation

Although feasible and potentially beneficial for patients without structural heart disease and monomorphic ventricular arrhythmias, radiofrequency catheter has questionable benefit to reduce adverse outcomes in patients with structural heart disease. This approach is really meant to prevent inducible, well-tolerated ventricular tachycardia from becoming a clinical problem in these patients, but not to prevent death (138–141).

Ablation may treat bundle-branch reentry and fascicular forms of ventricular tachycardia effectively (142–144). Ablation of Purkinje fibers may reduce the risk of idiopathic ventricular fibrillation initiated by a PVC (76) and some forms of ventricular tachycardia (145). Substrate modification can reduce specific forms of recurrent monomorphic ventricular tachycardias in patients with structural heart disease (138,146–149), particularly if the patient is having storms of tachycardia. Therefore, occasionally, ablation performed during electrophysiology testing can modify the ventricular tachycardia recurrences that might lead to frequent ICD activations. No study shows a survival benefit using ablation as treatment of ventricular tachycardia. No data show that ventricular tachycardia ablation can substitute for ICD therapy.

Implantable Cardioverter Defibrillator

Initial, nonrandomized studies demonstrated that the ICDs can detect ventricular fibrillation appropriately and discharge a shock to effectively stop ventricular fibrillation (150). The weight of evidence from observational studies, as well as single-site, multicenter, randomized, and controlled trials of ICD therapy indicate that life-threatening ventricular tachyarrhythmias can be prevented from causing death. The highly effective ICD simplifies and expedites management, can be cost-effective, shortens hospital stays, and might improve longevity and quality of life.

Although most single center studies showed advantages of the ICD, it was not clear to all investigators that the ICD could save lives, even for patients who had survived a previous cardiac arrest caused by ventricular fibrillation (151–154). Several investigators were concerned that the ICD may simply convert sudden deaths into not-so-sudden deaths because the basis of the ventricular fibrillation would inevitably lead to death in any instance (155–157). What did become clear from the initial trials was that the ICD prevented SCD, nearly eliminating it. The incidence of sudden arrhythmic death with the ICD was less than 2% per year, with the majority of patients receiving therapy from the ICD. Still, a group of vocal investigators and clinicians thought that the ICD would not prevent death and, therefore, would not be useful.

Skeptics have pointed to the continued high total mortality in the studies evaluating patients with ICDs. The risk of death in ICD patients was as high as 30% in some reports, and the expenses for the ICD implant were high. The benefits of the ICD remained clouded because it can be difficult to know the mode and mechanism of death with certainty and because early ICDs could not be interrogated. It was possible that the ICD was being activated for a nonfatal, benign, or nonsustained arrhythmia (ventricular or supraventricular). Proving benefit from ICD therapy challenged the electrophysiology community for more than 18 years.

A large body of clinical experience now supports these initial reports. As outlined in the following, large multicenter clinical trials have demonstrated the benefits of the ICD in certain patient populations. Based on these results, guidelines have been created to address the question of which patients benefit most from the ICD. The growing acceptance of ICD use by the medical community and the public is not to be underestimated (158,159). However, the ICD can be associated with potential psychological issues, especially in children (160), costs (161,162), adverse effects, complications (163–165), and does not prevent all sudden death (166,167).

Randomized Trials Evaluating ICDs

Randomized trials can be divided into two types: *primary prevention* trials, in which the ICD is prophylaxis for high-risk patients, and *secondary prevention* trials, in which the ICD treats sustained ventricular arrhythmias already present. The latter group was more extensively evaluated at first, although secondary prevention represents a smaller population. The chance of survival from a cardiac arrest or poorly tolerated ventricular tachycardia is low. Even in the best of circumstances, a 5% survival to the hospital and discharge is overly optimistic. In Chicago, the chance for a cardiac arrest victim to be resuscitated, admitted, and discharged without neurological deficit is < 2%. In New York, the chances of survival are even less (168,169). Efforts to identify high-risk patients and place an ICD before the cardiac arrest occurs (primary prevention trials make sense) resulted in much broader use as the population that was proven to benefit became much larger.

Important endpoints of ICD therapy are all-cause or total mortality (22). Surrogate endpoints such as "ICD shock" or "sudden death" are inadequate. Changing one form of death into another has little advantage. ICD shocks cannot be equated to survival benefit for an arrhythmia that may stop spontaneously or not even be life-threatening. The ICD may change the mode of death from sudden to not so sudden heart failure deaths. In any case, it can be difficult to determine the cause of death even with careful analysis of all available information.

Secondary Prevention Trials

The original intent of the ICD was to prevent recurrent cardiac arrest due to ventricular tachycardia and fibrillation. Secondary prevention of recurrent cardiac arrest was initially the prime reason for ICD implant. Five multicenter prospective randomized secondary prevention trials have been completed: AVID (Antiarrhythmics Versus Implantable Defibrillator), CASH (Cardiac Arrest Study Hamburg), CIDS (Canadian Implantable Defibrillator Study), DEBUT (Defibrillator versus beta-Blockers for Unexplained death in Thailand), and MAVERIC (The Midlands Trial of Empirical Amiodarone versus Electrophysiology-guided Interventions and Implantable Cardioverter-defibrillators) (Table 14.3) (77,118,121,149,170).

AVID

The AVID trial, a large multicenter prospective NIH-sponsored trial, compared antiarrhythmic drug (amiodarone or sotalol) therapy to ICD implant in patients who survived life-threatening hemodynamically destabilizing ventricular arrhythmias (ventricular tachycardia and ventricular fibrillation). One thousand sixteen patients were randomized (45% with ventricular fibrillation and 55% with poorly tolerated ventricular tachycardia). The mean ejection fraction was 0.32. Patients with sustained ventricular tachycardia who were enrolled had associated syncope or a left ventricular ejection fraction ≤ 0.40 (118). The AVID trial is the most persuasive and influential secondary prevention trial to date. At the time this trial was initiated, several centers refused to participate because of the belief that the ICD had already been shown to be the best therapy. Fifty-six U.S. and Canadian centers participated.

In those randomized to an ICD, 93% had a nonthoracotomy lead system, 5% had an epicardial system, and 2% had no device implanted. In those randomized to drug therapy, 356 immediately began empiric therapy with amiodarone. These patients were not considered candidates for sotalol because of concern about heart failure, a low ejection fraction, or both. Antiarrhythmic drug therapy was assigned to the remaining 153 patients randomized to drug therapy: 79 to amiodarone and 74 to sotalol. In 53 of the 74 patients assigned to

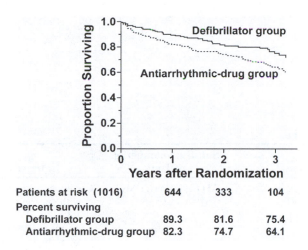

Fig. 14.1 Survival curves for patients in the AVID trial. A significant survival benefit was observed with defibrillator therapy. AA, antiarrhythmic drug group. (From AVID investigators. *N Engl J Med* 1997;337:1576–1583, with permission.)

sotalol, electrophysiology testing or Holter monitoring could guide sotalol therapy, but only 13 patients had adequate arrhythmia suppression to continue sotalol. The rest required amiodarone administration. The mean dose of amiodarone was 300 mg/day and the mean dose of sotalol was 250 mg/day. The crossover rate (ICD to drugs and vice versa) was low.

The study was stopped prematurely with a statistically significant benefit of the ICD (Fig. 14.1). The mean survival was 31 months with the ICD; it was 28.5 months with antiarrhythmic drugs. Survival in the ICD group was 89.3% at 1 year. At 2 years, the drug-treated group had a 25.3% mortality rate compared with an 18.4% mortality rate in the ICD-treated group. The ICD group had lower all-cause mortality ($p < 0.02$) and a lower risk for hospitalization ($p < 0.04$). The ICD group had a lower prevalence of congestive heart failure. Mortality reduction with the ICD was 39% at 1 year, 27% at 2 years, and 31% at 3 years. In a subgroup analysis, patients with left ventricular ejection fractions > 0.40 had less benefit from the ICD.

In AVID, 42% of the ICD patients were taking β-blockers compared to only 17% of the amiodarone patients (a possible explanation of the outcomes). The difference in mortality may, in part, be due to this difference. Costs in the ICD group, compared to the drug group, were high (over $100,000/life year saved). Cost-effectiveness, a parameter that is difficult to measure, was calculated to be as high in the ICD group as it was in the drug group. AVID, the definitive secondary prevention trial, showed that implanting an ICD was the best first strategy to manage patients with life-threatening ventricular arrhythmias. It is unlikely that any similar trial of this type will ever be performed again.

CIDS

CIDS assessed patients with prior cardiac arrest, poorly tolerated sustained ventricular tachycardia, or syncope associated with an electrophysiology test that was positive for sustained ventricular tachycardia (171). The study was

Table 14.3 Secondary prevention trials.

Trial/date of publication	Purpose	Substrate/number of patients	Entry criteria
AVID (antiarrhythmics versus implantable defibrillator, 1997)	ICD vs. amiodarone/sotalol for VT/VF	CAD (81%), prior MI (67%) 1,016 pts	Cardiac arrest; sustained VT with syncope or sustained VT with EF < 40% and symptomatic because of hemodynamic compromise from the arrhythmia
CIDS (Canadian Implantable Defibrillator Study, 1998)	ICD vs. amiodarone for VT/VF	Most CAD, prior MI (74%)	VT with syncope; VT > 150 bpm with EF < 35%, or inducible VT with syncope, VF
CASH (Cardiac Arrest Study, Hamburg 1994)	Metoprolol, amiodarone, propafenone vs. ICD for VT or VF	CAD	MI survivors: documented VT or VF unrelated to MI. EP testing before randomization

Treatment arms	Results	Clinical significance
(1) ICD or drug (2) Drug group received amiodarone (if not candidate for sotalol) or random assignment to amiodarone or sotalol (3) Amiodarone dose 3 yr: 256 ± 95 mg/d (4) Sotalol dose at 3 yr: 240 ± 113 mg/d	(1) 1,016 pts: 507 ICD group, 509 drug therapy (356 empiric amiodarone, 153 random assignment: 79 to amiodarone, 74 to sotalol – 13 suppressed on sotalol) (2) Fewer deaths in the ICD group than in the drug group	(1) ICDs prolong life compared to drug therapy in patients who have survived near-lethal arrhythmias (2) The absolute prolongation of life was modest, just > 3 mos (3) ICD is first-line therapy for pts with similar characteristics
Pts surviving near-fatal arrhythmia assigned to ICD or amiodarone	(1) 3-yr risk reduction 19.6% in ICD group (p = ns) (2) 22% of control group crossed over to ICDs (3) 30% of ICD group received appropriate shocks by 5 yr	(1) ICD benefit marginal, not significant (2) Results may be masked by high cross over rates
Pts randomly assigned to amiodarone propafenone, metoprolol, or ICD. Propafenone arm closed 1992	(1) 3/91, 230 pts randomized: 56 propafenone; 56 amiodarone; 59 metoprolol; 59 to ICD	(1) Propafenone associated with higher mortality than ICD

(continued)

Table 14.3 (continued)

Trial/date of publication	Purpose	Substrate/number of patients	Entry criteria
DEBUT	ICD vs. β-blockers (Propranolol)	Healthy subjects without structural heart disease	Unexpected arrest
MAVERIC	EP-guided interventions (anti-arrhythmic drugs, coronary revascularization, and ICD) vs. amiodarone therapy	Survivors of sustained VT, VF, or SCD in the absence of an MI in the last 48 h	

CAD, coronary artery disease; ICD, implantable cardioverter defibrillators; MI, myocardial infarction; Pts, patients; SD, sudden death; VF, ventricular fibrillation; VT, ventricular tachycardia; Yr, year; EF, ejection fraction; EP, electrophysiology; SCD, sudden cardiac death.

Treatment arms	Results	Clinical significance
	(2) 3/92, propafenone stopped because of excess mortality 12% incidence of SD and 23% incidence of MI recurrence of SD found in propafenone group vs. 0% in ICD arm ($p < 0.05$)	(2) Marginal benefit with ICD compared to drug (3) Numbers in each group were small (4) Prolonged enrollment
	(3) ICD group overall mortality reduced 37% ($p = 0.047$). ICD group 12.1% total mortality vs. 19.6% in drug group. No differences between amiodarone and metoprolol	
(1) ICD implantation (2) Propranolol 40 mg/d to up to 160 mg/d	Four deaths (out of 66 pts), all of which occurred in the β-blocker group (14% vs. 0%, $p = 0.02$)	ICD prevents death in healthy patients post sudden cardiac death
(1) EP-guided arm: arrhythmia suppression with either sotalol or amiodarone was first attempted (2) If unsuccessful, further treatment depended on haemodynamic status of the index event: (3) If haemodynamically unstable, the patient received an ICD; otherwise, various combinations of antiarrhythmic drugs (such as the combined use of sotalol or mexiletine with amiodarone) were tried	(1) No significant difference in survival between the two treatment arms (2) The survival of all trial patients who received an ICD was better than non-ICD recipients	No significant impact of EP study on the diagnosis or the prognosis of patients presenting with VT, VF, or SCD

designed to test the hypothesis that the ICD is an effective, first-line therapy compared to amiodarone for this patient population. Six hundred fifty-nine patients were enrolled; 328 randomized to ICD implant (33 thoracotomy ICD, 277 nonthoracotomy ICD, 18 no ICD) and 331 to amiodarone.

At 24 months, there was a 15% mortality rate in the ICD arm versus a 20% mortality rate in the amiodarone arm. At 36 months, the mortality rate in the ICD arm was 25% and for the amiodarone arm was 30%. Mortality reduction was 19.6% at 3 years with the ICD ($p = 0.072$) (Fig. 14.2). The conclusions were consistent with the AVID trial but CIDS did not show a statistically significant benefit of an ICD for this population. In the CIDS trial, similar to the AVID trial, β-blocker use was greater in patients randomized to ICD implantation. Older patients and less healthy patients derived the greatest benefit from an ICD. In CIDS, there was a high crossover rate: 30% of the patients in the ICD arm also received amiodarone and 22% in the amiodarone arm received an ICD implant (171).

CASH

In 1987, CASH began to assess which therapy would be most effective for patients with sustained ventricular tachycardia or ventricular fibrillation (170). There were four treatment arms: ICD, β-blocker (metoprolol), amiodarone, and propafenone. Three hundred forty-six patients were enrolled: 99 to ICD, 92 to amiodarone, 97 to metoprolol, and 58 to propafenone. Propafenone was stopped in 1992 because of increased mortality. The mortality in the ICD compared to propafenone was 11.5% versus 29.3% ($p = 0.01$). Sudden death mortality in the ICD limb was 2% versus 11% ($p < 0.001$) in the metoprolol or amiodarone limbs. ICD mortality versus amiodarone or metoprolol was 12% versus 19.6% ($p = 0.04$), a 37% reduction at 2 years (after 10 years accruing data). There was no significant difference between metoprolol and amiodarone. Although CASH was a small study with a long enrollment period, it provided further evidence for ICD therapy independent from β-blocker use.

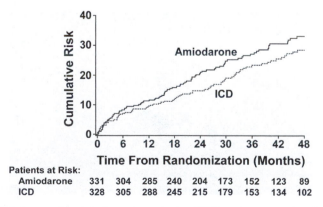

Fig. 14.2 Total mortality risk for patients in the CIDS study. A nonsignificant trend favoring defibrillator therapy (ICD) versus amiodarone therapy was observed. (From CIDS investigators, Circulation 2000;101:1297, with permission.)

DEBUT

DEBUT was a small multicenter, randomized, clinical trial that compared ICD implants (with or without amiodarone) to β-blockers (or amiodarone) in a different population – subjects without structural heart disease who had survived unexpected cardiac arrest (subjective symptoms of sudden death undocumented by electrocardiogram. Over a 3-year follow-up period, there were four deaths (out of 66 patients). All deaths occurred in the ß-blocker group (14 versus 0%, $p = 0.02$) (77).

MAVERIC

MAVERIC was a randomized trial that included survivors of sustained ventricular tachycardia, ventricular fibrillation, or SCD in the absence of an acute myocardial infarction. Electrophysiology-guided intervention (antiarrhythmic drugs, coronary revascularization, and ICD) was evaluated against empirical amiodarone therapy. In the electrophysiology-guided arm, stepwise suppression by an antiarrhythmic drug followed by ICD implantation was assessed. The study showed no advantage of an electrophysiology guided approach versus empiric amiodarone although survival with an ICD was statistically better without an ICD. However, ICD recipients were significantly younger and less likely to have diabetes. Electrophysiology testing had no role in ICD implantation for secondary prevention.

Primary Prevention Trials

Arguably, ICDs for primary prevention has greater benefit for the entire population than ICDs for secondary prevention. Several key primary prevention trials have been completed: MADIT, MUSTT, CABG-Patch (Coronary Artery Bypass Graft surgery), MADIT II, DINAMIT (Defibrillator in Acute Myocardial Infarction Trial), DEFINITE (Defibrillators in Non-Ischemic Cardiomyopathy Treatment Evaluation), SCD-HeFT, CAT (CArdiomyopathy Trial), and AMIOVERT (AMIOdarone VERsus implanv cardioverTer-defibrillator) trials (Table 14.4) (54,119,172–174).

MADIT

MADIT was the first randomized trial to show that the ICD, used as a prophylactic, can reduce the risk of death in "high-risk" patients. The MADIT assessed patients who had coronary artery disease and a prior Q-wave myocardial infarction. To be included, patients had to have: (a) asymptomatic nonsustained ventricular tachycardia recorded on a 24-h Holter monitor, (b) a left ventricular ejection fraction of ≤ 0.35 and, (c) inducible sustained monomorphic ventricular tachycardia or ventricular fibrillation not suppressed by procainamide at electrophysiology testing.

Treatment was randomized to "conventional" therapy or an ICD. "Conventional" therapy was not specified, but consisted initially of amiodarone in 74% of the patients (45% of these patients were taken off amiodarone within 6 months). More patients in the ICD arm received β-blockers. One hundred ninety-six patients (16 women, mean age 63 years) were enrolled from 32 centers over a 5-year period (slightly more than 1 year per center) with enrollment concentrated at two sites (63 patients, 32% of the population). The mean ejection fraction was 0.26. Seventy-five percent of patients were randomized more than 6 months after an acute myocardial infarction.

Table 14.4 Primary prevention trials.

Trial/date of publication	Purpose	Substrate/# pts
MADIT (Multicenter Automatic Defibrillator Implantation Trial, 1996)	Determine if ICD reduces death compared to "conventional" therapy in high-risk CAD pts	Post-MI 196 pts 5-year enrollment 32 centers
MADIT II	ICD as a primary prevention therapy in patient with CHF and low EF	CAD, 1,232 pts
CABG-Patch 1997	Determine if prophylactic ICD would reduce mortality in high-risk CABG pts	CAD/CABG 1,055 pts
MUSTT (Multicenter UnSustained Tachycardia Trial, 1999)	Determine if EP testing reduces risk of arrhythmic death and MI in CAD pts	CAD 2,202 pts 85 centers

Entry criteria	Treatment arms	Results
>3 wk after MI LVEF ≤ 0.35 New York Heart Association Class I–III Inducible VT/VF, not suppressed by procainamide	ICD or "conventional" therapy (conventional = antiarrhythmic drugs) NSVT: 3–30 beats > 120 bpm (nonsyncopal)	(1) ICD group had 54% reduction in overall mortality (2) Pts in "conventional" limb often received amiodarone (80%) (3) More in ICD arm received β-blocker than in the "conventional" arm (28% vs. 9%)
Prior myocardial infarction and a left ventricular ejection fraction of 0.30 or less	ICD (742 pts) or conventional medical therapy (490 pts).	Average follow-up of 20 months, hazard ratio for death from any cause in ICD group as compared with the conventional-therapy group was 0.69 (95% confidence interval, 0.51–0.93; $p = 0.016$)
Pts requiring CABG surgery EF ≤0.35 Abnormal SAECG	Pts randomized to ICD or control (both had CABG)	(1) 446 pts randomized to ICD and 454 to control (2) 52 in ICD group never received device or it was removed (3) Antiarrhythmic use was similar in both groups (4) 196 deaths: 101 in ICD group, 95 in control group (5) No benefit from ICD
EF ≤ 0.40 NSVT 3–30 s, > 100 bpm	If inducible, randomized "conservative" or EP-guided therapy (conservative = β-blocker and angiotensin converting enzyme inhibitor)	(1) 1,435 of 2,202 (65%) not inducible at EP testing (2) 767 (704 actually randomized) of 2,202 (35%) inducible were randomized to either EP test-guided antiarrhythmic therapy (353) or conservative therapy (351) (3) Trend toward improved survival in the EP test-guided group, with highest survival rates in those patients receiving an ICD

(continued)

Table 14.4 (continued)

Trial/date of publication	Purpose	Substrate/# pts
DEFINITE	ICD as a primary prevention therapy in patients with nonischemic cardiomyopathy (NICM) and nonsustained VT	Patients with NICM and NSVT. An angiogram or a stress test was used to confirm the absence of coronary artery disease
SCD-HeFT	Tests the hypothesis that adjunct antiarrhythmic therapies, including amiodarone and ICD implant, may improve total survival in high-risk congestive heart failure patients	2,521 pts with CHF
DINAMIT	Prophylactic implantation of an ICD s/p acute MI	S/P acute MI, 674 pts

CABG, coronary artery bypass graft surgery; CAD, coronary artery disease; CHF, congestive heart failure; EP, electrophysiology; MI, myocardial infarction; NSVT, nonsustained ventricular tachycardia; Pts, patients; LVEF, left ventricular ejection fraction; NYHA, New York Heart Association New York Heart Association; VT, ventricular tachycardia; VF, ventricular fibrillation; SAECG, signal averaged ECG.

Entry criteria	Treatment arms	Results
Nonischemic dilated cardiomyopathy NYHA Class I–III NSVT (3–15 beats)	ICD or to best therapy	Nonsignificant reduction in total mortality with ICD therapy
New York Heart Association Class II or III CHF and LVEF of 35% or less shock-only, single-lead ICD (829 pts)	(1) Conventional therapy for CHF plus placebo (847 pts) (2) Conventional therapy plus amiodarone (845 pts) (3) Conventional therapy plus a conservatively programmed, shock only, single-lead-ICD	(1) Median follow-up 45.5 months: 244 deaths (29%) in the placebo group (2) 240 deaths (28%) in the amiodarone group; similar risk of death as compared with placebo (hazard ratio, 1.06; 97.5% confidence interval, 0.86–1.30; $p = 0.53$) (3) 182 deaths (22%) in the ICD group; decreased risk of death of 23% (0.77; 97.5% confidence interval, 0.62–0.96; $p = 0.007$), an absolute decrease in mortality of 7.2 percentage points after 5 years in the overall population
(1) 1.6–40 days after a myocardial infarction (2) LVEF of 0.35 or less (3) Depressed heart-rate variability	Open-label comparison of ICD therapy (in 332 pts) and no ICD therapy (in 342 pts)	No difference in overall mortality between the two treatment groups: 120 pts died, 62 were in the ICD group and 58 in the control group (hazard ratio for death in the ICD group, 1.08; 95% confidence interval, 0.76–1.55; $p = 0.66$)

In MADIT, the relative risk reduction in total mortality with the ICD was 54% at 27 months compared to "conventional therapy," ($p = 0.009$, hazard ratio of 0.46, 95% confidence limits: 0.26–0.82). The fact that 50% of the ICD patients received an ICD shock made investigators suspect that the device was protecting the patients from death. The statistical methods used in MADIT allowed a relatively small number of patients to show a statistically significant result; however, these methods did not allow for multivariate analyses or subanalyses. Most of the benefit of the ICD occurred early after implantation.

The 24-month mortality rate was 32% in the "conventional arm." This high mortality rate may reflect selection bias. MADIT was a highly select population that was impossible to quantify. Were patients recently hospitalized or did they have an exacerbation of their heart disease? This population may not represent all patients who could satisfy the enrollment criteria (a potentially large population).

The common problem of nonsustained ventricular tachycardia in patients with structural heart disease can be a highly visible reminder of risk of death. Perhaps no study focused attention on this issue more than MADIT, but this issue is not laid to rest. As the first "randomized" trial on this issue, it provided a remarkable conclusion. Electrophysiologists have been quick to embrace the results of the MADIT, citing its randomized nature and the magnitude of the results, but without trying to dissect specific implications of the results. The provocative implications of this trial, however, are tempered by several important considerations: (a) nonsustained ventricular tachycardia is a nonspecific marker, especially in patients without coronary artery disease; (b) electrophysiology testing was not shown to enhance patient selection for ICDs; and (c) the applicability of these results remains questionable, even in patients with coronary artery disease.

MADIT is applicable to a small, highly select group and suggests that specific patient subgroups will benefit from ICD therapy. MADIT did not have a control group and was not designed to be a comparison between ICD therapy and other specific therapies. A more unbiased and global approach to the problem that addresses the issue of risk reduction in a larger patient cohort was necessary to define which patient will actually benefit from ICD prophylaxis.

MADIT II

The MADIT II trial addressed some of the issues raised by the MADIT. The MADIT II trial evaluated patients with ischemic cardiomyopathy (history of myocardial infarction ≥ 1 month before entry), New York Heart Association Functional Class I–III congestive heart failure, and left ventricular ejection fraction ≤ 0.30 (documented within 3 months), with or without ventricular ectopy. The study enrolled 1,232 patients to assess if an ICD improve total mortality compared to optimal therapy alone. No Holter or electrophysiology test criteria were required for enrollment. Optimal medical therapy included angiotensin-converting-enzyme inhibitors, beta-blockers, diuretics, and lipid-lowering statin drugs (172).

MADIT II was stopped early due to the lower mortality in the ICD arm based on a prespecified level of efficacy. There was a 31% reduction in mortality (HR 0.69) in the ICD arm compared to conventional-therapy. Divergence in survival began at 9 months. Intense subgroup analysis led to initial recommendations for ICDs in this population only if the QRS complex was wide. This was later rescinded. Of note, the ICD did not predict survival in women enrolled. A slightly higher (though nonsignificant) incidence of new or worsened heart failure was noted in the ICD group. Widespread prophylactic ICD implantation became recommended for ischemic cardiomyopathy.

CABG-Patch

ICD therapy does not benefit all high-risk patients The CABG-Patch trial assessed another high-risk group: patients with coronary artery disease, a positive signal-averaged electrocardiogram, and left ventricular dysfunction going for revascularization surgery (173). The potential survival benefit of a prophylactic ICD was determined at the time of coronary artery bypass graft surgery. Over a 5-year period, 37 centers screened patients scheduled for elective coronary artery bypass graft surgery. Patients were eligible to participate if they were < 80 years old, had a left ventricular ejection fraction ≤ 0.35, and had an abnormal signal-averaged electrocardiogram by at least one criterion.

Of 1,422 eligible patients, 1,055 were enrolled and 900 were randomized to an ICD implant by the thoracotomy approach (446 patients) or no ICD (454 patients) at time of CABG. The mean ejection fraction of the study population was 0.27. Frequent ventricular ectopy and nonsustained ventricular tachycardia were common findings. During a 32 ± 16-month follow-up, there were 101 deaths with the ICD and 95 with no ICD implant. The study was well balanced for β-blocker use. One-half of the ICD patients received a shock from their ICD, similar to the MADIT. There was no evidence for improved survival with the ICD in this high-risk cohort. The lack of benefit of the ICD in the CABG-Patch trial may be in part related to the positive benefits of revascularization. Nevertheless, patients recruited into CABG-Patch are a high-risk example: four times the mortality among all patients who undergo coronary artery bypass graft surgery. These data indicated that not all "high-risk" patients benefit from an ICD.

MUSTT

MUSTT assessed "high-risk" patients with coronary artery disease, left ventricular ejection fraction ≤ 0.40, and nonsustained ventricular tachycardia (69,175). The goal was to assess if an electrophysiology-guided therapeutic approach in these high-risk patients can reduce arrhythmic death and cardiac arrest (primary endpoints) and total death rate (secondary endpoint).

Of 2,202 patients enrolled, 1,435 (65%) were not inducible at electrophysiology testing. Of the 767 who were inducible, 351 were randomized to guided (by electrophysiology study) antiarrhythmic therapy in addition to an ACE inhibitor and a β-blocker as appropriate; 353 of those inducible were randomized to "best medical therapy" including an ACE inhibitor and a β-blocker. For patients randomized to electrophysiology-guided therapy, 48% ultimately had an ICD implanted; 45% received antiarrhythmic drugs. The risk of arrhythmic death or cardiac arrest in the inducible group that did not receive antiarrhythmic therapy was 18 and 32% at 2 and 5 years, respectively. Those randomized to antiarrhythmic therapy had a lower risk of arrhythmic and total deaths. Of importance, ICD therapy reduced arrhythmic or cardiac arrest by 50% compared to those in the electrophysiology-guided therapy group who did not receive ICDs. This is even more remarkable because the patients who received ICDs had failed antiarrhythmic therapy. ICD implantation conferred benefit compared with patients treated or not treated with an antiarrhythmic drug.

A controversial finding was that the mortality in MUSTT in the noninducible group was significantly lower than, but similar to, those with inducible ventricular tachycardia. The substantial mortality in the noninducible group, in contrast to previous reports, was a concern: electrophysiology testing was not as capable of predicting mortality as previous data suggested. Signal-averaged ECG abnormalities and impaired left ventricular ejection fraction < 0.30 were also predictors. High and low risks appear more a matter of opinion than an absolute distinction.

DEFINITE

DEFINITE was a prospective, randomized study that evaluated patients with nonischemic cardiomyopathy and nonsustained ventricular tachycardia. Patients were well treated medically for heart failure and cardiomyopathy. They were randomized to an ICD or to best therapy (the vast majority of patients were treated with Angiotensin Converting Enzyme Inhibitors and β-blockers) with a mean follow-up of 29.0 ± 14.4 months. The mortality rate at 2 years was 14.1% in the standard-therapy group and 7.9% in the ICD group ($p = 0.08$, i.e., nonsignificant) (159). This difference was almost entirely due to the reduction in deaths from arrhythmias in the ICD group as the hazard ratio for this type of death was 0.20. This reduction in total mortality might have failed to reach significance due to the benefits of optimized medical treatment, low overall mortality, and optimisms of relative risk reduction expected in this patient population.

SCD-HeFT

SCD-HeFT, a prospective NIH-sponsored, multicenter, randomized primary prevention trial enrolling high-risk, well treated, New York Heart Association Functional Class II and III heart failure patients tested the hypothesis that vamiodarone or ICD implant, compared to a placebo pill would improve survival. Patients with left ventricular ejection fractions ≤ 0.35 were enrolled, and randomized to a placebo pill, amiodarone, or an ICD. Patients ($n = 2,521$) were followed for a median of 45.5 months. ICDs decreased risk of death compared with placebo (hazard ratio, 0.77; $p = 0.007$). The curves deviated at 18 months. Amiodarone had a similar mortality outcome compared with placebo (hazard ratio, 1.06; $p = 0.53$) (Fig. 14.3). The absolute risk reduction at 5 years was 7.2%.

The interaction between ICD therapy and New York Heart Association Functional Class was significant but this subanalysis must be interpreted with caution as it was not the primary endpoint of the study and a post hoc analysis. Patients with New York Heart Association Class III heart failure had no apparent benefit from an ICD while patients with New York Heart Association Class II heart failure, there was a 46% relative risk reduction (54). These results were contrary to data from DEFINITE.

SCD-HeFT targeted the entire population of heart failure patients with ischemic and nonischemic cardiomyopathy with less bias than previous primary prevention trials. SCD-HeFT study raised the standard of care for many heart failure patients.

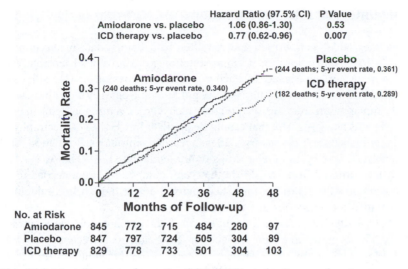

Fig. 14.3 Mortality data from the SCD-HeFT study. Improved outcomes were observed in the defibrillator group (ICD). (From Bardy, G.H., *N Engl J Med* 2005. 352(3): 225–37 with permission.)

DINAMIT

DINAMIT tested the hypothesis was that prophylactic ICDs reduce all-cause mortality in survivors of a recent myocardial infarction (within 6–40 days). These high risk survivors were selected based on left ventricular dysfunction (ejection fraction ≤ 0.35) as well as depressed heart-rate variability or an elevated 24-h heart rate. The annual all-cause mortality rates (7.5% for the ICD and 6.9% for the control arms) were not different. While fewer patients in the ICD arm died an arrhythmic death, this was offset by more nonarrhythmic deaths (174). This very ill group was likely too ill to benefit from an ICD. Based on these data, prophylactic ICDs are not currently recommended in high-risk patients who recently had a myocardial infarction.

Other Trials

CAT and AMIOVERT, smaller studies that examined use of prophylactic ICDs in nonischemic cardiomyopathy patients, failed to show benefit from ICDs. CAT was terminated early due to low 1-year mortality rates (5.6% as opposed to the anticipated rate of 30%). After 2-year follow-up, mortality rate was 26% in ICD group, 50% in controls ($p = 0.554$). Final conclusions cannot be derived from these small studies (148,176) and, in a meta-analysis, ICDs benefit patient with nonischemic cardiomyopathy(177).

Gender

Women have been under-represented in ICD trials and they have not fared as well. No study so far has shown significant improvement in outcomes for women who receive an ICD compared to control. It is not yet known whether the benefits and harms of ICDs differ by gender. The reason for the observation that women do not device the same benefit may be due to patient selection for studies, the age of the women, statistical factors, or that women have a different risk of mortality after ICD implant with similar heart disease (54,159,167,172). Further investigation is underway.

Guidelines for ICD Implantation

Guidelines have been written and rewritten to accommodate recent clinical data. In 1991, indications for ICD implantation were developed separately by the North American Society of Pacing and Electrophysiology (NASPE) and an ACC/AHA task force. The NASPE guidelines from 1991 recommended ICD implantation for: (a) ventricular tachycardia/ventricular fibrillation, spontaneous and sustained, that cannot be predicted by Holter or electrophysiology guidance, and (b) ventricular tachycardia/ventricular fibrillation, still inducible, despite best available drugs or after ablation (178). The ACC/AHA guidelines differed from NASPE in that ventricular tachycardia needed to be hemodynamically significant for ICD implant, whereas the NASPE guidelines did not mention a need for this criterion.

In 1998, the ACC/AHA guidelines for ICD implantation were revised (179). These guidelines were refined in 2002 and most recently in 2006 (180,181). Indications for ICDs can be expected to be modified further as large-scale trials are reported. ACC/AHA/ESC guidelines provide a consensus opinion about indications for ICD implantation but these data are not readily accepted in all venues and in all countries.

ACC/AHA/ESC indications for ICD therapy are based on a three-class scale. Class I indicates that there is evidence and/or general agreement that the ICD is beneficial, useful, and effective. Although this does not mean that this treatment must be used in all circumstances, there should be strong consideration for its use. Other therapies may be more appropriate for any individual patient and an attempt to use proper medical therapy for underlying cardiovascular conditions is expected. Class II indicates that there is conflicting evidence and/or a divergence of opinion about the usefulness and efficacy of the ICD. Class II has been further divided into Class IIa and IIb. Class IIa indicates that the weight of evidence and that the general opinion favors the usefulness of the ICD. Class IIb indicates that the usefulness of the ICD is less well established. Class III indicates that evidence and general opinion suggest that the ICD is not useful or effective, and may even be harmful.

The following are the conjoint ACC/AHA/ESC 2006 guidelines (76).

Class I Indications for an ICD: (1) Survivors of cardiac arrest secondary to ventricular tachycardia and ventricular fibrillation except when due to a reversible cause. (2) Sustained ventricular tachycardia associated with structural heart disease. (3) Syncope of unclear etiology with an inducible ventricular tachycardia or ventricular fibrillation at electrophysiology study. (4) Nonsustained ventricular tachycardia in patients with coronary artery disease, left ventricular dysfunction, and inducible ventricular tachycardia or fibrillation at electrophysiology study that is not suppressed will by an antiarrhythmic drug. (5) Spontaneous sustained ventricular tachycardia in patients without structural heart disease who are not amenable to medical therapy.

Class IIa Indications for an ICD: (1) Patients with a left ventricular ejection fraction of ≤ 0.35 at least 40 days after myocardial infarction and/or 3 months after coronary revascularization therapy. (2) ICD therapy combined with biventricular pacing in patients with New York Heart Association Functional Class III or IV receiving optimal medical therapy, in sinus rhythm with a QRS complex of at least 120 ms and who have reasonable (> 1 year) expectation of survival with a good functional status. (3) Patients with hypertrophic cardiomyopathy receiving chronic optimal medical therapy and remain at risk of SCD. (4) Patients with arrhythmogenic right ventricular cardiomyopathy, family history of SCD, or undiagnosed syncope. (5) Patients with long QT interval syndrome with syncope and/or ventricular tachycardia while receiving β-blockers and who have reasonable expectation of survival. (6) Patients with catecholaminergic polymorphic ventricular tachycardia with syncope and/or documented sustained ventricular tachycardia while receiving β-blockers and who have reasonable expectation of survival.

Class IIb indications for an ICD: (1) Patients optimally managed with New York Heart Association Functional Class I heart failure and nonischemic cardiomyopathy who have a left ventricular ejection fraction ≤ 0.35. (2) Syncope of unclear etiology and ECG evidence of Brugada syndrome. (3) Patients with congenital long QT interval syndrome who have reasonable expectation of survival.

Class III indications for an ICD: (i.e., NOT indicated): (1) Syncope of unclear etiology when an electrophysiology study fails to induce any ventricular arrhythmia. (2) Ventricular arrhythmias secondary to transient or reversible disorders. (3) Elderly patients with projected life expectancy less than 1 year due to major comorbidities. (4) Terminal illnesses with projected life expectancy < 12 months.

Combined Medicaid and Medicare Services Recommendations

In the United States, the Combined Medicare and Medicaid Services (CMS) carefully reviewed all of the data regarding prophylactic indication for implantable cardioverter defibrillators. In a well-written summary of all the data regarding the outcomes of studies in patients receiving ICDs, CMS provided recommendations for implantable cardioverter defibrillators in the United States (http://www.cms.hhs.gov/mcd/viewdecisionmemo.asp?id = 148). These recommendations are not necessarily followed in countries other than the US but they are reasonable recommendations based on the data. These recommendations were developed by a regulatory body that reimburses for medical procedures.

CMS found that ICDs for primary prevention purposes are *reasonable and necessary* for: (1) Patients with ischemic cardiomyopathy, myocardial infarction at least 40 days before, New York Heart Association Functional Class II and III heart failure, and left ventricular ejection fraction ≤ 0.35. (2) Patients with nonischemic cardiomyopathy treated for at least 9 months (although as short as 3 months is considered reasonable), Functional Class II or III heart failure and a left ventricular ejection fraction ≤ 0.35. (3). Patients with New York Heart Association Functional Class I heart failure, and a left ventricular ejection fraction ≤ 0.30. (4) Patients who have a QRS > 0.120, have New York Heart Association Functional Class IV heart failure, may benefit from cardiac resynchronization therapy and have a left ventricular ejection fraction ≤ 0.30.

The CMS has several criteria that excluded prophylactic ICD implantation: (1) Cardiogenic shock or symptomatic hypotension while in a stable baseline rhythm. (2) Coronary artery bypass graft or percutaneous transluminal coronary angioplasty within 3 months. (3) Acute myocardial infarction within the 40 days. (4) Symptoms or findings that would make them a candidate for coronary revascularization. (5) Irreversible brain damage from preexisting cerebral disease. (6) Any disease, other than cardiac disease (e.g., cancer, uremia, liver failure), associated with a likelihood of survival less than 1 year.

Practical Applications of the Guidelines

The ACC/AHA guidelines represent a consensus opinion and cannot address each individual patient. When faced with making a decision the choice about which patient requires an implant can be much more difficult than it might initially appear. Guidelines do not always pertain.

A patient with acute myocarditis and nonsustained ventricular tachycardia may be at high risk and may benefit from an ICD. A patient with a cardiac arrest who is found to have a poor ejection fraction and multivessel coronary disease, even if the ejection fraction improves somewhat may benefit form an ICD. A patient with congenital heart disease or a slight prolongation of the QT interval and a family history of sudden death are just some examples of the complexity in the decision making process. There is no one-percent mortality that is considered excess risk for which an ICD should be considered. An elderly patient with a 50% risk of dying suddenly in a year but with multiple severe medical problems that are likely to lead to death anyway may not benefit from an ICD, yet a younger otherwise healthy patient with a 5% risk of sudden death from long QT interval syndrome may be just the patient who would benefit most from an ICD.

A patient with transient electrolyte shift or a presumed cause for cardiac arrest, may or may not benefit from an ICD. Survivors of cardiac arrest due to ventricular arrhythmia should not be assumed as due to reversible cause unless this can be proven with high level of certainty. Consider the fact that it is often not clear what is the cause or the effect of a cardiac arrest. Hypokalemia and slight troponin elevation are two common findings after an arrest even if they are not the cause. Be careful not to jump to conclusions as to what caused a cardiac arrest. If the cause is not completely clear it is better to err on the side of an ICD implant rather than to rely on unfounded and potentially dangerous clinical assumptions.

It is important to recognize that an ICD should be considered for long-term rhythm management, not for acute treatment. As such, patients should not undergo implant of an ICD if ventricular arrhythmias are incessant or frequent or if supraventricular tachyarrhythmias are not well controlled. Any patient for whom an ICD implant is considered should have myocardial ischemia and heart failure controlled as best possible first. All other potential complicating medical problems should be addressed before delving into an implant.

The CMS recommendations are not part of a consensus document. They are designed to facilitate reimbursement in the US. Although there are some recommendations in the CMS recommendations guidelines regarding which patients might be appropriate for an ICD, this problem remains complex. For example, should there be an age limit for an ICD implant? How are these decisions to be made? How are the data regarding secondary prevention and slight increase in longevity to be interpreted with regard to the absolute need for an ICD? Now, a special form (http://www.accncdr.com/WebNCDR/ICD/ELEMENTS.ASPX), designed by the American College of Cardiology, and being used by CMS, is a potential deterrent for implanting defibrillators (and of no clear benefit). This involved form is extensive and requires information that is far beyond that mentioned in the indications for implantable defibrillators.

All therapies must be evaluated based on their effects on increasing longevity, to be sure, but other variables must be considered such as risk, hospitalization, heart failure, impact on other medical conditions, quality of life, and cost. ICDs tie a patient even more closely to the medical profession and take away some degree of autonomy. It is possible to have an integrated approach to the problem of SCD. No one therapy is always useful. The gain to prevent sudden death is attainable but the more important, the ultimate, yet complex, goal to prevent cardiac death, and extend meaningful life, may be achievable.

Unfortunately, many patients do not fit exactly into categories defined by the clinical trials. Extrapolations of data to specific patient conditions can be incorrect. With the changing guidelines, increased availability of technology and widespread publicity, enthusiasm for ICD use has spread to patients, often with complex medical problems for which the ICD may not extend their lives and may simply impair the quality of the remainder of their lives. Patients who have multisystem disease (e.g., renal failure, ongoing ischemia, or steroid use) may have problems that complicate the use of the ICD and increase the risk of device implantation.

Curiously, some clinical trials have had a large impact on clinical practice, whereas other trials have not. The MADIT II trial was considered substantial enough for the ACC/AHA guidelines to be changed and the population of patients who became candidates for an ICD literally doubled. Even so, many patients who may be candidates for and derive life-saving benefit from ICDs have not received them. Why the great majority of patients who may benefit from having an ICD implanted, had not had an ICD implant remains an open and disturbing issue.

While practical issues related to medical practice may be a limiting factor for referral for ICDs, there are concerns about small risks of ICD implants in the minds of physicians and patients that overshadow the possible benefits. It may be that many at risk of SCD may die anyway with or without an ICD (based on concomitant conditions and based on age) and these decisions are factored in by treating physicians. It is possible that physician bias or ignorance of the benefits of ICDs plays a role. The prejudices of the physicians caring for patients, in part, may be correct. It is possible that the MADIT II and SCD-HeFT trials do not reflect adequately the risk the average patient with impaired ventricular function has for SCD. Further, the real risk of SCD may be overemphasized. This, and the lack of consistent data in all populations, may affect the enthusiasm for patient referrals for ICDs.

Physicians caring for patients who have had a cardiac arrest have common biases. Patients and physicians alike often ascribe the cause of a cardiac arrest to etiologies that are either unrelated or simply associated with the event. Low potassium, for example, is a common sequel of a cardiac arrest. It is due to shifts in pH and due to a direct adrenergic effect on potassium transport into cells (182,183). Most patients who suffer a prolonged cardiac arrest will have low potassium. Another problem is the slight elevation in cardiac enzymes or electrocardiographic changes caused by the arrest itself. Such patients may be referred for coronary artery bypass graft surgery or angioplasty without even being considered for an ICD. Although this may be appropriate for a patient who has severe underlying coronary artery disease and normal left ventricular function, ischemia should not be considered the culprit in patients with impaired ventricular function, even when multivessel coronary disease is present unless it is clear that ischemia triggered the arrest.

Ironically, patients are frequently referred after a cardiac arrest when the etiology is clearly transient or due to correctable ischemia. In either case, an ICD alone will not improve the prognosis. A patient who has an ischemic cardiac arrest due to a left main lesion in the face of normal ventricular function will not derive substantial benefit from an ICD alone. An ICD may be of no benefit for a patient who has ventricular fibrillation or cardiac arrest due to an acute Q wave myocardial infarction.

Patients with syncope, heart failure, and impaired ventricular function are at high risk to die from SCD (184,185). We do not know, however, that an ICD will protect such patients from dying. With the recent wave of enthusiasm for ICD implants, temperance and prudent judgment must be employed. Not every event requires an ICD implant in a high-risk patient. It is even conceivable that a patient may trip on a rug at home only to find that a physician wants to top it off with an ICD implant. Risks of infection and inappropriate ICD discharge (a proarrhythmic effect of the ICD) may outweigh the benefit of implant in some patients. ICDs can transform an episode of nonsustained ventricular tachycardia into ventricular fibrillation, for example, and be proarrhythmic (186).

ICD placement in patient with nonsustained ventricular tachycardia, history of coronary artery disease, left ventricular dysfunction, and an inducible ventricular arrhythmia at an electrophysiology study is indicated as per MADIT criteria. However, these data are supplanted by SCD-HeFT which indicates that an ICD implant is appropriately independent of electrophysiology test results. A controversial area is ICD implantation in patients without structural heart disease who have spontaneous sustained ventricular tachycardia that is not amenable to medical therapy. We do not ascribe to this indication based on lack of data indicating the need for an ICD unless the ventricular tachycardia is polymorphic associated with evidence for a channelopathy such as long QT interval.

Primary drug therapy may be an acceptable alternative for a patient who has a slow, well-tolerated ventricular tachycardia in association with good ventricular function (ejection fraction > 0.40). Suppressing ventricular tachycardia with an antiarrhythmic drug, however, may not improve survival and may worsen the risk of SCD. The chance of recurrent ventricular tachycardia on an antiarrhythmic drug, based on ESVEM data, is high.

Ablation of ventricular tachycardia with complete cure is possible for idiopathic right ventricular outflow tract tachycardia, for idiopathic left ventricular tachycardia from the apical septum, for ventricular tachycardia due to Tetralogy of Fallot, and for bundle branch reentrant tachycardias. Ablation can be effective for ventricular tachycardia with other associated structural heart disease, but no evidence indicates that it will decrease the risk of death.

ICD implantation should be considered for this latter group. Idiopathic ventricular fibrillation is not a reason to consider drug therapy. An ICD should be implanted based on present data although emerging data now suggest that this may be an ablatable rhythm in some circumstances (187,188). On the other hand, patients with sustained ventricular tachycardia in association with structural heat disease remain at high risk for death despite medical treatment and are not usually amenable to ablation therapy.

Device Selection and Programing

Optimal ICD device selection (single chamber, dual chamber, triple chamber) remains an issue regarding patient outcomes and cost-effectiveness.

The Dual Chamber and VVI Implantable Defibrillator (DAVID) Trial was a single-blind, parallel-group, randomized clinical trial that aimed at determining the efficacy of dual-chamber pacing (DDDR 70–130) compared with backup ventricular pacing (VVI 40) in patients with standard indications for ICD implantation (and a left ventricular ejection fraction (≤0.40) but without indications for antibradycardia pacing. Patients had either primary prevention indications (47%) or secondary prevention indications (53%) for an ICD. Treatment with VVI-40 programming was associated with a better composite endpoint of death and heart failure hospitalization likely due to high degrees of right ventricular pacing in the DDDR arm (>50% right ventricular pacing) that caused "desynchronization therapy" (Fig. 14.4). Nevertheless, there are potential advantages to having an implanted atrial lead (82,189).

The Inhibition of Unnecessary RV Pacing with AV Search Hysteresis in ICDs (INTRINSIC RV) Trial was a prospective, multicenter; randomized trial evaluating similar outcomes in ICD recipients programmed VVI-40 or DDDR 60–130 with AV Search Hysteresis to reduce excessive right ventricular pacing. Those randomized had <20% right ventricular pacing after ICD implantation but before randomization. In this noninferiority trial, DDDR programming was associated with similar, if not better, outcomes measured as the combined endpoint of heart failure hospitalization and total mortality. The results indicated that right ventricular pacing as managed by AV search hysteresis, if it is ≤20%, is associated with acceptable, if not better, outcomes (Fig. 14.5) (190–192).

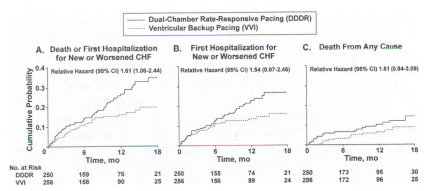

Fig. 14.4 Mortality and Morbidity data from the DAVID trial. Improved survival and heart failure hospitalization was observed in the VVI-40 programming. (From Wilkoff, B.L., et al., *JAMA* 2002. 288(24): 3115–23, with permission.)

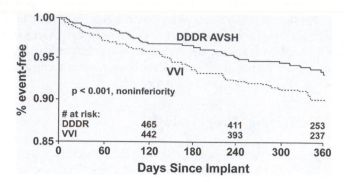

Fig. 14.5 Results of the INTRINSIC RV Trial (From Olshansky, B., et al. Circulation 2007;115(1): p. 9–16.

Needless to say that ICD programming for ventricular tachyarrhythmia detection and therapy is complex and requires high level of training. It might also influence outcomes like the frequency of shocks and patient morbidity. Recent data has proven that standardized empiric ICD programming for VT/VF settings is at least as effective as patient-specific, physician-tailored programming, as measured by these clinical outcomes. This implies that simplified and prespecified ICD programming is possible and maybe a favorable option in many situations (193).

Cardiac Resynchronization Therapy

Disordered electrical and mechanical ventricular activation can compromise cardiac function. Pacing technology has been used to attempt to correct the inter- and intraventricular conduction in an effort to optimize cardiac performance. The earliest attempts were performed during surgery when epicardial leads were placed over the lateral left ventricle free wall. Later, the coronary sinus was utilized to activate the left ventricle. Cardiac-resynchronization therapy (CRT) for treatment of patients with congestive heart failure and ventricular dyssynchrony can have a remarkable beneficial effect. Use of this technology continues to evolve.

The Cardiac Resynchronization in Heart Failure (CARE-HF) evaluated 813 patients with New York Heart Association Functional Class III or IV heart failure due to left ventricular systolic dysfunction and cardiac dyssynchrony (QRS interval ≥ 120 ms) who were receiving standard pharmacologic therapy. Patients were randomly assigned to receive medical therapy alone or with cardiac resynchronization. The primary end point (time to death from any cause or an unplanned hospitalization for a major cardiovascular event) was reached by 159 patients in the cardiac-resynchronization group, as compared with 224 patients in the medical-therapy group (39 versus. 55%; hazard ratio = 0.63; 95% CI 0.51–0.77; $p < 0.001$). There were 82 deaths in the cardiac-resynchronization group, as compared with 120 in the medical-therapy group (20 versus 30%; hazard ratio = 0.64; 95% CI 0.48–0.85; P < 0.002) (194,195).

The Comparison of Medical Therapy, Pacing, and Defibrillation in Chronic Heart Failure (COMPANION) trial was a randomized, open-label, 3-arm study of patients in New York Heart Association Functional Class III or IV with a left ventricular ejection fraction ≤ 0.35 and a QRS duration ≥ 120 ms. The study objectives were to determine whether optimal pharmacological therapy with (1) CRT therapy alone or (2) CRT with cardioverter-defibrillator capability is superior to optimal pharmacological therapy alone to reduce all-cause mortality and hospitalization The trial was terminated prematurely as it reached its primary endpoint with superiority in the device arms. Mortality was reduced by 40% in patients implanted with combined devices, while cardiac-resynchronization therapy alone gave an intermediate mortality of 15% (196,197).

The Multicenter InSync ICD Randomized Clinical Evaluation (MIRACLE ICD) trial was a randomized, double-blind, parallel-controlled trial of a high-risk population that included patients with left ventricular ejection fraction ≤ 0.35, QRS duration ≥ 130 ms and New York Heart Association Functional Class III or IV despite optimal medical treatment. Patients received devices with combined CRT and ICD capabilities and were randomized to the ICD therapy on or off. At 6 months, patients assigned to CRT had a greater improvement in median quality of life score and functional class as compared to controls. No significant differences were observed in changes in left ventricular size or function, overall heart failure status, survival, and rates of hospitalization. No proarrhythmia was observed and arrhythmia termination capabilities were not impaired (82).

The Multicenter InSync ICD Randomized Clinical Evaluation II (MIRACLE ICD II) was a follow-up randomized, double-blind, parallel-controlled clinical trial of CRT in New York Heart Association Functional Class II heart failure patients on optimal medical therapy with a left ventricular ejection fraction ≤ 0.35, a QRS ≥ 130 ms and a Class I indication for an ICD. Patients were randomized to control group (ICD activated, CRT off) and to CRT group (ICD activated, cardiac-resynchronization therapy on). No significant differences were noted in 6-min walk distance or quality of life scores or peak VO2. There were significant improvements in left ventricular diastolic and systolic volumes and in left ventricular ejection fraction (198).

In patients with heart failure and cardiac dyssynchrony, CRT improves symptoms and the quality of life and reduces complications and the risk of death. These benefits are in addition to those afforded by standard pharmacologic therapy.

Antiarrhythmic Drugs and ICDs

In approximately 50% of cases, antiarrhythmic drugs are required in patients with ICDs to reduce the frequency of recurrent ventricular arrhythmias (199). Antiarrhythmic drugs may also be necessary to suppress atrial arrhythmias, which may interfere with proper detection and lead to "inappropriate shocks" (200,201). In both situations, drugs must be used judiciously because of potential drug–device interactions. Drugs can: (a) slow ventricular tachycardia below the programmed rate cutoff, (b) increase energy threshold to defibrillate, (c) have an effect on pace termination of ventricular tachycardia, (d) be proarrhythmic, and (e) cause bradycardia and AV block. The process of drug selection is beyond the scope of this chapter; however, frequently used antiarrhythmic drugs with the ICD include amiodarone and sotalol.

Amiodarone is used in patients with impaired ventricular function and congestive heart failure to suppress atrial and ventricular arrhythmiass. If the patient is stable enough, amiodarone can be started on an outpatient basis. However, if ICD activations cause too many shocks or multiple activations in a very short time span, it is best to start any antiarrhythmic drug in the hospital.

After the drug is titrated and a steady state is reached, the patient needs to undergo an electrophysiology test, often known as a noninvasive programmed stimulation to assess inducibility and rate of ventricular tachycardia on the drug and the ICD response. The induced tachycardia may be at a slower rate and therefore will not be detected by the ICD unless it is properly programmed. Drugs can increase the energy needed to defibrillate although this is arguable even for patients taking moderate doses of amiodarone. The most potent drugs in this regard are amiodarone and Class I antiarrhythmic drugs. Sotalol is less likely to increase the defibrillation threshold and to slow the ventricular tachycardia rate. In a recently published study of patients with ICDs, sotalol was associated with a significant reduction in ICD shocks (sotalol: 1.43 ± 3.53 shocks per year versus placebo: 3.89 ± 10.65 shocks per year) (202). Drug therapy can facilitate pace termination of ventricular tachycardia (203,204).

ICD Malfunctioning

ICDs occasionally malfunction. FDA issues weekly Enforcement Reports that include recalls and safety alerts, a number of which have involved ICDs. Safety issues regarding ICDs can be divided into: (1) Lead problems and (2) Generator problems. These issues have been fairly well studied (205,206). Recognition of lead abnormalities, such as a tendency to fracture (205), have resulted in recalls, close follow-up, improvement in lead design, and also the development of safer methods of lead extraction. On the other hand, alerts and recalls involving ICD generators have not been as well characterized (186), although the risk of malfunction has been low and the risk of explants and a new device exceeds leaving them alone.

Maisel analyzed the weekly FDA Enforcement Reports issued between January 1990 and December 2000. They reported their assessment of 52 advisories involving 408,500 pacemakers and 114,645 ICDs. Hardware malfunctions and computer errors accounted for 95% of device recalls. This included about 1.3 million device checks and analyses and involved 36,187 device replacements at an approximate cost of $870 million (186).

In a follow-up study of 415,780 ICDs implanted in the United States between 1990 and 2002, 8,489 were explanted due to confirmed generator malfunction. Sixty-one deaths (31 ICD patients) were attributable to device malfunction. Battery/capacitor abnormalities (23.6%) and electrical issues (27.1%) accounted for half of the total device failures. The annual ICD malfunction replacement decreased between 1993 and 1996, but then increased markedly during the latter half of the study, peaking in 2001 at 36.4 per 1,000 (165).

Hauser searched the FDA database for ICD-devices-related deaths. Their search yielded 212 death events involving 100 ICD pulse generators and lead models from five manufacturers. Of 150 death events, 69% were associated with defective pulse generators or high-voltage leads. Apparently 81% of sudden or arrhythmic death events were associated with high-voltage lead failure; 19% of deaths were related to pulse generator failure caused by electronic component defects. Eleven death events occurred in patients whose pulse generators were found to be off or deactivated. These devices may have been deactivated either accidentally, by exposure to magnetic fields, or they were not reactivated after elective surgery (207). Therefore, careful monitoring of ICD performance is required especially with the advent of new technologies like transtelephonic monitoring.

Ethical Issues

As the rate of ICD implants has increased significantly, the number of sicker patients receiving this therapy also increased. In this population approaching the end of life, interventions become more complicated and less effective. Physicians play a central role in the decision to select sophisticated interventions versus palliative care. Unfortunately, physicians are not currently well prepared to face these issues.

Mueller described a series of terminally ill patients who requested (or whose surrogates requested) withdrawal of pacemaker or ICD support and the ethical issues that pertained. Potential interventions were an ethics consultation and subsequent withdrawal of pacemaker or ICD support. The study's main outcome measures were death and the context in which it occurred. Five had pacemakers; one had an ICD. While, five patients had advance directives that indicated a desire to withdraw medical interventions if death was inevitable, two patients and four surrogates requested withdrawal of pacemaker or ICD support. One patient died without withdrawal of support even though an ethics consultation had endorsed its permissibility. Another died while an ethics consultation was still in progress. The request to withdraw support was granted in four patients, all of whom died within 5 days of withdrawal of support (208). This study emphasizes that granting terminally ill patients' requests to withdraw unwanted medical support is both legal and ethical. It makes it clear that death after withdrawal of support is considered attributable to the patient's underlying pathology and is not the same as physician-assisted suicide or euthanasia. Thus, the clinician familiarity with these concepts is very critical as it will lead to more expeditious withdrawal of unwanted medical support from such terminally ill patients.

Cost-Effectiveness of ICD Therapy

Despite enthusiasm for ICD therapy, the cost of ICD implantation is a major concern because of the limited health care resources available. Although the ICD is very effective therapy, is it cost-effective?

Incremental cost-effectiveness compares the differences in total therapy cost and years lived between two alternative therapies and is usually expressed in units of cost per life year saved ($LYS). Cost per life year saved for the

ICD is calculated by the following equation, and incorporates clinical and economic outcomes to determine the extra cost incurred for an additional life year lived.

$$\frac{\text{ICD total cost } - \text{ drug total cost}}{\text{ICD life expectancy } - \text{ drug life expectancy}} = \text{ICD incremental cost-effectiveness}$$

Many incremental cost-effectiveness studies have been completed over the last 20 years. Several criteria have been proposed to judge the attractiveness of therapies based on their incremental cost-effectiveness.

Cost per life year saved can be: (a) cost savings ($0 or less), (b) highly cost-effective ($0 to $20,000), (c) cost-effective ($20,000 to $40,000), (d) borderline cost-effective ($40,000 to $60,000), (e) expensive ($60,000 to $100,000), and (f) unattractive (more than $100,000). Using these arbitrary categories, coronary artery bypass graft surgery in a patient with left main coronary artery disease is highly cost-effective ($8,000), angioplasty of a left anterior descending artery for single vessel disease is cost-effective ($26,000), and anticoagulation of a patient with mitral stenosis is very expensive or unattractive ($174,000).

With the large expansion of the indications for ICD implantation, especially after the several positive primary prevention trials came out, the cost–benefit ratio has significantly changed. After the initial public presentation of the SCD-HeFT results in March 2004, the CMS estimated that as many as 500,000 Medicare beneficiaries might be eligible to receive a prophylactic ICDs in the US (209). The economical sequelae of this shift in practice have been enormous as one might expect.

Before the era of primary implantation, ICD therapy generally used to fit in the cost-effective range of $20,000–$40,000 (136,210–213). Mushlin assessed incremental cost-effectiveness of ICD implant in the MADIT trial (214). After 4 years, ICD implants were associated with an incremental benefit of 0.8 years. Based on this survival benefit, the authors estimated that ICD cost was $22,800 for the 181 patients who received a transvenous device. The cost per life year saved for ICDs in the AVID trial was > $114,917. The reason for this extraordinarily high cost is, in part due to the short-term follow-up, and the short (2.9-month) survival advantage for the ICD group despite a 37% reduction in mortality.

Things have changed! The radical and relatively quick changes in guidelines, especially for primary prophylaxis therapy, have posed a dynamic challenge for both health care professionals and policymakers. The question was again whether this proven effective therapy is cost effective per the current standards of the society. Not surprisingly, multiple cost-effectiveness studies have emerged, trying to address this challenge. Using a Markov model of the cost, quality of life, survival, and incremental cost-effectiveness, and after analyzing the six positive prophylactic trials (MADIT I, MADIT II, MUSTT, DEFINITE, COMPANION, and SCD-HeFT), Sanders found that the cost-effectiveness of the ICD as compared with control therapy ranged from $34,000 to $70,200 per quality-adjusted life-years gained (213). The ICD cost was estimated at $27,975. Also a simple strategy like delaying the generator replacement to every 7 years improved the cost effectiveness to $30,800–$62,300 per QALY gained. A recent analysis of patients who satisfied MADIT

II criteria and who were enrolled in a Duke cohort cost effectiveness showed that reducing the cost of ICD placement and leads had much more effect on the cost-effectiveness ratios than changing the frequency of follow-up visits, complication rates, and battery replacements (215).

Data from the MADIT II trial indicated that the estimated cost/LYS by the ICD is relatively high at 3.5 years ($235,000) but is projected to be substantially lower over the course of longer time horizons ($78,600–114,000 in a projection to 12 years) (212). Their reason for these costs was likely due to the average survival gain for the defibrillator arm being only 2 months.

In SCD-HeFT, the lifetime cost effectiveness and cost utility ratios were estimated at $38 389/LYS and $41 530/quality adjusted LYS. A further analysis showed a cost-effectiveness ratio of $29 872/LYS for New York Heart Association Functional Class II but no incremental benefit for Functional Class III heart failure (216). Prophylactic use of single-lead, shock-only ICD seems attractive economically in patients with stable, moderately symptomatic heart failure and an ejection fraction ≤ 0.35.

Differences in the costs among analyses may be related to the types of patients enrolled in the trials but other factors also must be considered, including lack of accuracy of the cost analysis data, differences in mortality of the patients in the trials, difference in the benefit of the ICD, implant techniques, ICD longevity, patient longevity, and capabilities of the ICD to offset further problems, including readmission and need for follow-up.

The pressure to reduce costs has been particularly intense for high-technology interventions such as ICDs. Many US centers have now begun to use lower-cost practices for ICD implantation. These include elimination of a preimplant electrophysiology study, use of local anesthesia and/or conscious sedation, a shift in procedure site from the operating room to the electrophysiology laboratory or a procedure room, and reduced length of stay postimplant. Market pressures in the United State are forcing physicians and hospitals to update their practice patterns continually to provide higher quality, lower-cost care.

It appears that the ICD can now be cost-effective using modern, simpler implantation techniques, shorter hospitalizations, and better, longer-lasting devices requiring less follow-up even in the highest-risk patients who stand to derive a mortality benefit between 20 and 40%. It is not clear that any other therapies are less expensive or nearly as effective. With further streamlining of the implant approach and long-term follow-up, the costs should continue to come down even further. It is always important to keep cost-effectiveness analysis in clinical perspective. The worst possible alternative would be to deny any therapy and allow an unnecessary death. This approach is clearly unacceptable, even though it may save "resources."

Unexplored Areas

Patients waiting for heart transplant may be a potential population that would benefit from ICD implant (217–219). Up to 30% of patients on heart transplant lists die waiting for a transplant, and often the death is sudden and presumed arrhythmic. In one study of 978 patients from 12 institutions awaiting heart transplant, the ICD seemed to be helpful. This patient population included UNOS Status II patients (not in the intensive care unit on intravenous inotropic support), who are at risk for death while awaiting cardiac transplantation. The mean follow-up of survivors was 13 months (range 1–48 months). An ICD was placed a median of 8.1 months before heart transplant listing in 105 patients. A history of a confirmed or suspected arrhythmic event (ventricular tachycardia, cardiac arrest, syncope, or positive electrophysiologic study) was present in 406 patients and absent in 572 patients. At 18 months, the mortality in the ICD group was 11 versus 19% among patients without an arrhythmic event ($p = 0.09$) and 28% among those with arrhythmic events and no ICD ($p = 0.005$). These data suggested that patients awaiting transplantation are at significant risk of death and that ICD placement may improve survival. More data are needed to confirm the value of an ICD in this patient population.

Many other populations may benefit from ICD implantation perhaps even including the entire US population depending on what is considered high risks. High-risk patients such as those with heart failure may not always benefit as they may die of heart failure anyway. On the other hand, even a small risk in a young patient with congenital long QT syndrome may be too hard to accept. The concept of defining risk needs to be better clarified. Further, genetic screening may better identify patient at high risk.

Conclusion

ICD therapy has advanced tremendously within a short time span. The ICD simplifies management and improves patient outcome in properly selected patients. The ICD has become first-line therapy for patients with ventricular fibrillation, poorly tolerated ventricular tachycardia, patients with structural heart disease who have sustained ventricular tachycardia, and patients with syncope and induced ventricular tachycardia when other therapies are inappropriate. Prophylactic ICD implantation has revolutionized the treatment of patients at high risk for cardiac arrest, such as those with low ejection fraction and history of myocardial infarction or symptoms of heart failure. The ICD represents a major advancement in the treatment of high-risk patients with heart disease.

References

1. Thom, T., et al., Heart disease and stroke statistics – 2006 update: a report from the American Heart Association Statistics Committee and Stroke Statistics Subcommittee. Circulation, 2006. **113**(6): p. e85–151.
2. Rea, T.D., et al., Incidence of EMS-treated out-of-hospital cardiac arrest in the United States. Resuscitation, 2004. **63**(1): p. 17–24.
3. Lopshire, J.C. and D.P. Zipes, Sudden cardiac death: better understanding of risks, mechanisms, and treatment. Circulation, 2006. **114**(11): p. 1134–6.
4. Broadley, A.J., et al., Baroreflex sensitivity is reduced in depression. Psychosom Med, 2005. **67**(4): p. 648–51.
5. Liu, Y.B., et al., Dyslipidemia is associated with ventricular tachyarrhythmia in patients with acute ST-segment elevation myocardial infarction. J Formos Med Assoc = Taiwan yi zhi, 2006. **105**(1): p. 17–24.
6. James, A.F., S.C. Choisy, and J.C. Hancox, Recent advances in understanding sex differences in cardiac repolarization, 2007. **94**: p. 265–319.
7. Russo, A.M., et al., Influence of gender on arrhythmia characteristics and outcome in the Multicenter UnSustained Tachycardia Trial. J Cardiovasc Electrophysiol, 2004. **15**(9): p. 993–8.

8. Lampert, R., et al., Gender differences in ventricular arrhythmia recurrence in patients with coronary artery disease and implantable cardioverter-defibrillators. J Am Coll Cardiol, 2004. **43**(12): p. 2293–9.

9. Wolbrette, D., et al., Gender differences in arrhythmias. Clin Cardiol, 2002. **25**(2): p. 49–56.

10. Thorgeirsson, G., et al., Risk factors for out-of-hospital cardiac arrest: the Reykjavik Study. Eur Heart J, 2005. **26**(15): p. 1499–505.

11. Locati, E.H., et al., Age- and sex-related differences in clinical manifestations in patients with congenital long-QT syndrome: findings from the International LQTS Registry. Circulation, 1998. **97**(22): p. 2237–44.

12. Moise, N.S., et al., Age dependence of the development of ventricular arrhythmias in a canine model of sudden cardiac death. Cardiovasc Res, 1997. **34**(3): p. 483–92.

13. Goldenberg, I., et al., Current smoking, smoking cessation, and the risk of sudden cardiac death in patients with coronary artery disease. Arch Intern Med, 2003. **163**(19): p. 2301–5.

14. Diamond, J.A. and R.A. Phillips, Hypertensive heart disease. Hypertension research, 2005. **28**(3): p. 191–202.

15. Holzgreve, H., Benefits of antihypertensive treatment. How much damage does it really prevent? MMW Fortschritte der Medizin, 2006. **148**(14): p. 47, 49–50.

16. Bray, G.A. and T. Bellanger, Epidemiology, trends, and morbidities of obesity and the metabolic syndrome. Endocrine, 2006. **29**(1): p. 109–17.

17. Wheelan, K., et al., Sudden death and its relation to QT-interval prolongation after acute myocardial infarction: two-year follow-up. Am J Cardiol, 1986. **57**(10): p. 745–50.

18. Pagnoni, F., et al., Long-term prognostic significance and electrophysiological evolution of intraventricular conduction disturbances complicating acute myocardial infarction. Pacing and clinical electrophysiology, 1986. **9**(1 Pt 1): p. 91–100.

19. Kaufman, E.S., et al., "Indeterminate" microvolt T-wave alternans tests predict high risk of death or sustained ventricular arrhythmias in patients with left ventricular dysfunction. J Am Coll Cardiol, 2006. **48**(7): p. 1399–404.

20. Naccarelli, G.V. and M.A. Lukas, Carvedilol's antiarrhythmic properties: therapeutic implications in patients with left ventricular dysfunction. Clin Cardiol, 2005. **28**(4): p. 165–73.

21. Hagens, V.E., et al., Determinants of sudden cardiac death in patients with persistent atrial fibrillation in the rate control versus electrical cardioversion (RACE) study. Am J Cardiol, 2006. **98**(7): p. 929–32.

22. Pedersen, O.D., et al., Increased risk of sudden and non-sudden cardiovascular death in patients with atrial fibrillation/flutter following acute myocardial infarction. Eur Heart J, 2006. **27**(3): p. 290–5.

23. Underwood, R.D., J. Sra, and M. Akhtar, Evaluation and treatment strategies in patients at high risk of sudden death post myocardial infarction. Clin Cardiol, 1997. **20**(9): p. 753–8.

24. Middlekauff, H.R., W.G. Stevenson, and L.A. Saxon, Prognosis after syncope: impact of left ventricular function. Am Heart J, 1993. **125**(1): p. 121–7.

25. Vester, E.G., et al., Electrophysiological and therapeutic implications of cardiac arrhythmias in hypertension. Eur Heart J, 1992. **13**(Suppl D): p. 70–81.

26. Buxton, A.E., et al., Nonsustained ventricular tachycardia in patients with coronary artery disease: role of electrophysiologic study. Circulation, 1987. **75**(6): p. 1178–85.

27. Tan, H.L., et al., Sudden unexplained death: heritability and diagnostic yield of cardiological and genetic examination in surviving relatives. Circulation, 2005. **112**(2): p. 207–13.

28. Lind, J.M., C. Chiu, and C. Semsarian, Genetic basis of hypertrophic cardiomyopathy. Expert Rev Cardiovasc Ther, 2006. **4**(6): p. 927–34.

29. Kirchhof, P., G. Breithardt, and L. Eckardt, Primary prevention of sudden cardiac death. Heart, 2006. **92**(12): p. 1873–8.

30. Nishio, H., M. Iwata, and K. Suzuki, Postmortem molecular screening for cardiac ryanodine receptor type 2 mutations in sudden unexplained death: R420W mutated case with characteristics of status thymico-lymphatics. Circ J, 2006. **70**(11): p. 1402–6.

31. Bar-Cohen, Y. and M.J. Silka, Congenital long QT syndrome: diagnosis and management in pediatric patients. Curr Treat Options Cardiovasc Med, 2006. **8**(5): p. 387–395.

32. Postma, A.V., Z.A. Bhuiyan, and H. Bikker, Molecular diagnostics of catecholaminergic polymorphic ventricular tachycardia using denaturing high-performance liquid chromatography and sequencing. Methods Mol Med, 2006. **126**: p. 171–83.

33. Modell, S.M. and M.H. Lehmann, The long QT syndrome family of cardiac ion channelopathies: a HuGE review. Genet Med, 2006. **8**(3): p. 143–55.

34. Calkins, H., Arrhythmogenic right-ventricular dysplasia/cardiomyopathy. Curr Opin Cardiol, 2006. **21**(1): p. 55–63.

35. Podrid, P.J. and R.J. Myerburg, Epidemiology and stratification of risk for sudden cardiac death. Clinical cardiology, 2005. **28**(11 Suppl 1): p. I3–11.

36. Corrado, D., et al., Implantable cardioverter-defibrillator therapy for prevention of sudden death in patients with arrhythmogenic right ventricular cardiomyopathy/dysplasia. Circulation, 2003. **108**(25): p. 3084–91.

37. Spooner, P.M. and D.P. Zipes, Sudden death predictors: an inflammatory association. Circulation, 2002. **105**(22): p. 2574–6.

38. Burke, A.P., et al., Elevated C-reactive protein values and atherosclerosis in sudden coronary death: association with different pathologies. Circulation, 2002. **105**(17): p. 2019–23.

39. Biasucci, L.M., et al., C reactive protein is associated with malignant ventricular arrhythmias in patients with ischaemia with implantable cardioverter-defibrillator. Heart, 2006. **92**(8): p. 1147–8.

40. Bikkina, M., M.G. Larson, and D. Levy, Prognostic implications of asymptomatic ventricular arrhythmias: the Framingham Heart Study. Ann Intern Med, 1992. **117**(12): p. 990–6.

41. Buxton, A.E., et al., Prognostic factors in nonsustained ventricular tachycardia. Am J Cardiol, 1984. **53**(9): p. 1275–9.

42. Wilber, D.J., et al., Electrophysiological testing and nonsustained ventricular tachycardia. Use and limitations in patients with coronary artery disease and impaired ventricular function. Circulation, 1990. **82**(2): p. 350–8.

43. Bigger, J.T., Jr., et al., The relationships among ventricular arrhythmias, left ventricular dysfunction, and mortality in the 2 years after myocardial infarction. Circulation, 1984. **69**(2): p. 250–8.

44. Maggioni, A.P., et al., Prevalence and prognostic significance of ventricular arrhythmias after acute myocardial infarction in the fibrinolytic era. GISSI-2 results. Circulation, 1993. **87**(2): p. 312–22.

45. Schmidt, G., et al., Heart-rate turbulence after ventricular premature beats as a predictor of mortality after acute myocardial infarction. Lancet, 1999. **353**(9162): p. 1390–6.

46. Ghuran, A., et al., Heart rate turbulence-based predictors of fatal and nonfatal cardiac arrest (The Autonomic Tone and Reflexes After Myocardial Infarction substudy). Am J Cardiol, 2002. **89**(2): p. 184–90.

47. Barthel, P., et al., Risk stratification after acute myocardial infarction by heart rate turbulence. Circulation, 2003. **108**(10): p. 1221–6.

48. Smith, J.M., et al., Electrical alternans and cardiac electrical instability. Circulation, 1988. **77**(1): p. 110–21.

49. Estes, N.A., 3rd, et al., Electrical alternans during rest and exercise as predictors of vulnerability to ventricular arrhythmias. Am J Cardiol, 1997. **80**(10): p. 1314–8.

50. Rosenbaum, D.S., et al., Electrical alternans and vulnerability to ventricular arrhythmias. N Engl J Med, 1994. **330**(4): p. 235–41.

51. Narayan, S.M. and J.M. Smith, Exploiting rate-related hysteresis in repolarization alternans to improve risk stratification for ventricular tachycardia. J Am Coll Cardiol, 2000. **35**(6): p. 1485–92.

52. Bluzaite, I., et al., QT dispersion and heart rate variability in sudden death risk stratification in patients with ischemic heart disease. Medicina (Kaunas), 2006. **42**(6): p. 450–4.

53. Dinckal, M.H., et al., QT dispersion in the risk stratification of patients with unstable angina: correlation with clinical course, troponin T and scintigraphy. Acta Cardiol, 2004. **59**(3): p. 283–9.

54. Bardy, G.H., et al., Amiodarone or an implantable cardioverter-defibrillator for congestive heart failure. N Engl J Med, 2005. **352**(3): p. 225–37.

55. Iravanian, S., A. Arshad, and J.S. Steinberg, Role of electrophysiologic studies, signal-averaged electrocardiography, heart rate variability, T-wave alternans, and loop recorders for risk stratification of ventricular arrhythmias. Am J Geriatr Cardiol, 2005. **14**(1): p. 16–9.

56. Lander, P., et al., Critical analysis of the signal-averaged electrocardiogram. Improved identification of late potentials. Circulation, 1993. **87**(1): p. 105–17.

57. Rozanski, J.J. and M. Kleinfeld, Alternans of the ST segment of T wave. A sign of electrical instability in Prinzmetal's angina. Pacing Clin Electrophysiol, 1982. **5**(3): p. 359–65.

58. Bloomfield, D.M., et al., Microvolt T-wave alternans distinguishes between patients likely and patients not likely to benefit from implanted cardiac defibrillator therapy: a solution to the Multicenter Automatic Defibrillator Implantation Trial (MADIT) II conundrum. Circulation, 2004. **110**(14): p. 1885–9.

59. Gold, M.R., et al., T-Wave Alternans SCD HeFT Study: Primary Endpoint Analysis. Circulation, 2006. **114**: p. II-428–9.

60. Akhtar, M., et al., Sudden cardiac death: management of high-risk patients. Ann Intern Med, 1991. **114**(6): p. 499–512.

61. Olshansky, B., M. Mazuz, and J.B. Martins, Significance of inducible tachycardia in patients with syncope of unknown origin: a long-term follow-up. J Am Coll Cardiol, 1985. **5**(2 Pt 1): p. 216–23.

62. Mitchell, L.B., et al., A randomized clinical trial of the noninvasive and invasive approaches to drug therapy for ventricular tachycardia: long-term follow-up of the Calgary trial. Prog Cardiovasc Dis, 1996. **38**(5): p. 377–84.

63. Steinbeck, G., et al., A comparison of electrophysiologically guided antiarrhythmic drug therapy with beta-blocker therapy in patients with symptomatic, sustained ventricular tachyarrhythmias. N Engl J Med, 1992. **327**(14): p. 987–92.

64. Richards, D.A., et al., Ventricular electrical instability: a predictor of death after myocardial infarction. Am J Cardiol, 1983. **51**(1): p. 75–80.

65. Bourke, J.P., et al., Routine programmed electrical stimulation in survivors of acute myocardial infarction for prediction of spontaneous ventricular tachyarrhythmias during follow-up: results, optimal stimulation protocol and cost-effective screening. J Am Coll Cardiol, 1991. **18**(3): p. 780–8.

66. Zoni-Berisso, M., et al., Value of programmed ventricular stimulation in predicting sudden death and sustained ventricular tachycardia in survivors of acute myocardial infarction. Am J Cardiol, 1996. **77**(9): p. 673–80.

67. Behr, E.R., P. Elliott, and W.J. McKenna, Role of invasive EP testing in the evaluation and management of hypertrophic cardiomyopathy. Card Electrophysiol Rev, 2002. **6**(4): p. 482–6.

68. Kuck, K.H., et al., Programmed electrical stimulation in hypertrophic cardiomyopathy. Results in patients with and without cardiac arrest or syncope. Eur Heart J, 1988. **9**(2): p. 177–85.

69. Buxton, A.E., et al., Electrophysiologic testing to identify patients with coronary artery disease who are at risk for sudden death. Multicenter Unsustained Tachycardia Trial Investigators. New Engl J Med, 2000. **342**(26): p.1937–45.

70. Freedman, R.A., et al., Prognostic significance of arrhythmia inducibility or noninducibility at initial electrophysiologic study in survivors of cardiac arrest. Am J Cardiol, 1988. **61**(8): p. 578–82.

71. Mason, J.W., A comparison of electrophysiologic testing with Holter monitoring to predict antiarrhythmic-drug efficacy for ventricular tachyarrhythmias. Electrophysiologic Study versus Electrocardiographic Monitoring Investigators. New Engl J Med, 1993. **329**(7): p. 445–51.

72. Moss, A.J., et al., Improved survival with an implanted defibrillator in patients with coronary disease at high risk for ventricular arrhythmia. Multicenter Automatic Defibrillator Implantation Trial Investigators. New Engl J Med, 1996. **335**(26): p. 1933–40.

73. A comparison of antiarrhythmic-drug therapy with implantable defibrillators in patients resuscitated from near-fatal ventricular arrhythmias. The Antiarrhythmics versus Implantable Defibrillators (AVID) Investigators. New Engl J Med, 1997. **337**(22): p. 1576–83.

74. Brembilla-Perrot, B., et al., Programmed ventricular stimulation in survivors of acute myocardial infarction: long-term follow-up. Int J Cardiol, 1995. **49**(1): p. 55–65.

75. Bourke, J.P., et al., Does the induction of ventricular flutter or fibrillation at electrophysiologic testing after myocardial infarction have any prognostic significance? Am J Cardiol, 1995. **75**(7): p. 431–5.

76. Zipes, D.P., et al., ACC/AHA/ESC 2006 Guidelines for Management of Patients With Ventricular Arrhythmias and the Prevention of Sudden Cardiac Death-Executive Summary A Report of the American College of Cardiology/American Heart Association Task Force and the European Society of Cardiology Committee for Practice Guidelines (Writing Committee to Develop Guidelines for Management of Patients with Ventricular Arrhythmias and the Prevention of Sudden Cardiac Death). J Am Coll Cardiol, 2006. **48**(5): p. 1064–108.

77. Nademanee, K., et al., Defibrillator versus beta-blockers for unexplained death in Thailand (DEBUT): a randomized clinical trial. Circulation, 2003. **107**(17): p. 2221–6.

78. Gottlieb, S.S., R.J. McCarter, and R.A. Vogel, Effect of beta-blockade on mortality among high-risk and low-risk patients after myocardial infarction. N Engl J Med, 1998. **339**(8): p. 489–97.

79. The Cardiac Insufficiency Bisoprolol Study II (CIBIS-II): a randomised trial. Lancet, 1999. **353**(9146): p. 9–13.

80. Makikallio, T.H., et al., Frequency of sudden cardiac death among acute myocardial infarction survivors with optimized medical and revascularization therapy. Am J Cardiol, 2006. **97**(4): p. 480–4.

81. Bauer, A., et al., Reduced prognostic power of ventricular late potentials in post-infarction patients of the reperfusion era. Eur Heart J, 2005. **26**(8): p. 755–61.

82. Young, J.B., et al., Combined cardiac resynchronization and implantable cardioversion defibrillation in advanced chronic heart failure: the MIRACLE ICD Trial. JAMA, 2003. **289**(20): p. 2685–94.

83. Domanski, M.J., et al., Effect of angiotensin converting enzyme inhibition on sudden cardiac death in patients following acute myocardial infarction. A meta-analysis of randomized clinical trials. J Am Coll Cardiol, 1999. **33**(3): p. 598–604.

84. Fonseca, V.A., Insulin resistance, diabetes, hypertension, and renin-angiotensin system inhibition: reducing risk for cardiovascular disease. J Clin Hypertens (Greenwich), 2006. **8**(10): p. 713–20; quiz 721–2.

85. Susan, M., et al., Dual renin angiotensin system blockade in patients with acute myocardial infarction and preserved left ventricular systolic function. Rom J Intern Med = Revue roumaine de medecine interne, 2005. **43**(3–4): p. 187–98.

86. McMurray, J., et al., Antiarrhythmic effect of carvedilol after acute myocardial infarction: results of the Carvedilol Post-Infarct Survival Control in Left Ventricular Dysfunction (CAPRICORN) Trial. J Am Coll Cardiol, 2005. **45**(4): p. 525–30.

87. Pelargonio, G. and E.N. Prystowsky, Rate versus rhythm control in the management of patients with atrial fibrillation. Nature clinical practice, 2005. **2**(10): p. 514–21.

88. Taylor, F.C., H. Cohen, and S. Ebrahim, Systematic review of long term anticoagulation or antiplatelet treatment in patients with non-rheumatic atrial fibrillation. Br Med J (Clin Res Ed, 2001. **322**(7282): p. 321–6.

89. Peverill, R.E., Warfarin or aspirin: both or others? Med J Aust, 1999. **171**(6): p. 321–6.

90. Kottkamp, H., G. Hindricks, and G. Breithardt, Role of anticoagulant therapy in atrial fibrillation. J Cardiovasc Electrophysiol, 1998. **9**(8 Suppl): p. S86–96.

91. Cleland, J.G., et al., Update of clinical trials from the American College of Cardiology 2003. EPHESUS, SPORTIF-III, ASCOT, COMPANION, UK-PACE and T-wave alternans. Eur J Heart Fail, 2003. **5**(3): p. 391–8.

92. Chiu, J.H., et al., Effect of statin therapy on risk of ventricular arrhythmia among patients with coronary artery disease and an implantable cardioverter-defibrillator. Am J Cardiol, 2005. **95**(4): p. 490–1.

93. Effect of metoprolol CR/XL in chronic heart failure: Metoprolol CR/XL Randomised Intervention Trial in Congestive Heart Failure (MERIT-HF). Lancet, 1999. **353**(9169): p. 2001–7.

94. Dargie, H.J., Effect of carvedilol on outcome after myocardial infarction in patients with left-ventricular dysfunction: the CAPRICORN randomised trial. Lancet, 2001. **357**(9266): p. 1385–90.

95. Yusuf, S., et al., Effects of an angiotensin-converting-enzyme inhibitor, ramipril, on cardiovascular events in high-risk patients. The Heart Outcomes Prevention Evaluation Study Investigators. N Engl J Med, 2000. **342**(3): p. 145–53.

96. Teo, K.K., et al., Effect of ramipril in reducing sudden deaths and nonfatal cardiac arrests in high-risk individuals without heart failure or left ventricular dysfunction. Circulation, 2004. **110**(11): p. 1413–7.

97. Pitt, B., et al., The effect of spironolactone on morbidity and mortality in patients with severe heart failure. Randomized Aldactone Evaluation Study Investigators. N Engl J Med, 1999. **341**(10): p. 709–17.

98. Pitt, B., et al., Eplerenone, a selective aldosterone blocker, in patients with left ventricular dysfunction after myocardial infarction. N Engl J Med, 2003. **348**(14): p. 1309–21.

99. Zijlstra, F. and I.C. van der Horst, Sudden death in patients with myocardial infarction. N Engl J Med, 2005. **353**(12): p. 1294–7; author reply 1294–7.

100. Zaliunas, R., et al., Cardiac events and 5-year survival after acute coronary syndromes. Medicina (Kaunas), 2005. **41**(8): p. 668–74.

101. Antezano, E.S. and M. Hong, Sudden cardiac death. J Intensive Care Med, 2003. **18**(6): p. 313–29.

102. Germing, A., et al., Clinical and angiographic results of coronary artery stenting using PURA-VARIO (PUVA) stents. Int J Cardiovasc Intervent, 2003. **5**(3): p. 156–60.

103. Bradshaw, P.J., et al., Mortality and recurrent cardiac events after coronary artery bypass graft: long term outcomes in a population study. Heart, 2002. **88**(5): p. 488–94.

104. Elbaz, M., et al., Is direct coronary stenting the best strategy for long-term outcome? Results of the multicentric randomized benefit evaluation of direct coronary stenting (BET) study. Am Heart J, 2002. **144**(4): p. E7.

105. Every, N., et al., Risk of sudden versus nonsudden cardiac death in patients with coronary artery disease. Am Heart J, 2002. **144**(3): p. 390–6.

106. Mittal, S., et al., Prognostic significance of nonsustained ventricular tachycardia after revascularization. J Cardiovasc Electrophysiol, 2002. **13**(4): p. 342–6.

107. Uerojanaungkul, P., et al., Short and intermediate clinical outcome after late coronary stenting in myocardial infarction. J Med Assoc Thai, 2001. **84**(7): p. 948–57.

108. Jessup, M. and S. Brozena, Heart failure. N Engl J Med, 2003. **348**(20): p. 2007–18.

109. Bigger, J.T., Jr., Why patients with congestive heart failure die: arrhythmias and sudden cardiac death. Circulation, 1987. **75**(5 Pt 2): p. IV28–35.

110. Singh, S.N., et al., Amiodarone in patients with congestive heart failure and asymptomatic ventricular arrhythmia. Survival Trial of Antiarrhythmic Therapy in Congestive Heart Failure. New Engl J Med, 1995. **333**(2): p. 77–82.

111. Rogers, W.J., et al., Quality of life among 5,025 patients with left ventricular dysfunction randomized between placebo and enalapril: the Studies of Left Ventricular Dysfunction. The SOLVD Investigators. J Am Coll Cardiol, 1994. **23**(2): p. 393–400.

112. Segev, A. and Y.A. Mekori, The Cardiac Insufficiency Bisoprolol Study II. Lancet, 1999. **353**(9161): p. 1361.

113. Gheorghiade, M. and B. Pitt, Digitalis Investigation Group (DIG) trial: a stimulus for further research. American heart journal, 1997. **134**(1): p. 3–12.

114. Packer, M., et al., Effect of oral milrinone on mortality in severe chronic heart failure. The PROMISE Study Research Group. New Engl J Med, 1991. **325**(21): p. 1468–75.

115. De Sutter, J., et al., Lipid lowering drugs and recurrences of life-threatening ventricular arrhythmias in high-risk patients. J Am Coll Cardiol, 2000. **36**(3): p. 766–72.

116. Waldo, A.L., et al., Effect of d-sotalol on mortality in patients with left ventricular dysfunction after recent and remote myocardial infarction. The SWORD Investigators. Survival with oral d-Sotalol. Lancet, 1996. **348**(9019): p. 7–12.

117. Farre, J., et al., Amiodarone and "primary" prevention of sudden death: critical review of a decade of clinical trials. Am J Cardiol, 1999. **83**(5B): p. 55D–63D.

118. A comparison of antiarrhythmic-drug therapy with implantable defibrillators in patients resuscitated from near-fatal ventricular arrhythmias. The Antiarrhythmics versus Implantable Defibrillators (AVID) Investigators. N Engl J Med, 1997. **337**(22): p. 1576–83.

119. Buxton, A.E., et al., A randomized study of the prevention of sudden death in patients with coronary artery disease. Multicenter Unsustained Tachycardia Trial Investigators. N Engl J Med, 1999. **341**(25): p. 1882–90.

120. Capucci, A., D. Aschieri, and G.Q. Villani, The role of EP-guided therapy in ventricular arrhythmias: beta-blockers, sotalol, and ICD's. J Interv Card Electrophysiol, 2000. **4**(Suppl 1): p. 57–63.

121. Lau, E.W., et al., The Midlands Trial of Empirical Amiodarone versus Electrophysiology-guided Interventions and Implantable Cardioverter-defibrillators

(MAVERIC): a multi-centre prospective randomised clinical trial on the secondary prevention of sudden cardiac death. Europace, 2004. **6**(4): p. 257–66.

122. Julian, D.G., et al., Randomised trial of effect of amiodarone on mortality in patients with left-ventricular dysfunction after recent myocardial infarction: EMIAT. European Myocardial Infarct Amiodarone Trial Investigators. Lancet, 1997. **349**(9053): p. 667–74.

123. Cairns, J.A., et al., Randomised trial of outcome after myocardial infarction in patients with frequent or repetitive ventricular premature depolarisations: CAMIAT. Canadian Amiodarone Myocardial Infarction Arrhythmia Trial Investigators. Lancet, 1997. **349**(9053): p. 675–82.

124. Camm, A.J., et al., Mortality in patients after a recent myocardial infarction: a randomized, placebo-controlled trial of azimilide using heart rate variability for risk stratification. Circulation, 2004. **109**(8): p. 990–6.

125. Ruskin, J.N., The cardiac arrhythmia suppression trial (CAST). New Engl J Med, 1989. **321**(6): p. 386–8.

126. Anderson, J.L., et al., Interaction of baseline characteristics with the hazard of encainide, flecainide, and moricizine therapy in patients with myocardial infarction. A possible explanation for increased mortality in the Cardiac Arrhythmia Suppression Trial (CAST). Circulation, 1994. **90**(6): p. 2843–52.

127. Brooks, M.M., et al., Moricizine and quality of life in the Cardiac Arrhythmia Suppression Trial II (CAST II). Control Clin Trials, 1994. **15**(6): p. 437–49.

128. The Cardiac Arrhythmia Suppression Trial II Investigators, Effect of the antiarrhythmic agent moricizine on survival after myocardial infarction.. N Engl J Med, 1992. **327**(4): p. 227–33.

129. Greene, H.L., et al., The Cardiac Arrhythmia Suppression Trial: first CAST... then CAST-II. J Am Coll Cardiol, 1992. **19**(5): p. 894–8.

130. Impact Research Group, International mexiletine and placebo antiarrhythmic coronary trial: I. Report on arrhythmia and other findings. J Am Coll Cardiol, 1984. **4**(6): p. 1148–63.

131. Mason, J.W., A comparison of seven antiarrhythmic drugs in patients with ventricular tachyarrhythmias. Electrophysiologic Study versus Electrocardiographic Monitoring Investigators. New Engl J Med, 1993. **329**(7): p. 452–8.

132. Omoigui, N.A., et al., Cost of initial therapy in the Electrophysiological Study Versus ECG Monitoring trial (ESVEM). Circulation, 1995. **91**(4): p. 1070–6.

133. Burkart, F., et al., Effect of antiarrhythmic therapy on mortality in survivors of myocardial infarction with asymptomatic complex ventricular arrhythmias: Basel Antiarrhythmic Study of Infarct Survival (BASIS). J Am Coll Cardiol, 1990. **16**(7): p. 1711–8.

134. Doval, H.C., et al., Randomised trial of low-dose amiodarone in severe congestive heart failure. Grupo de Estudio de la Sobrevida en la Insuficiencia Cardiaca en Argentina (GESICA). Lancet, 1994. **344**(8921): p. 493–8.

135. Sim, I., et al., Quantitative overview of randomized trials of amiodarone to prevent sudden cardiac death. Circulation, 1997. **96**(9): p. 2823–9.

136. Steinberg, J.S., et al., Antiarrhythmic drug use in the implantable defibrillator arm of the Antiarrhythmics Versus Implantable Defibrillators (AVID) Study. Am Heart J, 2001. **142**(3): p. 520–9.

137. Camm, A.J., R. Karam, and C.M. Pratt, The azimilide post-infarct survival evaluation (ALIVE) trial. Am J Cardiol, 1998. **81**(6A): p. 35D–39D.

138. Stevenson, W.G., et al., Identification of reentry circuit sites during catheter mapping and radiofrequency ablation of ventricular tachycardia late after myocardial infarction. Circulation, 1993. **88**(4 Pt 1): p. 1647–70.

139. Hindricks, G., The Multicentre European Radiofrequency Survey (MERFS): complications of radiofrequency catheter ablation of arrhythmias. The Multicentre European Radiofrequency Survey (MERFS) investigators of the Working Group

on Arrhythmias of the European Society of Cardiology. European heart journal, 1993. **14**(12): p. 1644–53.

140. Morady, F., et al., Radiofrequency catheter ablation of ventricular tachycardia in patients with coronary artery disease. Circulation, 1993. **87**(2): p. 363–72.

141. Gonska, B.D., et al., Catheter ablation of ventricular tachycardia in 136 patients with coronary artery disease: results and long-term follow-up. J Am Coll Cardiol, 1994. **24**(6): p. 1506–14.

142. Blanck, Z., et al., Bundle branch reentrant ventricular tachycardia: cumulative experience in 48 patients. J Cardiovasc Electrophysiol, 1993. **4**(3): p. 253–62.

143. Lau, C.P., Radiofrequency ablation of fascicular tachycardia: efficacy of pace-mapping and implications on tachycardia origin. Int J Cardiol, 1994. **46**(3): p. 255–65.

144. Bennett, D.H., Experience with radiofrequency catheter ablation of fascicular tachycardia. Heart, 1997. **77**(2): p. 104–7.

145. Bogun, F., et al., Role of Purkinje fibers in post-infarction ventricular tachycardia. J Am Coll Cardiol, 2006. **48**(12): p. 2500–7.

146. Morady, F., et al., Concealed entrainment as a guide for catheter ablation of ventricular tachycardia in patients with prior myocardial infarction. J Am Coll Cardiol, 1991. **17**(3): p. 678–89.

147. Daoud, E. and F. Morady, Catheter ablation of ventricular tachycardia. Curr Opin Cardiol, 1995. **10**(1): p. 21–5.

148. Bansch, D., et al., Primary prevention of sudden cardiac death in idiopathic dilated cardiomyopathy: the Cardiomyopathy Trial (CAT). Circulation, 2002. **105**(12): p. 1453–8.

149. Della Bella, P., Canadian Implantable Defibrillator Study (CIDS): a randomized trial of the implantable cardioverter defibrillator against amiodarone. Ital Heart J Suppl, 2000. **1**(8): p. 1070–1.

150. Mirowski, M., et al., Termination of malignant ventricular arrhythmias with an implanted automatic defibrillator in human beings. New Engl J Med, 1980. **303**(6): p. 322–4.

151. Bocker, D., et al., Benefits of treatment with implantable cardioverter-defibrillators in patients with stable ventricular tachycardia without cardiac arrest. Br Heart J, 1995. **73**(2): p. 158–63.

152. Winkle, R.A., et al., Long-term outcome with the automatic implantable cardioverter-defibrillator. J Am Coll Cardiol, 1989. **13**(6): p. 1353–61.

153. Fogoros, R.N., et al., Efficacy of the automatic implantable cardioverter-defibrillator in prolonging survival in patients with severe underlying cardiac disease. J Am Coll Cardiol, 1990. **16**(2): p. 381–6.

154. Nisam, S., et al., AICD automatic cardioverter defibrillator clinical update: 14 years experience in over 34,000 patients. Pacing and clinical electrophysiology, 1995. **18**(1 Pt 2): p. 142–7.

155. Connolly, S.J. and S. Yusuf, Evaluation of the implantable cardioverter defibrillator in survivors of cardiac arrest: the need for randomized trials. Am J Cardiol, 1992. **69**(9): p. 959–62.

156. Epstein, A.E., AVID necessity. Pacing and clinical electrophysiology, 1993. **16**(9): p. 1773–5.

157. Kim, S.G., Implantable defibrillator therapy: does it really prolong life? How can we prove it? Am J Cardiol, 1993. **71**(13): p. 1213–8.

158. Luderitz, B., et al., Patient acceptance of the implantable cardioverter defibrillator in ventricular tachyarrhythmias. Pacing Clin Electrophysiol, 1993. **16**(9): p. 1815–21.

159. Kadish, A., et al., Prophylactic defibrillator implantation in patients with nonischemic dilated cardiomyopathy. N Engl J Med, 2004. **350**(21): p. 2151–8.

160. Eicken, A., et al., Implantable cardioverter defibrillator (ICD) in children. Int J Cardiol, 2006. **107**(1): p. 30–5.

161. Groeneveld, P.W., et al., Costs and quality-of-life effects of implantable cardioverter-defibrillators. Am J Cardiol, 2006. **98**(10): p. 1409–15.

162. Stevenson, L.W., Implantable cardioverter-defibrillators for primary prevention of sudden death in heart failure: are there enough bangs for the bucks? Circulation, 2006. **114**(2): p. 101–3.

163. Alter, P., et al., Complications of implantable cardioverter defibrillator therapy in 440 consecutive patients. Pacing Clin Electrophysiol, 2005. **28**(9): p. 926–32.

164. Gould, P.A. and A.D. Krahn, Complications associated with implantable cardioverter-defibrillator replacement in response to device advisories. JAMA, 2006. **295**(16): p. 1907–11.

165. Maisel, W.H., et al., Pacemaker and ICD generator malfunctions: analysis of Food and Drug Administration annual reports. JAMA, 2006. **295**(16): p. 1901–6.

166. Heller, S.S., et al., Psychosocial outcome after ICD implantation: a current perspective. Pacing Clin Electrophysiol, 1998. **21**(6): p. 1207–15.

167. Pires, L.A., et al., Clinical predictors and timing of New York Heart Association class improvement with cardiac resynchronization therapy in patients with advanced chronic heart failure: results from the Multicenter InSync Randomized Clinical Evaluation (MIRACLE) and Multicenter InSync ICD Randomized Clinical Evaluation (MIRACLE-ICD) trials. Am Heart J, 2006. **151**(4): p. 837–43.

168. Lombardi, G., J. Gallagher, and P. Gennis, Outcome of out-of-hospital cardiac arrest in New York City. The Pre-Hospital Arrest Survival Evaluation (PHASE) Study. JAMA, 1994. **271**(9): p. 678–83.

169. Becker, L.B., et al., Outcome of CPR in a large metropolitan area – where are the survivors? Ann Emerg Med, 1991. **20**(4): p. 355–61.

170. Kuck, K.H., et al., Randomized comparison of antiarrhythmic drug therapy with implantable defibrillators in patients resuscitated from cardiac arrest: the Cardiac Arrest Study Hamburg (CASH). Circulation, 2000. **102**(7): p. 748–54.

171. Connolly, S.J., et al., Canadian implantable defibrillator study (CIDS): a randomized trial of the implantable cardioverter defibrillator against amiodarone. Circulation, 2000. **101**(11): p. 1297–302.

172. Moss, A.J., et al., Prophylactic implantation of a defibrillator in patients with myocardial infarction and reduced ejection fraction. N Engl J Med, 2002. **346**(12): p. 877–83.

173. Bigger, J.T., Jr., Prophylactic use of implanted cardiac defibrillators in patients at high risk for ventricular arrhythmias after coronary-artery bypass graft surgery. Coronary Artery Bypass Graft (CABG) Patch Trial Investigators. N Engl J Med, 1997. **337**(22): p. 1569–75.

174. Hohnloser, S.H., et al., Prophylactic use of an implantable cardioverter-defibrillator after acute myocardial infarction. N Engl J Med, 2004. **351**(24): p. 2481–8.

175. Buxton, A.E., et al., Prevention of sudden death in patients with coronary artery disease: the Multicenter Unsustained Tachycardia Trial (MUSTT). Progress in cardiovascular diseases, 1993. **36**(3): p. 215–26.

176. Strickberger, S.A., et al., Amiodarone versus implantable cardioverter-defibrillator: randomized trial in patients with nonischemic dilated cardiomyopathy and asymptomatic nonsustained ventricular tachycardia–AMIOVIRT. J Am Coll Cardiol, 2003. **41**(10): p. 1707–12.

177. Desai, A.S., et al., Implantable defibrillators for the prevention of mortality in patients with nonischemic cardiomyopathy: a meta-analysis of randomized controlled trials. JAMA, 2004. **292**(23): p. 2874–9.

178. Lehmann, M.H. and S. Saksena, Implantable cardioverter defibrillators in cardiovascular practice: report of the Policy Conference of the North American Society

of Pacing and Electrophysiology. NASPE Policy Conference Committee. Pacing Clin Electrophysiol, 1991. **14**(6): p. 969–79.

179. Gregoratos, G., et al., ACC/AHA guidelines for implantation of cardiac pacemakers and antiarrhythmia devices: a report of the American College of Cardiology/American Heart Association Task Force on Practice Guidelines (Committee on Pacemaker Implantation). J Am Coll Cardiol, 1998. **31**(5): p. 1175–209.

180. Gregoratos, G., et al., ACC/AHA/NASPE 2002 Guideline Update for Implantation of Cardiac Pacemakers and Antiarrhythmia Devices–summary article: a report of the American College of Cardiology/American Heart Association Task Force on Practice Guidelines (ACC/AHA/NASPE Committee to Update the 1998 Pacemaker Guidelines). J Am Coll Cardiol, 2002. **40**(9): p. 1703–19.

181. Zipes, D.P., et al., ACC/AHA/ESC 2006 guidelines for management of patients with ventricular arrhythmias and the prevention of sudden cardiac death: a report of the American College of Cardiology/American Heart Association Task Force and the European Society of Cardiology Committee for Practice Guidelines (Writing Committee to Develop Guidelines for Management of Patients With Ventricular Arrhythmias and the Prevention of Sudden Cardiac Death). J Am Coll Cardiol, 2006. **48**(5): p. e247–346.

182. Flaker, G.C., In cardiac arrest: is a low K or a high K "okay?" J Cardiovasc Electrophysiol, 2001. **12**(10): p. 1113–4.

183. Todd, G.J. and G.F. Tyers, Potassium-induced arrest of the heart: effect of low potassium concentration. Surg Forum, 1975. **26**: p. 255–6.

184. Knight, B.P., et al., Outcome of patients with nonischemic dilated cardiomyopathy and unexplained syncope treated with an implantable defibrillator. J Am Coll Cardiol, 1999. **33**(7): p. 1964–70.

185. Middlekauff, H.R., et al., Syncope in advanced heart failure: high risk of sudden death regardless of origin of syncope. J Am Coll Cardiol, 1993. **21**(1): p. 110–6.

186. Maisel, W.H., et al., Recalls and safety alerts involving pacemakers and implantable cardioverter-defibrillator generators. JAMA, 2001. **286**(7): p. 793–9.

187. Weerasooriya, R., et al., Catheter ablation of ventricular fibrillation in structurally normal hearts targeting the RVOT and Purkinje ectopy. Herz, 2003. **28**(7): p. 598–606.

188. Haissaguerre, M., et al., Mapping and ablation of idiopathic ventricular fibrillation. Circulation, 2002. **106**(8): p. 962–7.

189. Wilkoff, B.L., et al., Dual-chamber pacing or ventricular backup pacing in patients with an implantable defibrillator: the Dual Chamber and VVI Implantable Defibrillator (DAVID) Trial. JAMA, 2002. **288**(24): p. 3115–23.

190. Olshansky, B., et al., Reduction of right ventricular pacing in patients with dual-chamber ICDs. Pacing Clin Electrophysiol, 2006. **29**(3): p. 237–43.

191. Olshansky, B., et al., Inhibition of Unnecessary RV Pacing with AV Search Hysteresis in ICDs (INTRINSIC RV): design and clinical protocol. Pacing Clin Electrophysiol, 2005. **28**(1): p. 62–6.

192. Olshansky, B., et al., Is dual-chamber programming inferior to single-chamber programming in an implantable cardioverter defibrillator? Results of the Intrinsic RV Study. Circulation, 2007. **115**(1): p. 9–16.

193. Wilkoff, B.L., et al., A comparison of empiric to physician-tailored programming of implantable cardioverter-defibrillators: results from the prospective randomized multicenter EMPIRIC trial. J Am Coll Cardiol, 2006. **48**(2): p. 330–9.

194. Cleland, J.G., et al., The effect of cardiac resynchronization on morbidity and mortality in heart failure. New Engl J Med, 2005. **352**(15): p. 1539–49.

195. Cleland, J.G., et al., Baseline characteristics of patients recruited into the CARE-HF study. Eur J Heart Fail, 2005. **7**(2): p. 205–14.

196. Salukhe, T.V., K. Dimopoulos, and D. Francis, Cardiac resynchronisation may reduce all-cause mortality: meta-analysis of preliminary COMPANION data with CONTAK-CD, InSync ICD, MIRACLE and MUSTIC. Int J Cardiol, 2004. **93**(2–3): p. 101–3.

197. Bristow, M.R., A.M. Feldman, and L.A. Saxon, Heart failure management using implantable devices for ventricular resynchronization: Comparison of Medical Therapy, Pacing, and Defibrillation in Chronic Heart Failure (COMPANION) trial. COMPANION Steering Committee and COMPANION Clinical Investigators. J Card Fail, 2000. **6**(3): p. 276–85.

198. Abraham, W.T., et al., Effects of cardiac resynchronization on disease progression in patients with left ventricular systolic dysfunction, an indication for an implantable cardioverter-defibrillator, and mildly symptomatic chronic heart failure. Circulation, 2004. **110**(18): p. 2864–8.

199. Carnes, C.A., A.A. Mehdirad, and S.D. Nelson, Drug and defibrillator interactions. Pharmacotherapy, 1998. **18**(3): p. 516–25.

200. Bardy, G.H., et al., Clinical experience with a tiered-therapy, multiprogrammable antiarrhythmia device. Circulation, 1992. **85**(5): p. 1689–98.

201. Rao, H.B. and S. Saksena, Implantable defibrillators configured for hybrid therapy of persistent and permanent atrial fibrillation: initial clinical experience with a novel lead system. Journal of interventional cardiac electrophysiology, 2005. **13 Suppl 1**: p. 79–86.

202. Pacifico, A., et al., Prevention of implantable-defibrillator shocks by treatment with sotalol. d,l-Sotalol Implantable Cardioverter-Defibrillator Study Group. New Engl J Med, 1999. **340**(24): p. 1855–62.

203. Mason, J.W., et al., Programmed ventricular stimulation in predicting vulnerability to ventricular arrhythmias and their response to antiarrhythmic therapy. Am Heart J, 1982. **103**(4 Pt 2): p. 633–9.

204. Podczeck, A., et al., Termination of re-entrant ventricular tachycardia by subthreshold stimulus applied to the zone of slow conduction. Eur Heart J, 1988. **9**(10): p. 1146–50.

205. Kawanishi, D.T., et al., Cumulative hazard analysis of J-wire fracture in the Accufix series of atrial permanent pacemaker leads. Pacing Clin Electrophysiol, 1998. **21**(11 Pt 2): p. 2322–6.

206. Saksena, S., Antiarrhythmic device advisories and recalls: managing an increasingly vulnerable process. Pacing Clin Electrophysiol, 1999. **22**(6 Pt 1): p. 950–2.

207. Hauser, R.G. and L. Kallinen, Deaths associated with implantable cardioverter defibrillator failure and deactivation reported in the United States Food and Drug Administration Manufacturer and User Facility Device Experience Database. Heart Rhythm, 2004. **1**(4): p. 399–405.

208. Mueller, P.S., C.C. Hook, and D.L. Hayes, Ethical analysis of withdrawal of pacemaker or implantable cardioverter-defibrillator support at the end of life. Mayo Clin Proc, 2003. **78**(8): p. 959–63.

209. McClellan, M.B. and S.R. Tunis, Medicare coverage of ICDs. N Engl J Med, 2005. **352**(3): p. 222–4.

210. Kuppermann, M., et al., An analysis of the cost effectiveness of the implantable defibrillator. Circulation, 1990. **81**(1): p. 91–100.

211. Kupersmith, J., et al., Evaluating and improving the cost-effectiveness of the implantable cardioverter-defibrillator. Am Heart J, 1995. **130**(3 Pt 1): p. 507–15.

212. Zwanziger, J., et al., The cost effectiveness of implantable cardioverter-defibrillators: results from the Multicenter Automatic Defibrillator Implantation Trial (MADIT)-II. J Am Coll Cardiol, 2006. **47**(11): p. 2310–8.

213. Sanders, G.D., M.A. Hlatky, and D.K. Owens, Cost-effectiveness of implantable cardioverter-defibrillators. N Engl J Med, 2005. **353**(14): p. 1471–80.

214. Mushlin, A.I., et al., The cost-effectiveness of automatic implantable cardiac defibrillators: results from MADIT. Multicenter Automatic Defibrillator Implantation Trial. Circulation, 1998. **97**(21): p. 2129–35.

215. Al-Khatib, S.M., et al., Clinical and economic implications of the Multicenter Automatic Defibrillator Implantation Trial-II. Ann Intern Med, 2005. **142**(8): p. 593–600.

216. Mark, D.B., et al., Cost-effectiveness of defibrillator therapy or amiodarone in chronic stable heart failure: results from the Sudden Cardiac Death in Heart Failure Trial (SCD-HeFT). Circulation, 2006. **114**(2): p. 135–42.

217. Actuarial risk of sudden death while awaiting cardiac transplantation in patients with atherosclerotic heart disease. DEFIBRILAT Study Group. Am J Cardiol, 1991. **68**(5): p. 545–6.

218. Uretsky, B.F. and R.G. Sheahan, Primary prevention of sudden cardiac death in heart failure: will the solution be shocking? J Am Coll Cardiol, 1997. **30**(7): p. 1589–97.

219. Dreifus, L.S., et al., Guidelines for implantation of cardiac pacemakers and antiarrhythmia devices. A report of the American College of Cardiology/American Heart Association Task Force on Assessment of Diagnostic and Therapeutic Cardiovascular Procedures (Committee on Pacemaker Implantation). J Am Coll Cardiol, 1991. **18**(1): p. 1–13.

15

Cardiac Device Therapy in Children

George F. Van Hare

Introduction

It is ironic that the first transistorized, wearable pacemaker was designed by Earl Bakken specifically to make open heart surgery in children possible (1). Despite their pediatric origins, however, current heart rhythm control devices and leads are not designed or manufactured for children. Instead, they are designed with adults in mind, with respect to device size and lead length, as well as to the indications that prompt pacemaker implantation in adults. For this reason, the clinician who implants pacemakers in children and who follows such children must adapt the technology to the unique requirements of children. These requirements include the need for small size, but they also include flexibility in programmability, to take into account potentially higher levels of activity, higher natural heart rates, and the wide spectrum of problems encountered with congenital heart disease.

Indications for Pacing

The indications for placement of a permanent pacemaker in a child are not substantially different than those that are published for adults. Children deserve special consideration, however, because of their smaller size, the different disease processes that lead to a need for pacing, and the effect of growth, development, and the simple passage of time on these disease processes. Because the risks of pacemaker implantation are affected by the size of the patient, it should not be surprising that patient size influences the indications for pacing.

The special considerations in children can be grouped into several main categories: (a) those relating to sinus node dysfunction which is secondary to surgical palliation or repair of congenital heart disease, often with concomitant atrial tachyarrhythmias; (b) those relating to postsurgical atrioventricular block; and (c) those relating to congenital atrioventricular block. In addition, all the indications listed for adults are applicable to children, with perhaps a revision when the indication is based on rate. For example, when considering sinus node dysfunction, baseline rates should be evaluated in the context of the patient's age, and one would use age-inappropriate bradycardia correlated with symptoms, rather than the adult criterion of 40 beats per minute, as a Class I indication for pacing in the child. The recently updated guidelines from the American College of Cardiology, the American Heart Association, and the Heart Rhythm Society included a list of specific pediatric indications and these have been summarized in Table 15.1 (2).

Table 15.1 Indications for permanent pacing in children and adolescents.

Class I

1. Advanced 2nd or 3rd degree AV block associated with symptomatic bradycardia, ventricular dysfunction, or low cardiac output
2. Sinus node dysfunction with correlation of symptoms during age-inappropriate bradycardia. The definition of bradycardia depends on age
3. Postoperative advanced 2nd or 3rd degree AV block that is not expected to resolve or persists >7 days after cardiac surgery
4. Congenital 3rd degree AV block with a wide QRS escape rhythm, complex ventricular ectopy, or ventricular dysfunction
5. Congenital 3rd degree AV block in infant with ventricular rate <50–55 or with congenital heart disease and ventricular rate <70.
6. Sustained pause-dependent VT, with or without prolonged QT, in which the efficacy of pacing is documented

Class IIa

1. Bradycardia–tachycardia syndrome with the need to long-term antiarrhythmic treatment with drugs other than digoxin
2. Congenital 3rd degree AV block beyond 1 year of age with average heart rate <50, abrupt pauses in ventricular rate of 2–3 times the basic cycle length, or associated with symptoms due to chronotropic incompetence
3. Long QT syndrome with 2:1 2nd degree or 3rd-degree AV block
4. Asymptomatic sinus bradycardia with complex congenital heart disease and resting heart rate <40, or pauses >3 s.
5. Congenital heart disease and impaired hemodynamics due to sinus bradycardia or loss of AV synchrony

Class IIb

1. Transient postoperative 3rd degree AV block which resolves with residual bifascicular block
2. Congenital 3rd degree AV block in asymptomatic infant, child, adolescent, or young adult with acceptable rate, narrow QRS, and normal ventricular function
3. Asymptomatic sinus bradycardia in the adolescent with congenital heart disease and resting heart rate <40 or pauses >3 s
4. Neuromuscular diseases with any degree of AV block (including 1st degree) due to risk of unpredictable progression of AV conduction disease

Class III

1. Transient postoperative AV block with return of normal AV conduction
2. Asymptomatic postoperative bifascicular block with or without 1st degree AV block and without prior 3rd degree AV block
3. Asymptomatic Wenckebach 2nd degree AV block
4. Symptomatic sinus bradycardia in the adolescent with longest RR interval <3 s and lowest heart rate >40

Adapted from Gregoratos G, Abrams J, Epstein AE, et al. ACC/AHA/NASPE 2002 guideline update for implantation of cardiac pacemakers and antiarrhythmia devices: summary article. A report of the American College of Cardiology/American Heart Association Task Force on Practice Guidelines (ACC/AHA/NASPE Committee to Update the 1998 Pacemaker Guidelines). J Cardiovasc Electrophysiol 2002;13:1183–99.

Postsurgical Sinus Node Dysfunction, With or Without Atrial Tachyarrhythmias

This indication for pacing is a special case of the broader adult indications related to sinus node dysfunction and to the bradycardia–tachycardia syndrome. Surgery for congenital heart disease often involves large incisions in the right atrium, and in particular types of operations, the sinus node can be damaged (3–5). The sinus node may be damaged directly by suturing, incision, or clamping, or damage may be a result of interruption of the blood supply to the sinus node. Whatever the actual mechanism, certain types of surgery are commonly associated with early and late postsurgical sinus node dysfunction, and the degree of sinus node dysfunction can be profound. Both the Mustard and the Senning procedure for atrial redirection in D-transposition of the great vessels involve extensive atrial suture lines, and the incidence of sinus rhythm in such patients progressively decreases as they are followed into adulthood. In the study by Flinn et al., by the of the first year following surgery, sinus rhythm was present in 76%, but had dropped to 57% by the 8th postoperative year, and 33% by the 14th year (6). These operations are, for the most part, no longer performed, as transposition is now managed in nearly all cases by the arterial switch procedure. Still, thousands of children and adults are alive today following the Mustard or Senning procedure, and most have some elements of sinus node abnormality. Another operation that is commonly associated with sinus node dysfunction is the Fontan procedure, which is a form of palliation for single ventricle and its variants. The Fontan procedure has been performed using several methods and modifications since its introduction more than 20 years ago. More recently, different methods of completing the Fontan procedure have been developed, and in particular, the so-called hemi-Fontan is associated with a higher incidence of postsurgical sinus node dysfunction (7), most likely due to suture lines which are placed close to the sinus node region of the right atrium.

The loss of sinus rhythm with subsequent junctional escape rhythm leads to AV asynchrony, which may well have greater adverse consequences for the patient with Fontan circulation, or the patient with significant systemic ventricular dysfunction, that would be the case in a patient with an otherwise normal heart. In a patient with borderline hemodynamic function, it is reasonable to consider permanent pacing to restore AV synchrony, even if a more obvious indication such as syncope or chronotropic incompetence is not present.

Due to the presence of extensive atrial incisions and suture lines, such patients are also at risk for the development of atrial tachyarrhythmias, and in particular, intra-atrial reentrant tachycardia (8). The coexistence of these tachyarrhythmias with significant sinus node dysfunction is important. While episodes of tachycardia can certainly lead to hemodynamic instability and syncope, the sudden spontaneous termination of an episode of atrial tachycardia may be followed by a very prolonged asystolic episode in patients with profound sinus node dysfunction, leading to syncope. The medications used to suppress atrial arrhythmias can have serious negative chronotropic effects. While drugs such as sotalol and amiodarone may have little serious effect in the presence of a normal sinus node, when they are given to patients with preexisting sinus node disease, profound abnormalities of sinus node function may result (9). Thus, antiarrhythmic agents may cause a previously asymptomatic patient with sinus node dysfunction to become symptomatic. Therefore, when instituting such drugs in patients with documented preexisting sinus node disease, many clinicians electively implant a permanent pacemaker, even if the patient has not previously been symptomatic due to bradycardia. If one chooses not to implant a pacemaker in such an asymptomatic patient, the clinician must diligently follow the patient for the subsequent development of more severe sinus node dysfunction.

Postsurgical Atrioventricular Block

The surgical repair of most forms of congenital heart disease entail some risk of damage to either the compact AV node or the distal conduction system. Such damage may occur as a result of the proximity of the conducting system to the defect being repaired. For example, in patients with perimembranous ventricular septal defect (VSD), the bundle of His perforates the central fibrous body to emerge on the margin of the defect, before branching into right and left fascicles (10,11). This is also the situation for tetralogy of Fallot, as well as truncus arteriosus. Placement of the patch requires pacing deep sutures into myocardium, and the conduction system is at risk. The surgeon is often able to avoid the conducting system by altering the placement of these sutures, but there is still a substantial incidence of complete AV block following surgery. For all surgery at all ages, this incidence is 1–2% (12,13) but may well be higher in patients operated during the first year of life (14). Patients with AV septal (canal) defects are at even higher risk, as are those who have enlargement of their VSD as part of certain complex repairs. Postoperative AV block may also be seen following repair of simple defects in the atrium, such as secundum atrial septal defects, but in these situations, it is likely that it is the compact AV node which is damaged, rather than the distal conduction system. Finally, transient block may be seen due to injury relating to suction catheters or mechanical traction on these structures.

Post-operative AV block often resolves spontaneously within several days of surgery, and such resolution may allow one to avoid placing of the pacemaker (12,15). Of those that eventually resolve, most will do so by 8–11 days (16), and complete AV block persisting beyond 14 days is a clear indication for pacing. This is related to the poor prognosis of such patients and the potential for syncope and sudden death. It should be noted here that the observation of a seemingly adequate heart rate in the presence of post-surgical complete AV block should not be seen as reassuring, as such escape rhythms are notoriously unreliable, particularly those with a wide QRS complex.

There are several uncertainties inherent in this recommendation. First, when a patient has resumption of AV conduction quite late, for example 13 days after surgery, one may question the adequacy of the AV conduction, particularly when there is bifascicular block and/or a prolonged PR interval (17). Noninvasive conduction studies using temporary epicardial wires and/or exercise testing may be helpful. Second, if a pacemaker is implanted, and AV conduction returns later, one is often in the situation of needing to decide whether to proceed with pulse generator change when the initial generator reaches end-of-life, versus pulse generator removal. Again, the quality of AV conduction is an issue is this situation, and formal electrophysiologic evaluation of AV conduction may be needed.

Complete Congenital Atrioventricular Block

Most cases of complete congenital AV block are related to maternal mixed connective tissue disease and/or systemic lupus erythematosis (18,19). Mothers of affected infants have abnormally high titers of antibodies to the factors SS-A and SS-B (anti-Ro and anti-La). A second group of infants have congenital heart disease, especially including L-transposition of the great vessels (ventricular inversion, so-called congenitally corrected transposition). Finally, there is a large group in whom the disease is idiopathic, some of whom may carry the NKX2.5 mutation (20). Patients are considered to have congenital complete AV block if AV block is present at birth or develops during the first year of life, and infants born to mothers with lupus may progress from second degree to complete AV block during infancy (21).

Some infants with complete congenital AV block will present in utero with hydrops fetalis. If they are born alive, pacing is clearly indicated. Others may present with symptoms related to low heart rates, such as syncope, near-syncope, or documented exercise intolerance. They also should clearly have pacemaker implantation. The difficulty is in developing indications for, and recommendations for timing of, pacemaker implantation in those that are completely asymptomatic. We have no prospective studies in such patients, and must rely on a few large retrospective studies involving mainly adults. These studies are contradictory, with one suggesting that average daytime rates >50 are reassuring and not associated with adverse outcomes (22), and another suggesting that there are no factors that are reassuring and outcomes such as syncope and sudden death may occur even in the absence of daytime rates <50 or long pauses on the Holter monitor (23). In addition, these studies do not really take into account the normal developmental changes in heart rate. While one might be reassured by an average daytime rate of 55 in an adolescent with complete congenital AV block, the same rate in a newborn would potentially be of greater concern.

Most (but not all) clinicians agree that daytime rates <50 in children older than 1 year, or long ventricular pauses (defined recently as at least twice the basic escape cycle length) are indications for pacemaker implantation in asymptomatic individuals. Some also feel that all asymptomatic patients with complete congenital AV block should undergo implantation. The older the patient, the more reasonable this recommendation would be, due to the easier and safer the implant procedure in larger patients.

Lead and Generator Selection in the Pediatric Patient

The application of pacing system hardware designed for adult anatomy and adult indications to the pediatric population often requires that the clinician make compromises in the choice of leads, generator, and implantation technique to obtain an optimal result.

Epicardial Approach vs. Transvenous Approach

There are several anatomic situations that dictate the choice of an epicardial system over a transvenous system with endocardial leads. The most obvious is the situation of the Fontan procedure, in which there is no venous access to the ventricular mass. There are many variations of the Fontan procedure, and some authors have proposed the placement of pacing leads in the coronary sinus or middle cardiac vein by a transvenous approach as a way of pacing the ventricle in such patients (24), but these techniques have not been well developed. Furthermore, modern Fontan operations include a bidirectional Glenn anastomosis, in which the superior vena cava is anastomosed directly to the main pulmonary artery, preventing direct access to the heart from the subclavian vein. Finally, patients with the Fontan procedure are prone to the formation of intra-atrial thrombi, and introduction of a transvenous pacing lead could be thrombogenic.

The second situation that dictates an epicardial approach is when there is no reasonable venous access to the heart from the superior venous structures. This is most commonly encountered in patients who have undergone a Senning or Mustard procedure with subsequent development of obstruction at the junction of the superior vena cava and the intra-atrial baffle. In such patients, superior vena cava syndrome is possible, with elevated SVC pressures and concomitant additional problems, but more often, venous return from the upper body diverts to the inferior vena cava by azygous connections. In the latter situation, there is no elevation of SVC pressures and no hemodynamic consequences of the obstruction, but one cannot pass a pacing lead from the subclavian vein into the heart. This situation may also exist in any patient who has had numerous prior operations and who lacks adequate subclavian vein caliber.

Epicardial lead implantation may be preferred over a transvenous approach due to patient size. While transvenous leads and pulse generators are now very small, and it is technically possible to implant a transvenous system in children as small as 5 kg in weight (25), in practice the epicardial approach should be preferred for children less than 15 or 20 kg in weight, due to a high likelihood of subclavian vein thrombosis. Such thrombosis may well render the subclavian system unsuitable for further use in the future. Small patients will undergo rapid linear growth, and placement of transvenous leads at such a small size means that these leads will either have to be advanced, or replaced, in the future. If such patients have had only a single lead placed, it may be difficult or impossible to add a second lead. For these reasons, this author prefers to place epicardial systems in children who are less than 20 kg in weight, and to only consider transvenous systems in smaller children for reasons such as epicardial lead failure or infectious issues such as mediastinitis. Some implanters use a model based on fluid dynamics to predict the feasibility of transvenous leads in small patients (26) and the recent development of a lumen-less 4.1 French lead may alter these considerations in the future (27).On the other hand, the general availability of steroid-eluting epicardial leads which minimize the problem of late exit block (28,29) has allowed excellent dual-chamber pacing systems to be placed by the epicardial route. In most cases, by the time the pulse generator reaches end-of-life, these small patients will have grown large enough to be converted to a transvenous system at very low risk.

Unipolar vs. Bipolar Leads

Given a choice, one nearly always prefers bipolar leads in children for transvenous implants. The advantages of bipolar leads include a lower incidence of inappropriate sensing of noncardiac electrical activity such as muscle artifact, no possibility of muscle stimulation, and higher lead impedance resulting in potentially better longevity of the pulse generator. The principal advantage of a unipolar transvenous lead is a smaller French size of the lead body, and perhaps a lower likelihood of lead fracture. These potential advantages may well have been nullified by the recent development of new bipolar lead technologies which allow placement of bipolar leads which have very small lead bodies (27,30).

Active vs. Passive Lead Fixation

There is no general agreement on the preferred method of lead fixation for transvenous leads in children. Both active and passive fixation leads have advantages in the pediatric population.

Passive fixation leads are available that provide a high lead impedance, thereby minimizing current used for pacing and battery drain (31). This is an attractive concept, considering the fact that the typical pediatric patient will need many pulse generator changes during their lifetime.

Passive fixation leads are often easier and fast to place in larger children and adolescents. In particular, a tined lead with a preformed J for placement in the right atrial appendage yields a stable position with excellent long-term performance. In smaller children, however, the J bend in the lead may be to large, actually making stable positioning more difficult rather than less. Furthermore, many pediatric candidates for permanent pacing are postoperative patients with congenital heart disease, and most of these patients lack an atrial appendage, as it has been amputated in the process of achieving cardiopulmonary bypass. Another disadvantage of passive fixation leads is that they are very limited in the number of potential sites where they can be placed. This is potentially a problem in patients with congenital heart disease who may have poor atrial or ventricular myocardium at the potential pacing sites, or may have patch material that must be avoided. For these reasons, in patients who have had cardiac surgery, active fixation leads should always be used in the atrium. In addition, certain anatomic situations dictate the use of active fixation leads in the ventricle, namely those conditions in which the ventricle to be paced is morphologically a left ventricle. These conditions are D-transposition following a Senning or Mustard procedure, in which systemic venous return is routed via a baffle to the mitral annulus and left ventricle, and L-transposition (ventricular inversion, congenitally corrected transposition) in which the right atrium is connected to a right-sided morphologically left ventricle. The morphologic left ventricle is a smooth-walled ventricle, and tined leads are therefore not ideal, as the ventricle lacks the heavy trabeculations in which the tines need to be trapped.

Active fixation leads are now available which provide a steroid-eluting electrode, thereby minimizing the incidence of late exit block (32). With appropriate lead stylets which may be shaped for the specific clinical situation, they can be directed to anywhere in the atrium or ventricle, and one available lead-sheath system allows for placement via a deflectable sheath (27). One advantage specific to small and growing children is the ability of feed extra lead into the heart to allow for future growth, without having to be concerned that the lead may dislodge to a poor position for sensing and pacing, as can happen with passive fixation leads.

With the advent of lead extraction techniques that promise the prospect of lead removal and replacement at low risk (33,34), one needs to consider whether the choice of lead fixation might influence the difficulty of future extraction procedures. It is not clear whether passive fixation leads are more or less difficult to extract, with some practitioners reporting equal success with either type, and at least one experienced pediatric laboratory reporting more difficulty with passive fixation leads (35). More experience is needed with lead extraction before a clear answer can be provided to this question.

Rate-Responsive vs. Non-Rate-Responsive Pacing

The majority of pacemakers placed in children are programmed to a rate-responsive mode, for good reason. Certainly, for patients with sinus node dysfunction, rate-responsive pacing is clearly indicated. Patients with complete AV block can be programmed to higher upper tracking limits by the use of sensor-driven adaptive AV delay. Atrial electrodes are less likely to provide long-term stable thresholds, particularly when placed epicardially, and particularly if placed in patients with a great deal of scar tissue from prior cardiac surgery. Should the patient develop inadequate pacing or sensing from the atrial lead, the patient can be reprogrammed to pace in the ventricle in rate-responsive mode. Finally, there is an increased incidence of the development of atrial arrhythmias in the population of patients with congenital heart disease and sinus node dysfunction, and atrial pacing at rates above the junctional escape rate maintains AV synchrony and may decrease the incidence of atrial tachycardia.

Pacemaker Implantation Technique in the Pediatric Patient

Epicardial Pacing System Implantation

Exposure of the heart: Epicardial pacing systems are placed by cardiac surgeons, and may involve limited or wide access to the heart. One approach is the transdiapragmatic approach, in which a pocket is formed in the subcostal region and the diaphragmatic surface of the heart is exposed without making a sternotomy. While this approach is most convenient for the placement of ventricular leads, the atrium may be reached as well (36). Access to the heart can be also accomplished by standard or a short sternotomy or by a left lateral thoracotomy (for those whose heart is in the left chest.)

With whatever method of exposure, the surgeon should avoid tunneling the leads between the rib cage and the skin, as this leaves the leads much more exposed and at greatly increased risk of lead fracture.

Pocket location: With placement of the pocket for the pulse generator in the subcostal region, there are two common approaches used. The pocket may be placed in the fascial plane just superficial to the rectus abdominus muscle, between the muscle and the subcutaneous fat, or it may be placed deep to the rectus muscle. The former approach has the advantage of convenience for subsequent pulse generator changes, but the generator is more exposed and the result is less appealing cosmetically. When the generator is placed deep to the rectus muscle, it is more protected against the complication of erosion and separation of the wound, but there have been reports of migration of such generators to the abdominal cavity (37).

Lead selection: Steroid-eluting bipolar leads are nearly always preferable for pacemakers, and are now available, but are bulky due to their bifurcation and take up some room on the heart surface, and so may not be feasible in small hearts. Unipolar leads work fairly well, but problems such as local muscle stimulation and far-field sensing of myopotentials may be seen. The use of steroid-eluting leads has decreased the incidence of late exit block in patients following implantation (28,29,38). They have a "button" configuration and are sewn to the epicardial surface.

Also available are the so-called stab-on unipolar epimyocardial leads, which have a small barb that allows fixation to the myocardium, as well as the so-called screw-in unipolar leads, which have a corkscrew-like fixation mechanism and are fixed to the heart by 2–3 turns. The former lead is best suited to the atrium, and to the ventricle in very small hearts, while the latter cannot be used in the atrium and should be used with extreme caution in smaller hearts because of the depth to which they penetrate. These leads may be obtained with platinized electrodes, which may minimize subsequent threshold rise.

Transvenous Pacing System Implantation

The correct method for transvenous pacemaker implantation in children will be dictated by the patient's size, the presence or absence of congenital heart disease, and the presence or absence of other venous abnormalities. A complete listing of all the possible congenital abnormalities that can be encountered in pediatric cardiology is, of course, beyond the scope of this chapter. Interested readers should consult a pediatric cardiology textbook. The most commonly confronted situations are listed here.

Structurally Normal Heart

Sedation and anesthesia. In adult patients, one may often implant a pacemaker using excellent local anesthesia and light conscious sedation. This approach is often not appropriate in the pediatric patient. Younger children (<12 or 13 years) are usually not cooperative enough to tolerate the amount of discomfort involved, and may have trouble holding still. One may consider deeper sedation for such patients, remembering that excellent local anesthesia is just as essential with deep sedation and such patients must be carefully monitored for respiratory depression as a result of the use of sedative agents. When in doubt, the implanting physician should arrange for the attendance of an anesthesiologist.

Pocket location. First, it must be decided whether to place the pocket on the left or right chest. In general, one chooses right-handed pockets for left-handed patients, and left-sided pockets for right-handed patients, to minimize the amount of stress on the pacing system related to activity and thereby limit the risk of lead fracture in the future. Activity levels in children may be very high, considering involvement with sports and other activities. There are several exceptions, however. Patients who have fractured their clavicle in the past should in general not have a pacemaker placed on this side, as entry into the subclavian vein may be more difficult. Second, there may be other venous anatomic problems related to prior congenital heart disease surgery. One may observe complete nonpatency of the subclavian vein on one side, as this vein is often used for prolonged hemodynamic monitoring and may become thrombosed as a result. It is also possible that the vein has been ligated at surgery.

The pacemaker pocket may be placed either in the prepectoral fascia or sub-pectorally. The subpectoral approach has the advantage of a better cosmetic result, and a lower likelihood of erosion. The latter issue is particularly impor-tant in patients with little or no subcutaneous tissue or who are very small. It has the disadvantage of being somewhat more difficult to enter when the pulse generator needs to be replaced, but experienced pacemaker implanters find that this is not a significant impediment.

Venous access. In adult pacemaker practice, it is common to obtain a cut-down on the cephalic vein that will accommodate one or two leads. However, in children, because of the size of the vein, this is less likely. Still, the cephalic approach is preferable to the subclavian approach, when avail-able, as it completely avoids the complication of subclavian crush injury to the lead (39,40). Subclavian crush injury results from entrapment of the lead between the clavicle and the first rib, where it is subject to great stress with patient movement.

The implanting cardiologist or surgeon must take all necessary measures to insure that if a pocket is made, it is used and not abandoned due to lack of venous access. In practice, the most common cause of this problem is in patients with congenital heart disease who have developed obstruction of the superior vena cava (below). In patients with structurally normal hearts, it is also possible to fail at obtaining venous access, due to the patient's small size. One approach that may be used to insure that a pocket is not made and then abandoned is to place the guide wire percutaneously in the subclavian vein prior to forming the pocket. This insures that the leads will be placed on this side. One must take particular care when using this approach that the wire is brought down through dissection to the level of the pacemaker pocket, and not left more superficially. It is best if the wire entry site is included in the initial incision and then carried down as part of the process of forming the pocket. The use of a guide wire in the subclavian vein does not prevent the use of the cephalic vein; indeed, one should always attempt to isolate and utilize the cephalic vein in all cases.

Another approach is the placement of a catheter in the subclavian vein via the femoral vein, which may be used to perform a radiographic contrast injec-tion for outlining the venous structures, and may also be left as a target for subclavian needle entry. The catheter is advanced far laterally to the junction between the subclavian and axillary veins, and the use of this as a target allows for a very lateral entry and thereby avoids the problem of subclavian crush injury to the leads (41). The use of such a catheter for angiograms will also identify venous abnormalities, such as a persistent left superior vena cava prior to creation of the pacemaker pocket.

When the subclavian vein is used, one may use a simple peel-away sheath, retaining a guide wire. This approach will allow some back bleeding from the subclavian entry site. This back bleeding will be more prominent when two leads are introduced through the same subclavian entry site. This bleeding is usually not a problem, when the patient is large and when lead placement can be completed quickly. However, in pediatric patients, there is a lower total blood volume, so the amount of bleeding will always be larger in comparison to the total blood volume. Furthermore, when there are anatomic abnor-malities, one can expect lead placement to take longer, thereby increasing the likely blood loss. For these reasons, one may consider the use of hemostatic

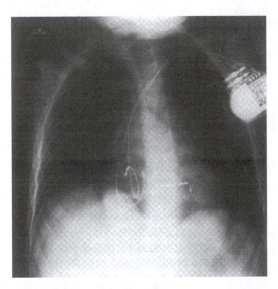

Fig. 15.1 Typical transvenous active-fixation lead placement in a 5-year-old child with complete congenital AV block. Note the large amount of extra lead that was introduced to allow for future growth, as well as the placement of the ventricular lead high in the ventricle to minimize the effect of future growth.

sheaths with side-ports that can be peeled away once the lead positioning is completed.

Lead positioning. In the atrium, preformed J leads, either passive or active fixation, may be too large in terms of the J loop for use in smaller children. Therefore, in small children, active fixation leads are preferred. These leads can be placed anywhere, but targeting the right atrial appendage is best, as it provides a stable site far away from the right phrenic nerve. Should the lead be placed along the lateral wall of the right atrium, one must take particular care to pace at maximum output to test for phrenic stimulation. One should advance a fair amount of lead into the atrium to allow for changes in position, deep breathing, and future growth (Fig. 15.1).

In the ventricle, one may choose the right ventricular apex with an active or passive fixation lead, or a site higher in the ventricle, for example in the right ventricular outflow tract or on the septum, where an active fixation lead will be needed. The outflow tract site has the advantage of minimizing the possibility of needing to revise the lead in the future due to growth (Fig. 15.1). This is because the vertical distance from the subclavian entry site to the lead tip will be small and not subject to a great amount of linear growth on the part of the child. There is, however, a somewhat higher likelihood of lead dislodgment when the lead is placed high in the right ventricular outflow tract. If the lead is placed at the right ventricular apex, the implanting physician should advance a fair amount of extra lead to allow for future growth, as well as for deep breathing and change of position. One should also carefully test for diaphragmatic stimulation at high output, which may occur simply due to proximity of the diaphragm to the lead position.

Lead tie-down. Some authors have advocated the use of absorbable sutures for lead fixation to the pectoralis muscle, asserting that the use of absorbable suture allows the leads to advance with growth (25). However, to date no data has been presented to support this contention, and it is unclear whether this approach offers any advantages.

D-Transposition Following the Mustard or Senning Procedure

There are several issues that must be considered by the physician who plans to place a transvenous system in a patient with the Mustard or Senning procedure. First, as discussed above, venous anomalies may be found. The most important of these is the possibility of stenosis or complete obstruction at the junction between the superior vena cava and the atrium, due to fibrosis of the baffle (42). Collateral venous return often develops in such patients, allowing unobstructed return to the heart via the azygous system and inferior vena cava, but these channels cannot be used for passage of a pacing lead. This problem must be demonstrated in advance of making the incision. In this author's experience, echocardiography is not adequate to rule out this problem, and injection of contrast through an arm vein does not provide adequate opacification to rule out partial or complete obstruction. Finally, simply passing a wire from the subclavian vein to the heart is inadequate, as it does not rule out a significant stenosis. One may demonstrate the area angiographically by passing an angiographic catheter from the femoral vein into the subclavian vein and performing an injection. One may also place a small sheath into the subclavian vein percutaneously prior to the incision, using it for a contrast injection, and then exchanging it for a guide wire which is incorporated into the pocket and used for eventual introduction of the pacing leads.

Should a complete obstruction between the superior vena cava and right atrium be documented, it is likely that the only reasonable approach for pacing will be an epicardial system, although there is at least one report of the use of the transhepatic approach for placement of a permanent pacing lead in such a patient (43). However, if there is stenosis without complete obstruction, one may consider balloon dilation with or without placement of an expandable stent (44). If a stent is placed, one should not cross the site immediately with a pacemaker lead because of the chance of dislodging the stent. If a stent is not placed, one should still wait until the area has healed to avoid the possibility of disrupting an area with a fresh intimal tear.

The atrial lead must be passed into the systemic venous atrium, which is composed mostly of artificial material in the Mustard procedure. Areas of left atrial tissue are incorporated into the systemic venous atrium and are available for pacing. The ideal location for placement of an active fixation atrial lead is in the roof of the left atrial portion of the systemic venous atrium, with the lead pointed directly superior. The tendency of the lead as it crosses the baffle is to be directed against the lateral wall of the left atrium just above the mitral annulus, but placement of the lead here almost always allows phrenic stimulation. Directing the lead superiorly avoids the phrenic nerve (45).

The ventricular lead crosses the baffle and passes through the mitral valve and into the left ventricle. It is quite easy in most patients to direct the lead to the apex, but one must also be careful to avoid diaphragmatic pacing.

L-transposition (Congenitally Corrected Transposition)

Patients with so-called congenitally corrected transposition (L-transposition of the great vessels, ventricular inversion) develop atrioventricular block at a rate of about 2% per year (46). The principal problem that L-transposition poses is recognition. While most patients with associated defects such as ventricular septal defect and single ventricle will be already diagnosed, those with isolated L-transposition may be asymptomatic from the cardiac standpoint and may have few if any abnormal findings on physical examination. L-transposition may be suspected by the finding of a single second heart sound on auscultation, and may be further suspected by the finding of abnormal initial forces on the electrocardiogram, with a lack of normal Q-waves in the lateral precordial leads. It is diagnosed by echocardiography. In L-transposition, the ventricles are inverted, and the chamber to be paced is a right-sided morphologically left ventricle. Therefore, the ventricular lead must be an active fixation lead, as passive leads with tines may not be adequately stable in the ventricle. In addition, the septum is in the sagittal plane rather than the oblique plane, and so the lead will not be as far to the left on anteroposterior fluoroscopy as one would normally expect.

Persistent Left Superior Vena Cava

The presence of a persistent left superior vena cava is easily documented by echocardiography (47), but it must be suspected first. In nearly all cases with L-SVC, the vessel carries left subclavian and left internal jugular venous return and connects to the coronary sinus, which is enlarged due to increased flow. The isolated persistent left superior vena cava to coronary sinus connection is quite unusual, and nearly all patients with this venous anomaly have associated congenital heart disease. Still, one may encounter this abnormality in otherwise normal children, and therefore it is important to diagnose the condition prior to placement of an incision for the pocket. When encountered, in general it should not be used for the introduction of leads to the heart. First, the angle of entry into the right atrium makes lead positioning much more difficult, especially in the ventricle. Second, and more importantly, there is little or no experience with extraction of leads introduced via the coronary sinus, and there may be a higher risk of venous damage and perforation in this situation. Should the L-SVC and coronary sinus be the only available approach for a transvenous lead, then the smallest possible lead should be chosen (30).

Pacemaker Follow-Up in the Pediatric Patient

Pacemaker follow-up in the pediatric patient is similar to that performed in the adult, with the addition of the issue of growth. Lead dislodgment is possible if the transvenous lead has inadequate extra slack and the patient goes through an episode of rapid growth. For this reason, it is appropriate to follow patients using periodic chest radiographs, for assessment of the amount of extra lead still available for subsequent growth. Radiographs may be obtained every several years, but should be done more frequently during the adolescent growth spurt and when the lead seems to have little extra length.

Transtelephonic pacemaker follow-up is also appropriate in children, especially in those who have epicardial leads which function at low lead impedance and often with high thresholds. When such pacemakers are reaching end of service, the progression can be rapid. The provision of a transtelephonic monitor to pediatric pacemaker patients also makes it possible for the family to send transmissions after such events as collisions and other sports injuries, when families often need reassurance that the pacemaker is working normally.

Implantable Cardioverter-Defibrillators in Children

Consensus statements that include specific indications for implantation of ICDs in children and patients with congenital heart disease have yet to be developed, and in the absence of these, adult indications are generally followed. There are several special points to be made, however. Some diagnoses are similar in many respects. For example, ICDs have found wide use in children with dilated cardiomyopathy and are employed as a bridge to transplant, as in adults (48) and the rate of appropriate defibrillator therapy is high. Certain forms of congenital heart disease are associated with an increased incidence of sudden death, especially transposition of the great vessels following the Mustard and Senning procedures (49), and tetralogy of Fallot late after repair (50). While indications for ICD implantation in these groups are not well agreed-upon due to the lack of prospective date, factors such as arrhythmia inducibility, spontaneous arrhythmias, and ventricular function are important considerations.

Transvenous ICD implantation techniques are similar to those stated above for transvenous pacemakers, with the proviso that the larger lead body diameter and larger pulse generator volume have the potential to complicate implantation procedures to a greater extent than in the adult population (51). A group of patients exist, however, for whom transvenous implantation is not feasible, either due to size or anatomy. In such patients, novel lead systems have been developed at several centers (52). Such systems involve conventional epicardial pacing lead placement or the use of transvenous leads tunneled to a subcostal pocket, for rate sensing. Defibrillation is accomplished via subcutaneous coils or arrays, often using the pulse generator as one of the high-voltage conductors in a "hot-can" arrangement.

Cardiac Resynchronization Therapy

As in the situation with ICDs, there are no agreed-upon indications at this time for the use of CRT pacing in children and those with congenital heart disease, and so the adult indications are used, with some exceptions. As reflected in a recent multicenter survey of the use of CRT in pediatric centers, the great majority of patients coming to CRT implantation have nonstandard indications and most have an epicardial approach to implantation, either due to heart size or, more often, anatomic issues (53). One area of great interest is the use of "biventricular pacing" in patients with failing single ventricles. A great deal of work remains to be done to delineate the indications and optimal pacing sites in such patients.

Conclusions

Although current pacemaker and ICD systems are not specifically designed for children, the great diversity of pulse generators and leads, and the increasing degree of programmability, mean that most children can have a very good result of device implantation. The clinician who implants devices in children and follows them must have a good knowledge of the special needs of children, as well as the technical skill needed for working with smaller anatomy and a good understanding of congenital heart disease.

References

1. Lillehei CW, Gott VL, Hodges PC, Jr., Long DM, Bakken EE. Transitor pacemaker for treatment of complete atrioventricular dissociation. JAMA 1960;172:2006–10.
2. Gregoratos G, Abrams J, Epstein AE, et al. ACC/AHA/NASPE 2002 guideline update for implantation of cardiac pacemakers and antiarrhythmia devices: summary article. A report of the American College of Cardiology/American Heart Association Task Force on Practice Guidelines (ACC/AHA/NASPE Committee to Update the 1998 Pacemaker Guidelines). J Cardiovasc Electrophysiol 2002;13:1183–99.
3. Lewis AB, Lindesmith GG, Takahashi M, et al. Cardiac rhythm following the Mustard procedure for transposition of the great vessels. J Thorac Cardiovasc Surg 1977;73:919–26.
4. Bharati S, Molthan ME, Veasy LG, Lev M. Conduction system in two cases of sudden death two years after the Mustard procedure. J Thorac Cardiovasc Surg 1979;77:101–8.
5. Saalouke MG, Rios J, Perry LW, Shapiro SR, Scott LP. Electrophysiologic studies after mustard's operation for d- transposition of the great vessels. Am J Cardiol 1978;41:1104–9.
6. Flinn CJ, Wolff GS, Dick M, et al. Cardiac rhythm after the Mustard operation for complete transposition of the great arteries. N Engl J Med 1984;310:1635–8.
7. Cohen MI, Wernovsky G, Vetter VL, et al. Sinus node function after a systematically staged Fontan procedure. Circulation 1998;98:II-352–8.
8. Kalman JM, VanHare GF, Olgin JE, Saxon LA, Stark SI, Lesh MD. Ablation of 'incisional' reentrant atrial tachycardia complicating surgery for congenital heart disease. Use of entrainment to define a critical isthmus of conduction. Circulation 1996;93:502–12.
9. Garson A, Jr. Medicolegal problems in the management of cardiac arrhythmias in children. Pediatrics 1987;79:84–8.
10. Ho SY, Gerlis LM, Toms J, Lincoln C, Anderson RH. Morphology of the posterior junctional area in atrioventricular septal defects. Ann Thorac Surg 1992;54:264–70.
11. Anderson RH, Wilcox BR. The surgical anatomy of ventricular septal defect. J Card Surg 1992;7:17–35.
12. Goldman BS, Williams WG, Hill T, et al. Permanent cardiac pacing after open heart surgery: congenital heart disease. Pacing Clin Electrophysiol 1985;8:732–9.
13. Bonatti V, Agnetti A, Squarcia U. Early and late postoperative complete heart block in pediatric patients submitted to open-heart surgery for congenital heart disease. Pediatr Med Chir 1998;20:181–6.
14. Kuribayashi R, Sekine S, Aida H, et al. Long-term results of primary closure for ventricular septal defects in the first year of life. Surg Today 1994;24:389–92.
15. Vetter VL, Horowitz LN. Electrophysiologic residua and sequelae of surgery for congenital heart defects. Am J Cardiol 1982;50:588–604.
16. Weindling SN, Saul JP, Gamble WJ, Mayer JE, Wessel D, Walsh EP. Duration of complete atrioventricular block after congenital heart disease surgery. Am J Cardiol 1998;82:525–7.

17. Yabek SM, Jarmakani JM, Roberts NK. Diagnosis of trifasicular damage following tetralogy of fallot and ventricular septal defect repair. Circulation 1977;55:23–7.

18. Chameides L, Truex RC, Vetter V, Rashkind WJ, Galioto FM, Jr., Noonan JA. Association of maternal systemic lupus erythematosus with congenital complete heart block. N Engl J Med 1977;297:1204–7.

19. Litsey SE, Noonan JA, O'Connor WN, Cottrill CM, Mitchell B. Maternal connective tissue disease and congenital heart block. Demonstration of immunoglobulin in cardiac tissue. N Engl J Med 1985;312:98–100.

20. Benson DW, Silberbach GM, Kavanaugh-McHugh A, et al. Mutations in the cardiac transcription factor NKX2.5 affect diverse cardiac developmental pathways. J Clin Invest 1999;104:1567–73.

21. Geggel RL, Tucker L, Szer I. Postnatal progression from second- to third-degree heart block in neonatal lupus syndrome. J Pediatr 1988;113:1049–52.

22. Dewey RC, Capeless MA, Levy AM. Use of ambulatory electrocardiographic monitoring to identify high-risk patients with congenital complete heart block. N Engl J Med 1987;316:835–9.

23. Michaelsson M, Jonzon A, Riesenfeld T. Isolated congenital complete atrioventricular block in adult life. A prospective study. Circulation 1995;92:442–9.

24. Rosenthal E, Qureshi SA, Crick JC. Successful long-term ventricular pacing via the coronary sinus after the Fontan operation. Pacing Clin Electrophysiol 1995;18:2103–5.

25. Gillette PC, Zeigler VL, Winslow AT, Kratz JM. Cardiac pacing in neonates, infants, and preschool children. Pacing Clin Electrophysiol 1992;15:2046–9.

26. Figa FH, McCrindle BW, Bigras JL, Hamilton RM, Gow RM. Risk factors for venous obstruction in children with transvenous pacing leads. Pacing Clin Electrophysiol 1997;20:1902–9.

27. Gammage MD, Lieberman RA, Yee R, et al. Multi-center clinical experience with a lumenless, catheter-delivered, bipolar, permanent pacemaker lead: implant safety and electrical performance. Pacing Clin Electrophysiol 2006;29:858–65.

28. Cutler NG, Karpawich PP, Cavitt D, Hakimi M, Walters HL. Steroid-eluting epicardial pacing electrodes: six year experience of pacing thresholds in a growing pediatric population. Pacing Clin Electrophysiol 1997;20:2943–8.

29. Beaufort-Krol GC, Mulder H, Nagelkerke D, Waterbolk TW, Bink-Boelkens MT. Comparison of longevity, pacing, and sensing characteristics of steroid-eluting epicardial versus conventional endocardial pacing leads in children. J Thorac Cardiovasc Surg 1999;117:523–8.

30. Tang C, Yeung-Lai-Wah JA, Qi A, Mills P, Clark J, Tyers F. Initial experience with a co-radial bipolar pacing lead. Pacing Clin Electrophysiol 1997;20:1800–7.

31. Ellenbogen KA, Wood MA, Gilligan DM, Zmijewski M, Mans D. Steroid eluting high impedance pacing leads decrease short and long-term current drain: results from a multicenter clinical trial. CapSure Z investigators. Pacing Clin Electrophysiol 1999;22:39–48.

32. Crossley GH, Brinker JA, Reynolds D, et al. Steroid elution improves the stimulation threshold in an active-fixation atrial permanent pacing lead. A randomized, controlled study. Model 4068 Investigators. Circulation 1995;92:2935–9.

33. Smith HJ, Fearnot NE, Byrd CL, Wilkoff BL, Love CJ, Sellers TD. Five-years experience with intravascular lead extraction. U.S. Lead Extraction Database. Pacing Clin Electrophysiol 1994;17:2016–20.

34. Wilkoff BL, Byrd CL, Love CJ, et al. Pacemaker lead extraction with the laser sheath: results of the pacing lead extraction with the excimer sheath (PLEXES) trial. J Am Coll Cardiol 1999;33:1671–6.

35. Friedman RA, Van Zandt H, Collins E, LeGras M, Perry J. Lead extraction in young patients with and without congenital heart disease using the subclavian approach. Pacing Clin Electrophysiol 1996;19:778–83.

36. Ott DA, Gillette PC, Cooley DA. Atrial pacing via the subxyphoid approach. Texas Heart Inst J 1982;9:149–52.

37. Salim MA, DiSessa TG, Watson DC. The wandering pacemaker: intraperitoneal migration of an epicardially placed pacemaker and femoral nerve stimulation. Pediatr Cardiol 1999;20:164–6.

38. Horenstein MS, Hakimi M, Walters H, 3rd, Karpawich PP. Chronic performance of steroid-eluting epicardial leads in a growing pediatric population: a 10-year comparison. Pacing Clin Electrophysiol 2003;26:1467–71.

39. Magney JE, Flynn DM, Parsons JA, et al. Anatomical mechanisms explaining damage to pacemaker leads, defibrillator leads, and failure of central venous catheters adjacent to the sternoclavicular joint. Pacing Clin Electrophysiol 1993;16:445–57.

40. Jacobs DM, Fink AS, Miller RP, et al. Anatomical and morphological evaluation of pacemaker lead compression. Pacing Clin Electrophysiol 1993;16:434–44.

41. Spencer WH, 3rd, Zhu DW, Kirkpatrick C, Killip D, Durand JB. Subclavian venogram as a guide to lead implantation. Pacing Clin Electrophysiol 1998;21:499–502.

42. Stark J, Tynan MJ, Ashcraft KW, Aberdeen E, Waterston DJ. Obstruction of pulmonary veins and superior vena cava after the Mustard operation for transposition of the great arteries. Circulation 1972;45:I116–20.

43. Fishberger SB, Camunas J, Rodriguez-Fernandez H, Sommer RJ. Permanent pacemaker lead implantation via the transhepatic route. Pacing Clin Electrophysiol 1996;19:1124–5.

44. Bu'Lock FA, Tometzki AJ, Kitchiner DJ, Arnold R, Peart I, Walsh KP. Balloon expandable stents for systemic venous pathway stenosis late after Mustard's operation. Heart 1998;79:225–9.

45. Gillette PC, Wampler DG, Shannon C, Ott D. Use of cardiac pacing after the Mustard operation for transposition of the great arteries. J Am Coll Cardiol 1986;7:138–41.

46. Huhta JC, Maloney JD, Ritter DG, Ilstrup DM, Feldt RH. Complete atrioventricular block in patients with atrioventricular discordance. Circulation 1983;67:1374–7.

47. Snider AR, Ports TA, Silverman NH. Venous anomalies of the coronary sinus: detection by M-mode, two-dimensional and contrast echocardiography. Circulation 1979;60:721–7.

48. Dubin AM, Berul CI, Bevilacqua LM, et al. The use of implantable cardioverter-defibrillators in pediatric patients awaiting heart transplantation. J Card Fail 2003;9:375–9.

49. Kammeraad JA, van Deurzen CH, Sreeram N, et al. Predictors of sudden cardiac death after Mustard or Senning repair for transposition of the great arteries. J Am Coll Cardiol 2004;44:1095–102.

50. Harrison DA, Harris L, Siu SC, et al. Sustained ventricular tachycardia in adult patients late after repair of tetralogy of Fallot. J Am Coll Cardiol 1997;30:1368–73.

51. Cooper JM, Stephenson EA, Berul CI, Walsh EP, Epstein LM. Implantable cardioverter defibrillator lead complications and laser extraction in children and young adults with congenital heart disease: implications for implantation and management. J Cardiovasc Electrophysiol 2003;14:344–9.

52. Stephenson EA, Batra AS, Knilans TK, et al. A multicenter experience with novel implantable cardioverter defibrillator configurations in the pediatric and congenital heart disease population. J Cardiovasc Electrophysiol 2006;17:41–6.

53. Dubin AM, Janousek J, Rhee E, et al. Resynchronization therapy in pediatric and congenital heart disease patients: an international multicenter study. J Am Coll Cardiol 2005;46:2277–83.

16

Cardiac Pacing in the Critical Care Setting

Richard H. Hongo and Nora F. Goldschlager

Cardiac pacing can play an integral role in the management of critically ill patients. This role is not limited to the appropriate implementation of temporary cardiac pacing, but also includes maximizing therapies already available through a patient's previously implanted permanent pacemaker or implantable cardioverter-defibrillator (ICD). Complications related to the implanted device can also lead to a need for management within the critical care setting. Finally, a permanent cardiac device can interact, and at times interfere, with therapies such as intravenous monitoring line placement, and external cardioversion and defibrillation.

Temporary Cardiac Pacing

The critical care or the cardiac care units are the settings where temporary cardiac pacing therapy is implemented. The main indications for temporary heart rate support can be divided into three broad categories. First, temporary pacing is used to support the heart rate in patients with hemodynamically unstable bradycardias, either while awaiting resolution of the bradycardia, or as a bridge to permanent pacemaker insertion. Second, prophylactic temporary pacemaker insertion can be considered for patients at high-risk for sudden severe bradycardias, such as prolonged sinus arrest or complete atrio-ventricular (AV) block, that would not be expected to be well tolerated. Finally, overdrive pacing the heart above the intrinsic heart rate can provide rhythm or hemodynamic stabilization in specific circumstances.

Indications for Temporary Cardiac Pacing

Chronotropic Support. Temporary pacing should be considered in patients who demonstrate hemodynamic compromise due to bradycardia. Unstable bradycardia is usually caused by either severe sinus node dysfunction or complete AV conduction block, but even mild sinus bradycardia or second-degree AV block can result in instability if there are underlying conditions such as severe dilated cardiomyopathy or critical aortic stenosis. In some patients, the bradycardia is due to intrinsic conduction system disease and temporary pacing is merely a bridge to permanent pacemaker insertion. In others, a reversible cause for the bradycardia is present and temporary chronotropic support is sufficient. However, it is not always clear if a condition is permanent, and patients are often observed for a period of time to see if reversible causes can be identified.

The most common reversible cause of bradyarrhythmias is medication. Bradycardia-producing agents include beta-adrenergic blockers, and nondihydropyridine calcium-channel blockers (diltiazem, verapamil). These medications cause bradyarrhythmia by slowing automaticity of intrinsic pacemaker cells such as the sinus node and sites of escape rhythms, and by slowing conduction through the AV node. Antiarrhythmic drugs such as Class IC (flecainide, propafenone) and Class III agents (sotalol, amiodarone) have additional effects on myocardial and His-Purkinje system conduction. Patients with conduction system and myocardial disease are particularly susceptible to the effects of these agents. Permanent withdrawal of the offending drug may result in restoration of an adequate heart rate, thus avoiding the need for rate support with cardiac pacing. Frequently, however, the medication causing bradyarrhythmia is a necessary treatment and permanent pacemaker implantation is needed to facilitate therapy with these drugs. A common example of this would be beta-adrenergic blocker therapy for the treatment of angina, or congestive heart failure due to ischemic or nonischemic dilated cardiomyopathy.

Various types of AV block can occur during acute myocardial infarction. AV block that occurs early in the course of a myocardial infarction is thought to be due to parasympathetic activation that is provoked by pain, anxiety, or by direct stimulation of intracardiac vagal afferent receptors. The latter is known as the Bezold-Jarisch reflex and tends to occur during inferoposterior and right ventricular infarcts, possibly related to the high concentration of vagal receptors in these territories (1). The AV block is usually limited to a first-degree block (PR interval >200 ms) but can progress to a second- or third-degree AV block. This type of block usually responds to atropine (2,3), or to infusions of other positive dromotropic agents such as dopamine, and resolves within 48–72 h. Temporary cardiac pacing is required only if there is persistent symptomatic bradycardia or hypotension that is not responsive to atropine. AV sequential pacing is preferred because the additional hemodynamic benefit over ventricular pacing alone can be important in the setting of a myocardial infarction.

In contrast, direct ischemic damage to the AV node or the His-Purkinje conduction system can result in complete AV block. Third-degree AV block has been found to occur in 8% to 13% of patients with acute myocardial infarctions, usually involving the inferior wall (4–7). The occurrence of complete AV block during inferior myocardial infarction is associated with higher in-hospital mortality (20% versus 4%, $p < 0.001$) even after appropriate fibrinolytic therapy (8). The AV node is almost exclusively supplied by the AV nodal artery, although collateral flow from the first septal perforator of the left anterior descending artery is sometimes present. The AV nodal artery arises from either the distal right coronary artery (90%) or the distal left circumflex artery (10%), and is determined by whether or not the artery goes on to become the posterior descending artery that supplies the inferior wall of the left ventricle. When complete AV block results from interrupted blood flow to the AV nodal artery, an escape rhythm usually arises from the AV node (distal to the level of block), and is a narrow QRS complex rhythm that retains responsiveness to autonomic tone, helping to maintain a heart rate (40–60 beats/min) sufficient to protect against hemodynamic collapse. Temporary pacing is indicated in the setting of profound bradycardia (<45 beats/min), persistent hypotension from bradycardia, or bradycardia-dependent ventricular tachyarrhythmias.

Although less common, ischemic damage to the His-Purkinje conduction system can result in complete AV block, and usually signals a more extensive infarction. The His-bundle and left anterior fascicle are supplied by the first septal perforator and the proximal diagonal branches of the left anterior descending artery, respectively. The left posterior fascicle is supplied by both anterior and posterior septal perforators. Complete AV block from His-Purkinje system damage is therefore typically associated with a large anterior wall myocardial infarction involving the proximal left anterior descending artery. The escape rhythm originates from the distal Purkinje system or ventricular myocardium, and is thus a wide QRS complex rhythm that is usually slow (20–40 beats/min) with unpredictable stability. The escape rhythm is typically not sufficient to maintain necessary cardiac output and temporary pacing is invariably necessary. With current therapies of acute myocardial infarction that achieve early revascularization, the extent of myocardial damage is typically limited and complete AV block occurring during acute anterior wall myocardial infarctions have become rare. Persistent AV block is rarer still and permanent pacemaker insertion is nowadays only occasionally required.

Vagally mediated episodes of bradyasystole are commonly seen in the critical care setting. The bradyasystolic events are typically sudden and transient, and can manifest as sinus bradycardia, sinus arrest, and high-degree AV block. The response can be predominantly cardioinhibitory, resulting in a slowing of the heart rate below 30 beats/min and in pauses >3 s. There may also be a vasodepressor component to the episode, resulting in acute vasodilatation and hypotension that is not corrected by cardiac pacing. Triggers for these events include coughing, gagging, pharyngeal or gastroesophageal manipulation during endoscopic or endotracheal intubation, and gastric distension. The episodes are typically fleeting and responsive to atropine, and are not always reproduced by the same triggers. Backup transcutaneous pacing can be considered in selected cases, but temporary transvenous pacing is rarely needed.

Prophylactic Temporary Pacemaker Insertion. Approximately 1% of patients with acute myocardial infarction develop a Type II second-degree AV block. Although this rhythm is often tolerated hemodynamically, because there can be sudden progression to complete AV block, temporary pacing should be considered. New bundle-branch block (BBB) has been associated with an 18% risk of transient complete AV block (9–11). The development of BBB usually signifies an extensive infarction, typically involving the anterior wall. Death in these patients usually results from left ventricular pump failure, although 9% of deaths have been attributable to complete AV block (9).

In the prefibrinolytic era, BBB of new or indeterminate age occurred in 6% to 15% of patients with acute myocardial infarction (9,10,12). The most common forms were left BBB (38%) and right BBB with left anterior fascicular block (34%), followed by isolated right BBB (11%), right BBB with left posterior fascicular block (10%), and alternating BBB (6%). In the current era, the incidence of new or indeterminate-age BBB is still 10% to 13% overall

(7,13). Bifascicular block appears to be less frequent, however, and right BBB is more likely to be transient, suggesting that reperfusion therapy may reduce ischemic damage to the bundle branches (14).

In the prefibrinolytic era, alternating BBB (or right BBB with alternating fascicular block), or first-degree AV block with either left BBB or bifascicular block predicted one-third of patients progressing to complete AV block (10,15). The actual risk of developing complete AV block during acute myocardial infarction in the current era of early revascularization with fibrinolysis and primary percutaneous intervention and is not entirely clear. Nevertheless, prophylactic pacing should be considered for patients with acute myocardial infarction who present with alternating BBB or first-degree AV block with BBB.

The bleeding risks associated with fibrinolytic therapy raise concern over the safety of transvenous pacing. Fibrinolytic therapy, when appropriate, should not be delayed in order to place a prophylactic transvenous pacing system. Development of complete AV block can be managed initially with a transcutaneous pacing system, with placement of a transvenous system only if reliable or better tolerated pacing becomes necessary. With the high potential for vascular complications in fibrinolysed patients, venous access for transvenous pacing should be limited to approaches that are more readily controlled in the event of bleeding, such as the femoral, external jugular, or brachial approaches.

In patients who have a preexisting left BBB, manipulation of catheters or guidewires within the right ventricle can result in traumatic injury to the right bundle branch, resulting in complete AV block. Because the block occurs below the level of the AV node, the escape rate is usually < 40 beats/min and causes significant hemodynamic compromise. This type of block is typically transient (minutes), but can be prolonged (hours), necessitating temporary pacing support. Routine placement of a temporary pacing catheter prior to right heart catheterization (such as with a Swan-Ganz catheter), however, is not recommended because the risk of right bundle branch trauma is low. Although earlier studies estimated the risk to be as high as 10%, more recent reports have suggested a rate less than 3% (16–19). Transcutaneous pacing should be made available prior to the procedure, and patch electrodes can be placed if desired. Equipment necessary for transvenous cardiac pacing should also be readily available, so that, if needed, rapid catheter insertion can be accomplished. Placement of either the right-heart catheter or the temporary pacing catheter in this setting is best done under fluoroscopic guidance.

Complete AV block in a patient undergoing a left heart catheterization with a preexisting right BBB is rare, owing to a shorter and broader left-bundle branch (20). Transient AV block can also occur during coronary angiography, percutaneous coronary intervention, and during percutaneous valvuloplasty, but the risks are as low as 0.06%, 0.4%, and 2.5%, respectively (21). Routine placement of a temporary pacing catheter is therefore not recommended for patients undergoing left-heart catheterization with or without a preexisting right BBB.

Prophylactic temporary pacing catheter placement is not necessary for patients scheduled to undergo surgery and general anesthesia. Even in patients with evidence of advanced AV conduction disease (such as bifascicular block and prolonged PR interval suggesting trifascicular disease), AV block occurring during surgery is rare (22). Moreover, patients with fascicular block have not been found to be at increased risk for vagally mediated bradycardia compared with those with normal intraventricular conduction.

Infectious processes can result in AV conduction block. Acute bacterial endocarditis, particularly if due to *Staphylococcus aureus*, has been reported to lead to complete AV block in 2–4% of cases, typically through the formation of perivalvular ring abscesses that extend into the AV node or proximal His-bundle (23). The risk is especially high with aortic valve endocarditis, and with involvement of the noncoronary cusp, as this lies closest to the AV node. Second- or third-degree AV block has been reported to be as high as 17% in patients with aortic valve ring abscesses (24). When first-degree AV block occurs in a patient with aortic valve endocarditis, progression to complete AV block has been reported to occur in up to 22% of cases (25). Prophylactic temporary pacing should therefore be considered once there is PR interval prolongation beyond 200 ms, while patients await definitive treatment with surgical debridement and valve replacement.

The most common manifestation of acute Lyme myocarditis, caused by the tick-borne spirochete *Borrelia burgdorferi*, is AV block. The AV block can be exacerbated by the suppression of ventricular escape rhythms that also occurs with Lyme myocarditis. The risk for developing complete AV block is highest in those presenting with a PR interval more than 300 ms, and when it occurs, the block can last for more than a week (26). Prophylactic temporary pacing should therefore be considered for patients with Lyme myocarditis that develop a new first-degree AV block measuring > 300 ms.

Overdrive Pacing. The most common therapeutic use of overdrive pacing in the critical care setting is for the management of *torsade de pointes* ventricular tachycardia (VT). This specific polymorphic VT occurs in the setting of delayed ventricular repolarization that manifests as a prolonged QT interval (frequently > 500 ms), and is characterized by a constantly changing QRS polarity, giving the appearance on the electrocardiogram (ECG) of QRS twisting, or "turning on a point." The rhythm is triggered by afterdepolarizations, or abnormal myocardial cell activations that occur when oscillations in voltage across cellular membranes reach a critical voltage threshold. These afterdepolarizations are caused by a decrease in outward potassium current, or by an increase in late residual currents from incomplete inactivation of sodium and L-type calcium channels (27). Hypokalemia promotes afterdepolarizations by depressing outward potassium current and enhancing inward L-type calcium current. Slow ventricular rates accentuate abnormal refractoriness and facilitate afterdepolarizations. The initiation of *torsade de pointes*, therefore, is frequently bradycardia- or pause-dependent (Fig. 16.1). Medications that are known to prolong the QT interval should be avoided in patients with abnormally prolonged QT intervals (corrected QT > 440 ms).

Intravenous magnesium is the initial therapy of choice, regardless of preexisting serum magnesium levels, because of its immediate effect in suppressing afterdepolarizations (28). The effects of intravenous magnesium will rapidly wane, however, and attention should be directed to suppressing the bradycardia- or pause-dependent initiation of this arrhythmia by increasing the heart rate. This is most readily achieved with temporary pacing. In the absence of AV conduction block, either atrial or ventricular pacing can be used. The pacing rate is increased till there is a shortening of QT interval and effective suppression of ventricular ectopy, typically between 80 and 110 beats/min, although

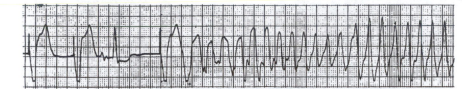

Fig. 16.1 Pause-dependent polymorphic ventricular tachycardia occurring in a patient with acute myocardial infarction, normal electrolytes, and a previously implanted single-chamber ventricular pacemaker. The first two paced QRS complexes are followed by a sinus P-wave and conducted QRS complex. The relative pause following this QRS complex (compared to the RR interval preceding it) is terminated by a paced QRS complex at the programmed lower rate interval, which initiates the arrhythmia. These tachycardias can be managed by eliminating the pauses and by intravenous magnesium; intravenous lidocaine may also be useful. Elimination of short pauses such as that seen here can be difficult, but is best managed by increasing the pacing rate. After cardioversion and increasing the pacing rate, this patient remained arrhythmia-free and recovered from an otherwise uncomplicated myocardial infarction.

higher pacing rates are not infrequently required. While the arrhythmia is suppressed by temporary pacing, reversal of identifiable causes of QT prolongation must be sought. Overdrive pacing is continued, sometimes for days, until ventricular ectopy is no longer observed. If temporary pacing is delayed or is not feasible, intravenous isoproterenol can be used to increase the heart rate in the absence of ischemic heart disease. If isoproterenol is used, the patient should be monitored closely for a potential paradoxical increase in ventricular arrhythmia. Potassium-channel blockers such as Class IA and III antiarrhythmic agents will further prolong the QT interval and should be avoided. Even though amiodarone rarely causes *torsade de pointes* (0.7% incidence) (29), and has even been reported to successfully treat a patient with *torsade de pointes* despite further prolongation of QT interval (30), because there remains the potential for proarrhythmia, it should be avoided. By blocking the late inward sodium current, pure sodium-channel blockers such as lidocaine (Class IB) can be effective, although this effect can be inconsistent (31).

Temporary cardiac pacing at rapid rates can be used to stabilize patients with acute aortic insufficiency while awaiting valve replacement. Rapid pacing shortens the time during which valve regurgitation and associated diastolic closure of the mitral valve occurs; consequently, forward cardiac output is augmented and left ventricular end-diastolic pressure and volume are reduced (32). The optimal pacing rate can be adjusted to coincide with the closure of the mitral valve during diastole using echocardiography (33).

Methods of Temporary Cardiac Pacing

The temporary pacing lead is a bipolar electrode catheter that is advanced into the venous system through a vascular sheath. The right internal jugular vein is most commonly used for vascular access because of its direct approach into the heart. The subclavian and femoral veins can be considered if the internal jugular vein approach is not possible. The left subclavian vein is preferred because the left brachiocephalic vein and superior vena cava create a single large arch that naturally directs a curved catheter into the right ventricle. The transfemoral vein approach is considered to have a higher risk of infection as well as of deep vein thrombosis (34). A single-chamber temporary pacing system is usually employed, and the pacing lead is ideally positioned at or near the right ventricular apex because of the relative stability of this position; right ventricular outflow tract or right atrial positions are prone to dislodgment and loss of capture. The lead is guided into position using fluoroscopy. Appropriate tension on the lead should be gauged carefully using fluoroscopy. There should be sufficient tension to keep the lead from floating within the heart chamber or falling out of the right ventricle, but not so much as to threaten penetration or perforation through the myocardium.

Complications tend to occur when pacing catheters are left in place for longer then 72h (35). Infections can track down the catheter and care should be taken whenever the catheter or vascular sheath is manipulated. The catheter should be left within a sterile sleeve that allows for subsequent advancement and withdrawal. Acute thrombosis of the vein can occur, leading to extremity engorgment and to thromboembolic events. Routine anticoagulation, however, is not considered to be necessary unless there is a septal defect that could allow a venous thrombus to cause a stroke (paradoxical embolism).

When the temporary pacing catheter is in stable contact with tissue, the capture threshold is typically <1.0–2.0mA. The capture threshold should be verified daily to ensure reliable pacing support, and is done by gradually decreasing the current output during pacing; the current output value just before capture is lost is the "capture threshold." High capture thresholds may signal either lead dislodgment, or penetration of the lead into or through the myocardium. Overexposed upright chest radiographs should be performed to assess the slack or tension on the lead, and to look for any change in lead position compared with prior radiographs. If the lead appears to have advanced toward or through the cardiac border, an echocardiogram should be performed to determine if the lead has perforated into the pericardial space. If lead perforation is evident, the lead should be pulled back using echocardiographic guidance. Pericardial tamponade can occur after pulling the lead back out of the perforation track created through the myocardium, and equipment necessary for emergent pericardiocentesis should be readily available.

The use of an active fixation permanent pacemaker lead can be a solution for several unique clinical scenarios. When longer periods of temporary pacing are anticipated, such as during antibiotic therapy after extraction of an infected device from a pacemaker-dependent patient, an active fixation lead allows relative freedom of movement for the patient while minimizing the risk of lead migration. An active fixation lead is also ideal for patients with significant tricuspid regurgitation that threatens to prolapse the temporary catheter back into the right atrium. The permanent pacemaker lead is connected to a nonsterile pacemaker generator that is then secured to the chest wall surface.

There are times when a multichamber temporary pacing system is indicated. Ventricular pacing alone can result in "pacemaker syndrome," or the development of fatigue, weakness, dyspnea, mitral regurgitation, and even frank pulmonary edema, due to AV dissociation or 1:1 retrograde VA conduction (36,37). Hemodynamic instability can also result, especially in patients with cardiomyopathy in whom the atrial contribution to stroke volume can be substantial; dual-chamber temporary pacing should be considered for these patients. After open-heart surgery, patients are usually left with temporary epicardial wires as a safeguard against postsurgical AV block and bradycardia. An increasing number of surgeons are placing both atrial and ventricular wires in order to maintain AV synchrony during pacing, and, more recently, multiple ventricular wires to accomplish biventricular pacing for further hemodynamic benefit.

Cardiac Device Related Complications Encountered in the Critical Care Setting

Complications Related to Device Implantation

Infection. It has been estimated that 1% of implanted cardiac devices become infected. Infections can range from device pocket infections to endocarditis. Infections usually occur early after implantation and are caused by introduction of bacteria into the surgical wound, but can also occur years after implantation (38,39). The usual organisms in both device pocket and systemic infections are *Staphylococcus aureus* and *Staphylococcus epidermidis*, the latter more often the cause in late infections. Unusual organisms, however, are not rare.

Infection of the pocket is first suspected by erythema, swelling, warmth, and fluctuance overlying the device. On occasion, it is difficult to ascertain if swelling of the device pocket is an infection or a simple hematoma or seroma. Although it is suggested by some that sterile needle aspiration can produce a definitive diagnosis, there are potential complications that can arise from advancing a needle into a device pocket. Normally, the device body, or the pulse generator, is placed over the pacing leads at the time of implant in order to protect them from inadvertent injury during subsequent generator exchanges. Blind needle aspiration of the pocket can result in laceration of the lead insulation, or even damage to the lead body. There is also concern that despite sterile technique, bacteria can be introduced creating an infection even if there was none before. It is therefore our practice to closely observe pocket fluctuance without needle aspiration, as it is expected that an underlying infection will become clearly evident with time.

Intravenous antibiotics that effectively cover Staphylococcal species (or the actual organism grown from blood cultures) should be started immediately. Although a pocket infection may occasionally respond to antibiotic therapy alone, in the majority of cases the entire pacing system needs to be removed (38,40). Frequently, explanted lead tips come back culture-positive even if the infection appears to be limited to the pocket cavity. Because all but a few lead designs have an open track within the lead for stylets or guidewires that are used during lead positioning, an infection within the pocket has the potential to track down the lead into the heart itself (41).

Infective endocarditis is suggested by fever, chills, and positive blood cultures, and is confirmed by new murmurs of tricuspid or pulmonary valve insufficiency, signs of septic pulmonary emboli, and echocardiographic findings of vegetations on the tricuspid valve or the pacemaker leads (42). Although the echocardiographic presence and severity of tricuspid regurgitation is increased when a pacemaker lead crosses the tricuspid valve (43), clinically apparent tricuspid regurgitation is relatively uncommon. Therefore, when tricuspid regurgitation is accompanied by prominent V-waves in the neck, pulsations in the liver, or evidence of right heart failure, infective endocarditis should be strongly considered.

After total pacing system explantation, and once bacteremia is suppressed with intravenous antibiotic therapy, a new system is implanted on the contralateral side, sometimes within a week if appropriate. The duration of antibiotic therapy prior to implantation of a new system is dependent on the identification of the organism and its sensitivity to antibiotic therapy, healing and the lack of any residual infection of the wound site, and by the level of the patient's dependency on the cardiac device. Antibiotic therapy is continued after implantation of the new system until an appropriate course is completed, usually a total of 3–6 weeks. If the patient is pacemaker-dependent, a secure temporary pacing system is placed on the contralateral side and the patient is observed with continuous ECG monitoring until the new system is implanted. If an ICD is explanted, the patient is either monitored in the hospital or sent home with an external defibrillator vest until a new device can be placed.

Venous Thromboses and Pulmonary Emboli. Although the incidence of venous thrombosis diagnosed by ultrasound has been estimated to be as high as 23%, only approximately 2% of patients experience symptomatic venous thrombosis (44). If axillary or subclavian vein occlusion occurs, ipsilateral arm edema with associated pain becomes readily apparent. Superior vena cava obstruction from pacemaker leads is rare, with an estimated incidence between 0.03% and 0.4%, and results in bilateral arm, facial, and chest edema (45–47). With time, venous drainage of the extremity is rerouted through recruitment and dilation of collateral vessels, and the edema gradually subsides. Anticoagulation is instituted for at least 3 months to inhibit further thrombus formation and propagation, and to prevent thromboembolic events.

Although it has been thought that deep vein thrombosis of the upper extremities rarely results in pulmonary embolism, accumulating evidence suggests that this risk has been underestimated (48,49). Not only can pulmonary emboli lead to dyspnea and hypoxemia, but pulmonary hypertension and right-sided heart failure can also develop, albeit rarely (50). Obstructive intracardiac thrombosis involving pacemaker leads has been reported (51). Computed tomographic angiography and venography can diagnose the pulmonary embolism. Echocardiography can assess pulmonary hypertension and right ventricular dysfunction. When pulmonary embolism results in significant hemodynamic compromise, thrombolytic therapy or surgical thrombectomy should be considered. Thrombolysis using streptokinase and urokinase has been reported, with good results (52). Lead removal may also become necessary. A hypercoagulability evaluation should be considered in patients with clinically significant venous thromboses.

Device Malfunctions and Pseudomalfunctions

Following the highly publicized pacemaker and ICD recalls of 2005, there has been growing concern regarding the safety of cardiac devices. The most prominent problem involved a dual-chamber ICD that developed circuitry failure due to wire insulation degradation, leading to failure to deliver therapy during cardiac arrest (53). Other pacemaker and ICD component failures occurred in several devices from multiple manufacturing companies, and ranged from premature battery depletion to magnet mode problems. The overall occurrence of these malfunctions was found to be in the order of 1 per 10,000 devices. A review of cardiac device reports sent to the Food and Drug Administration

(FDA) between 1990 and 2002 found the mean annual pacemaker and ICD malfunction replacement rate to be 4.6 and 20.7 per 1000 implants, respectively (54). This rate is higher than what is encountered in many clinical practices, and the true scope of the problem is yet to be defined. This experience, however, has started a process involving industry, the FDA, and professional societies that will hopefully lead to tighter quality control of these devices that so often life depends upon. The failure to deliver therapy can be life threatening in a patient that is pacemaker-dependent, and can be due to both delivery stimulus problems as well as sensing problems. Pacemaker malfunctions fall into four broad categories: (1) failure of output, (2) failure to capture, (3) oversensing, and (4) undersensing.

Failure of Output. When there is either complete battery depletion or a component failure in the pulse generator, failure to deliver stimulus output results. The absence of an expected pacing artifact on the ECG suggests failure of output, but this can also occur with oversensing of unwanted electrical signals, and with inability of current to reach myocardial tissue as occurs with lead fracture. If placement of a magnet over the pulse generator (which disables sensing function and delivers stimulus outputs at the magnet rate) results in pacing, the problem is due to output inhibition from oversensing, and output failure is excluded. Lead fracture is confirmed by high lead impedance measurements obtained during interrogation of the pacemaker. If there is no pacing after magnet placement and the lead impedance is normal, the diagnosis of failure of output is made. Management of failure of output is the replacement of the pulse generator. Temporary pacing may be necessary to stabilize the patient prior to this procedure.

Failure to Capture. The absence of myocardial depolarization despite appropriate stimulus delivery from the pulse generator defines failure to capture. Failure to capture is usually diagnosed from the ECG by the occurrence of visible pacing artifact without resultant paced P-waves or QRS complexes (Fig. 16.2). Failure to capture can, however, result in no visible stimulus artifact despite stimulus output from the generator when there is complete lead fracture (see above). Failure to capture results from lead failure, lead-tissue interface problems, and increases in myocardial stimulation threshold (Fig. 16.3).

Lead failure can result from lead fracture or insulation break. The incidence of lead fracture has been reported to be as high as 4%, and most often results from repeated mechanical stress from clavicular movement, also known as "clavicular crush." The most common site of fracture is within the soft tissue between the clavicle and first rib (55) and tends to occur when the subclavian vein approach is used. When the lead passes between these two bones within the vein and not the soft tissue, as with the axillary and cephalic vein approaches, lead fracture is rare. An extremely high lead impedance (>2000–3000 ohms) is conclusive evidence for a lead fracture. If only one of the conductor wires within a bipolar lead is fractured, reprogramming the lead to function in unipolar configuration will result in restored function. Because the underlying mechanical stress can eventually lead to further degradation of the lead, including fracture of the other conductor wire or insulation, conversion to unipolar mode of function should be considered a temporary solution, especially in pacemaker-dependent patients.

The only other situation that mimics lead fracture in both failure to capture and high lead impedance is a faulty connection between the lead connector

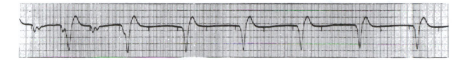

Fig. 16.2 Failure to capture due to insufficient current delivery in a patient with a pulse generator at end of life. The first and third QRS complexes are paced; the second complex represents true fusion (the QRS complex resulting from both the pacing stimulus and spontaneous depolarization); the fourth complex represents pseudofusion (the QRS complex resulting from spontaneous depolarization despite pacing stimulus output); the remaining complexes are spontaneous.

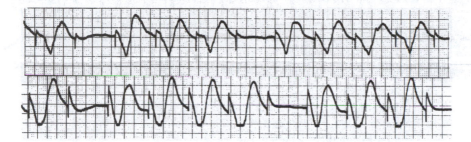

Fig. 16.3 Intermittent failure to capture and episodes of pacemaker Wenckebach in a patient with hyperkalemia and acidosis. Pacing stimuli are being delivered at a rate of about 83 per minute. There is intermittent failure to capture, as reflected in the occurrence of some output stimuli without accompanying QRS complexes. The QRST complexes are broad and bizarre, at times approaching a sine wave pattern. In the top strip, pacing stimuli are followed by QRS complexes, which occur at increasing intervals from the stimulus, eventuating in failure to capture. The increasing stimulus-to-paced complex intervals, followed by failure of conduction from the stimulus to surrounding myocardial tissue, constitute a Wenckebach type of pacemaker exit block. Pacemaker exit block is not rare in patients with hyperkalemia and acidosis, but is commonly an agonal rhythm. Treatment is of the underlying condition. This patient did not survive.

pin and the pulse generator header (loose setscrew). Although this problem generally becomes apparent shortly after the implant procedure, backward movement of the connector pin can gradually occur over time, and can thus manifest late. On occasion, connection between the pulse generator and the lead connector pin can be temporarily restored by manipulating the pacemaker pocket so as to bring the two back into contact; lead impedance will temporarily normalize. Lead fracture may also be sensitive to pocket manipulation or ipsilateral arm position if the fracture is partial and a "make-break" circuit is present (Fig. 16.4); a partial lead fracture can also result in malfunction due to oversensed electrical potentials that are generated across the partial fracture (see below).

Lead insulation breaks also result from mechanical stresses such as "clavicular crush." A break in the outer insulation will result in current leak into the surrounding tissue. A break in the inner insulation that separates the conducting wires in a bipolar lead will result in a short circuit. In either case, insufficient current reaches the myocardium and failure to capture results.

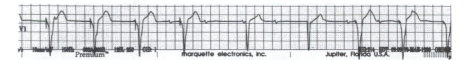

Fig. 16.4 Lead V1 rhythm strip from a patient who had a permanent VVI pacing system implanted 2 months previously, and who was admitted with recurrent syncope. The first four and the last three QRS complexes are paced. Pacing stimulus artifacts are absent from the middle of the rhythm strip; their absence is not explained by normal inhibition because no spontaneous QRS complexes occur prior to termination of the escape interval of the pacemaker. The absence of pacing artifacts occurs at about four times the interstimulus interval, suggesting that output from the pulse generator is continuing to occur at the programmed rate, but that current is not reaching body tissues. Interrogation revealed high lead impedance. These observations are most compatible with conductor wire fracture, or a loose connection between the lead and pulse generator. Oversensing can also cause absence of pacing stimuli, in which case the interrogated lead impedance would be normal and magnet application over the pulse generator would restore pacing stimulus output by eliminating sensing (and therefore also oversensing).

Insulation failure is confirmed by documenting a decrease in lead impedance. If the break is in the inner insulation of a bipolar lead, programming the lead to function in unipolar mode will restore capture and sensing function. Again, unipolar programming should be considered a temporary solution since the underlying mechanical stress can result in further insulation degradation or lead fracture. Placement of a new lead using an approach that avoids the problematic mechanical stresses is the recommended management strategy for all lead failures.

Lead-tissue interface problems include a maturation process following lead implantation, lead dislodgment, and myocardial penetration or perforation. When the lead first comes into contact with endocardial tissue, there is an immediate local tissue reaction that causes an acute rise in myocardial capture threshold. This reaction is more pronounced with active fixation leads compared with passive fixation leads. Over the subsequent 6–8 weeks, a fibrous cap forms at the interface, and this coincides with stabilization and improvement in (lowering of) the capture threshold. Corticosteroid-eluting lead tips minimize the initial local tissue reaction and reduce chronic capture thresholds by as much as 50% (56,57). Pulse generator outputs are typically programmed to 2–3 times the initial capture threshold for the first 2 to 3 months, before they are reduced to maximize battery longevity. In some devices, automatic capture algorithms can be programmed that will continuously measure the capture threshold and automatically adjust the output to stay just above the measured threshold.

Lead dislodgment occurs in approximately 2% of cases despite the use of active fixation leads, and myocardial penetration or perforation occurs in approximately 1% of cases (58). Movement of the lead tip is detected by changes in lead performance and by changes in the paced QRS complex morphology on the surface ECG. The typical paced QRS complex has a left BBB-like pattern with either a superior (with a right ventricular apex position) (Fig. 16.5) or an inferior (with a right ventricular outflow tract position) (Fig. 16.6) mean frontal plane axis. A right BBB-like pattern may indicate perforation of the lead into the left

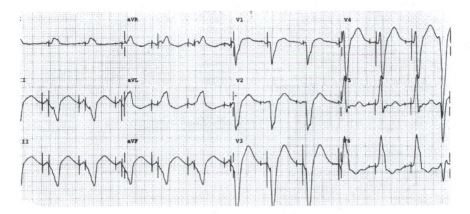

Fig. 16.5 AV pacing is present in this 12-lead ECG. The paced QRS complexes have a superiorly directed mean frontal place axis, and a left bundle branch block pattern. This is the expected configuration when ventricular pacing is initiated from the right ventricular apex.

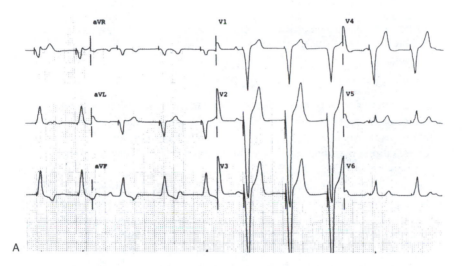

Fig. 16.6 The paced QRS complexes in this 12-lead ECG have an inferiorly directed mean frontal plane axis, and a left bundle branch block pattern. This suggests that pacing is occurring in the right ventricle, from the area of the outflow tract or high septum. This position is not associated with pacing function instability in permanent systems; in temporary pacing systems, however, right ventricular outflow tract lead position is not stable and revision is required.

ventricle or the pericardial space overlying the left ventricle. If the pacing system is biventricular, the paced QRS complex morphology depends on the position of the LV lead and the relative timing between the stimulus output of the two ventricular leads. A paced 12-lead ECG recorded immediately after device implantation, which should always be obtained, can be used as a comparison if lead dislodgment is suspected. If the lead has migrated into the pericardial space, chest pain, a pericardial friction rub or effusion, and, or stimulation capture of the diaphragm or intercostal musculature can occur.

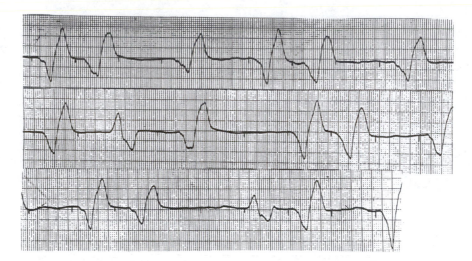

Fig. 16.7 Continuous MCL1 rhythm strip recorded from a patient with hyperkalemia, acidosis, and multiorgan failure. The serum potassium at this time was 7.6 mEq/dL. All QRS complexes are broad and bizarre, and resemble sine waves compatible with hyperkalemia. Pacing stimuli are occurring at a rate of 70 per minute. None can be ascertained to be capturing ventricular tissue. Pacing cannot be restored without correction of the underlying abnormality.

There are a variety of conditions that can increase the myocardial capture threshold. These include metabolic derangements, medications, and traumatic events such as inadvertent conduction of current down the lead during direct current cardioversion or defibrillation that results in tissue injury at the lead–tissue interface. Metabolic disturbances that increase the myocardial capture threshold include myocardial ischemia and infarction, hyperkalemia, hypoxemia, hypercarbia, acidemia, alkalemia, hyperglycemia, and hypothyroidism (59–62). Hyperkalemia is the most common electrolyte abnormality that can leads to failure to capture (Fig. 16.7), and the threshold typically increases when the serum potassium concentration exceeds 7.0 mEq/L (63–65). Increasing the stimulus output is only variably successful and should not be relied on. Immediate reversal of hyperkalemia should be the first priority.

Medications that can increase myocardial capture threshold include insulin, mineralocorticoids, and certain antiarrhythmic agents (59,60,62,66,67). The more potent sodium-channel blockers (Class IC agents), such as flecainide and propafenone, are the most likely to cause a clinical problem. This adverse effect is potentiated by hyperkalemia and can be effectively treated with sodium bicarbonate infusion. Hemodialysis is not effective because of the extensive tissue distribution. Beta-adrenergic receptor blockers (Class II agents) and potassium-channel blockers (Class III agents) such as amiodarone have not been shown to appreciably impact myocardial capture thresholds (68). Appropriate increase in the programmed stimulus output along with the withdrawal of the offending medication is usually sufficient management.

Oversensing. Inappropriate inhibition of output due to sensing of unwanted electrical signal by the pulse generator constitutes oversensing. The sources of oversensed signals include electrical noise from a partial lead fracture, skeletal

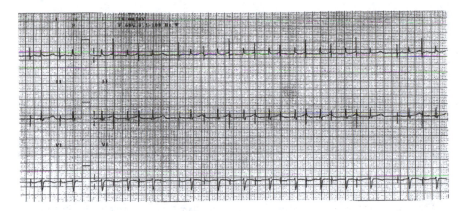

Fig. 16.8 Intermittent pauses in atrial paced rhythm. Atrial pacing is occurring at a rate of about 95 per minute; the AR interval (interval between paced P waves [A] and spontaneous QRS complexes [R]) is about 0.33 s. All QRS complexes are spontaneous. There are two longer AA intervals that constitute the intermittent pauses. Applying the shorter AA interval to the pause indicates that it is the QRS complex that is intermittently sensed, inhibiting the atrial output and resetting the atrial escape interval (far-field oversensing). This patient was asymptomatic. The problem was corrected by programming a lower sensitivity.

muscle activation (myopotentials), electromagnetic interference from the environment, and "far-field oversensing" between cardiac chambers (P-wave sensing by the ventricular lead, or R-wave sensing by the atrial lead). T-wave sensing by the ventricular lead is rare, and oversensing of concealed extrasystoles (local nonpropagating ectopic depolarizations) is rarer still.

When the pacemaker is programmed in AAI or VVI mode, oversensing results in the absence of pacing stimulus delivery when it is otherwise expected (Fig. 16.8). In DDD mode, in addition to output inhibition within each chamber, oversensing by the atrial lead can result in triggered pacing in the ventricle. This manifests as paced ventricular complexes that occur earlier than expected based on programmed parameters, without discernible preceding atrial events, and often at high rates (see below). The application of a magnet over the pulse generator will disable the sensing function of the pacemaker, and the initiation of asynchronous pacing will confirm the diagnosis of oversensing.

In a pacemaker-dependent patient, oversensing can result in prolonged episodes of asystole. Placement of a magnet over the pulse generator will immediately restore function until programming changes can be made through the programmer. It is important to point out that an ICD responds to magnet application by suspending tachyarrhythmia therapies (or shocks) only, and does not institute asynchronous pacing. Because inappropriate shocks can occur when oversensed signals by the ventricular lead are perceived as ventricular tachyarrhythmias, a magnet may be useful to suspend inappropriate shocks, but restoration of pacing can only be accomplished by changing to an asynchronous pacing mode using the programmer (Fig. 16.9).

Oversensing can usually be managed by reprogramming. By making the lead less sensitive, or by extending blanking or refractory periods, the unwanted oversensed signal can be "hidden" from the pulse generator.

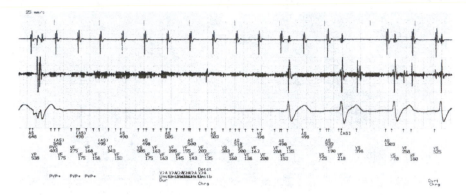

Fig. 16.9 Ventricular asystole caused by oversensing electrical noise from a partial ventricular lead fracture. This electrogram was retrieved from a dual-chamber ICD in a patient with complete AV block and dilated cardiomyopathy that presented with three days of recurrent syncope and intermittent shocks. The top tracing shows a rapid atrial rhythm detected by the atrial lead; the first atrial event appropriately triggers a ventricular paced event. The middle tracing shows electrical noise that is sensed by the bipolar ventricular electrode, resulting in inappropriate inhibition of ventricular pacing. The bottom tracing shows ventricular electrical signals detected by the shocking coil. Oversensed signal in the ventricular channel is also detected (designated as "Detect") as ventricular fibrillation (designated as "VF") and the capacitor starts to charge (designated as "Chrg") in the middle of the strip. Towards the end of the strip, the amplitude of the electrical noise drops below the sensing threshold and the shock is diverted (designated as "Dvrt Chrg"); this coincides with the onset of a ventricular escape rhythm. The internal log confirmed a sudden increase in right ventricular lead impedance (>3000 ohm) three days prior. A magnet was placed over the device to suppress inappropriate shocks; the sensing threshold was increased through the programmer until the electrical noise was no longer oversensed. The lead was revised without incident.

Unipolar leads are more susceptible to environmental and myopotential oversensing since sensing is achieved between the lead tip (cathode) and pulse generator (anode); the larger separation between the poles (centimeters) compared with that of bipolar leads (millimeters) results in detection of signal over a larger area ("antenna effect"). If environmental or myopotential oversensing occurs in a bipolar pacing system that is functioning in unipolar lead configuration, programming the lead sensing to bipolar configuration should be tried. If oversensing cannot be avoided in a unipolar lead system, a bipolar pacing system can be implanted. In the case of partial lead fracture, reprogramming is not sufficient and a new lead should be placed. When far-field oversensing cannot be eliminated with reprogramming, the lead can be moved to a position that no longer senses the other chamber.

Undersensing. Inappropriate delivery of pacing stimuli when the pacemaker system fails to sense P-waves or QRS complexes defines undersensing. Delivery of stimuli can be harmful if they occur during the atrial and ventricular relative refractory periods that are predisposed to tachyarrhythmia induction. Of particular concern is the induction of ventricular tachycardia or fibrillation when ventricular pacing occurs on the terminal portion of the T-wave ("R-on-T"), especially in the critical care setting where concomitant ischemia, metabolic and electrolyte abnormalities are frequently present.

Undersensing occurs when the electrical activity detected by the lead electrode falls below the programmed sensitivity value. A decrease in sensed signal amplitude can occur with movement of the lead tip (dislodgment, myocardial penetration or perforation), lead electrode–tissue interface abnormality (fibrosis surrounding the lead tip), or hemodynamic and metabolic derangements that directly alter the electrical signal quality. These derangements include congestive heart failure, acute myocardial ischemia or infarction, hyperkalemia, and drug toxicities.

In most cases, the sensitivity parameters can be programmed to better sense intracardiac electrical activity (by decreasing the sensitivity mV value). Care must be taken, however, to avoid oversensing. If the lead has moved early after an implant procedure, lead repositioning should be considered. Before lead repositioning is performed, however, the possibility of "functional undersensing" should be excluded. Functional undersensing is not a malfunction, and occurs because a P-wave or QRS complex falls within programmed refractory intervals. Functional undersensing can be avoided by adjusting refractory intervals noninvasively through the programmer.

Because ectopic ventricular complexes activate the heart differently from normal ventricular depolarizations, they can result in poor electrical signals that are undersensed by the lead electrode. Not infrequently, an increase in ventricular ectopy in a critical care patient can result in repetitive ventricular arrhythmias due to "R-on-T" pacing stimulus output following undersensed ventricular ectopic complexes. The pacemaker can be reprogrammed to either better sense the ventricular ectopy or discontinue pacing altogether. The latter can be accomplished by programming the pacemaker to OOO mode, or by decreasing the ventricular stimulus output to subthreshold values so that myocardial depolarization does not occur despite stimulus output. These measures should only be attempted if the patient has an underlying rhythm.

Pseudomalfunctions. In order to avoid inappropriate management, pacemaker pseudomalfunction must be distinguished from true malfunction. The most common causes of pseudomalfunction include pacemaker stimulus outputs that do not depolarize myocardium because they are delivered during periods of myocardial tissue refractoriness ("functional noncapture"), and nonrecognition of native P-waves or QRS complexes that fall within the refractory intervals programmed into the pacemaker ("functional undersensing").

A common example of pseudomalfunction is "pseudofusion." Pseudofusion is recognized by a stimulus output that is delivered just after the onset of either a P-wave or QRS complex that remains identical to a nonpaced native complex. Not only does the pacemaker appear to undersense the onset of the complex and inappropriately deliver a stimulus, but the stimulus output also appears not to capture. Pseudofusion of QRS complexes occurs because the programmed AV interval is just long enough to allow conduction from the atria down the AV node-His-Purkinje system, but just short enough to "time out" before the depolarization wavefront reaches the right ventricular lead tip. By the time the pacemaker delivers a stimulus output, the depolarization wavefront has passed over the lead tip and rendered the tissue interface refractory (Fig. 16.10).

Rapid Paced Ventricular Rates

DDD and VDD pacing modes ensure AV synchrony by providing either AV sequential pacing (only with DDD mode), or triggered ventricular pacing in response to sensed P-waves. On occasion, these modes of function can result in

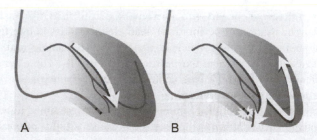

Fig. 16.10 Mechanism of QRS complex pseudofusion. A. Although normal depolarization of the ventricle has started, it has not reached the right ventricular apex. No signal is sensed at the right ventricular lead tip at the end of the programmed AV interval. B. Stimulus output is delivered but does not capture the ventricle because local myocardium is now refractory after the normal depolarization wavefront has progressed over it.

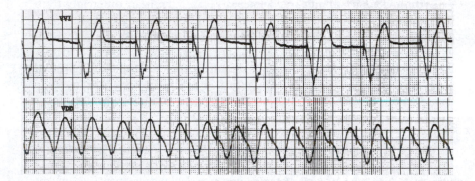

Fig. 16.11 Ventricular pacing in the setting of atrial fibrillation. The top strip illustrates atrial fibrillation with ventricular pacing in VVI mode. In the bottom strip, the mode of function is VDD mode, in which sensed atrial signals trigger ventricular stimulus outputs. Atrial fibrillatory impulses are sensed, leading to ventricular pacing at a rate of 100 per minute; note the increased QRS duration due to rate-dependent intraventricular conduction delay. Based on this ECG, an erroneous diagnosis of hyperkalemia could be entertained.

rapid ventricular pacing that is uncomfortable, and at times hemodynamically unstable. The rapid ventricular rate is due to triggered pacing in response to rapid sensed atrial activity. These sensed atrial events include atrial oversensing, atrial tachyarrhythmias such as atrial fibrillation (Fig. 16.11), atrial flutter (Fig. 16.12) and atrial tachycardia, and retrograde P-waves during pacemaker-mediated tachycardia (PMT).

Rapid ventricular pacing due to atrial oversensing may be eliminated through reprogramming the atrial sensitivity (by increasing the sensitivity mV value). If the pacemaker is tracking an atrial tachyarrhythmia, changing the mode to a nontracking mode such as VVI or DDI will reduce the ventricular rate to the programmed base rate. "Mode Switch" is a programmable function that automatically changes the pacing mode from DDD (or VDD) to either VVI or DDI when rapid atrial rates are detected. If the atrial arrhythmia persists, sinus rhythm should be restored with either antiarrhythmic agents or

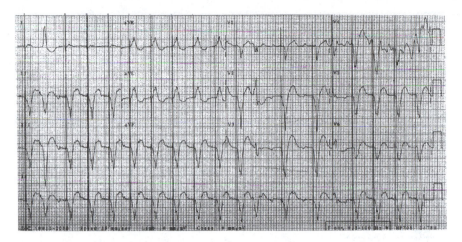

Fig. 16.12 Rapid paced ventricular rate caused by tracking of atrial flutter. The flutter waves are best seen in lead V1. The atrial rate is about 250 per minute. The paced ventricular rate is about 120 per minute, indicating that every alternate flutter wave is sensed, triggering a ventricular paced output. Ventricular sensing is normal, as indicated by the sensed premature ventricular complex in the third panel. Rapid ventricular rates are potentially detrimental to hemodynamic function, and require correction. The best option is to temporarily program to VVI mode of function, thus eliminating atrial sensing and tracking, until the atrial arrhythmia can be converted to sinus rhythm. If reprogramming capability is not immediately available, placing a magnet over the pulse generator will eliminate sensing and produce asynchronous dual-chamber output (DOO) at the magnet rate. Importantly, the magnet rate may be higher than the programmed rate, is manufacturer-specific, and is not programmable.

external cardioversion. If atrial oversensing cannot be avoided or if persistent atrial arrhythmias recur, the paced ventricular rate can be limited by either decreasing the programmed upper rate limit or by permanently changing the pacemaker function to a nontracking mode.

PMT is most commonly initiated by a premature ventricular complex that conducts retrograde through the AV node and capture the atrium. The retrograde P-wave is sensed, and a paced ventricular complex is triggered. If the paced ventricular complex generates another retrograde P-wave, an electronic ventriculo-atrial "reentrant circuit" is established. Less commonly, a paced ventricular complex that is not preceded by atrial depolarization (failure to capture in the atrium during AV sequential pacing, or atrial oversensing with triggered ventricular complex) allows retrograde atrial depolarization and initiates PMT. Disabling sensing function with placement of a magnet over the pulse generator terminates this tachycardia. PMT is prevented by extending the postventricular atrial refractory period (PVARP) beyond the timing of the retrograde P-wave; because the generator will not respond to atrial events that fall within this postventricular refractory period, PMT cannot be initiated. Failure of atrial capture or atrial oversensing can be remedied by reprogramming atrial output or sensitivity, respectively. Current pacemakers have algorithms that recognize and automatically terminate most occurrences of PMT.

Management of the Critical Care Patient with a Preexisting Cardiac Device

Identification of Device Type. It is necessary to know the manufacturer of the implanted device when choosing the appropriate programmer for device interrogation and programming. Most patients carry their device identification card with them that will list the manufacturer, device model number, and other information such as implant date and following physician. Calls to the "patient registration" personnel of the device manufacturers (for example, Medtronic, Inc. 1–800–328–2518, St Jude Medical 1–800–722–3423, Boston Scientific/Guidant 1–800–227–3422) can rapidly verify a device type and specifications. A magnified look at the pulse generator on chest radiograph may reveal a manufacturer-specific logo (Fig. 16.13) if the radiograph is sufficiently penetrated.

Monitoring Catheters and Lead Dislodgment Risk. Even with the use of active fixation leads, within the first 3–6 months after implantation there is a significant risk for lead dislodgment when catheters are introduced into the right heart. In patients with biventricular pacing systems that incorporate a left ventricular lead placed within a coronary sinus vein branch, the dislodgment risk is higher yet, even if the lead is chronic. The current coronary sinus leads are fixed passively within veins that do not develop fibrosis over the lead tip to the same degree as endocardium. Fluoroscopic guidance should be used whenever possible during right-heart catheterization in patients with recently implanted or biventricular pacing systems. If a balloon-tipped monitoring catheter is used, the balloon should always be deflated before pulling back so that entanglement with the pacemaker leads is avoided (Fig. 16.14). Whenever a central venous line or catheter is inserted, prophylactic antibiotics that adequately cover Staphylcoccal species should be considered in order to minimize the chance of lead infection.

Termination of Tachyarrhythmias. In patients with a preexisting cardiac device, termination of reentrant tachyarrhythmias such as atrial flutter and

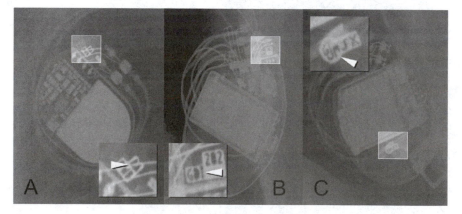

Fig. 16.13 Manufacturer identification logos of pacemaker and implantable cardioverter defibrillators can be found on chest radiography. A. Medtronic, Inc. logo, "M." B. Boston Scientific/Guidant logo, "GDT." C. St Jude Medical logo, "SJM."

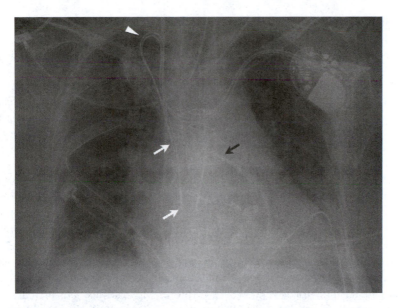

Fig. 16.14 Dislodgment of newly implanted atrial and ventricular pacemaker leads (white arrows) during placement of a Swan-Ganz catheter (black arrow). Both leads are looped up into the right internal jugular vein (white arrowhead) revealing the mechanism of dislodgment; the balloon at the tip of the Swan-Ganz catheter was left inflated while it was pulled back towards the venous sheath.

monomorphic ventricular tachycardias can sometimes be achieved through overdrive pacing. The chamber of origin of the rhythm is paced at a rate just above (typically by 10–20%) that of the tachyarrhythmia. Depending on the properties of the reentrant circuit and the position of the pacemaker lead relative to the location of the reentry circuit, capture of the circuit can occur, in which case the circuit will be "entrained" or synchronized to the pacemaker rate. By gradually increasing the pacing rate, the paced cycle length will eventually encroach on the refractory period of the circuit and the tachyarrhythmia can block and terminate. Alternatively, abrupt cessation of pacing after tachycardia entrainment can result in termination of the tachyarrhythmia.

Although generally safe, overdrive pacing of atrial flutter and ventricular tachycardia can induce atrial fibrillation and ventricular fibrillation, respectively. In patients with atrial flutter, induction of atrial fibrillation may actually be desirable because ventricular response in atrial fibrillation is easier to control than in atrial flutter. Because induction of ventricular fibrillation must be treated immediately, preparation for external defibrillation should be made prior to initiating ventricular overdrive pacing. Appropriate sedation should also be considered in the event that a shock will become necessary. This is especially important if the patient has an ICD that is active, since the programmed time interval from arrhythmia detection to shock typically is not long enough to allow the patient to lose consciousness.

External Cardioversion or Defibrillation. The energy surge from direct current external cardioversion or defibrillation has the potential to damage the pulse generator or cause a burn at the electrode–tissue interface due to flow of current through the leads (69,70). Protective measures, such as serially placed diodes, have been incorporated into pulse generators to decrease the chance of pulse generator damage (71). The most important measure to minimize pulse generator damage is to place the external cardioverter pads or paddles away from the device as much as possible. If the initial shock is not successful, a period of time (approximately 5 min) should elapse between successive shocks, if feasible, so as to cool the protective diodes (72). In order to decrease the chance of current flow through the leads, the shock vector should not be parallel to the lead-generator axis. Cardioverter pads or paddles placed in the anterior-posterior configuration are ideal because it positions the shock vector perpendicular to the lead-generator axis.

Despite these precautions, increases in capture thresholds do still occur from electrode–tissue interface burn (72). This becomes especially important in patients who are pacemaker-dependent since a rise in stimulation threshold may result in loss of capture (73). In pacemaker-dependent patients who are to undergo external cardioversion, baseline capture thresholds should be assessed and outputs increased temporarily prior to the procedure. Following the cardioversion, capture thresholds should be reassessed for any change. Leaving the outputs high for several weeks to protect against any late increases in threshold can be considered (72). In patients with an ICD, this complication can potentially be avoided by attempting cardioversions through the device.

Diagnostic Studies. Magnetic resonance imaging (MRI) scans are currently contraindicated in patients with either a pacemaker or an ICD. The concern arises from a variety of responses that these devices can have to the strong magnetic and radiofrequency forces generated during an MRI scan. These responses have ranged from rapid ventricular pacing due to oversensing or inappropriate rate response, to actual reprogramming or damage to the device. At least 10 cases of death have been reported in patients with pacemakers and ICDs that underwent MRI scan; all were poorly supervised (74). It is anticipated that newer devices will have circuitry that is better protected so that MRI scanning will be safe. A number of studies have suggested that with certain device models and specific scanning protocols, MRI scanning is safe (75–78). At this time, however, there is insufficient evidence to support even limited use of MRI scanning in patients with a cardiac device. If MRI must be performed, tachyarrhythmia therapies, magnet mode function, and sensor functions should be programmed off prior to scanning; the pacemaker mode should be changes to a nontracking mode. A full device check should be performed after the scan to ensure that lead and generator function is unchanged, and all previous parameters are reinstated. The patient's ECG should be continuously monitored during and after the scan.

Management of a Biventricular Device. It has been estimated that up to 38% of patients with moderate to severe congestive heart failure due to left ventricular systolic dysfunction have intraventricular conduction delays with wide QRS complexes and ventricular dyssynchrony (79). Cardiac resynchronization therapy using a biventricular pacemaker is now a Class I indication therapy for systolic heart failure in patients with a QRS complex $\geq$ 120 ms and left ventricular ejection fraction $\leq$ 35% (80). Although cardiac resynchronization therapy decreases heart failure hospitalizations (81,82), as the overall number of patients with biventricular pacemakers and ICDs increase, more critical care patients will present with implanted biventricular devices, and familiarity with the management of these devices will become increasingly important.

The left ventricular lead is what is unique about the biventricular system when compared with a conventional pacemaker or ICD. The left ventricular lead is implanted in a distal vein branch of the coronary sinus. The distal portion of the lead has a fixed bend that passively secures itself within the vein branch. The body of the lead courses along the lateral wall and anterior floor of the right atrium before it enters the coronary sinus os. This lead is susceptible to dislodgment with minimal catheter manipulation within the right atrium. Unlike leads that are implanted against the endocardium in the right atrium and right ventricle, there is less fibrosis over the left ventricular lead within a vein branch, and lead stability is a concern even with chronic leads. Right-heart catheterization should be performed under fluoroscopic guidance in a patient with a biventricular pacemaker or ICD, and stability of lead thresholds and position should be verified after catheterization.

Left ventricular pacing, when fused with right ventricular pacing, typically results in a narrower QRS complex than what would be expected with conventional right ventricular pacing. The left BBB pattern seen with right ventricular pacing is replaced by a nonspecific pattern that depends on the position of the left ventricular lead and the relative timing of stimulus output between the two ventricular leads (either lead can be programmed to deliver its output first by 0–80 ms). When a change in the paced QRS complex morphology from baseline is detected, loss of left ventricular lead capture due to an increase in capture threshold, or loss of biventricular pacing due to fusion from native AV nodal conduction should be suspected. An increase in left ventricular stimulus output, or shortening of the AV interval, respectively, will restore biventricular pacing. If the left ventricular lead tip is close to the phrenic nerve that courses over the lateral left ventricular wall, higher stimulus outputs may result in phrenic nerve stimulation.

The timing intervals between the three leads (AV interval and VV interval) can be optimized using echocardiographic measures for stroke volume or myocardial synchronization (such as using tissue Doppler imaging). Because the optimal timing parameters change with fluid status and loading conditions, echocardiography-guided optimization of pacemaker parameters, when aimed at prevention of future heart failure exacerbations, should be performed after adequate therapy with intravenous diuretics or inotropic agents.

References

1. Mark AL. The Bezold-Jarish reflex revisited: clinical implications of inhibitory reflexes originating in the heart. *J Am Coll Cardiol* 1983;1:90–102.
2. Feigl D, Ashkenazy J, Kishon Y. Early and late atrioventricular block in acute inferior myocardial infarction. *J Am Coll Cardiol* 1984;4:35–38.
3. Sclarovsky S, Strasberg B, Hirshberg A, Arditi A, Lewin RF, Agmon J. Advanced early and late atrioventricular block in acute inferior wall myocardial infarction. *Am Heart J* 1984;108:19–24.
4. Tan AC, Lie KI, Durrer D. Clinical setting and prognostic significance of high grade atrioventricular block in acute inferior myocardial infarction. *Am Heart J* 1980;99:4–8.
5. Nicod P, Gilpin E, Dittrich H, Polikar R, Henning H, Ross J Jr. Long-term outcome in patients with inferior myocardial infarction and complete heart block. *J Am Coll Cardiol* 1988;12:589–594.

6. Gupta PK, Lichstein E, Chadda KD. Heart block complicating acute inferior wall myocardial infarctions. *Chest* 1976;69:599–604.

7. Berger PB, Ruocco NA Jr, Ryan TJ, Frederick MM, Jacobs AK, Faxon DP. Incidence and prognostic implications of heart block complicating inferior myocardial infarction treated with thrombolytic therapy: results from TIMI II. *J Am Coll Cardiol* 1992;20:533–540.

8. Clemmensen P, Bates ER, Califf RM, et al. Complete atrioventricular block complicating inferior wall acute myocardial infraction treated with reperfusion therapy. *Am J Cardiol* 1991;67:255–230.

9. Hindman MC, Wagner GS, JaRo M, et al. The clinical significance of bundle branch block complicating acute myocardial infarction. 1. Clinical characteristics, hospital mortality, and one-year follow-up. *Circulation* 1978;58:679–688.

10. Hindman MC, Wagner GS, JaRo M, et al. The clinical significance of bundle branch block complicating acute myocardial infarction. 2. Indications for temporary and permanent pacemaker insertion. *Circulation* 1978;58:689–699.

11. Jones ME, Terry G, Kenmure AC. Frequency and significance of conduction defects in acute myocardial infarction. *Am Heart J* 1977;94:163–167.

12. Kyriakidis MK, Kourouklis CB, Papaioannou JT, Christakos SG, Spanos GP, Avgoustakis DG. Sinus node coronary arteries studied with angiography. *Am J Cardiol* 1983;51:749–750.

13. Go AS, Barron HV, Rundle AC, Ornato JP, Avins AL. Bundle-branch block and in-hospital mortality in acute myocardial infarction. National Registry of Myocardial Infarction 2 Investigators. *Ann Intern Med* 1998;129:690–697.

14. Melgarejo-Moreno A, Galcerá-Toms J, García-Alberola A, et al. Incidence, clinical characteristics, and prognostic significance of right bundle-branch block in acute myocardial infarction; a study in the thrombolytic era. *Circulation* 1997;96:1139–1144.

15. Lamas GA, Muller JE, Turi ZG, et al. A simplified method to predict occurrence of complete heart block during acute myocardial infarction. *Am J Cardiol* 1986;57:1213–1219.

16. Thomson IR, Dalton BC, Lappas DG, Lowenstein E. Right bundle-branch block and complete heart block caused by the Swan-Ganz catheter. *Anesthesiology* 1979;51:359–362.

17. Luck JC, Engel TR. Transient right bundle branch block with "Swan-Ganz" catheterization. *Am Heart J* 1976;92:263–264.

18. Morris D, Mulvihill D, Lew WY. Risk of developing complete heart block during bedside pulmonary artery catheterization in patients with left bundle-branch block. *Arch Intern Med* 1987;147:2005–2010.

19. Sprung CL, Elser B, Schein RM, et al. Risk of right-bundle branch block and complete heart block during pulmonary artery catheterization. *Crit Care Med* 1989;17:1–3.

20. Stein PD, Mahur VS, Herman MV, Levine HD. Complete heart block induced during cardiac catheterization of patients with pre-existent bundle-branch block. The hazard of bilateral bundle-branch block. *Circulation* 1966;34:783–791.

21. Harvey JR, Wyman RM, McKay RG, Baim DS. Use of balloon flotation pacing catheters for prophylactic temporary pacing during diagnostic and therapeutic catheterization procedures. *Am J Cardiol* 1988;62:941–944.

22. Bellocci F, Santarelli P, Di Gennaro M, Ansalone G, Fenici R. The risk of cardiac complications in surgical patients with bifascicular block. A clinical and electrophysiologic study in 98 patients. *Chest* 1980;77:343–348.

23. DiNubile MJ, Calderwood SB, Steinhaus DM, Karchmer AW. Cardiac conduction abnormalities complicating native valve active infective endocarditis. *Am J Cardiol* 1986;58:1213–1217.

24. Arnett EN, Roberts WC. Valve ring abscess in active infective endocarditis. Frequency, location, and clues to clinical diagnosis from the study of 95 necropsy patients. *Circulation* 1976;54:140–145.

25. Roberts NK, Somerville J. Pathological significance of electrocardiographic changes in aortic valve endocarditis. *Br Heart J* 1969;31:395–396.
26. Steere AC, Batsford WP, Weinberg M, et al. Lyme carditis: cardiac abnormalities of Lyme disease. *Ann Intern Med* 1980;93:8–16.
27. el-Sherif N, Zeiler RH, Craelius W, Gough WB, Henkin R. QTU prolongation and polymorphic ventricular tachyarrhythmias due to bradycardia-dependent early afterdepolarizations. Afterdepolarizations and ventricular arrhythmias. *Circ Res* 1988;63:286–305.
28. Tzivoni D, Banai S, Schuger C, et al. Treatment of torsade de pointes with magnesium sulfate. *Circulation* 1988;77:392–397.
29. Hohnloser SH, Klingenheben T, Singh BN. Amiodarone-associated proarrhythmic effects. A review with special reference to torsade de pointes tachycardia. *Ann Intern Med* 1994;121:529–535.
30. Rankin AC, Pringle SD, Cobbe SM. Acute treatment of torsade de pointes with amiodarone: proarrhythmic and antiarrhythmic association of QT prolongation. *Am Heart J* 1990;119:185–186.
31. Nguyen PT, Scheinman MM, Segar J. Polymorphous ventricular tachycardia: clinical characterization, therapy, and the QT interval. *Circulation* 1986;74:340–349.
32. Firth BG, Dehmer GJ, Nicod P, Willerson JT, Hillis LD. Effect of increasing heart rate in patients with aortic regurgitation. Effect of incremental atrial pacing on scintigraphic, hemodynamic and thermodilution measurements. *Am J Cardiol* 1982;49:1860–1867.
33. Meyer TE, Sareli P, Marcus RH, Patel J, Berk MR. Beneficial effect of atrial pacing in severe acute aortic regurgitation and role of M-mode echocardiography in determining the optimal pacing interval. *Am J Cardiol* 1991;67:398–403.
34. Pandian NG, Kosowsky BD, Gurewich V. Transfemoral temporary pacing and deep vein thrombosis. *Am Heart J* 1980;100:847–851.
35. Austin JL, Preis LK, Crampton RS, Beller GA, Martin RP. Analysis of pacemaker malfunction and complications of temporary pacing in the coronary care unit. *Am J Cardiol* 1982;49:301–306.
36. Fleischmann KE, Orav EJ, Lams GA, et al. Pacemaker implantation and quality of life in the Mode Selection Trial (MOST). *Heart Rhythm* 2006;3:653–659.
37. Heldman D, Mulvihill D, Nguyen H, et al. True incidence of pacemaker syndrome. *Pacing Clin Electrophysiol* 1990;13:1742–1750.
38. Choo MH, Holmes DR Jr, Gersh BJ, et al. Permanent pacemaker infections: characterization and management. *Am J Cardiol* 1981;48:559–564.
39. Ruiter JH, Degener JE, Van Mechelen R, Bos R. Late purulent pacemaker pocket infection caused by staphylococcus epidermidis: serious complication of in situ management. *Pacing Clin Electrophysiol* 1985;8:903–907.
40. Goldman B, MacGregor DC. Management of infected pacemaker systems. *Clin Prog Pacing Electrophysiol* 1989;2:220ff.
41. Klug D, Wallet F, Kacet S, Courcol RJ. Detailed bacteriologic tests to identify the origin of transvenous pacing system infections indicate a high prevalence of multiple organisms. *Am Heart J* 2005;149:322–328.
42. Arber N, Pras E, Copperman Y, et al. Pacemaker endocarditis. Report of 44 cases and review of the literature. *Medicine* 1994;73:299–305.
43. Paniagua D, Aldrich HR, Lieberman EH, Lamas GA, Agatston AS. Increased prevalence of significant tricuspid regurgitation in patients with transvenous pacemaker leads. *Am J Cardiol* 1998;82:1130–1132.
44. van Rooden CJ, Molhoek SG, Rosendaal FR, Schalij MJ, Meinders AE, Huisman MV. Incidence and risk factors of early venous thrombosis associated with permanent pacemaker leads. *J Cardiovasc Electrophysiol* 2004;15:1258–1262.
45. Goudevenos JA, Reid PG, Adams PC, Holden MP, Williams DO. Pacemaker-induced superior vena cava syndrome: report of four cases and review of the literature. *Pacing Clin Electrophysiol* 1989;12:1890–1895.

46. Chamorro H, Rao G, Wholey MH. Superior vena cava syndrome: a complication of transvenous pacemaker implantation. *Radiology* 1978;126:377–378.

47. Mazzetti H, Dussaut A, Tentori C, Dussaut E, Lazzari JO. Superior vena cava occlusion and/or syndrome related to pacemaker leads. *Am Heart J* 1993;125:831–837.

48. Hingorani A, Ascher E, Marks N, et al. Morbidity and mortality associated with brachial vein thrombosis. *Ann Vasc Surg* 2006;28:245–247.

49. Black MD, French GJ, Rasuli P, Bouchard AC. Upper extremity deep venous thrombosis. Underdiagnosed and potentially lethal. *Chest* 1993;103:1887–1890.

50. Reynolds J, Anslinger D, Yore R, Paine R. Transvenous cardiac pacemaker, mural thrombosis, and pulmonary embolism. *Am Heart J* 1969;78:688–691.

51. Nicolosi GL, Charmet PA, Zanuttini D. Large right atrial thrombosis. Rare complication during permanent transvenous endocardial pacing. *Br Heart J* 1980;43:199–201.

52. Bradof J, Sands MJ Jr, Lakin PC. Symptomatic venous thrombosis of the upper extremity complicating permanent transvenous pacing: reversal with streptokinase infusion. *Am Heart J* 1982;104:1112–1113.

53. Meier B. Maker of heart device kept flaw from doctors. *New York Times,* May 24, 2005.

54. Maisel WH, Moynahan M, Zuckerman BD, et al. Pacemaker and ICD generator malfunctions: analysis of Food and Drug Administration annual reports. *JAMA* 1006;295:1944–1946.

55. Alt E, Völker R, Bölmer H. Lead fracture in pacemaker patients. *Thorac Cardiovasc Surg* 1987;35:101–104.

56. Wish M, Swartz J, Cohen A, Cohen R, Fletcher R. Steroid-tipped leads versus porous platinum permanent pacemaker leads: a controlled study. *Pacing Clin Electrophysiol* 1990;13:1887–1890.

57. Radovsky AS, Van Vleet JF. Effects of dexamethasone elution on tissue reaction around stimulating electrodes of endocardial pacing lead in dogs. *Am Heart J* 1989;117:1288–1298.

58. Link MS, Estes NA III, Griffin JJ, et al. Complications of dual chamber pacemaker implantation in the elderly. Pacemaker Selection in the Elderly (PASE) Investigators. *J Interv Card Electrophysiol* 1998;2:175–179.

59. Preston TA, Fletcher RD, Lucchesi BR, Judge RD. Changes in myocardial threshold. Physiologic and pharmacologic factors in patients with implanted pacemakers. *Am Heart J* 1967;74:235–242.

60. Dohrmann ML, Goldschlager NF. Myocardial stimulation threshold in patients with cardiac pacemakers: effect of physiologic variables, pharmacologic agents, and lead electrodes. *Cardiol Clin* 1985;3:527–537.

61. Hughes JC Jr, Tyers GF, Torman HA. Effects of acid-base imbalance on myocardial pacing thresholds. *J Thorac Cardiovasc Surg* 1975;69:743–746.

62. Westerholm CJ. Threshold studies in transvenous cardiac pacemaker treatment. Direct measurement with special reference to short and long term stimulation and influence of certain metabolic, respiratory and pharmacological factors. *Scand J Thorac Cardiovasc Surg* 1971;8(Suppl):1–35.

63. Gettes LS, Shabetai R, Downs TA, Surawicz B. Effect of changes in potassium and calcium concentrations on diastolic threshold and strength-interval relationships of the human heart. *Ann NY Acad Sci* 1969;167:693–705.

64. Lee D, Greenspan K, Edmands RE, et al. The effect of electrolyte alteration on stimulus requirement of cardiac pacemakers [abstract]. *Circulation* 1968;38(Suppl): VI–124.

65. Surawicz B, Chlebus H, Reeves JT, Gettes LS. Increase of ventricular excitability threshold by hyperpotassemia. *JAMA* 1965;191:1049–1054.

66. Mohan JC, Kaul U, Bhatia ML. Acute effects of anti-arrhythmic drugs on cardiac pacing threshold. *Acta Cardiologica* 1984;39:191–201.

67. Brandfonbrener M, Kronholm J, Jones HR. The effect of serum potassium concentration on quinidine toxicity. *J Pharmacol Exp Ther* 1966;154:250–254.

68. Khastgir T, Lattuca J, Aarons D, et al. Ventricular pacing threshold and time to capture postdefibrillation in patients undergoing implantable cardioverter-defibrillator implantation. *Pacing Clin Electrophysiol* 1991;14:768–772.

69. Guarnieri T, Datorre SD, Bondke H, Brinker J, Myers S, Levine JH. Increased pacing threshold after an automatic defibrillator shock in dogs: effect of class I and class II antiarrhythmic drugs. *Pacing Clin Electrophysiol* 1988;11:1324–1330.

70. Dahl CF, Ewy GA, Warner ED, Thomas ED. Myocardial necrosis from direct current countershock: effect of paddle electrode size and time interval between discharges. *Circulation* 1974;50:956–960.

71. Lau FYK, Bilitch M, Wintrob HJ. Protection of implanted pacemakers from excessive electrical energy of DC shock. *Am J Cardiol* 1969;23:244–249.

72. Waller D, Callies F, Langenfeld H. Adverse effects of direct current cardioversion on cardiac pacemakers and electrodes. Is external cardioversion contraindicated in patients with permanent pacing systems? *Europace* 2004;6:165–168.

73. Altamura G, Bianconi L, Lo Bianco F, et al. Transthoracic DC shock may represent a serious hazard in pacemaker dependent patients. *Pacing Clin Electrophysiol* 1995;18:194–198.

74. Martin ET. Can cardiac pacemakers and magnetic resonance imaging systems co-exist? *Eur Heart J* 2005;26:325–327.

75. Del Ojo JL, Moya F, Villalba J, et al. Is magnetic resonance imaging safe in cardiac pacemaker recipients? *Pacing Clin Electrophysiol* 2005;28:274–278.

76. Nazarian S, Roguin A, Zviman MM, et al. Clinical utility and safety of a protocol for noncardiac and cardiac magnetic resonance imaging of patients with permanent pacemakers and implantable-cardioverter defibrillators at 1.5 Tesla. *Circulation* 2006;114:1277–1284.

77. Gimbel JR, Kanal E, Schwartz MK, Wilkoff BL. Outcome of magnetic resonance imaging in selected patients with implantable cardioverter defibrillators. *Pacing Clin Electrophysiol* 2005;28:270–273.

78. Martin ET, Coman JA, Shellock FG, Pulling CC, Fair R, Jenkins K. Magnetic resonance imaging and cardiac pacemaker safety at 1.5-Tesla. *J Am Coll Cardiol* 2004;43:1315–1325.

79. Aaronson KD, Schwartz JS, Chen TM, et al. Development and prospective validation of a clinical index to predict survival in ambulatory patients referred for cardiac transplant evaluation. *Circulation* 1997;95:2660–2667.

80. Hunt SA, ACC/AHA Task Force. ACC/AHA guideline update for the diagnosis and management of chronic heart failure in the adult. *J Am Coll Cardiol* 2005;46:1–82.

81. Abraham WT, Fisher WG, Smith AL, et al for the MIRACLE Study Group. Cardiac resynchronization in chronic heart failure. *N Engl J Med* 2002;346:1845–1853.

82. Cleland JG, Daubert JC, Erdmann E, et al. For the CARE-HF Study Investigators. The effects of cardiac resynchronization on morbidity and mortality in heart failure. *N Engl J Med* 2005;352:1539–1549.

Section IV

Evaluation and Follow-up of Implantable Devices

17

Environmental Effects on Cardiac Pacing Systems

Louise Cohan, Fred M. Kusumoto, and Nora F. Goldschlager

Early artificial pacemakers delivered asynchronous pulses at a fixed rate regardless of the intrinsic activity of the heart. As pacemaker technology improved, devices were developed that not only delivered pacing stimuli but also sensed intrinsic cardiac electrical activity. However, the circuitry used to detect small amplitude (1–20 mV) intracardiac electrical signals generated by the atrium and ventricle can also detect signals generated from both internal and external sources (1–3). Internal sources of signals include extracardiac muscle depolarization and other implanted devices such as ICDs and spinal cord stimulators. External sources of signals can arise from a variety of sources and are collectively referred to as electromagnetic interference (EMI).

Methods for Reducing the Potential Effects of Interference

Manufacturers have taken a number of steps to reduce the influence of interference on pacing system function. First, modern pacemakers are relatively immune to most common sources of EMI because the circuitry is shielded inside a hermetically sealed titanium or stainless steel case that often has an additional insulative coating. The body tissues also provide some degree of additional protection by acting as a barrier to signal transmission. Interference at field strengths that can cause abnormal pacing system behavior during bench testing frequently does not affect in vivo pacing system function (4,5). It is important for the clinician to distinguish between laboratory and clinical studies for evaluating the clinical relevance of various environmental sources of interference.

Second, the increased use of bipolar leads has further decreased the susceptibility of pacing systems to external interference. The initial designs of pacing leads used a single distal electrode located on the tip (cathode). The circuit was completed by the pulse generator itself, which served as the anode. This system is called a unipolar system since only one electrode is located in the heart. Although this design is reliable it is more susceptible to environmental signals because of the large antenna-like effect owing to the separation between cathode and anode. Most pacing leads implanted today have a bipolar design with two pacing electrodes located at the distal portion of the lead. The small

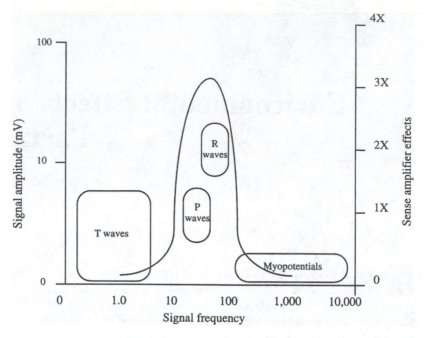

Fig 17.1 Signal amplitude and frequency from various sources. Modern sense amplifiers employ bell-shaped response curves that amplify signals within the 10–100 Hz range while attenuating signals below and above these frequencies. In this way signals from ventricular depolarization (R waves) and atrial depolarization (P waves) can be amplified and the effects from spurious signals, such as T waves and myopotentials, can be minimized.

space between the electrodes (2–3 cm) provides a relatively small antenna when compared to a unipolar system.

Third, the pacemaker is designed to filter out noncardiac signals by using filters that attenuate signals outside a narrow range of frequencies (bandpass filters). Cardiac depolarization has a frequency range of 10–50 Hz (Fig. 17.1). All pacing systems use electronic sensing amplifiers that attenuate signals outside this range and amplify signals within this range. Although this sophisticated circuitry reduces the potential for interference from outside sources, it does not eliminate interference with frequencies between 5 and 100 Hz. More recently, feed-through filters are routinely placed between the pacemaker electronics and the connector block to prevent unwanted signals from entering the pacemaker circuitry.

Finally, manufacturers have developed various algorithms such as noise-sampling periods and safety pacing to decrease the possibility that signals sensed from environmental sources will lead to inappropriate inhibition or triggering of the pacing system. In general, most noise-sensing algorithms scan for signals during a period when intrinsic ventricular depolarization would generally not be expected (the terminal portion of the P wave or after the T wave); if signals are sensed during this period the signals are defined as "noise" by the pacemaker, which then begins delivering pacing stimuli at some specified noise-reversion or interference rate. These algorithms are discussed fully in Chapter 3.

Internal Sources

Musculoskeletal

Throughout the 1970s several investigators reported inappropriate pacemaker sensing ("oversensing") of skeletal muscle myopotentials; the incidence of myopotential oversensing has ranged from 11 to 85% in pacing systems using unipolar leads and from 5 to 10% in pacing systems with bipolar leads (6–9). Sophisticated sensing amplifiers and bandpass filters have reduced, but not eliminated, the frequency of myopotential oversensing in the current generation of pacing systems. Myopotential oversensing in single-chamber pacing systems usually causes inhibition of pacing stimuli, whereas myopotential oversensing in dual-chamber pacing systems can lead to both inhibition (if oversensing occurs in the ventricular channel) or triggering of ventricular output (if oversensing occurs in the atrial channel). The sensitivity of modern pulse generators usually can be adjusted to minimize myopotential oversensing even if a unipolar lead is employed. In a recent study, myopotential oversensing was present in 50% of patients with unipolar systems and 5% of patients with bipolar pacing systems using "standard" sensitivity settings ranging from 0.625 to 1.5 mV (9). However, optimal programming of the sensitivity in unipolar systems has reduced the incidence of myopotential oversensing to 5%.

Myopotential oversensing can also occur in implantable cardioverter defibrillator (ICD) systems (10–12). In one study of 227 patients with ICDs, myopotential interference occurred in 10% (12). Myopotential interference is more commonly observed in ICD lead systems that use an integrated bipolar design where a large surface shocking coil is also used as the anode for sensing and pacing (Fig. 17.1). Myopotential oversensing in ICDs can cause both inappropriate shocks and inappropriate inhibition of pacing. Because ICDs require some type of sensitivity circuitry in which myopotential oversensing may become more prevalent in the newest generation of ICDs, which are used as primary therapy for both bradycardia and tachycardia. In order to detect rapid low amplitude ventricular activity sometimes associated with ventricular fibrillation, all defibrillators use some type of signal amplification or adjustable sensitivity algorithm. Smaller electrical signals from myopotentials may be inappropriately defined as ventricular activity. In general, inappropriate myopotential sensing by defibrillators is rare.

Periodic provocative tests should be performed to evaluate for myopotential oversensing in patients with pacing systems or ICDs. While the surface ECG, intracardiac electrograms, and marker channels are monitored through the programmer, the patient should be asked to perform various maneuvers such as Valsalva, deep inspiration and expiration, and coughing. In addition, isometric and isotonic exercises using skeletal muscle adjacent to the pulse generator should be performed; for example, a patient with a pectorally implanted device should push and pull with his or her arms against variable resistance.

Implanted Devices

In the past, 1–5% of patients with ICDs also had separate implanted pacing systems since earlier generations of ICDs (prior to 1997–1999) were not designed to provide extended periods of pacing (13). There are several possible interactions between devices: ICD oversensing of pacing stimuli, ICD underdetection of ventricular arrhythmias owing to the presence of pacing stimuli (which in turn result from undersending of the arrhythmia), and direct damage to the pacing system or myocardium by an ICD discharge (14–16). Currently patients with two devices should have the pacing system removed and a new ICD with pacing capability placed.

Other implanted medical devices such as spinal cord stimulators and skeletal muscle stimulators can interact with permanent pacing systems (13,17). Output from the stimulator can be sensed by the pacing system and cause inhibition of pacing stimulus output. Using bipolar stimulators, minimizing stimulator output, or programming the pacing system to a higher sensing threshold can usually eliminate these unwanted interactions.

External Medical Sources

The hospital environment has many potential sources of high energy that can interact with pacing systems. These energy sources include electrocautery, external cardioversion, magnetic resonance imaging cameras, therapeutic ionizing radiation, and other therapeutic medical equipment. However, with some basic precautions most potential problems owing to interaction with these sources of EMI can be avoided.

Electrocautery

In common use since the 1900s for multiple types of surgery, electrocautery uses radiofrequency current to cut or coagulate tissues. In most electrocautery units, radiofrequency current having frequencies of 100–5,000 kHz and power levels of 10–500 W is delivered between a cauterizing instrument (cathode) and an indifferent electrode attached to the skin. Electrocautery can produce electrical signals that can cause unwanted inhibition of pacing stimuli or triggered ventricular pacing owing to atrial oversensing. In patients with ICDs, electrical signals generated by electrocautery can be sensed by the ICD and be incorrectly defined as a ventricular tachyarrhythmia, resulting in delivery of a shock (13,18). The frequency of interaction between ICDs and electrocautery has varied widely. In one study of 45 patients with ICDs undergoing surgery no episodes of oversensing, reprogramming, or ICD damage were detected (18). However, in a survey of dermatologic surgeons only 15% of respondents reported routine deactivation of ICDs and 25 complications were reported, including four inappropriate ICD discharges (19). In addition to oversensing, current produced by electrocautery can be concentrated at the pacing or ICD electrode–tissue interface by inductive coupling or if shunting by the protective Zener diode circuits occurs. Concentration of current can cause myocardial burns and acute and chronic increases in pacing threshold with loss of capture. If the indifferent electrode of the electrocautery inadvertently becomes disconnected, the pacing electrode can become the active anode for the electrocautery circuit; in this situation, induction of atrial fibrillation in patients with atrial leads and ventricular fibrillation in patients with ventricular leads can occur.

Specific issues that must be considered for patients with implanted pacing systems or ICDs include the distance between the surgical site where electrocautery is being used and the implanted device, the orientation of the electrocautery electrodes relative to the pacing system electrodes, the frequency of electrocautery applications, and the pacemaker dependency of the patient.

Very high current densities are generated at the site where electrocautery is being applied. Use of the electrocautery tip near the implanted pacemaker may induce current of sufficient strength to cause the pulse generator to revert to a fixed-rate (noise-reversion) mode of function or totally inhibit output in response to the oversensed signals. Currents at the electrocautery tip disperse rapidly so that effects on the pulse generator are significantly reduced at a distance of only a few centimeters. Electrocautery should not be used in the vicinity of a pacing system or ICD. The current effects of electrocautery are reduced if the current flow from the electrocautery system is perpendicular to the lead(s) of the pacemaker system (2). Because of the wide spacing of the electrodes in unipolar pacing systems, in which one electrode is in the heart and the other is in the pulse generator, it is more important to maintain a perpendicular orientation in these systems.

Pacing system inhibition from interference is more important in the pacemaker-dependent patient. If inhibition is observed in a pacemaker-dependent patient, electrocautery application should be limited to 1–2 s with a rest period of approximately 10 s. This will allow the pacemaker to function properly for a greater portion of the time. In some cases back-up temporary transvenous or transcutaneous pacing will be required, or the pacemaker can be programmed to the asynchronous mode of function.

Recommendations

- A comprehensive assessment of the pacemaker function and patient pacemaker dependency is recommended prior to the surgical procedure. Pacer dependency can be determined by programming the pacemaker to the VVI mode and gradually reducing the pacing rate. Gradual reduction in pacing rate is preferred to abrupt reduction in rate to avoid overdrive suppression of intrinsic cardiac rhythm. If no consistent intrinsic ventricular activity is noted in the pacing rate when decreased to 35 bpm the patient probably does not have a reliable "backup" rhythm and can be classified as pacemaker dependent (20,21).
- Rate response and any special algorithms should be programmed "off" prior to the surgical procedure. It is also important to ascertain ahead of time specific characteristics of that manufacturer's magnet response since magnet application may be required during the surgical procedure (20,21).
- The pacemaker can be programmed to an asynchronous pacing mode (VOO, AOO, or DOO) just prior to surgery. Programming the pacemaker to an asynchronous mode may be preferable to placing a magnet over the device particularly if there is little or no intrinsic ventricular activity since the manufacturers' magnet rates may be higher than desired (e.g., 100/min St. Jude devices). However, problems can arise during asynchronous pacing if the pacemaker competes with the patient's intrinsic rhythm. This can result in the induction of tachyarrythmias.
- Use bipolar cautery if possible. This type of system has a short current path, which greatly reduces the area of significant electrical signal generation to roughly a 6-in. circle centered on the site of electrocautery application. In addition, an ultrasonic scalpel may reduce EMI (22). If a unipolar cautery

system must be used, the indifferent electrode (grounding pad) should be placed such that the current flow between it and the cautery tip will not intersect the pacing system. For example, the thigh ipsilateral to the surgical site can be used in abdominal procedures (13). Good contact between the indifferent electrode and the skin must be maintained to reduce the chance of loss of contact, resulting in the pacing lead becoming a current sink for the electrocautery.

- Do not use electrocautery within 6 in. of the pulse generator.
- Use the minimum power settings required for adequate electrocautery.
- Use short bursts (preferably less than 1 s in duration) spaced more than 5 s apart. If electrocautery is causing inhibition of the pacemaker, a longer time between bursts will minimize hemodynamic effects.
- Monitor the patient for signs of pacemaker inhibition or triggering. If the ECG tracing is not clear because of interference from the use of cautery, the patient should be monitored manually or by some other means, such as ear or finger plethosgraphy or arterial pressure display. Provisions for alternative pacing and defibrillation should be readily available in the operating suite.
- Verify function of the pacemaker after the procedure with a complete pacing system interrogation and threshold determinations.

The same general guidelines apply for patients with ICDs. In addition, ICD therapies and tachycardia detection algorithms must be programmed off during the surgical procedure. In contrast to the effects on pacemakers, magnet application in patients with ICDs should be avoided since in some cases magnet application will deactivate the ICD. The ICD must be interrogated after the surgical procedure and tachycardia detection and therapies must be turned "on."

Transthoracic Cardioversion and Defibrillation

Transthoracic cardioversion uses relatively high voltages (up to 3.5 kV) delivered by cutaneous patches. Modern pacemakers and ICDs employ specialized protective circuitry that minimizes the harmful effects of high energy. Despite this protective circuitry, several specific problems may be observed after transthoracic cardioversion or defibrillation: reversion of the pacemaker to the "backup" mode (under unusual conditions such as potential component failure or exposure to extreme temperatures some pacemakers will revert to a backup pacing mode at a specified rate): transient increases in capture thresholds; and actual destruction of the pacemaker circuitry (23–31).

Recommendations

- Interrogate the pacing system prior to elective cardioversion.
- Determine the pacemaker dependency of a patient. If the patient is pacemaker dependent, increasing stimulus output prior to the procedure may compensate for post cardioversion transient elevated pacing thresholds, should they occur.
- Place paddles or cutaneous electrodes using an anterior–posterior configuration, more than 5 cm from the pacemaker. When two anterior paddles are used, paddle

placement should be greater than or equal to 13 cm from the axis formed by the pulse generator and lead electrodes.

- Reinterrogate the pacing system after defibrillatation or cardioversion. A programmed parameter, such as a mode of function, should be programmed to confirm that the pacemaker actually performs telemetered instructions.

In addition to the same guidelines that apply for pacemakers, ICD reinterrogation should include verification of the charge time, battery voltage, and appropriate capacitor formation. If the charge time is elevated, a manual capacitor formation is needed (Chapter 20, ICD follow-up) (24,25).

Magnetic Resonance Imaging

Of available imaging techniques, Magnet resonance imaging (MRI) is the best for delineating soft tissue structures, and is often the preferred imaging method for the head, neck, brain, spine, and musculoskeletal system. Historically, the presence of pacemakers and ICDs have been absolute contraindications for MRI. With the growing importance of MRI it has been estimated that there will be a 50–75% probability that over the lifetime of the patient's implanted device there will be an indication for an MRI (32–36). With more widespread use of implanted cardiac devices, there has been intense pressure on clinicians to develop protocols that provide "safe" use of MRI in these patients.

An MRI is performed by first producing a static magnetic field, which is followed by application of rapidly varying magnetic fields (100–200 Hz) and electromagnetic radiofrequency (RF) fields (60–70 MHz). Pacing system and ICD behavior are affected by all three components of MRI (32).

The static magnetic field exerts its effects on the reed switch of the pacemaker. The reed switch on most pacemakers will be closed by a 10-G or greater constant magnetic field. Magnetic fields generated from permanent magnets and electromagnets are measured in Tesla (T); 1 T equals 10,000 G. Older studies have shown that the reed switch will be closed by exposure to the constant or static magnetic field of the MRI. With the reed switch closed, the pacemaker functions in the magnet (asynchronous) mode and rate, which varies among pacemaker manufacturers (32–40). Some pacemakers provide the option of turning off the magnet response to the closure of the reed switch (32). Asynchronous pacing should pose little problem in most otherwise stable pacemaker patients but can be associated with the development of ventricular and atrial arrhythmias (1). In a recent study using the current generation of pacemakers and MRI scanners, reed switch closure was observed in only approximately 50% of cases. The static magnetic field of the MRI may exert a significant torquing effect on the pacemaker pulse generator. Some pacemakers are constructed with sufficient amounts of ferromagnetic materials that allow stray magnetic fields outside the MRI to impose significant rotational and attractive forces upon them. Inside the MRI only the rotational force is experienced. One study reported attractive forces of 5 N (Newtons) in a 1.5-T magnetic field and 1.7 N in a 0.5-T magnetic field for an older pacemaker pulse generator (as a comparison, the force of gravity is 0.5 N) (32). However, no significant physical movement has been reported in newer pacemakers that do not use large amounts of ferromagnetic material in their battery construction (32–34).

Inappropriate pacemaker function may be induced by the alternating magnetic fields and rapid radiofrequency pulses emitted during each scan (41–49). Rapid pacing in unipolar systems exposed to the pulsing radiofrequency field owing to the "antenna" effect of the electrode separation has been demonstrated (41). Another potential problem that can arise from the alternating magnetic fields and radiofrequency pulses is electrode heating. In a laboratory study, a 1.5-T MRI caused a greater than 15°C temperature increase at the electrode–tissue interface, with myocardial burns resulting (44). Other studies have described "acceptable" increases in tissue temperature (<1–4°C) using endocardial leads and standard MRI protocols, with higher temperatures recorded in MRI protocols that used higher specific absorption rates (SAR). In one in vitro study, substantial heating (up to 35°C) was observed in experiments where the lead was embedded deeply into a gel, emphasizing the importance of the cooling effect of blood flow through heart tissue and at the lead–endocardial tissue interface.

Several clinical studies have evaluated the use of MRI in selected patients with implanted cardiac devices using very specific protocols. In one study, a total of 115 clinically urgent MRI examinations were performed in 82 patients with pacemakers (37). Important points included limiting the SAR to 1.5 W/kg, using pacemakers from a single manufacturer, and excluding pacemaker-dependent patients and thoracic MRI examinations. All MRI examinations were completed safely and no arrhythmias were observed. A ≥ 1.0 V increase in capture threshold was observed in six (3%) pacing systems and two of the increases were detected only at a 3 month follow-up visit. Heating and subsequent alteration of the electrode tissue interface is the most likely cause of the increase in capture threshold. Activation of the reed switch was observed in only 55% of examinations, and seven examinations (6.1%) resulted in electrical reset. As emphasized in an accompanying editorial, this combination could be clinically significant in the pacemaker-dependent patient due to inhibition of pacing therapy if the factory reset is the VVI pacing mode (38). In a second study 68 MRI examinations were performed in 31 patients with pacemakers and 24 patients with ICDs (including 7 patients with left ventricular leads) (35). Patients with epicardial, superior vena cava coil, or abandoned leads were excluded; studies were limited to devices that had been evaluated by in vitro testing; and SAR was limited to <2.0 W/kg. All examinations were completed safely and at follow-up no alterations in lead characteristics or unexpected programming changes were observed. Importantly, diagnostic questions were answered by the MRI examination in all patients who had nonthoracic imaging. Significant imaging artifacts due to the implanted device were observed in patients requiring thoracic images; these were most pronounced in the inversion-prepared gradient echo and steady state free-precession cine sequences, but nevertheless the diagnostic question was answered in 93% of patients. There have been several reports of possible adverse events associated with MRI in patients with cardiac devices. Complete loss of ICD programmability due to memory corruption has been reported and a survey of German hospitals identified six patients with pacemakers who died during MRI examinations although specific causes of death were not specified (46).

To summarize, while limited data suggest MRI can be performed in selected patients with pacemakers and ICDs, in general, MRI imaging is contraindicated. If MRI is clinically required and no adequate alternative exists, the following recommendations should be kept in mind.

Recommendations

- Recently implanted devices (<2–3 months), devices with epicardial leads, abandoned leads, or long leads (>70 cm) generally should not be imaged since they have not been included in any studies to date.
- Obtain informed consent with an emphasis on potential hazards, including death, particularly in those patients that are pacemaker dependent.
- An MRI physician as well as personnel trained in pacemaker/ICD function should be present during the scan (36).
- A full resuscitation team should be available.
- Before MRI, evaluate the pacing system thoroughly. Determine both pacing and sensing thresholds and print the current programmed parameters. Consult with the manufacturer to verify magnet function (mode, rate, and intervals) of the implanted device. Evaluate and document the patient's underlying rhythm in case the pacemaker fails completely.
- Special programming features such as rate adaption, magnet response algorithms to suppress atrial fibrillation, mode switch response, and premature ventricular contraction responses should be programmed "off."
- ICDs should have monitoring and therapies programmed "off."
- In nonpacemaker-dependent patients, program the pacemaker to the OOO mode, if it is available in the particular device. Alternatively, the stimulus amplitude may be programmed to a (subthreshold) value that will not result in myocardial capture in case rapid stimulus output does occur in response to the alternating magnetic field (40). Pacemaker-dependent patients should be programmed to the VOO or DOO pacing mode.
- MRI equipment that uses a low magnetic field (0.5 T) is preferred where possible. The SAR must be limited to less than 2.0 W/kg, and preferably to less than 1.5 W/kg. For extremity MRI examinations, a 0.2-T extremity MR system should be used if available.
- The patient should be continuously monitored during the scan by pulse oximetry, ECG (although this may be distorted to some degree), blood pressure, and visually by personnel trained in paced ECG interpretation.
- After the procedure, reinterrogate the pacemaker and reprogram it to its original parameters. ICD therapies must be programmed "on" and back to the original parameters. Perform a complete evaluation including threshold testing. Testing and documentation of pacing thresholds should be repeated at 3 month follow-up.

Lithotripsy

Extracorporeal shock wave lithotripsy (ESWL) is a commonly used method for treating kidney stones. In this technique, pressure waves are generated by the lithotriptor's electrical discharges (18–30 KV) between two electrodes submersed in water. The electrical discharge causes an abrupt expansion and collapse of a gas bubble that in turn generates a pressure wave that is focused by a lens, ellipsoid reflectors, or shaped array, and transmitted through the body to a focal point approximately 2 cm in diameter. The energy delivered from this pressure wave ranges from 20 to 40 J. Serial pressure wave pulses are delivered, with a typical treatment requiring 1,000–1,500 pulses.

Patients with pacemakers have been successfully and safely treated with ESWL, although there have been reported cases of induced supraventricular and ventricular tachycardias (47–49). Current lithotriptors are designed to deliver the shock wave 20 ms after a sensed QRS complex, during the ventricular refractory period, to minimize the risk for induction of sustained ventricular arrhythmias.

There is little likelihood of damage to pacemakers that have been implanted in the pectoral area; however, an abdominal implant (pacemaker or ICD) is subject to damage (47, 50–52). In vitro studies have documented that pacemakers can be damaged during ESWL. If the shock wave is aimed directly at a pacemaker that employs a piezoelectric crystal sensor for rate response function, the crystal can be damaged.

The delivery of the shock wave should be timed to the ventricular stimulus output in patients who are paced, to avoid pacemaker inhibition owing to oversensing of the shock wave. Dual-chamber pacemakers may need to be programmed to a single-chamber ventricular pacing mode: should the lithotriptor synchronize off an atrial pacing stimulus, the ensuing electrical discharge between the spark plug electrodes may be sensed in the ventricular channel and inhibit the ventricular output (51).

One study has addressed the use of lithotripsy in patients with ICDs. This issue is particularly important because many older ICDs have been implanted in the abdomen and are closer to the pressure waves. Lithotripsy can be performed if padding is used over the device (52). However, the device must be thoroughly evaluated after the lithotripsy procedure; loosening of the setscrew holding the lead in place has been reported in one case series (52).

Recommendations

- Place the lithotriptor focal point greater than or equal to 6–10 inches away from the pacemaker. There are no conclusive studies that have quantified the likelihood of damage to an implanted pacemaker; the greater the distance of the focal point from the pacemaker the greater the margin of safety.
- Reprogram dual-chamber pacemakers to the VVI mode of function to avoid having the lithotriptor trigger off the atrial stimulus.
- Interrogate the pacemaker after the procedure and reprogram the device back to the original parameters.
- Interrogate ICDs fully before and after ESWL treatment. All detection algorithms and therapies should be disabled during ESWL.

Radiation

Diagnostic radiation has no important effect on pacemakers. However, high-energy radiation used for the treatment of many types of malignancies can cause potentially catastrophic problems for patients with pacemakers or ICDs (53–65). Adverse effects that have been reported can be either transient, owing to the electromagnetic field of a linear accelerator or betatron, or permanent, owing to direct damage of the pacemaker circuitry. Older pacemakers were relatively resistant to the effects of ionizing radiation; unfortunately, advances in semiconductor technology have reduced most of that resistance. As a result, today's pacemakers are more advanced, but are also more susceptible to damage by very high-energy radiation from the gamma rays, electrons, protons, or neutrons produced by cobalt radiators, linear accelerators, and betatrons (53,54).

Modern pacemakers use complementary metal oxide semiconductor (CMOS) circuitry, which is very reliable, energy efficient, and space efficient. Radiation can cause damage to the thin oxide layers and transistors because of accumulation of positive charge inside the CMOS circuitry. The resulting damage can be seen in alteration of the transistor parameters or in creation of undesired electrical shorts or leakage currents between adjacent circuits, leading to failure of various battery components or accelerated battery depletion. The problems are transient in some cases, but most commonly the damage is permanent (60). The amount of damage to the device is unpredictable, but depends, in part, on the type of radiation, cumulative dose, and location of the device. Unfortunately, there is no consistent way to predict how a device will fail or at what radiation dose failure will occur (53). Pacing system malfunctions have included reprogramming, changes in sensing capability, failure of telemetry function (ability to communicate with the pacemaker), changes in rate (including runaway), and complete shutdown (56,64). The sensitivity of a CMOS circuit is proportional to the thickness of the metal oxide layer. The most recent generation of pacemakers uses thinner (3-μm) CMOS circuits, which are more resistant to radiation damage. The effects of therapeutic radiation on ICDs are essentially unknown.

Recommendations

- Evaluate the patient for pacemaker dependency.
- Contact the manufacturer to determine the susceptibility and response of the specific device to radiation.
- Position the field of radiation at an angle oblique to the pacemaker in order to minimize the amount of radiation delivered at the pacemaker site. The pacemaker will receive some radiation even when it is outside the edge of the collimated radiation beam. It has been recommended that a total accumulated dosage limit of 2 rad be estimated, using either luminescent dosimeters or a diode dose measurement system (63). Additional shielding of the pacemaker with a 1-cm margin may be required (64). A 3-cm distance from the edge of the unblocked collimator to the device should be maintained (53). Direct irradiation of the pacemaker must be avoided. If this is not possible, the pacemaker should be explanted and moved to another suitable site.
- Carefully monitor the patient with ECG and pulse oximetry for pacemaker function during radiation therapy. It may be necessary to have temporary pacing capability available in case the pacing system malfunctions during the treatment.
- Evaluate pacing system function following the radiation treatment.

Radiofrequency Catheter Ablation

Radiofrequency catheter ablation has emerged as an effective method for treating various tachyarrhythmias. Radiofrequency generators produce unmodulated signals with frequencies between 400 and 500 kHz and a strength of 5–50 W. In an experimental study in dogs, abnormal pacing function was observed if ablation was performed within 1 cm from the pacing lead electrode (66). No abnormal pacing system behavior was observed if the ablation was performed more than 4 cm from the pacing electrode. In a clinical study involving 25 patients with implanted pacing systems undergoing radiofrequency catheter ablation, eight pacing systems functioned at the noise-reversion rate and four exhibited transient loss of capture during radiofrequency energy application (67). Rapid pacing at the programmed upper rate during radiofrequency energy application has been described in a patient with a minute ventilation rate adaptive pacing system (68). Finally, elevated pacing thresholds after radiofrequency catheter ablation has been reported (69). In 59 patients with permanent implanted devices undergoing AV nodal ablation, a twofold increase in pacing thresholds was detected in 13% of patients with pacing leads and 46% of ICDs at 24 h (69). At follow-up, the threshold generally decreased, but lead revision was required in 4% of patients with pacing leads and 15% of patients with ICDs. ICD leads may be more susceptible to dispersed radiofrequency energy during ablation due to the large distal coil used as the anode for pacing in some lead designs. Finally, in a study of 86 patients with implanted devices undergoing pulmonary vein ablation for atrial fibrillation, no changes in capture thresholds or lead impedances were detected, but two patients had atrial lead dislodgment (70). Generally, radiofrequency catheter ablation can be performed in patients with pacing systems if several simple precautions are followed and the risk for subsequent pacemaker revision due to increased capture thresholds or lead dislodgement is acknowledged.

Recommendations

- Have temporary pacing available.
- Turn off rate-adaptive functions.
- If the patient is not pacemaker dependent, program the pulse generator to the OOO pacing mode (if available) or to subthreshold stimulus output. Pacemaker runaway, observed in one experimental study, is probably due to radiofrequency energy entering the output circuits, as described above for pacemaker–MRI interactions.
- Reinterrogate the pacing system after completion of the ablation procedure and evaluate all prior programmed parameters.
- Disable ICD therapies and detection algorithms in patients with these devices and have standard transthoracic defibrillation methods readily available. Perform full interrogation of ICD function including threshold testing and measurement of lead impedances. It is imperative to confirm that tachycardia therapies have been reinstituted after the procedure.

Transcutaneous Electrical Nerve Stimulation

Transcutaneous electrical nerve stimulation (TENS) is a treatment for relief of acute or chronic pain. A TENS unit consists of several electrodes placed on the skin and connected to an external pulse generator, applying pulses of 0–60 mA at a frequency of 20–100 Hz. To provide maximum pain relief, the patient adjusts the output and frequency of stimulation. Stimulation pulses are usually bipolar and of short duration, with a frequency content that is usually filtered by the sense amplifiers of the pulse generator. In rare cases, the stimuli from a TENS unit can be sensed by a pacing system. Studies have shown that TENS rarely causes output inhibition in bipolar pacing systems, although transient inhibition in unipolar pacing systems is more commonly seen; abnormal pacing system behavior can usually be corrected by reprogramming the sensitivity of the pacemaker generator (71,72). TENS does not cause direct damage to the pacemaker pulse generator and any unwanted effects on pacing system function will end when the TENS unit is turned off or disconnected. Clinical studies have shown that TENS units can be used safely in pacemaker patients (72).

Recommendations

- Use a bipolar pacing system whenever possible, as they are much less likely than unipolar systems to be affected by EMI.
- Place the TENS electrodes as close together as possible.
- In rare instances, cardiac monitoring may be required in pacemaker-dependent patients with a unipolar pacemaker.

Hyperbaric Therapy

Hyperbaric treatments are used for treatment of carbon monoxide poisoning, bacterial infections, and burns. They typically utilize the physiological effects of 100% oxygen at a pressure of 2–3 atmospheric pressure absolute (ATA). The high static pressure generated during hyperbaric therapy can potentially cause mechanical deformation of the pacemaker "can" and damage the internal circuits. However, one study of four pacemaker models tested for up to 4 h at a pressure equivalent to 165 ft. of seawater or 5 ATA reported no adverse effects (73). Testing of pacemaker rate response function showed diminished rate responsive pacing at pressures in excess of approximately 45 psi (3 ATA), which caused the devices to pace at the programmed lower rate. The loss of rate responsive pacing was temporary, with return of expected function at lesser pressures. At pressures approaching 5 ATA deformation of the titanium can began to occur; however, the pacemakers continued to perform within specification (73).

Other Medical Sources of EMI

A number of isolated cases of pacemaker interaction with a variety of medical sources have been described. Certain cardiac monitoring systems used for recording continuous electrocardiograms in hospitalized patients can cause inappropriate rate changes in patients with rate-adaptive pacing systems that use a minute ventilation sensor (74,75). For example, electrical signals generated by the monitoring system (Hewlett Packard, Palo Alto, CA) used by the pacemaker for "loose-lead" detection and respiratory monitoring can be inappropriately defined as increased respiratory effort, leading to increased pacing rates (75). In one report, EMI from the hospital paging system occurred during pacemaker telemetry and led to inaccurate battery voltage, current, and impedance measurements (76). The paging system used in that hospital employed a frequency of 36 kHz, which was similar to the frequencies used by some pacemaker programmers. The study authors recommended using hospital-paging systems with high carrier frequencies (in the mHz range) since the programmers used by most manufacturers utilize carrier frequencies that range from 32 to 175 kHz.

Electromagnetic energy generated from a variety of dental instruments, including ultrasound scalers and cleaners, and electrosurgical instruments can cause transient inhibition of pacemaker output (77).

Nonmedical Sources

Cellular Phones

The cellular telephone is one of the most pervasive technologies in the world to date; industry estimates suggest that currently over 500 million cellular phones are in use worldwide. Depending on the type of cellular telephone system and the country, power requirements for transmission and reception of phone calls range from 0.6 to 3 W. Signals are transmitted in two ways. In older analog systems, signals are emitted as waves of varying frequency; in newer digital systems signals are sent as a series of rapid on/off pulses. In the early 1990s several in vitro studies and small in vivo studies suggested the possibility of adverse interactions between cellular phones and pacemakers, particularly with the newer digital systems (78–86). These early studies found that cellular phones could cause inhibition of pacing output, asynchronous pacing, and triggering of ventricular stimulus outputs due to oversensing. Interaction between pacing systems and cellular phones is greatest when the antenna of the phone is located near the pulse generator header. The header provides the connection between the pacing leads and the circuitry and battery located within the pacemaker can. In the header, the electrical connection between the leads and circuitry is maintained by a ceramic feedthrough (a wire surrounded by glass or sapphire). The intense radiofrequency fields near the base of the cell phone antenna can generate spurious voltages in the feedthrough wires that can lead to interference in the pacemaker circuitry. Interference occurs almost exclusively when the phone is in the calling or receiving mode. In addition to proximity and orientation of the cellular phone and method of signal transmission, lead configuration (unipolar versus bipolar) and filtering methods used by the pacing system can also affect the occurrence of cellular phone–pacemaker interactions (78–83). In the present generation of pacemakers, manufacturers have employed specialized capacitive filters on the feedthrough wires that are designed to minimize the high-frequency signals generated during transmission and reception of cellular phone calls before they are carried on to the sensing circuitry.

The effects of five cellular phones (1 analog and 4 digital) on a wide range of pacing systems have been evaluated by a large multicenter clinical study (79). In 980 patients, more than 5,000 specific tests for cell phone–pacemaker interaction were performed. The incidence of all types of interference was 20%. Ventricular "tracking" of signals sensed on the atrial channel (overall incidence 14%), noise reversion or asynchronous pacing (overall incidence 7%), and inhibition of ventricular output (overall incidence 6%) were the most commonly observed types of interference. The incidence of "definitely clinically significant" interference (presence of symptoms, ventricular asystole for more than 3 s) was 1.7%. Interference was more common in dual-chamber systems (25%) than in single-chamber systems (7%), and in digital telephones (24%) compared to analog telephones (3%). The incidence of interference in this multicenter study was similar in unipolar and bipolar pacing systems. Interference was most commonly observed when the phone was placed directly over the implanted device. No clinically significant interference was observed when the phone was used in normal fashion. One experimental study found no interactions between pacemakers and cell phones using a Bluetooth protocol.

Cell phones can potentially cause interference in patients with ICDs (84,85). In in vitro studies, inhibition of pacing and inappropriate high-voltage discharge can be observed if the cellular phone is in proximity (<16 cm) to the ICD (84–86). Although limited in vitro data suggest that cellular phone interactions with ICDs are uncommon, we consider it prudent to use the cell phone more than 6 in. (15 cm) from the ICD implant site, contralateral to a pectoral ICD implant.

Recommendations

- Advise use of an analog-type cellular phone system, particularly in patients who are pacemaker dependent.
- Do not carry the cell phone in a breast or shirt pocket on the ipsilateral side of the body as the implanted pacemaker.
- Use the ear opposite the implanted pacemaker when making or receiving calls, maintaining a minimum separation of 6 cm between the hand-held cellular phone's antenna and the pacemaker or ICD implant site.

Antitheft Devices

Recently there has been publicity surrounding the possible interaction between pacemakers and antitheft devices (87,88). National news organizations as well as local newspapers have run lead stories on this new "health issue" for pacemaker patients citing potential interactions between pacemakers and electronic article surveillance (EAS) devices (89). More than 400,000 EAS devices are in use worldwide, as this technology has become a universal tool to combat the increasing frequency and cost of theft. Technology employed in EAS devices involves the production of varying levels of radiant energy between transmitter and receiver pedestals (the "gates" at store entrances). The emitted field is designed to interact with a "tag" in an unpurchased item, such that the tag emits a signal of its own that is detected by the EAS receiver. A "tag deactivator" is placed near the cashier so that a properly purchased item will not trigger the alarm as it passes through the gate. In the United States there are three common methods used by EAS systems to interact with the tagged article: magnetic audiofrequency systems that use extremely low frequency (ELF) signals (200–500 Hz), acoustomagnetic systems that use low frequency signals (60 kHz), and swept radiofrequency systems (2–9 mHz). In one study in which 50 patients with pacemakers were exposed to all three types of EAS systems, no pacemaker–EAS interactions were observed for swept radiofrequency systems, two interactions were observed with ELF systems, and 48 interactions were observed with acoustomagnetic systems (90). The predominant pacemaker interactions with EAS fields were reversion to asynchronous pacing (noise reversion mode), and rapid triggered ventricular pacing owing to tracking of high-frequency EMI signals sensed in the atrial channel. The only potential clinically relevant adverse interaction was ventricular oversensing with inhibition of output (91). All of the interference was transient, with normal pacemaker function returning once the patient was removed from the EAS field. The same study evaluated the effects of EAS systems in 25 patients with ICDs and found no ICD–EAS interactions with any type of EAS technology (90). There has been a case report of a patient with an ICD who received multiple shocks during prolonged standing within 1 ft. of an EAS device (92).

The paucity of published reports suggests that the overall incidence of clinically meaningful device-EAS interactions is low given the large number of patients with pacing systems and ICDs and the virtual universal presence of EAS gates. Although physicians should advise their patients with pacing systems or ICDs to walk normally through EAS systems and not linger near an EAS "gate," they should also emphasize the very low probability of a significant adverse interaction.

Another type of security device are metal detectors used in airport terminals, courthouses, and other public sites. These detectors, in compliance with the National Institute of Law Enforcement and Criminal Justice standards for weapons detection, generate relatively small amplitude magnetic fields, which are unlikely to affect implanted pacing systems. Independent testing performed on 103 pacemakers from various manufacturers showed no inhibition of pacemaker output, inappropriate pacing, or reprogramming in any of the units tested (93). A more recent study of 348 patients (200 pacemaker and 148 ICD patients) found no EMI due to airport medical detectors (94). Passing a hand-held detector wand over the pacemaker can result in transient ventricular oversensing and short pauses in paced rhythm. More frequent movement of the wand over the pacemaker can potentially cause increased interference; a spurious ICD shock due to use of a handheld metal detector has been reported (93). A pacemaker patient walking through an archway metal detector can trigger its alarm because the pacemaker is a metallic object; therefore, a hand search of the patient may be required for security clearance. Patients should inform security personnel that they have an implanted pacemaker by presenting their pacemaker identification card.

Recommendations

- Instruct patients not to linger at store entrances with EAS devices.
- Notify security officials on the presence of an implanted cardiac device. In general it is safe for patients with cardiac devices to walk through airport security gates.

Arc Welding

Electrical arc welders are a frequent source of interference. The interference is caused by the electrical fields generated by the welding electrode and magnetic fields generated by the large current flowing through the welding electrode or cable. One recent study found no effects on bipolar pacemaker systems when patients used arc welders or if the patient was standing within 2–3 m of the equipment (95). The welding cables were not coiled, and the welding site and the power generator were kept away from the pacemakers. Larger arc welding equipment with currents exceeding 1,000 A did inhibit pacemakers during an in vitro test in which the pacemakers were placed within 1–2 m of the machines or the weld site.

In a small study that involved ten patients with ICDs from a single manufacturer and arc welders from six different manufacturers, no significant effects on ICD function were found (96). Although the magnetic field measured at the surface of the arc welder cable was 40 G, the magnetic field at 2 ft. from the cable was 1.2 G, which is less than the 10-G field required to activate the magnet response of the ICD. The investigators recommended that patients with

ICDs could perform arc welding if the sensitivity of the device is increased to 0.6 mV, the number of signals required to detect tachycardia is increased, and the precautions listed below are followed.

Recommendations

- Use acetylene welding if possible.
- Wear nonconductive (leather, fireproof cloth, or rubber) gloves to reduce the chance for inadvertent direct contact with electrical currents generated by the arc welder.
- Connect the "ground" clamp to the metal as close to the point of welding as possible to reduce the generated electromagnetic field.
- Keep the cables close together by twisting them around each other to reduce the effects of generated electromagnetic fields.
- Position the welding machine and excess cable more than 2 ft. away from the implanted pacemaker or ICD.
- Arrange work such that the cables extend away from the patient.
- Do not weld with rapidly repeated short bursts. Wait about 10 s between each weld. When having difficulty starting a weld, do not strike the rod in a rapidly repeated manner. Wait about 10 s between each strike.
- Advise the patient to stop operating the equipment if he feels light-headed, dizzy, or faint, lay the welding rod down, and move away from the welding machine.
- Do not work alone.

Miscellaneous EMI Sources

Normal operation of household appliances and electrical devices generally does not affect pacing system function. However, there have been numerous reports of sprurious shocks from ICDs due to improperly grounded appliances or current leak (97–111). One in vitro study found potential interactions between unipolar pacemakers and induction ovens when the devices were within 34 cm of the ovens (103). However, a study of 19 patients with ICDs found no oversensing with normal use of an induction oven (104). Since 1976, microwave ovens that have greater leakage protection have been manufactured; these ovens have better shielding and will not operate if the oven door is ajar. These changes have virtually eliminated the risk of pacemaker interactions, even when used at full power.

During daily life, transient reversion to magnet mode pacing has been estimated to occur at a rate of up to 11% per patient per year (106). All contemporary ICDs will suspend therapy while exposed to a magnetic field, and some ICDs can be programmed to permanently "turn off" with magnet application. There have been isolated case reports of accidental ICD deactivation from a variety of sources (106,107). More widespread use of powerful small magnets made from neodymium–iron–boron may increase the risk for inadvertent magnet exposure (108).

Radiofrequency energy with a range of 10–3,000 MHz is widely used for communications and radar equipment. The peak electric field strengths in public areas close to the transmitter source are less than 200 V/m, except for those of ham radios, which can be 325 V/m, and microwave radar, which is estimated to be as high as 1,400 V/m. Aircraft radio communication transmitters and radar have caused pacemaker output inhibition during in vitro testing, but such responses have not been observed in patients (97). One recent study found no interaction between cardiac devices and wireless local area networks (98).

Patients involved with automobile repair should not work on a car ignition while it is running. Transient inhibition or reversion to asynchronous pacing can occur if the patient comes in contact with current from the ignition caused by faulty insulation on the ignition wire. Moving away from the wire or having someone turn the engine off will immediately restore normal pacemaker function. Finally hybrid cars that use both electric and gasoline powered engines can potentially interact cardiac devices although there have been no published reports.

Tests at high-voltage substations in the vicinity of 110 and 400 kV/m power lines have been conducted in 12 different pacemakers (95). Several unipolar systems were shown to oversense the electromagnetic field signals at moderate (1.2–2.7 kV/m) and strong (7–8 kV/m) fields. Only one bipolar pacing system showed output inhibition in the strongest field and only when the pacemaker sensitivity was programmed to the most sensitive setting (0.5–1.0 mV).

Stun guns produce electrostatic voltage pulses up to 100 kV at 5–20 pulses/s (110). In one recent case report, EMI due to stun gun application led to inappropriate detection of ventricular fibrillation but therapy was not delivered because the energy delivery stopped before reconfirmation of the arrhythmia (111).

Testing of implanted pacing systems with electric blankets, razors, drills, and citizen band radios have been conducted. In these reports, older unipolar pacing systems could inhibit a single output pulse (13). A case series involving four patients of inappropriate ICD shocks due to slot machines has been reported (112). Recently, potential interaction between pacing systems and an Apple i-Pod has been reported (113).

The same guidelines and precautions that have been outlined for pacemaker patients and hyperbaric therapy apply to recreational diving. Testing of several rate-adaptive pacemakers to determine maximum safe depths for recreational scuba diving has shown that devices operate normally in up to 60 ft. of seawater, and the can begins to deform at pressures near 132 ft. of seawater (5 ATA) (113). Therefore, recreational scuba diving depths should not exceed 100 ft. (4 ATA). No loss or degradation of output operation was observed for any of the devices tested. However, rate-adaptive pacing response began to diminish at pressures in excess of 60 ft. of seawater (approximately 45 psi, 3 ATA), causing eventual pacing at the programmed lower rate. The loss of rate-adaptive pacing was temporary; normal pacing function returned as pressures were decreased to baseline.

We would like to acknowledge editing provided by Janet Hite for this chapter.

References

1. Barold SS, Falkoff MD, Ong LS, Heinle RA. Interference in cardiac pacemakers: Exogenous sources. In: El-Sherif N, Samest P, eds. *Cardiac pacing and electrophysiology*, 3rd ed. Philadelphia: WB Saunders, 1991:608–632.
2. Irnich W. Interference in pacemakers. *Pacing Clin Electrophysiol* 1984;7: 1021–1048.

3. Furman S, Parker B, Krauthammer J, Esher DJ. The influence of electromagnetic environment on the performance of artificial cardiac pacemakers. *Ann Thorac Surg* 1968;6:90.

4. Olson WH. The effects of external interference on implanted cardioverter defibrillators and pacemakers. In: Estes M III, Manolis AS, Wang PJ, eds. *Implantable cardioverter-defibrillators*. Boston: Marcel Dekker, 1994:139–152.

5. Toff WD, Edhag OK, Camm AJ. Cardiac pacing and aviation. *Eur Heart J* 1992;13(Suppl H):162–175.

6. Barold SS, Ong LS, Falkoff MD, Henle RA. Inhibition of bipolar demand pacemaker by diaphragmatic myopotentials. *Circulation* 1977;56:679–683.

7. Gialafus J, Maillis A, Kalogeropoulos C, Kalikazaros J, Basiakos L, Avqoustakis D. Inhibition of demand pacemakers by myopotentials. *Am Heart J* 1985;109:984.

8. Fetter J, Bobeldyk GL, Engman FJ. The clinical incidence and significance of myopotential sensing with unipolar pacemakers. *Pacing Clin Electrophysiol* 1984;7:871–881.

9. Exner DV, Rothschild JM, Heal S, Gillis AM. Unipolar sensing in contemporary pacemakers: using myopotenial testing to define optimal sensitivity settings. *J Interv Card Electrophysiol* 1998;2:33–40.

10. Sandler MJ, Kutalek SP. Inappropriate discharge by an implantable cardioverter defibrillator: recognition of myopotential sensing using telemetered intracardiac electrograms. *Pacing Clin Electophysiol* 1994;17:665–671.

11. Deshmukh P, Anderson K. Myopotential sensing by a dual chamber implantable cardioverter defibrillator: two case reports. *J Cardiovasc Electrophysiol* 1998;9:767–772.

12. Neuzner J, Dursch M, Sperzel J, Konig S, Pitschner HF. Myopotential sensing: cause of inappropriate arrhythmia detection and device discharges in implantable defibrillator therapy. *Pacing Clin Electrophysiol* 1997;20:Pt II:1225A.

13. Kusumoto FM, Goldschlager N. Unusual complications of cardiac pacing. In: Barold SS, Mugica J, eds. *Recent advances in cardiac pacing: Goals for the 21st century*, vol. 4. Armonk, NY: Futura Publishing, 1998:237–279.

14. Glikson M, Trusty JM, Grice SK, Hayes DL, Hammill SC, Stanton MS. A stepwise testing protocol for modern cardioverter defibrillator systems to prevent pacemaker-implantable cardioverter defibrillator interactions. *Am J Cardiol* 1999;83:360–366.

15. Cohen AI, Wish MF, Fletcher RD, Miller FC, McCormick D, Shuck J, Shapira N, Delnegro AA. The use and interaction of permanent pacemakers and the automatic implantable cardioverter-defibrillator. *Pacing Clin Electrophysiol* 1988;11:704–711.

16. Slepian M, Levine JH, Watkins L, Brinker J, Guarnieri T. Automatic implantable cardioverter defibrillator/pacemaker interaction: loss of pacemaker capture following ICD discharge. *Pacing Clin Electrophysiol* 1987;1;1194–1197.

17. Monahan K, Casavant D, Rasmussen C, Hallet N. Combined use of a true-bipolar sensing implantable cardioverter defibrillator in a patient having a prior implantable spinal cord stimulator for intractable pain. *Pacing Clin Electrophysiol* 1998;12:2669–2672.

18. Fiek M, Dowarth U, Durchlaub I, Janko S, VonBary C, Steinbeck G, Hoffman E. Application of radiofrequency energy in surgical and interventional procedures: are there interactions with ICDs? *Pacing Clin Electrophysiol* 2004;27:293–298.

19. El-Gamal HM, Dufresne RG, Saddler K. Electrosurgery, pacemakers and ICDs: a survey of precutions and complications experienced by cutaneous surgeons. *Dermatol Surg* 2001;27:385–390.

20. American Society of Anesthesiologists Task Force on Perioperative Management of Patients with Cardiac Rhythm Management Devices. *Anesthesiology* 2005;103:186–198.

21. Rastogi S, Goel S, Tempe D, Virmani S. Anaesthetic management of patients with cardiac pacemakers and defibrillators for noncardiac surgery. *Ann Card Anaesth* 2005;8:21–32.

22. Epstein MR, Mayer JE, Duncan BW. Use of an ultrasonic scalpel as an alternative to electrocautery in patients with pacemakers. *Ann Thorac Surg* 1998;65:1802–1804.

23. Das G, Eaton J. Pacemaker malfunction following transthoracic countershock. *Pacing Clin Electrophysiol* 1981;4:487–490.

24. Waller C, Callies F, Langenfeld H. Adverse effects of direct current cardioversion on cardiac pacemakers and electrodes. *Eurospace* 2004;165–168.

25. McPherson C, Manthous C. Permanent pacemakers and implantable defibrillators. *Am J Respiratory Crit Care Med.* 2004; 170:933–940.

26. Aylward P, Blood R, Tonkin A. Complications of defibrillation with permanent pacemaker in situ. *Pacing Clin Electrophysiol* 1979;2:462–464.

27. Furman S. External defibrillation and implanted cardiac pacemakers. *Pacing Clin Electrophysiol* 1981;4:485–486 (editorial).

28. Aylward P, Blood R, Tonkin A. Complications of defibrillation with permanent pacemaker in situ. *Pacing Clin Electrophysiol* 1979;2:462–464.

29. Levine PA, Barold SS, Fletcher RD, Talbot T. Adverse acute and chronic effects of electrical defibrillation and cardioversion on implanted unipolar cardiac pacing system. *J Am Coll Cardiol* 1983;1:1413–1422.

30. Altamura G, Bianconi L, Lo Bianco F, Toscaro S, Ammarati F, Pandozi C, Castro A, Cardinale M, Mennuni M, Santini M. Transthoracic DC shock may represent a serious hazard in pacemaker dependent patients. *Pacing Clin Electrophysiol* 1995;18:194–198.

31. Gould L, Patel S, Gomes GI, Chokshi AB. Pacemaker failure following external defibrillation. *Pacing Clin Electrophysiol* 1981;4:575–577.

32. Tobisch RJ, Irnich W. Electromagnetic compatibility of pacemakers and magnetic resonance imaging. In: Aubert AD, Ector H, Stroobandt R, eds. EURO-PACE '93; 6th European Symposium on Cardiac Pacing. Ostend, Belgium, June 6–9, 1993. Bologna, Italy. *Monduzzi Eitore* 1993;215–218.

33. Nair P, Roguin A. Magnetic Resonance Imaging in patients with ICDs and pacemakers. *Indian Pacing Electrophysiol J* 2005;5(3):197–209.

34. Loewy J, Loewy A, Kendall E. Reconsideration of pacemakers and MR imaging. Radiographics 2004;24:1257–1268.

35. Nazarian S, Roguin A, Zviman MM, Lardo AC, Dickfeld TL, Calkins H, Weiss RG, Berger RD, Bluemke DA, Halperin HR. Clinical utility and safety of a protocol for noncardiac and cardiac magnetic resonance imaimg of patients with permanent pacemakers and implantable-cardioverter defibrillators at 1.5 Tesla. *Circulation* 2006;114:1277–1284.

36. Roguin A, Zviman M, Meininger GR, Rodrigues ER, Dickfeld TM, Bluemke DA, Lardo A, Berger RD, Calkins H, Halperin HR. Modern pacemaker and implantable cardioverter defibrillator systems can be magnetic resonance imaging safe. Arrhythmia/electrophysiology. *Circulation* 2004;110:475–482.

37. Sommer T, M.D., Vahlhaus C, Lin H, Skowasch D, Naehle CP, Yang A, Schild H, Zeijlemaker V, Strach K, Hackenbroch M, Schmeidel A, Mayer C. Strategy for safe performance of extrathoracic magnetic resonance imaging at 1.5 Tesla in the presence of cardiac pacemakers in non-pacemaker-dependent patients. *Circulation* 2006;114:1285–1292.

38. Faris OP, Shein MJ. Government viewpoint; U.S. Food and Drug Administration; pacemakers, ICD's, and MRI. *Pacing Clin Electrophysiol* 2005;28:268–269.

39. Fiek M, Remp T, Reithmann C, Steinbeck G. Complete loss of ICD programmability after magnetic resonance imaging. *Pacing Clin Electrophysiol* 2004;27:1002–1004.

40. Holmes DR Jr, Hayes DL, Gray JE, Merideth J. The effects of magnetic resonance imaging on implantable pulse generators. *Pacing Clin Electrophysiol* 1986;9:360–370.

41. Hayes DL, Holmes DR Jr, Gray JE. Effect of 1,5 Tesla nuclear magnetic resonance imaging scanner on implanted permanent pacemakers. *J Am Coll Cardiol* 1987;10:782–786.

42. Lauck G, von Smekal A, Wolke S, Seelos KC, Jung W, Manz M, Luderritz B. Effects of nuclear magnetic resonance imaging on cardiac pacemakers. *Pacing Clin Electrophysiol* 1995;18:1549–1555.

43. Iberer F, Justich E, Tscheliessnigg KH, Wasler A. Nuclear magnetic resonance imaging in pacemaker patients. In: Atlee JL, Gombots H, Tscheliessnigg KH, eds. *Perioperative management of pacemaker patients*. New York: Springer-Verlag, 1992:86–90.

44. Achenbach S, Moshage W, Diem B, Bieberle T, Schibqilla V, Bachmann K. Effects of magnetic resonance imaging on cardiac pacemakers and electrodes. *Am Heart J* 1997;134:467–473.

45. Shellock FG, O'Neil M, Ivans V, Kelly D, O'Connor M, Toay L, Crues JV. Cardiac pacemakers and implantable cardioverter defibrillators are unaffected by operation of an extremity MR imaging system. *Am J Roentgenol* 1999;172:165–170.

46. Irnich W, Irnich B, Bartsch C, Stertmann WA, Gufler H, Weiler G. Do we need pacemakers resistant to magnetic resonance imaging? *Europace* 2005;7:353–365.

47. Drach GW, Weber C, Donovan JM. Treatment of pacemaker patients with extracorporeal shock wave lithotripsy: experience from 2 continents. *J Urol* 1990;143:895–896.

48. Jocham D, Brandl H, Chaussy C, Schmiedt E. Treatment of nephrolithiasis with ESWL. In: Gravenstein JS, Peter K, eds. *Extracorporeal Shock Wave Lithotripsy for renal stone disease: Technical and clinical aspects*. Boston: Butterworth, 1986:35–60.

49. Carlson CA, Gravenstein JS, Gravenstein N. Ventricular tachycardia during ESWL: etiology, treatment, and prevention. In: Gravenstein JS, Peter K, eds. *Extracorporeal Shock Wave Lithotripsy for renal stone disease: Technical and clinical aspects*. Boston: Butterworth, 1986:119–123.

50. Cooper D, Wilkoff B, Masterson M, Castle M, Belco K, Simmons T, Morant V, Streem S, Maloney J. Effects of extracorporeal shock wave lithotripsy on cardiac pacemakers and its safety in patients with implanted cardiac pacemakers. *Pacing Clin Electrophysiol* 1988;11:1607–1616.

51. Langberg J, Abber J, Thuroff JW, Griffin JC. The effects of extracorporeal shock wave lithotripsy on pacemaker function. *Pacing Clin Electrophysiol* 1987;10:1142–1146.

52. Chung MK, Streem SB, Ching E, Grooms M, Mowrey KA, Wilkoff B. Effects of extracorporeal shock wave lithotripsy on tiered therapy implantable cardioverter defibrillators. *Pacing Clin Electrophysiol* 1999;22:738–742.

53. Souliman SK, Christie J. Pacemaker failure induced by radiotherapy. *Pacing Clin Electrophysiol* 1994;17:270–273.

54. Rodriguez F, Filimonov A, Henning A, Coughlin C, Greenberg. Radiation-induced effects in multiprogrammable pacemakers and implantable defibrillators. *Pacing Clin Electrophysiol* 1991;14:2143–2153.

55. Raitt MH, Stelzer KJ, Laramore GE, Bardy GH, Dolack GL, Poole JE, Kudenchuk DJ. Runaway pacemaker during high-energy neutron radiation therapy. *Chest* 1994;106:955–957.

56. Lee RW, Huang SK, Mechling E, Bazqan I. Runaway atrioventricular sequential pacemaker after radiation therapy. *Am J Med* 1986;81:883–886.

57. Venselaar JLM, Van Kerkoerle HLMJ, Vet AJTM. Radiation damage to pacemakers from radiotherapy. *Pacing Clin Electrophysiol* 1987;10:538–542.
58. Venselaar JLM. The effects of ionizing radiation on eight cardiac pacemakers and the influence of electromagnetic interference from two linear accelerators. *Radiother Oncol* 1985;3:81.
59. Lewin AA, Serago CF, Schwade JG, Arbitol AA, Margolis SC. Radiation induced failures of complementary metal oxide semiconductor containing pacemakers: a potentially lethal complication. *Int J Radiat Oncol Biol Physiol* 1984;10:1967–1969.
60. Maxted KJ. The effects of therapeutic x-radiation on a sample of pacemaker generators. *Phys Med Biol* 1984;29:1143–1146.
61. Quertermous T, Megahy MS, Das Gupta DS, Griem ML. Pacemaker failure resulting from radiation damage. *Radiology* 1983;148:257–258.
62. Shehata WM, Daoud GL, Meyer RL. Radiotherapy for patients with cardiac pacemakers: possible risks. *Pacing Clin Electrophysiol* 1986;9:919.
63. Mellenberg DE Jr. A policy for radiotherapy in patients with implanted pacemakers. *Med Dosim* 1991;16:221–223.
64. Muller-Runkel R, Orswolini G, Kalokhe UP. Monitoring the radiation dose to a multiprogrammable pacemaker during radical radiation therapy: a case report. *Pacing Clin Electrophysiol* 1990;12:1466–1470.
65. Ngu SL, O'Meley P, Johnson N, Collins C. Pacemaker function during irradiation: *in vivo* and *in vitro* effect. *Australas Radiol* 1993;37:105–107.
66. Chin MC, Rosenqvist M, Lee MA, Griffin JC, Lanberg JJ. The effect of radiofrequency catheter ablation on permanent pacemakers: an experimental study. *Pacing Clin Electrophysiol* 1990;13:23–29.
67. Pfeiffer B, Tebbenjohanns J, Schumacher B, Jung W, Luderitz B. Pacemaker function during radiofrequency catheter ablation. *Pacing Clin Electrophysiol* 1995;18:1037–1044.
68. van Gelder BM, Bracke FA, el Gamal MIH. Upper rate pacing after radiofrequency catheter ablation in a minute ventilation rate adaptive DDD pacemaker. *Pacing Clin Electrophysiol* 1994;17:1437–1440.
69. Burke MC, Kopp DE, Alberts M, Patel A, Lin AC, Kall JG, Arrida M, Mazeika P, Wilber DJ. Effect of radiofrequency current on previously implanted pacemaker and defibrillator ventricular lead systems. *J Electrocardiol* 2001;34s:143–148.
70. Lakireddy D, Patel D, Ryschon K, Bhateja R, Bhakru M, Thal S, Chung M, Wilkoff B, Tchou P, Natale A, Verma A, Wazni O, Kilcaslan F, Kondur A, Prasad S, Cummings J, Belden W, Burkhardt D, Saliba W, Schweikert R, Bhargava M. Safety and efficacy of radiofrequency catheter ablation of atrial fibrillation in patients with pacemakers and implantable cardiac defibrillators. *Heart Rhythm* 2005;2:1309–1316.
71. Chen D, Philip M, Philip PA, Monga TN. Cardiac pacemaker inhibition by transcutaneous electrical nerve stimulation. *Arch Phys Med Rehabil* 1990;71:27–30.
72. Rasmussen MJ, Hayes DL, Vlietstra RE, Thorsteinsson G. Can transcutaneous electrical nerve stimulation be safely used in patients with permanent pacemakers? *Mayo Clin Proc* 1988;63:443.
73. Eichers P. Hyperbaric chamber and pressure vessel tests. *Medtronic Design Assurance Rep* 1992;PE92–292.
74. Duru F, Lauber P, Klaus G, Candinas R. Hospital pager systems may cause interference with pacemaker telemetry. *Pacing Clin Electrophysiol* 1998;21:2353–2359.
75. Lau W, Corcoran SJ, Mond HG. Pacemaker tachycardia in a minute ventilation rate-adaptive pacemaker induced by electrocardiographic monitoring. *Pacing Clin Electrophysiol* 2006; 29: 438–440.
76. Agarval A, Hewson J, Redding V. Ultrasound dental scalers and demand pacing. *Pacing Clin Electrophysiol* 1988;11(6):853.

77. Miller CS, Leonelli FM, Latham E. Selective interference with pacemaker activity by electrical dental devices. *Oral Surg Oral Med Oral Pathol* 1998;85:33–36.

78. Barbaro V, Bartolini P, Donato A, Militello C, Atamura G, Ammirati F, Santini M. Do European GSM mobile cellular phones pose a potential risk to pacemaker patients? *Pacing Clin Electrophysiol* 1995;18:1218–1224.

79. Hayes DL, Wang PJ, Reynolds DW, Estes M 3rd, Griffith JL, Stephens RA, Carlo GL, Finday GK, Johnson CM. Interference with cardiac pacemakers by cellular phones. *N Engl J Med* 1997;336:1473–1479.

80. Irich W, Batz L, Muller R, Tobisch R. Electromagnetic interferences of pacemaker by mobile phones. *Pacing Clin Electrophysiol* 1996;19:1431–1446.

81. Chen WH, Lau CP, Leung SK, Ho DS, Lee IS. Interference of cellular phones with implanted permanent pacemakers. *Clin Cardiol* 1996;19:881–886.

82. Altamura G, Toscano S, Gentilucci G, et al. *Eur Heart J* 1997;18:1632–1641.

83. Yousef J, Lars AN. Validation of a real-time wireless telemedicine system using a Bluetooth protocol and a mobile phone, for remote monitoring patient in clinical practice. *Eur J Med Res* 2005;10:254–262.

84. Bassen HI, Moore HJ, Ruggera PS. Cellular phone interference testing of implantable cardiac defibrillators in vitro. *Pacing Clin Electrophysiol* 1998;21:1709–1715.

85. Barbaro V, Bartolini P, Bellocci F, Caruso F, Donato A, Gabrielli D, Militello C, Montenaro AS, Zecchi P. Electromagnetic interference of digital and analog cellular telephones with implantable cardioverter defibrillators: *in vitro* and *in vivo* studies. *Pacing Clin Electrophysiol* 1999;22:626–634.

86. Trigano A, Blandeau O, Dale C, Wong MF, Wiary J. Reliability of electromagnetic filters of cardiac pacemakers tested by cellular phone ringing. *Heart Rhythm* 2005;2:837–841.

87. Dodinot B, Godenir JP, Costa AB. Electronic article surveillance: a possible danger for pacemaker patients. *Pacing Clin Electrophysiol* 1993;16:46–53.

88. Lucas E, Johnson D, McElroy BP. The effects of electronic article surveillance systems on permanent pacemakers: an *in vitro* study. *Pacing Clin Electrophysiol* 1994;17(Pt II):2021–2026.

89. Pacemaker patients in department stores: anti-theft security systems are dangerous. *Med Tribune* 1991;40:28–29.

90. McIvor ME, Reddinger J, Floden E, Sheppard RC. Study of Pacemaker and Implantable Cardioverter Defibrillator Triggering by Electronic Article Surveillance Devices (SPICED TEAS). *Pacing Clin Electrophysiol* 1998;21:1847–1861.

91. Harthorne JW. Theft deterrent systems: a threat for medical device recipients or an industry cat fight? *Pacing Clin Electrophysiol* 1998;21:1845 (editorial).

92. Santucci PA, Haw J, Trohman RG, Pinski SC. Interference with an implantable defibrillator by an electronic antitheft surveillance device. *N Engl J Med* 1998;339:1371–1374.

93. Cooperman Y, Zarafti D, Laniado S. The effect of metal detector gates on implanted permanent pacemakers. *Pacing Clin Electrophysiol* 1988;11:1386–1387.

94. Kolb C, Schmieder S, Lehmann G, Zrenner B, Karch MR, Plewan A, Schmitt C. Do airport metal detectors interfere with implantable pacemakers and cardiac defibrillators? *J Am Coll Cardiol* 2003;41:2054–2059.

95. Marco D, Eisinger G, Hayes DL. Testing work environments for electromagnetic interference. *Pacing Clin Electrophysiol* 1992;15:2016–2022.

96. Fetter JG, Benditt DG, Stanton MS. Electromagnetic interference from welding and motors on implantable cardioverter-defibrillators as tested in the electrically hostile work site. *J Am Coll Cardiol* 1996;28:423–427.

97. Toff WD, Edhag OK, Camm AJ. Cardiac pacing and aviation. *Eur Heart J* 1992;13(Suppl H):162–175.

98. Tri JL, Trusty JN, Hayes DL. Potential for personal digital assistant interference with implantable cardiac devices. *Mayo Clin Proc* 2004;79:1527–1530.

99. Chan NY, Ho LWL. Inappropriate implantable cardioverter-defibrillator shock due to external alternating current leak; Report of two cases. *Europace* 2005;7:193–196.

100. Al Khadra AS, Al Jutaily A, Al Shuhri S. Detection of refrigerator associated 60 Hz alternating current as ventricular fibrillation by an implantable defibrillator. *Europace* 2006;8:175–177.

101. Kolb C, Schmieder S, Schmitt C. Inappropriate shock delivery due to interference between a washing machine and an implantable cardioverter defibrillator. *J Interv Card Electrophysiol* 2002;7:255–256.

102. Vlay SC. Fish pond electromagnetic interference resulting in an inappropriate implantable cardioverter defibrillator shock. *Pacing Clin Electrophysiol* 2002;25:1532.

103. Hirose M, Hida M, Sato E, Kokubo K, Nie M, Kobayashi H. Electromagnetic interference of implantable unipolar cardiac pacemakers by an induction oven. *Pacing Clin Electrophysiol* 2005;28:540–548.

104. Binggelli C, Rickli H, Ammann P, Bingelli C, Brunkhorst C, Hufschmid V, Luechinger R, Duru F. Induction ovens and electromagnetic interference: What is the risk for patients with implantable cardioverter defibrillatos? *J Cardiovasc Electrophysiol* 2005;16:399–401.

105. Kolb C, Deisenhofer I, Weyerbrock S, Schmeider S, Plewan A, Zrenner B, Schmitt C. Incidence of antitachycardia therapy suspension due to magnet reversion in implantable cardioverter defibrillators. *Pacing Clin Electrophysiol* 2004;27:221–223.

106. Bonnet CA, Elson JJ, Fogoros RN. Accidental deactivation of the automatic implantable cardioverter defibrillator. *Am Heart J* 1990;120:696–697.

107. Ferrick KJ, Johnston D, Kim SG, Roth J, Brodman R, Zimmerman J, Fisher JD. Inadvertent AICD inactivation while playing bingo. *Am Heart J* 1991;121:206–207.

108. Wolber T, Ryf S, Binggeli C, Holzmeister J, Brunkhorst C, Luechinger R, Duru F. Potential interference of small neodymium magnets with cardiac pacemakers and implantable cardioverter-defibrillators. *Heart Rhythm* 2007;4:1–4.

109. Toivonen L, Valjus J, Hongisto M, Metso R. The influence of elevated 50 Hz electric and magnetic field on implanted cardiac pacemakers: the role of the lead configurations and programming of the sensitivity. *Pacing Clin Electrophysiol* 1991;14(12):2114–2122.

110. Roy OZ, Podgorshi AS. Tests on a shocking device: the stun gun. *Med Biol Eng Comput* 1989;27:445–448.

111. Haegeli LM, Sterns LD, Adam DC, Leather RA. Effect of a Taser shot to the chest of a patient with an implantable defibrillator. *Heart Rhythm* 2006;3:339–341.

112. Madrid A, Sanchez A, Bosch E, Fernandez E, Morro Serrano C. Dysfunction of implantable defibrillators caused by slot machines. *Pacing Clin Electrophysiol* 1997;20:212–214.

113. Patel MB, Thaker JP, Punnam S, Jongnarangsin K. Pacemaker interference with an i Pod. *Heart Rhythm* 2007;4:781–784.

114. Trignano A, Lafav V, Blandeau O, Levy S, Gardette B, Micoli C. Activity-based rate-adaptive pacemakers under hyperbaric conditions. *J Interven Card Electrophysiol* 2006;15:179–183.

Radiography of Implantable Arrhythmia Management Devices

David L. Hayes

Abbreviations

CRT, cardiac resynchronization therapy
ICD, implantable cardioverter-defibrillator
PA, posteroanterior

Introduction

Radiographic evaluation is often helpful after placement of pacemakers, implantable cardioverter-defibrillators (ICDs), and devices for cardiac resynchronization therapy (CRT). Important information may be missed if the chest radiograph is reviewed in a cursory fashion for adequacy of lead placement and for a pneumothorax following venous puncture for lead placement. Radiographic inspection of an implantable cardiac device system, whether pacemaker, ICD, or CRT device, should be performed in an organized manner (Table 18.1). Without an orderly approach, essential information may be overlooked. Posteroanterior (PA) and lateral chest radiographs from any patient with a permanent pacemaker or ICD should be obtained and reviewed by the implanting physician or follow-up team. Oblique views do not commonly provide a great deal of additional data for most pacemakers and ICDs but may be helpful for better assessment of left ventricular lead placement in some patients with CRT devices.

Although any order of evaluation can be used (i.e., the order presented in this chapter may be altered), every portion of the pacing or ICD system must be evaluated systematically. If, at the end of the evaluation, the clinical question being investigated remains unanswered, the chest radiograph should then be approached in a problem-focused fashion.

A few references exist that may serve as general sources of information on radiographic evaluation of an implanted device (1,2). The approach used and examples provided throughout the chapter are based largely on the experience of a single institution.

Table 18.1 Systematic approach to radiographic assessment of pacemakers and implantable cardioverter-defibrillators.

Systematic approach	Clinical considerations
Determine the pulse generator site.	Any suggestion that there has been a notable shift from intended position? For example, a displaced generator could be associated with lead dislodgment or twiddler syndrome.
Determine the pulse generator manufacturer, model, and polarity if possible.	Radiographic identifiers allow determination of the manufacturer, which is helpful if the patient comes without an identification card. The polarity of the pulse generator should be determined and compared with the polarity of the leads.
Inspect the connector block.	Is connector pin (or pins) completely through the connector block? A loose connection could explain intermittent or complete failure to output or intermittent failure to capture.
Consider the venous route used.	This is especially important if a pacemaker system revision is being considered. Can the same venous route be accessed, and how many leads are already placed in a single vein?
Determine the lead polarity.	Does the lead polarity match the pulse generator polarity, or has some type of adapter been used to allow the system hardware combination?
Determine the lead position.	Determine where the lead was positioned. Is the ventricular lead in the apex, outflow tract, septal position, or coronary sinus? Is the atrial lead in the atrial appendage, lateral wall, septal position, or coronary sinus?
Does the lead position appear radiographically acceptable?	Inadequate lead position may explain failure to capture or sense. Compare current and previous radiographs if possible. Is ventricular lead redundancy, or slack, adequate? Is atrial J adequate?
Inspect the entire length of the lead for lack of integrity, such as fracture, compression, or crimp.	Intermittent or complete failure to capture or sense or output could be secondary to lead conductor coil fracture or loss of insulation integrity. Attempt to follow each lead along its course, assessing the conductor coil. Also, inspect for any crimping of the lead as it passes under the clavicle.
Is any other chest radiographic abnormality potentially related?	For a recent implantation, be certain there is no pneumothorax or hemopneumothorax. For the patient with an implantable cardioverter-defibrillator who has a change in defibrillation thresholds, whether acute or chronic, remember that a pneumothorax can be responsible for alterations in thresholds.
If no abnormality is appreciated radiographically but there is a clinical abnormality, reassess the chest radiograph in a problem-oriented fashion.	For example, if the patient has intermittent failure to output, the differential diagnosis includes a problem with the connector pin, such as a loose set screw or fracture of the conductor coil. Go back once again and inspect these elements of the pacing system.

Normal Pacing System

The radiographic appearance of a normal implantable cardiac device should be understood before radiographic abnormalities can be appreciated. A radiographically normal pacing system is reviewed in its entirety for reference throughout this chapter. Almost all implantable cardiac device systems are interpretable radiographically if a systematic approach is followed carefully. Although the process described here is primarily for radiographic evaluation of a permanent pacing system, the same principles can be applied to radiographic evaluation of an ICD or CRT system.

Pulse Generator

Position

The site of the pulse generator is a good place to begin radiographic assessment. This starting point allows systematic attention to each component of the pacing or ICD system, moving from the most peripheral portion, the device, to the tip electrode or electrodes.

Normally, the pulse generator is located in the prepectoral position (Fig. 18.1). For most transvenous implantations, the pulse generator is visible on

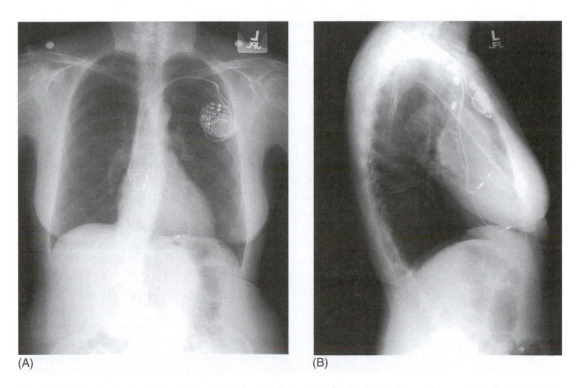

(A)   (B)

Fig. 18.1 Posteroanterior (*A*) and lateral (*B*) chest radiographs of a dual-chamber pacing system. The pulse generator is located in a left prepectoral position. The position of both atrial and ventricular leads is acceptable. The J on the atrial lead is adequate. The ventricular lead is not positioned in a true apical position but is well seated with adequate slack.

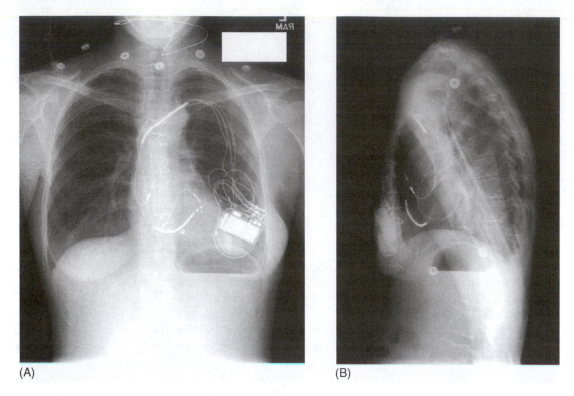

Fig. 18.2 Posteroanterior (*A*) and lateral (*B*) chest radiographs of a dual-chamber pacing system with the pulse generator located in a retromammary position.

the chest radiograph, usually high in the pectoral region, away from the axilla, well inferior to the clavicle, and relatively medial, either right or left. The appearance of a device in the subpectoral position may be similar to that of a device in the prepectoral position.

If the pulse generator is not in a pectoral position, the leads should be traced to the point of the pulse generator. For example, the pacemaker or ICD may be placed in the abdomen, and the path of the leads on the chest radiograph should make this location obvious.

Other uncommon pulse generator placements are retromammary and axillary positions. Retromammary placement has been advocated as a cosmetic approach to minimize chest deformity from the pacemaker (Fig. 18.2). However, with the increasingly smaller size of pulse generators, this location is rarely necessary. In addition, a retromammary implant may obscure breast tissue, making subsequent mammography suboptimal. Axillary positioning of the pulse generator is almost never done because of the potential discomfort from placement in this position.

Comparison of previous and current radiographs for pulse generator position is useful. The clinical concern when pulse generator migration occurs is that tension may be placed on the lead, causing possible dislodgment or fracture. Whether the patient is a "twiddler" cannot be determined from a radiograph. However, without notable migration of a device, a twisted appearance of the lead is usually attributed to twiddler syndrome (Fig. 18.3). Although a twisted

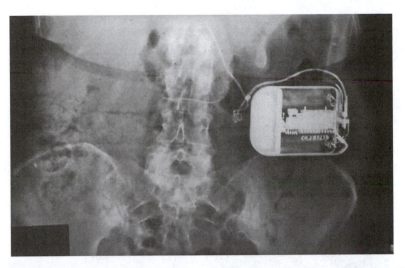

Fig. 18.3 Abdominal scout CT image in a patient with a malfunctioning implantable cardioverter-defibrillator. Inspection demonstrated a tight twisting of the lead, which resulted in device malfunction. The most likely diagnosis was twiddler syndrome. (From Hayes DL. Complications; and Lloyd MA, Hayes DL. Pacemaker and ICD radiography. In: Hayes DL, Lloyd MA, Friedman PA, editors. Cardiac pacing and defibrillation: a clinical approach. Armonk [NY]: Futura Publishing, 2000:453–84, 485–517. Used with permission of Mayo Foundation for Medical Education and Research.)

lead may occur because the patient has manipulated the pulse generator, more commonly the device has rotated repeatedly within the pocket, an outcome of a large pocket in a patient with relatively lax tissues.

Identification

All pulse generators can be identified radiographically to some degree. Historically, the position of the cell or battery and the position of the radiopaque circuit components were unique to each model. However, as the shape of pulse generators has become less distinctive, identification of the manufacturer from these characteristics alone is not usually possible. Most pacemakers have an identification code visible on radiographic views of the generator. Once the radiographic code and manufacturer have been identified, the company can be contacted via a toll-free telephone number and the company's technical service staff should be able to assist in pacemaker identification.

Figure 18.4 shows several different types of identification. A Guidant pulse generator is distinguished by the notation GDT 204, the actual model number of the generator. A St Jude Medical, Inc, pacemaker shows the company logo and the letters MM. A Medtronic pulse generator has the company logo and the letters PKM.

Polarity

The polarity of the device should be identified during examination of the pulse generator. This is important for complete pacing system identification and may also be important if lead compatibility is a question. It is possible to identify a unipolar, bifurcated bipolar, or in-line bipolar pulse generator. Because the

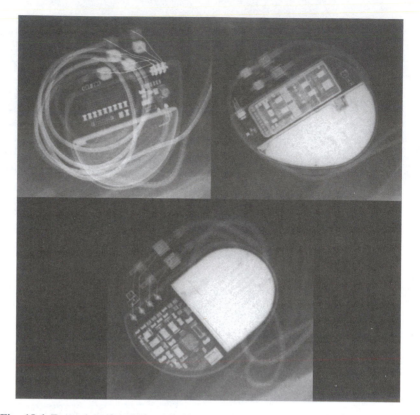

Fig. 18.4 Examples of radiographic identification of the pacemaker by radiographic codes embedded in the device.

polarity of the pacemaker may be programmable, identification of the device as bipolar does not necessarily mean that it is functioning in the bipolar configuration.

Figure 18.5 shows pulse generators with three different polarities. In *A*, a single connector pin identifies the device as unipolar. In *B*, the two connector pins indicate either a unipolar dual-chamber pacemaker or an older single-chamber pacemaker that accepts a bifurcated bipolar lead. (Although these leads are no longer implanted, some are still in service.) In *C*, two leads with two pins each represent a bipolar in-line lead and therefore a dual-chamber bipolar generator.

A connector block that appears to have two leads, but only one lead is seen to emerge from the pulse generator, indicates one of two situations. Older bifurcated bipolar leads, widely used before coaxial in-line leads were available, had separate pins for the positive and negative poles. Also, single-lead VDD systems, now rarely used, generally had a bifurcated connection of the lead with the ventricular pacing portion in the bottom port and the atrial pin in the upper port, which allowed sensing via atrialized floating electrodes. If three leads are present when the header is inspected, the device is most likely a CRT system.

At some point during inspection of the chest radiograph, lead polarity should also be determined. This could be done simultaneously with inspection

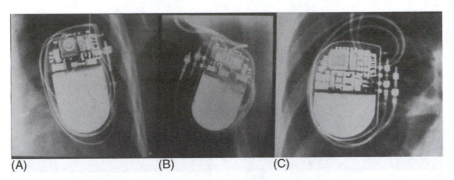

Fig. 18.5 Examples of three pulse generator polarity configurations, as described in the text. (From Hayes DL (1). Used with permission of Mayo Foundation for Medical Education and Research.)

of the pulse generator's polarity or later when lead integrity is inspected. It is important to remember that the cathode is always within the heart, and in the unipolar system, the anode is the metallic housing of the pulse generator; on the radiograph only the radiopafue electrode at the tip of the catheter is seen. In a bipolar system, both the radiographic electrode at the lead tip and a more proximal ring electrode can be seen. On occasion, a bipolar lead is converted to a unipolar configuration to accommodate a unipolar pulse generator or to take advantage of superior unipolar sensing or pacing. For this, an upsizing sleeve is placed over the positive terminal of the lead and insulates this terminal from the pacing system. This would not be detectable radiographically.

Connector Block

The purpose of inspecting the connector block is to determine that the connector and pin are firmly in contact. If the pin of the pacing lead is not firmly in the connector block, intermittent or permanent disruption of the circuit occurs. In Figure 18.6, the chest radiograph demonstrates a dual-chamber pacemaker with a lower pin that is only partially advanced. At presentation, the patient had intermittent failure to capture the ventricle and intermittent failure to deliver a ventricular pacing output.

Lead Placement

The first aspect of lead assessment is vascular access, that is, the venous route used. Identification of the venous route used is not critical, but there are two clinical reasons for attempting to identify the venous route. First, different stresses on the lead system exist at different venous sites. Second, if lead revision is planned, the options for new lead placement should be clear. Adjunctive dye studies may be helpful in determining vein patency or accessibility. Figure 18.7 demonstrates peripheral dye injection to determine the patency of the vein.

Radiographic differentiation of the venous route used for lead placement, e.g., axillary, subclavian, and cephalic veins, may be difficult if not impossible. With implantation of the lead in an axillary or cephalic vein, the approach

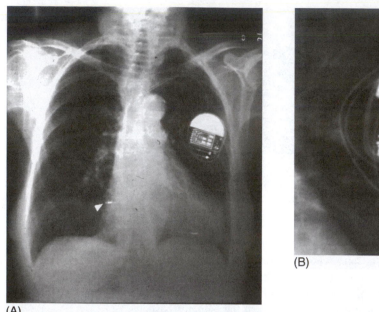

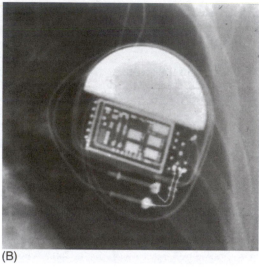

(B)

(A)

Fig. 18.6 Posteroanterior radiograph (*A*) and close-up view (*B*) from a patient with intermittent failure to pace. Comparison of the upper and lower pins reveals that the lower of the two unipolar leads is not completely advanced. This difference is more evident on the close-up view. By convention, the lower of the two leads in the connector block is the ventricular lead, so that this patient must have had intermittent or permanent ventricular failure to output. An unrelated observation (arrowhead on 6 *A*) is the shallow positioning of the atrial lead, i.e., the "J" is much wider than 90°. (From Hayes DL. Pacemaker radiography. In: Furman S, Hayes DL, Holmes DR Jr, editors. A practice of cardiac pacing, third edition. Mount Kisco [NY]: Futura Publishing, 1993:361–400. Used with permission of Mayo Foundation for Medical Education and Research.)

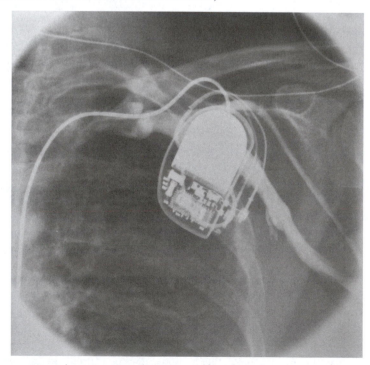

Fig. 18.7 Contrast material injection before a pacemaker system revision demonstrates that the contrast material essentially stops, indicating extensive, if not total, obstruction of the subclavian vein.

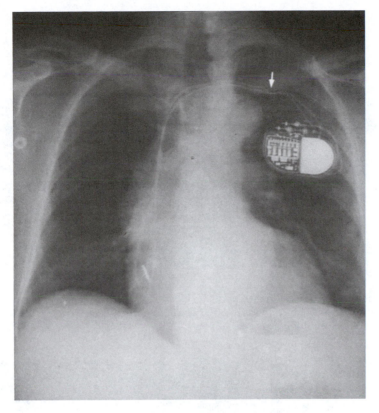

Fig. 18.8 Pacing lead entering via the subclavian vein. Note indentation (arrow) of the lead as it passes under the clavicle, signifiying compression of the lead.

is more lateral than if the subclavian vein is used. In Fig. 18.8, the lead is placed via the subclavian vein. This approach is more medial, and lead compression is seen where the lead passes under the clavicle.

Right Ventricular Lead

The right ventricular lead is most commonly positioned in the right ventricular apex. Radiographically, the end of the ventricular lead appears on the PA projection to be between the left border of the vertebral column and the cardiac apex. The position of the heart, whether vertical or relatively more horizontal, largely determines the position of the lead in relation to the cardiac apex, and this characteristic varies among patients. The lateral view is necessary to differentiate an apical position, in which the lead tip is anterior and caudally directed, from a coronary sinus position, in which the lead is directed posteriorly in the right ventricle or is on the posterior surface of the heart. When the lead is placed in a right ventricular apical position, the ventricular lead should have a gentle curve along the lateral wall of the right atrium and cross the tricuspid valve to the ventricular apex (Figs. 18.1 and 18.9).

Other right ventricular positions may be used. In the radiograph shown in Fig. 18.10, the lead is positioned in the right ventricular outflow tract. Previous inferior right ventricular myocardial infarction in this patient resulted in high

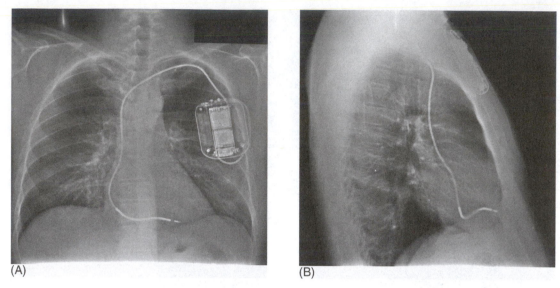

Fig. 18.9 Posteroanterior (*A*) and lateral (*B*) chest radiographs of an older implantable cardioverter-defibrillator (ICD) system. The ICD is connected to a single-coil ventricular lead. Single-coil leads are now used less commonly for initial implants, but a number are still in use.

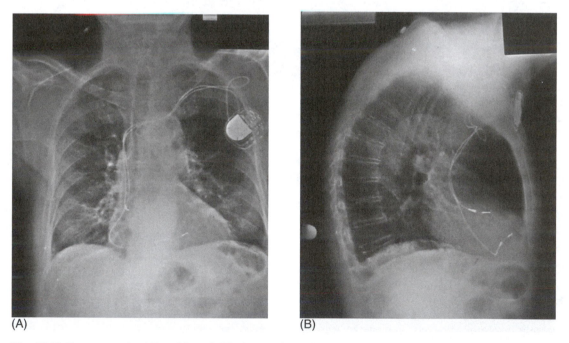

Fig. 18.10 Posteroanterior (*A*) and lateral (*B*) chest radiographs in a patient with the ventricular lead positioned in the right ventricular outflow tract. The lateral view is necessary for absolute determination of the position of this lead.

pacing thresholds when the lead was positioned in the right ventricular apex. The PA projection suggests coronary sinus positioning, but in the lateral radiograph, anterior positioning of the ventricular lead excludes coronary sinus positioning.

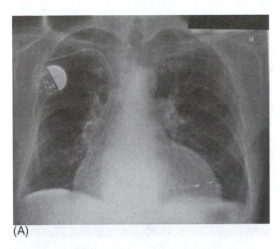
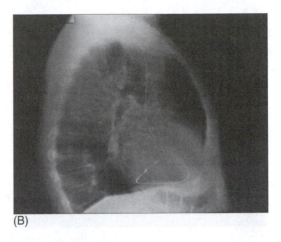

(A)   (B)

Fig. 18.11 Posteroanterior (*A*) and lateral (*B*) chest radiographs demonstrating a ventricular lead that courses posteriorly in the coronary sinus and into a cardiac vein, probably a tributary of the posterior cardiac vein. This determination cannot be made from the posteroanterior view only.

In the radiograph shown in Fig. 18.11, ventricular lead placement could be compatible with apical lead placement. However, the lateral view shows a nonapical position, and the lead is in fact positioned in a tributary of the posterior cardiac vein.

Undesirable positions for the ventricular lead are in the left ventricular cavity, that is, through perforation of the ventricular septum, the lead having inadvertently crossed a patent foramen ovale, atrial septal defect, or ventricular septal defect during transvenous placement, and in the pericardial space as a result of perforation (Fig. 18.12). A lead could be inadvertently placed in the left side of the heart by a direct puncture of the arterial system (Fig. 18.13). If a lead has been placed inadvertently in the left atrium or left ventricle and this positioning is recognized shortly after placement, the lead should be withdrawn and repositioned in the right side of the heart.

Atrial Lead

The atrial lead is most commonly positioned in the right atrial appendage (other atrial positions are considered later in this chapter). Regardless of whether a preformed J or a straight lead is implanted in the atrium, if implantation is in the right atrial appendage, the J portion of the lead is slightly medial on the PA projection and anterior on the lateral projection. Optimally, the limits of the J should be no more than approximately 80° apart.

The atrial lead may be positioned anywhere in the atrium where thresholds are adequate and the lead is stable. Conventionally, the atrial appendage is the most common site (Fig. 18.1), but other atrial positions may be used (Fig. 18.14). Interest in the potential superiority of placing the lead in a septal position is increasing (Fig. 18.15).

For both atrial and ventricular leads, it is important that the lead not be too shallow. For ventricular leads, this means that slack left in the lead is inadequate, and a shallow atrial lead implies that the angle of the J is much greater than 90°. In Fig. 18.16, placement of both leads is too shallow. The atrial lead

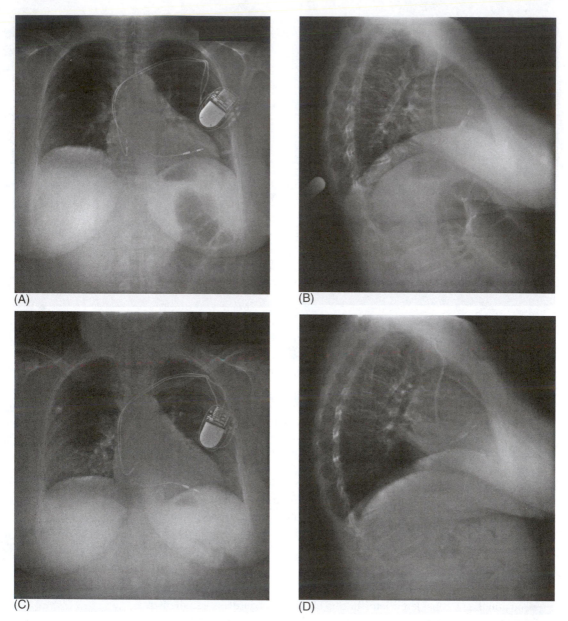

Fig. 18.12 Unusual course of the ventricular lead. In posteroanterior (*A*) and lateral (*B*) chest radiographs obtained the day after pacemaker implantation, the lead has a "high take-off," as it begins to cross to the left from the atrial position. This lead had been passed across an unknown patent foramen ovale and positioned in the left ventricle. Posteroanterior (*C*) and lateral (*D*) chest radiographs obtained the day after the lead had been withdrawn and repositioned in the right ventricular apex. (*A*, *C*, From Hayes DL. Complications; and Lloyd MA, Hayes DL. Pacemaker and ICD radiography. In: Hayes DL, Lloyd MA, Friedman PA, editors. Cardiac pacing and defibrillation: a clinical approach. Armonk [NY]: Futura Publishing, 2000:453–84, 485–517. Used with permission of Mayo Foundation for Medical Education and Research.)

is most likely in the right atrial appendage. The atrial lead is not optimally positioned and is best appreciated on the lateral view. The angle of the J is much wider than 90°. The ventricular lead is also much too shallow, and this can be appreciated in both views.

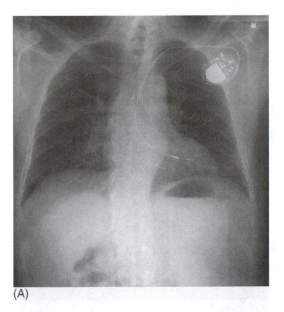

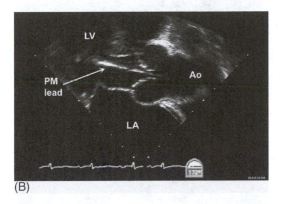

Fig. 18.13 Posteroanterior chest radiograph (*A*) demonstrating a ventricular lead that courses over the spine, is relatively straight, and is positioned in an unusually high position when viewed on the posteroanterior film. On a still frame from the two-dimensional echocardiogram (*B*), the lead is seen crossing the aortic valve and residing in the left ventricle. The lead had been placed inadvertently via the subclavian artery.

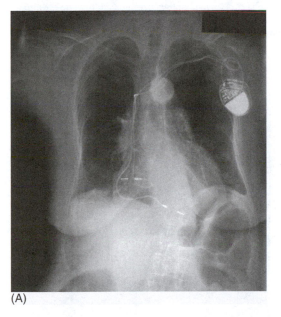

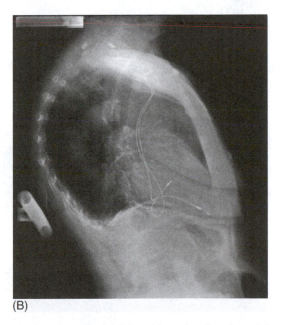

Fig. 18.14 Posteroanterior (*A*) and lateral (*B*) chest radiographs demonstrate an atrial position other than the atrial appendage. The lead is positioned laterally. Also noted on the lateral view is a loop in the ventricular lead.

Coronary Sinus Lead

Coronary sinus lead placement was used many years ago but lost favor because of the high rate of lead dislodgment. However, with the advent of CRT, placing a permanent lead in the coronary venous system has become

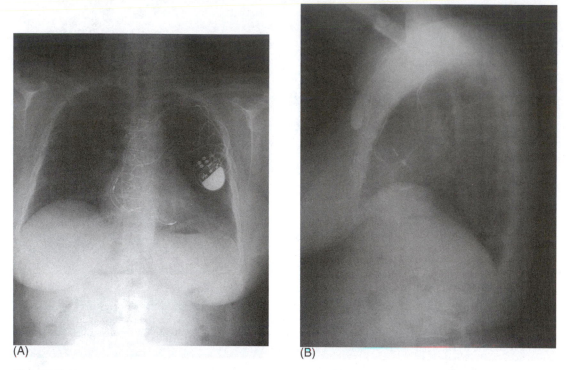

(A)   (B)

Fig. 18.15 Posteroanterior (*A*) and lateral (*B*) chest radiographs of a dual-chamber pacing system. The atrial lead is positioned in a septal position (arrow). This patient had extremely long intra-atrial conduction times, and septal placement was the only way to maintain effective atrioventricular synchrony.

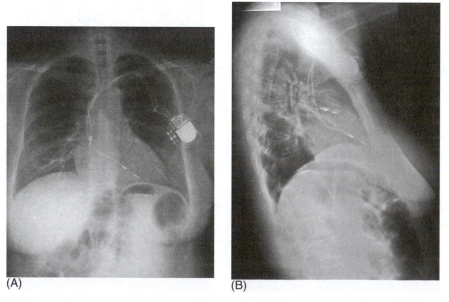

(A)   (B)

Fig. 18.16 Posteroanterior (*A*) and lateral (*B*) chest radiographs of a dual-chamber pacing system. Both the atrial and the ventricular leads have inadequate redundancy, which may result in poor pacing thresholds or lead dislodgment.

commonplace. Atrial pacing can also be achieved via the coronary venous system, but this is not commonly done.

The ventricle or atrium can be paced, depending on where in the coronary sinus the lead is positioned. Figures 18.17–18.19 demonstrate coronary sinus lead placement in the lateral coronary, anterior interventricular, and middle cardiac veins.

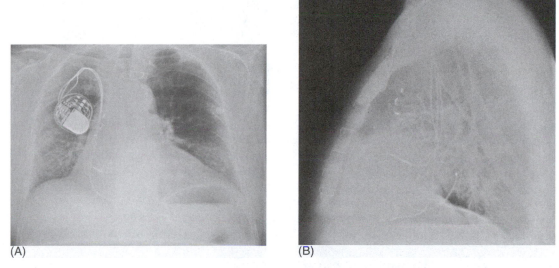

(A)   (B)

Fig. 18.17 Posteroanterior (A) and lateral (B) chest radiographs from a patient with right atrial, right ventricular, and coronary sinus leads. The coronary sinus lead is positioned in the lateral cardiac vein.

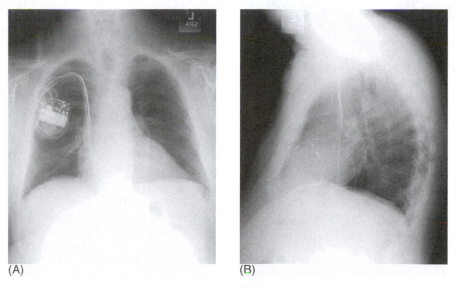

(A)   (B)

Fig. 18.18 Posteroanterior (A) and lateral (B) chest radiographs from a patient with right atrial, right ventricular, and coronary sinus leads. The coronary sinus lead is positioned in the anterior interventricular cardiac vein.

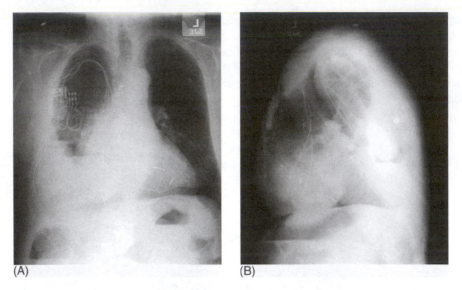

Fig. 18.19 Posteroanterior (*A*) and lateral (*B*) chest radiographs from a patient with right atrial, right ventricular, and coronary sinus leads. The coronary sinus lead is positioned in the middle cardiac vein.

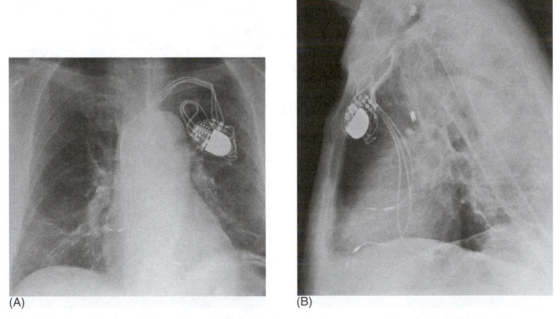

Fig. 18.20 Posteroanterior (*A*) and lateral (*B*) chest radiographs in a patient with a dual-site atrial pacing system for the prevention of paroxysmal atrial fibrillation. Leads are positioned in the right atrium, coronary sinus, and right ventricular apex.

Figure 18.20 depicts dual-site atrial pacing used to decrease paroxysmal atrial fibrillation. In this example, one lead is positioned in the right ventricular apex, another in the right atrial appendage, and a third in the posterior portion of the right atrium near the coronary sinus ostium.

Anatomic Variations

Anatomic variations can alter the placement of the pacing system and therefore the radiographic appearance. It is not possible to discuss all potential anatomic variations. However, one anatomic variation does merit discussion – a persistent left superior vena cava. A permanent pacing system can be implanted via a persistent left superior vena cava (Fig.18.21). (If this anatomic variation is noted before pacemaker implantation, it is easier to implant the system via the right side if the patient has a normal right superior vena cava.) If pacing leads are implanted through a persistent left superior vena cava, the lead in the PA projection descends within the left side of the cardiac shadow and enters the atrium and then the ventricle by communication of the left superior vena cava and the coronary sinus. On the lateral projection, the ventricular lead is seen on the posterior cardiac wall within the coronary sinus.

Lead Type

Although the specific type of transvenous lead often cannot be identified, it may be helpful to determine whether the lead is active or passive fixation. Specifically, this may be helpful when lead extraction is being contemplated and the lead model and manufacturer are unknown.

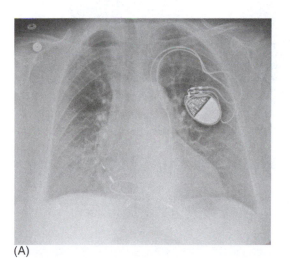
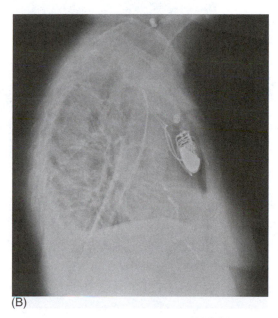

(A)   (B)

Fig. 18.21 Posteroanterior (*A*) and lateral (*B*) chest radiographs of a DDD pacing system in a patient with a persistent left superior vena cava. The atrial lead courses through the left superior vena cava and the coronary sinus and into the right atrium. The ventricular lead follows the same path but is then looped into the right ventricle. (From Hayes DL. Implantation techniques. In: Hayes DL, Lloyd MA, Friedman PA, editors. Cardiac pacing and defibrillation: a clinical approach. Armonk [NY]: Futura Publishing, 2000:159–200. Used with permission of Mayo Foundation for Medical Education and Research.)

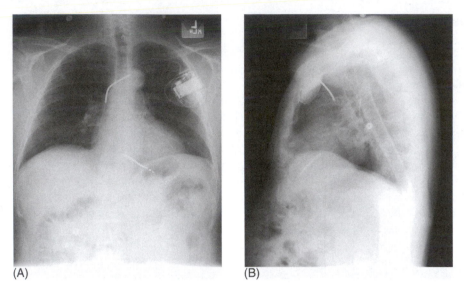

Fig. 18.22 Posteroanterior (*A*) and lateral (*B*) chest radiographs of an implantable cardioverter-defibrillator (ICD) system in the left prepectoral position. The ICD is connected to a dual-coil ventricular lead.

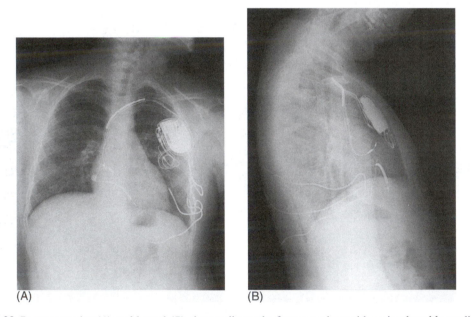

Fig. 18.23 Posteroanterior (*A*) and lateral (*B*) chest radiographs from a patient with an implantable cardioverter-defibrillator. Unacceptable defibrillation thresholds necessitated placement of a subcutaneous array.

When an ICD system is inspected radiographically, it is possible to determine whether the ICD lead has a single coil (Fig. 18.9) or a dual coil (Fig. 18.22) and whether any additional leads are associated with the ICD. Although additional leads are not commonly used, they may include a superior vena cava lead, subcutaneous array (Fig. 18.23), or subcutaneous patch.

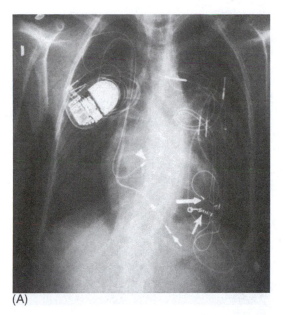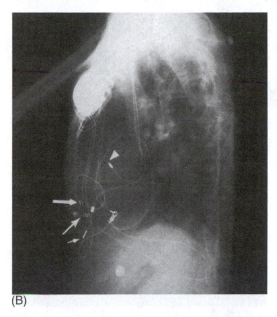

(A)   (B)

Fig. 18.24 Posteroanterior (A) and lateral (B) chest radiographs demonstrating several kinds of pacing leads, as described in the text. The arrowhead indicates active fixation of the atrial endocardial lead; large arrow, an abandoned stab-in epicardial lead; medium arrow, an abandoned screw-in epicardial lead; and small arrow, a passive fixation transvenous lead.

Numerous epicardial active fixation devices are available but are not commonly used. The radiograph in Fig. 18.24 shows four different types of leads in one patient: two epicardial leads and two endocardial leads. In this patient, previous epicardial pacing did not have long-term success. Two types of leads had been used, including a "stab-in" epicardial-myocardial lead and a screw-in epicardial-myocardial lead. A transvenous ventricular passive fixation lead and an active fixation atrial lead are also visible. Details of these leads are also seen on the lateral view.

At times, a combination of atrial endocardial and ventricular epicardial leads may be used because a prosthetic tricuspid valve prevents placing a transvenous ventricular lead (Fig. 18.25) or because, in certain congenital cardiac anomalies, transvenous access to a nonsystemic ventricle is not possible.

Lead Integrity

The entire length of the lead should be inspected for integrity. An insulation break usually cannot be identified radiographically, but occasionally, the radiograph suggests that the conductor coil is intact, yet it has the radiographic appearance of insulation disruption (Fig. 18.26). A lead fracture can sometimes be identified, depending on the location of the fracture. Any position that involves an acute angle of the lead or applies constant pressure or friction on the lead increases the chance of fracture or insulation failure at that point.

In Fig. 18.27, placement of the atrial lead is too shallow, and close observation reveals that the conductor coil of the atrial lead has separated. Atrial pacing was not possible, but surprisingly, atrial sensing remained intact, probably

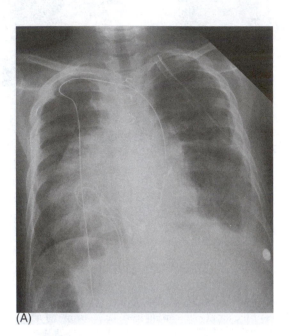
(A)

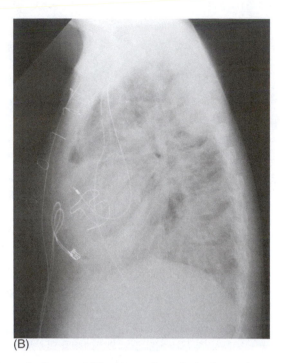
(B)

Fig. 18.25 Posteroanterior (*A*) and lateral (*B*) chest radiographs from a child with a univentricular heart after a septation procedure and implantation of a dual-chamber pacemaker. The ventricular lead has been placed in an epicardial position, and the atrial lead is transvenously positioned. (From Lloyd MA, Hayes DL. Pacemaker and ICD radiography. In: Hayes DL, Lloyd MA, Friedman PA, editors. Cardiac pacing and defibrillation: a clinical approach. Armonk [NY]: Futura Publishing, 2000:485–517. Used with permission of Mayo Foundation for Medical Education and Research.)

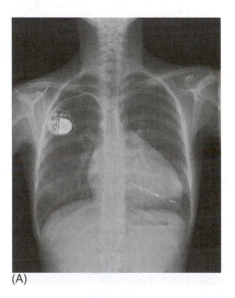
(A)

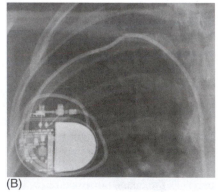
(B)

Fig. 18.26 Posteroanterior (*A*) chest radiograph and close-up (*B*) of a portion of the posteroanterior film demonstrating a disruption of the outer portion of the lead, presumably the insulation, with the appearance that the conductor coil is intact. In this patient, chronic pacing thresholds were considered acceptable and unchanged.

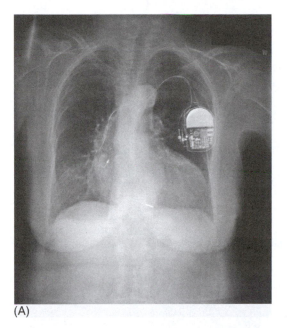
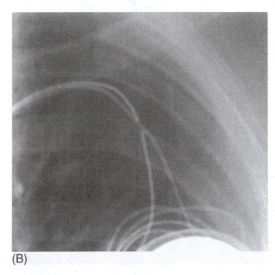

(A)   (B)

Fig. 18.27 Posteroanterior chest radiograph (*A*) and close-up view (*B*) in a patient with a dual-chamber pacemaker and separation of the atrial conductor coil.

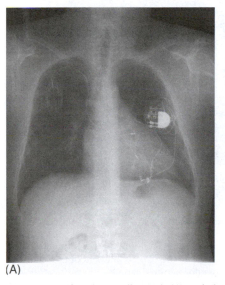
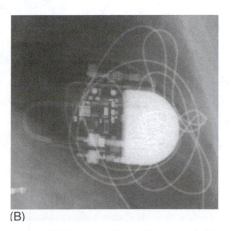

(A)   (B)

Fig. 18.28 Posteroanterior chest radiograph (*A*) and close-up view (*B*) from a patient with congenital heart disease and an abandoned dual-chamber endocardial pacing system. Two ventricular epicardial leads are connected with a Y connector to a single chamber ventricular pacemaker. On the close-up view (*B*) the arrow notes a defect in the lead adaptor just as it exits the connector block.

because a fluid column within the lead maintained some degree of conduction between the fractured ends of the conductor coil. Close inspection of the chest radiograph in Fig. 18.28 identifies a fracture of the lead adaptor. Complete separation of the conductor coil of the ventricular lead is noted in Fig. 18.29.

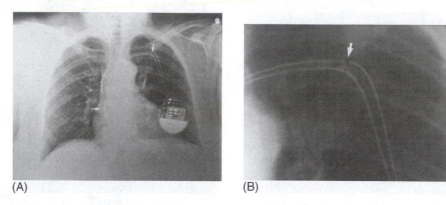

(A)   (B)

Fig. 18.29 Posteroanterior chest radiograph (*A*) demonstrating complete separation of the conductor coil of the ventricular lead as it passes below the clavicle (upper arrow). (Lower arrow, a suboptimally positioned atrial lead that is too shallow.) In the close-up view (*B*), the arrow again denotes the separation of the conductor coil.

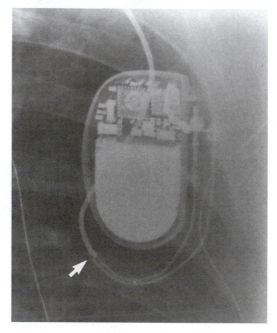

Fig. 18.30 Close-up from a posteroanterior radiograph of a bifurcated bipolar pacing lead. The appearance of a fracture where the two conductors of the lead come together is designated as a radiographic pseudofracture (arrow).

In older bifurcated bipolar leads, the intact lead gives the appearance of discontinuity at the point of bifurcation (Fig. 18.30). This radiographic finding is designated a pseudofracture. This is not a fracture but rather the normal radiographic appearance of this lead, which simply reflects the two conductors of a bipolar lead coming together. The term "pseudofracture" has also been applied inappropriately to a different circumstance: the indentations caused by ligatures compressing the insulating material of a lead (Fig. 18.31).

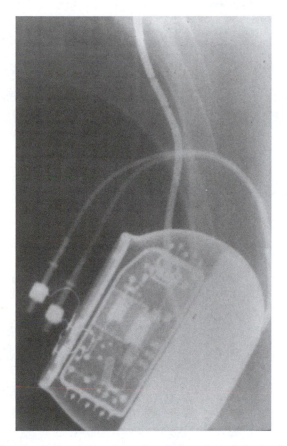

Fig. 18.31 Close-up radiographic view of an indentation of the insulation material caused by excessive tightening of the ligature around the sleeve. (From Hayes DL (1). Used with permission of Mayo Foundation for Medical Education and Research.)

Lead Dislodgment or Abnormality

Lead dislodgment is a common cause of failure to pace or to sense. Dislodgment may be obvious, that is, "macrodislodgment." Such dislodgment can be anywhere other than the original position of the lead, for example, the pulmonary artery, coronary sinus, ventricular cavity, or superior or inferior vena cava. Dislodgment may not be identifiable radiographically. This form has been labeled "microdislodgment," but without radiographic documentation, the diagnosis is one of exclusion. A macrodislodged atrial lead is shown in Fig. 18.32.

In Fig. 18.33, a chest radiograph of a system implanted several years earlier shows that the ventricular lead has a large loop. The patient's long-term thresholds were excellent, and no problems had been encountered. Even though positioning is suboptimal, no intervention is necessary if function is normal.

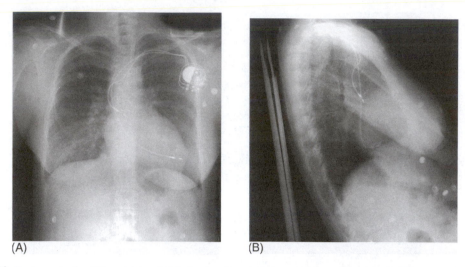

(A)   (B)

Fig. 18.32 Posteroanterior (*A*) and lateral (*B*) chest radiographs in a patient with gross dislodgment of the atrial lead. The ventricular lead position is also inadequate; i.e., too little slack has been left on the lead.

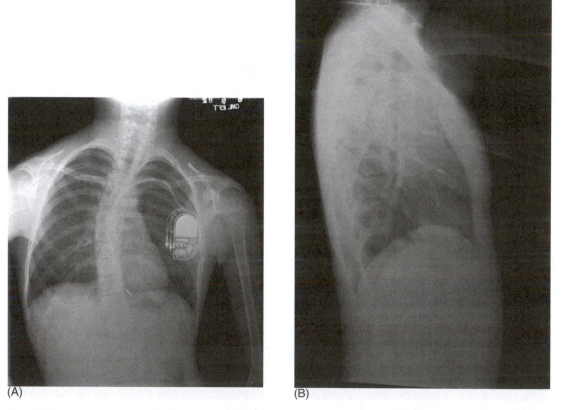

(A)   (B)

Fig. 18.33 Lateral chest radiograph in a patient with a large loop in the ventricular lead. If this appearance is noted early after implantation, repositioning should be considered. If it is found later and the lead is functioning normally, no action is necessary. (From Hayes DL (1). Used with permission of Mayo Foundation for Medical Education and Research.)

Multiple Leads

When multiple leads or, less commonly, multiple devices are visible on the chest radiograph, an attempt should be made to trace each lead from its origin in the pacemaker to its intracardiac or intravascular position. An abandoned lead should be traced on the radiograph to prove that it is freestanding and not connected to the pulse generator. With multiple leads, the radiographic appearance can become confusing, and individual leads can be difficult to trace.

Implantation Complications

Pneumothorax may occur as a complication of the subclavian puncture technique, and when this technique is used, the radiograph obtained after device placement should be inspected specifically for this complication (Fig. 18.34). A potentially more important complication is hemothorax, with or without an associated pneumothorax.

Hematoma may occur as a result of inadvertent arterial puncture and bleeding into the subcutaneous tissues. Rarely is this identifiable radiographically (Fig. 18.35).

In patients being upgraded from an existing pacemaker or ICD to a CRT system, venous access and venous narrowing may hamper placement of the additional coronary sinus lead. One potential complication with difficult passage of a lead is venous perforation. In Fig. 18.36, the sheath used for introduction of the coronary sinus lead has perforated the vein, and dye was injected to determine the sheath position. The dye is shown in the mediastinum. In this patient, the sheath was withdrawn and redirected into the lumen of the vein, and the patient remained hemodynamically stable.

During positioning of a coronary venous lead, the coronary venous system may be perforated or dissected. In the event of a dissection, a blush of dye is characteristic, and the blush may remain present for hours to days (Fig. 18.37).

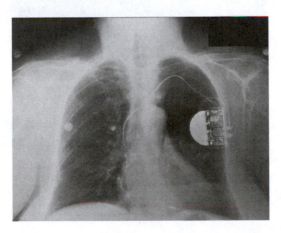

Fig. 18.34 Posteroanterior chest radiograph obtained immediately after pacemaker insertion shows a pneumothorax on the left as a complication of subclavian vein puncture. (From Hayes DL. Pacemaker complications. In: Furman S, Hayes DL, Holmes DR Jr, editors. A practice of cardiac pacing, third edition. Mount Kisco [NY]: Futura Publishing, 1993:537–69. Used with permission of Mayo Foundation for Medical Education and Research.)

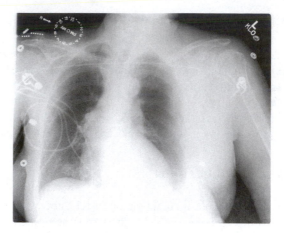

Fig. 18.35 Posteroanterior chest radiograph from an elderly patient on dipyridamole and aspirin at the time of attempted implant in the left prepectoral region. Attempted venous puncture was complicated by axillary artery puncture and bleeding. The procedure was abandoned, and a pacemaker was placed several days later via the left axillary vein. However, on this posteroanterior radiograph obtained after the left-sided implant attempt, a very large hematoma was indicated by the marked soft tissue expansion on the left thorax. In addition, an area of greater opacity in the left prepectoral region is consistent with hematoma formation in the pectoral muscle and prepectoral tissues.

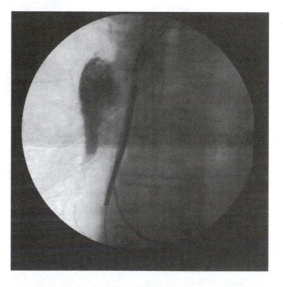

Fig. 18.36 Posteroanterior chest radiograph obtained after the prior device was upgraded to a cardiac resynchronization therapy defibrillator system. During the course of the upgrade, the central venous circulation was perforated, and when dye was injected to determine the position of the sheath, the contrast material was seen in the mediastinum.

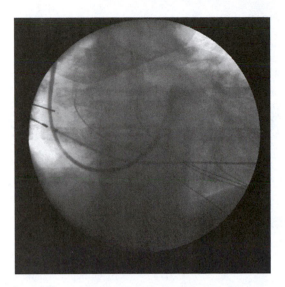

Fig. 18.37 Still-frame from a cineangiogram following coronary venous injection. A catheter is positioned in the coronary sinus. The faint "blush" that can be appreciated distal to the catheter tip represents a small amount of contrast material that has extravasated into the myocardial tissue.

Summary

Careful radiographic examination of a pacing or ICD system can yield a great deal of information and be critical in troubleshooting a clinical problem. A definite step-by-step approach to radiographic evaluation should be adopted to prevent overlooking information on the radiograph.

References

1. Hayes DL. Pacemaker radiography. In: Furman S, Hayes DL, Holmes DR Jr., editors. A practice of cardiac pacing, second edition. Mount Kisco (NY): Futura Publishing, 1989:323–68.
2. Condon B, Hadley D. Cardiac pacing systems and implantable cardiac defibrillators (ICDs): a radiological perspective of equipment, anatomy and complications. Clin Radiol 2004;59:1145.

19

Follow-up Management of the Paced Patient

Paul A. Levine and Dale M. Isaeff

Introduction

The recommendation and subsequent implantation of a pacemaker constitutes a therapeutic prescription with the same long-term responsibility for the periodic assessment of the continued appropriateness of that therapy as with the prescription of any pharmacologic agent. The multiplicity of programmable options available in the modern pacemaker allows the physician to titrate the dose of pacing in a manner similar to the periodic adjustment of the dose of a medication. A prime example is renal failure which commonly requires a decrease in the dose of some medications necessitated by a reduction in renal clearance, this same condition may require an increase in the programmed output of the pacemaker if the patient is prone to hyperkalemia because of associated rises in the capture threshold.

This chapter will review multiple aspects and techniques associated with the routine follow-up of the pacing system including biventricular systems.

The Pacing System

A common misconception by both patients and the medical community is that the periodic evaluations are solely for the purpose of evaluating the pacemaker. This has been promulgated, in part, by the Centers for Medicare and Medical Services (CMS) which has focused its recommended and thus reimbursable follow-up schedule on the need to detect signs of battery depletion in a timely manner warranting elective replacement of the pulse generator. If the primary goal was the treatment of the pacemaker or achieving the maximal longevity for the pacemaker, then the physician should program it to the lowest output possible or even to an "off" setting. In this manner, the pacemaker will last virtually forever. Unfortunately, this approach will not help the patient for whom the therapy was prescribed.

Physicians treat patients and for those individuals who have been implanted with a permanent pacemaker for a symptomatic bradycardia or pharmacologically refractory congestive heart failure with cardiac resynchronization therapy (CRT), it is necessary to periodically determine whether or not the present

Table 19.1 Components of the pacing system.

Patient
Pulse generator
Programmable settings of the pulse generator
Lead(s)

settings in the pacemaker continue to be both appropriate for the patient and provide the optimal level of support. The purpose of the follow-up evaluation is to evaluate the patient and the continued effectiveness of the present therapeutic regimen (1–3). At the time of this evaluation, all components of the pacing system need to be evaluated. This requires an assessment of the clinical status of the patient along with the mechanical integrity of the lead(s) which connect the pulse generator to the patient's heart in addition to the status of the battery. The pacing system is comprised of four components (Table 19.1). The periodic evaluations are intended to assess the performance of the pacing system and not just the pulse generator.

Follow-Up Objectives

There are multiple objectives associated with each follow-up evaluation. These may vary from one session to another and will determine the relative complexity of the particular session; whether ancillary testing such as an echo-Doppler evaluation or chest x-ray is indicated or if the sole test that is required is a simple ECG rhythm strip.

In the course of pacing therapy, long before these devices could have their various parameters noninvasively reset, a prime purpose for periodic patient evaluation was the identification of signs of battery depletion. This continues to be important but with devices expected to function properly for at least 5 years and, in many cases, closer to 10 years or longer, other goals have assumed a greater importance during the usual follow-up visit. Given the significant longevity associated with the modern pacemaker, the underlying indication for pacing therapy is likely to evolve during that period of time and in the presence of progression of concomitant disease processes may necessitate periodic changes in the pacing prescription. Thus a primary objective at each detailed follow-up evaluation is an assessment of the appropriateness of the present programmed parameters for the patient (Table 19.2). As a subset of this, capture and sensing thresholds should be assessed and appropriate safety margins established. This evaluation is facilitated by the extensive telemetry capabilities in the pacemakers including event markers, telemetered electrograms, and diagnostic event counters. The status of the patient's chronotropic status needs to be assessed and a determination made as to whether or not rate modulation is required. If rate modulation as well as any special algorithms had been enabled, it is appropriate to determine the degree to which these have been utilized since the last evaluation and on an overall basis, whether the pacemaker had been functioning in a manner thought to be appropriate based on the physician's knowledge about the clinical status of the patient. As part of this evaluation, one should also assess the degree of pacemaker dependency.

Table 19.2 Objectives of the follow-up evaluation.

Assessment of patient status

    Symptoms – palpitations, congestive heart failure, syncope, vital signs

    Examination of the pacemaker pocket site

    Edema of the arm, venous collaterals, cannon A waves, rales, varying S1

Status of intrinsic rhythm

    Pacemaker dependency

Appropriateness of the current pacemaker prescription

    Capture thresholds and safety margin

    Sensing thresholds and safety margin

    Rate modulation

    Special algorithms

    Battery status

Need for ancillary testing

    PA and lateral chest x-ray

    Echo-Doppler studies

    Invasive hemodynamic monitoring

    Ambulatory electrocardiographic monitoring

Integral to the above evaluation is an assessment of the mechanical integrity of the leads and the electrical integrity of the pulse generator including battery status. This evaluation need not be performed very frequently but when performed, it should be comprehensive. The results of these periodic detailed assessments will also provide a baseline for an evaluation should a pacing system problem be suspected (4). As such, meticulous documentation in the medical record including copies of the printouts documenting the capture and sensing thresholds as well as other evaluations is essential. As this may entail a significant volume of printouts, some practices have elected to maintain a separate device chart for these records. The programmed settings can often be downloaded to electronic medical records systems and in the future, this will also be possible with the electrograms and other pacing system diagnostics.

As the pacing system advances in age, it is appropriate to perform more frequent evaluations looking for signs of battery depletion as well as assessing lead integrity. In the office, this may be easily accomplished with interrogation of the pacemaker which will often report the battery status and an estimate of remaining longevity or a demand and magnet rhythm strip recorded during a transtelephonic evaluation.

For the detailed periodic pacing system evaluation, the results of the capture and sensing threshold assessments, review of the event counter diagnostics, and focused history and physical allow the physician to guide the need for additional testing as well as determine if any changes in the programmed settings are required. The result of this evaluation is a prescription with respect to the pacing system.

Symptom Review and Physical Examination

There is more to the pacing system than just the electrical performance of the pacemaker and leads. Although the review of symptoms and physical examination does not need to be extensive, a screening review for the recurrence of any symptoms that were present prior to the implantation of the pacemaker is warranted along with symptoms which may suggest a potential problem. For example, the new onset of palpitations may suggest a new intrinsic arrhythmia, a pacemaker mediated tachycardia, possible pacemaker syndrome due to the loss of appropriate AV synchrony, or an inappropriate rate in response to the sensor. It is also prudent to screen for symptoms that may be associated with other cardiovascular disease such as dyspnea, angina, and congestive heart failure which becomes even more important with the increase role of CRT in the management of congestive heart failure.

Standard vital signs such as blood pressure, pulse rate, respiratory rate, and if the symptoms or physical findings suggest an infection, temperature are indicated. It is important to examine the pocket looking for signs of infection, pressure necrosis, or overt erosion (Fig. 19.1). Examination of the anterior chest wall for dilated veins and the ipsilateral arm for swelling may identify venous obstruction which will be important information if and when central venous access or a lead revision is required. This is an aspect of the pacing system evaluation that cannot be performed via transtelephonic monitoring and a problem may be present even when the system is electronically normal.

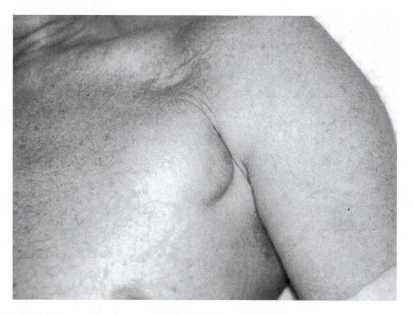

Fig. 19.1 Photograph of pressure necrosis. The subcutaneous tissue over the lateral aspect of the pulse generator is thinned due to the resorbtion of the adipose tissue while the overlying skin is molded to the pulse generator and developing a blue-red discoloration. The area is also tender.

Pacemaker Dependency

There is no standard definition of pacemaker dependency although the concept has significant potential implications with respect to patient management (5). Some physicians consider a patient to be dependent if the rhythm is totally paced each time the patient is seen where as others require that the patient be virtually asystolic without the presence of the pacemaker before labeling the individual as being dependent upon the pacemaker. With respect to the latter definition, the duration of asystole has not been well defined. The authors would suggest a practical definition. In our practice, a patient is considered pacemaker dependent if the abrupt failure of the pacing system, for whatever reason, whether this be loss of capture due to a mechanical failure of the lead, oversensing with pacemaker inhibition, or a component failure in the pulse generator, results in significant symptoms such as syncope or presyncope. As a practical test, we reduce the pacing rate to 30 bpm in a nontracking mode and if the rhythm remains paced or the patient develops symptoms at the escape rhythm, the patient is considered to be pacemaker dependent. Our testing is performed with the patient lying supine on an examination table. If the routine evaluation is performed with the patient sitting in a geriatric chair and is partially or totally upright, it might not be prudent to reduce the rate as low as 30 bpm. Once a patient is identified as being pacemaker dependent, the pacemaker chart and medical record are appropriately flagged. An individual who receives the pacemaker for intermittent asystole whether it be due to complete heart block associated with Stokes–Adams syncope or marked sinus node dysfunction would also be treated as pacemaker dependent even if the pacemaker is being inhibited on most of the office and transtelephonic evaluations.

Knowing whether or not the patient is pacemaker dependent is essential to the patient's management when the patient or referring physician calls with a concern about the system or the physician receives notification of a manufacturer's advisory or safety alert. A patient who has never demonstrated asystole, who has always had a stable although slow intrinsic rhythm can be managed on an elective basis if a problem is suspected where as one who is even intermittently pacemaker dependent warrants a relatively urgent evaluation if not further intervention.

Once the patient has been labeled as being pacemaker dependent, it is no longer necessary to decrease the rate to look for an intrinsic rhythm at each follow-up visit. For the patient who is being paced but who has not previously been identified as being pacemaker dependent, there are a number of simple bedside techniques that can be used. One is to totally inhibit the pacemaker using the inhibit function available in some programmers while another is to reduce the base rate of the pacemaker to a very slow rate such as 30 bpm in a nontracking mode (Fig. 19.2). This testing is safest when performed with the patient lying on an examination table rather than sitting. A totally paced rhythm for 5–10 s at the low programmed rate or symptoms at the patient's intrinsic escape rhythm is our working definition of pacemaker dependency.

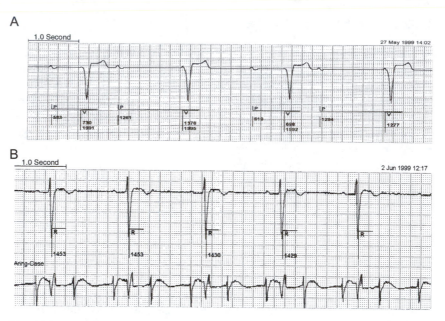

Fig. 19.2 Assessment of pacemaker dependency. (a) Totally paced ventricular rhythm when the base rate is reduced to 30 ppm in a nontracking (DDI) mode in a patient who has asystolic complete heart. The P waves that occur during the atrial alert period are identified by event markers as are all the ventricular paced complexes. (b) Underlying 2:1 block rhythm is identified in a patient with a DDD pacemaker whose ventricle is normally totally controlled by the permanent pacemaker. To show this, the mode was temporarily changed to VVI and the pacing rate reduced to 30 ppm. The simultaneously telemetered unipolar atrial electrogram is shown along the bottom demonstrating the atrial activity as well as far-field ventricular signals.

Pacemaker Diagnostics

The present generation pacemakers are capable of providing detailed measured data reporting lead and battery status in addition to a listing of all the current programmed settings (3,6–8). Some even include additional information that can be entered into the implanted pulse generator by the clinician. To facilitate an evaluation of the paced rhythm and behavior, many devices have event marker and electrogram telemetry (9–24). An event marker is telemetered directly from the pulse generator to the programmer and will be displayed on the programmer screen. If external electrocardiographic (ECG) leads are connected to the patient, the event markers will coincident with a simultaneously recorded electrocardiogram (ECG). The event markers report the real-time behavior of the implanted pacemaker with respect to paced and sensed events using a variety of cryptic alphanumeric labels (9–14). These vary in complexity and differ between manufacturers. Although there are differences, most systems utilize a two-letter combination where atrial events are identified with an "A" while a "V" is used to represent a ventricular event. The second letter is "S" for a sensed event and "P" for a paced event. Most systems today can also identify events coinciding with the refractory period and here, there are differences between the three major manufacturers. Medtronic utilizes an "R" for a sense refractory event where as Boston Scientific still uses the "S" but places the two-letter code within parentheses, and St. Jude Medical places the two-letter code within a box. One needs to be cautious in interpreting these event markers since they only report what the pacemaker was doing. Release of a ventricular output does not mean that there was ventricular capture. Detection of a native event, be it in the atrium or in the ventricle does not mean that this was a true P wave or R wave but simply that a signal of sufficient amplitude was detected on the respective channel of the pacing system. Hence, it is imperative to record a surface ECG rhythm with the simultaneously telemetered event markers. Most programmers which provide a channel for event markers and telemetered electrograms also provide a separate cable to connection to skin leads allowing for a standard ECG rhythm strip although leadless ECG systems are being developed.

The system may also be capable of telemetering and displaying the intracardiac electrical signal from either the atrium, the ventricle, or both as detected by the pacemaker (15–24). A signal recorded from inside the heart is called an electrogram (EGM) while the signal recorded from the surface of the body is termed an electrocardiogram. The morphology of EGM displayed on the programmer may vary depending on whether it is transmitted to the programmer before or after it has been processed by the sensing circuit of the pacemaker (4). Both the telemetered EGMs and event markers are real-time events requiring that the programmer be in active communication with the pacemaker at the time of the evaluation.

The event marker technology also allows the pacemaker to "know" when it has paced or sensed on a given channel. Pacemakers incorporate a microprocessor with significant random access memory. This allows the implanted device to store this information for retrieval at a later time. The result is a variety of event counter diagnostics being capable of reporting device system behavior, both overall and with respect to specific unique algorithms, since the last detailed evaluation. The event counter data should be retrieved at the beginning of the pacing system evaluation as the temporary programming of selected parameters that might be required to complete the evaluation may force the clearing of these counters (25–35).

Capture Thresholds

The capture threshold is the lowest output of the pacemaker which results in consistent capture (36–39). Capture is the induction of an electrical depolarization of the cardiac chamber which is being stimulated. In order to assess the capture threshold, it is essential to first confirm the presence of pacing. While this is preferably achieved by monitoring the surface ECG, there are occasions when an indirect marker of capture will need to be utilized. Depending on the lead which is being monitored during this evaluation, the pacemaker-induced complex, also called an evoked response, may or may not be visible on the ECG. This is most common when assessing atrial capture as the evoked P wave tends to be significantly smaller than the paced QRS complex (Fig. 19.3). It may be necessary to examine a number of surface ECG leads to determine which one provides the best visualization of the effective depolarization. Another technique that has been effective in the confirmation

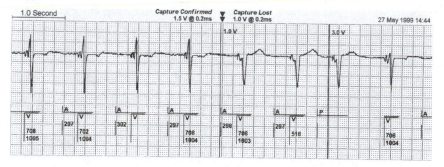

Fig. 19.3 ECG recording during an atrial capture threshold test in a patient with first-degree AV block sinus node dysfunction. The P wave is not visible on the surface ECG lead which is being monitored. Although the ventricular depolarization is labeled as a paced ventricular beat by the event markers shown below the rhythm strip, the QRS complex is narrow suggesting that it is really a fusion beat. With loss of capture associated with a progressive decrement in the pulse amplitude to 1.0 V, there is a marked change in the paced QRS morphology confirming that at the higher output, there had to be atrial capture in order for conduction to occur to cause the fusion beats even though a "P" wave is not seen on the surface ECG lead which was being monitored.

of capture is to look at the known electrophysiologic events that should be associated with a specific phenomenon (40). For example, if there is atrial pacing and AV nodal conduction is intact, each atrial output, when capture is present, will be followed by a conducted QRS complex at an interval that approximates the normal PR interval even if a "P" is not visible in the ECG lead which is being monitored. In the case of ventricular pacing, a visible T wave representing repolarization means that there had to have been an effective depolarization, even if the evoked QRS complex is isoelectric in the given lead which is being monitored. With respect to cardiac resynchronization therapy, it is sometimes helpful to change the surface lead being monitored during the evaluation of the left ventricular capture threshold and the right ventricular capture threshold. In those patients who are receiving CRT in the presence of intact AV nodal conduction, their intrinsic QRS complex usually has a left bundle branch block (LBBB) pattern. In that dedicated RV pacing also results in a LBBB pattern, it is helpful to monitor a superior–inferior lead such as Lead II where as evaluation of the left ventricular capture threshold, a Lead I with its right–left orientation allows for a readily identified change in QRS morphology with loss of capture. With pure LV capture, a Lead I has a right bundle branch block pattern while loss of LV capture is associated with the restoration of the intrinsic LBBB pattern.

If the entire pacemaker or a specific channel of the pacemaker is being inhibited, it will be necessary to reprogram the pacemaker to demonstrate capture in order to assess the capture threshold. With respect to atrial pacing in either a dual- or single-chamber pacing system, it may be necessary to increase the rate. It is recommended that the rate be increased at least 20 bpm above the intrinsic rate to minimize the chance of a waxing and waning sinus arrhythmia confusing the evaluation by periodic inhibition of the pacemaker. For ventricular capture in a dual-chamber system with intact AV nodal conduction, shortening the paced or sensed AV delay until there is a clear change in the morphology of the ventricular complex will confirm the presence of capture, even if this is a fusion beat. Once this is achieved, the output can

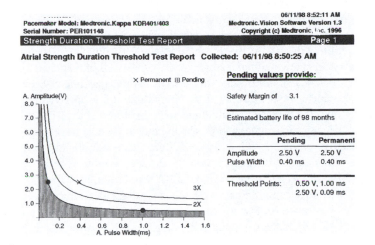

Fig. 19.4 Strength–duration curve created based on a pulse duration threshold at 2.5 V amplitude and a pulse amplitude threshold at a 1.0 ms pulse duration. This curve is automatically constructed by the Medtronic programmer based on testing with the Medtronic Kappa® 400 pacemaker. If the output were to fall within the shaded area, it would be subthreshold. The two times and three times safety margin curves are also provided along with the location of the current programmed parameters (X). The curve, based on two data points, is generated from a library of templates which resides within the 9790 programmer.

be either manually or semiautomatically decreased until loss of capture is observed on the ECG, the test sequence terminated, and the output returned to an appropriate level. In this setting, the capture threshold is commonly taken as the last output setting at which there was stable capture. The capture threshold determined by a progressive decrease in the output (down-threshold) may be lower than the capture threshold measured when starting from a loss of capture and progressively increasing the output (up-threshold) due to phenomenon called the Wedensky effect (39). Although these two values are commonly very close, a rare patient shows a marked difference between the two values with the up-threshold being higher than the down-threshold.

The capture threshold is not a fixed number. Rather, it may wax and wane during the course of the day (41–46). The measurement that is made in the office reflects the minimal amount of energy that is required to be delivered to the heart to assure effective capture at that moment in time. Energy is a function of current, voltage, and pulse duration (time). The two parameters that can be independently controlled and programmed by the physician are pulse amplitude (voltage) and pulse duration. As such, capture is usually reported in terms of either voltage or pulse duration. This should be reported as the voltage threshold at a given pulse duration or the pulse duration threshold as measured at a predefined pulse amplitude. The relationship between these two parameters can be defined by a "strength-duration" curve (Fig. 19.4). At a very narrow pulse duration, a very high pulse amplitude will be required. As the pulse duration is progressively increased, the required voltage decreases but not in a linear manner. The relative rate of decrease progressively slows until a pulse duration is achieved where the pulse voltage which is required for capture will not decrease further. If the pulse duration continues to be increased, the pulse voltage will remain at this fixed level. This is called the rheobase while the pulse duration threshold at twice the rheobase is called the chronaxie point.

The chronaxie point with present generation leads commonly ranges between 0.3 and 0.5 ms with many pacemakers being shipped by the manufacturer at a pulse duration of 0.4 ms. As the threshold fluctuates, both on a daily basis with changing sympathetic and parasympathetic tone as well in response to disease processes, it tends to follow parallel curves. Some pacemaker-programmer systems provide a graphic display of the strength–duration curve with a 2:1 and 3:1 safety margin curve being simultaneously displayed (Fig. 19.3).

Marked changes in capture and/or sensing threshold may be an early marker for mechanical problems with a lead or reflect changes at the electrode–tissue interface associated with progression of disease. Minor changes over the course of the day ranging between 1 and 2 programming steps are normal. As of 2006, most recently released models have algorithms that automatically monitor the presence or absence of ventricular capture and adjust the output based on detected changes may minimize the need to perform capture thresholds. Some devices even automatically evaluate the atrial capture threshold although these capabilities are not available in older generation devices that are still in service. In pacing systems without an automatic capture or threshold measurement algorithm, it is essential to periodically assess the threshold levels allowing the pacemaker to be programmed with an appropriate safety margin, particularly if one has reduced the output level in an effort to increase pulse generator longevity. The capture safety margin is a ratio defined by the programmed output divided by the measured threshold level.

In a pacemaker-dependent patient, the usual recommendation for a pacemaker which cannot automatically monitor the status of capture and adjust its output is to set the pacemaker to provide a 2:1 safety margin with respect to the voltage threshold. This is a voltage that is 100% above the measured threshold voltage although Danilovic and Ohm (44) have recommended a 150–200% safety margin to protect the patient from unexpected late threshold rises that may occur even with the present generation of steroid-eluting leads.

The concept of safety margin is not a guarantee that the capture threshold will not rise above the programmed output of the pacemaker. If the goal is to maximize patient safety, the output of the pacemaker should be programmed to its highest allowed level. This, however, will increase the battery current drain and accelerate the rate of battery depletion. If the capture threshold is stable at a very low level, a high output is wasteful and will unnecessarily shorten the pulse generator longevity. The concept of safety margin attempts to weigh the anticipated waxing and waning of capture thresholds once the capture threshold is stable in an effort to protect the patient while maximizing the longevity of the implanted pulse generator by reducing the output thus reducing the battery current drain. Hence, in the pacemaker-dependent patient, a 2:1 or higher safety margin has been recommended (44,45). For the patient in whom pacemaker dependency has never been demonstrated, it may be safe to set the pacemaker to a lower output and a narrower safety margin.

The decision as to the degree to which the output should be reduced is directly impacted by the effective reduction in the battery current drain associated with the lower outputs. If the reduction is minimal and will not significantly increase the projected longevity of the implanted unit, there is little to be gained by a marked reduction in the output. On the other hand, if the projected increase in longevity is by a year or more, it is reasonable to decrease the output consistent with patient safety.

Table 19.3 Comparison of battery current drains at a multiplicity of output voltages at rate 60 ppm, DDDR mode, and similar pulse duration and lead impedances.

Mgf/Device	St. Jude Medical	Medtronic	St. Jude Medical
Output voltage (V)	Pacesetter synchrony II 2022 (μA)	Thera DRi 7960i (μA)	Pacesetter Affinity DR 5330 (μA)
1.0	16	9.6	6
1.5	17	10.9	7
2.0	18	11.6	8
2.5	19	13.0	9
3.0	23	14.9	15
3.5	25	16.9	17
4.0	26	19.4	21
5.0	30	22.5	25
7.5	48	38.6	46

Measurements as actually recorded at the time of follow-up. Synchrony II 2022 – 27919 collected 18 Jan, 1993, Thera DRi 7960i – PDB128693 collected 27 May, 1999 and Affinity DR 5330 – 13927 collected 27 May, 1999. The SJM Pacesetter devices round-off the reported battery current drain to the nearest whole number.

Continued refinements in the output circuit of the pacemaker have enabled a marked reduction in battery current drain associated with progressive reductions in the output setting. Until recently, reducing the output of the pacemaker below "2.5" V had a minimal impact on battery current drain in earlier generation devices while increasing it above this level significantly increased battery current drain thus compromising device longevity. In these earlier units, the goal, as long as patient safety was the priority, was to reduce the output to at least 2.5 V but not worry about going to lower levels. The rationale behind this decision was based on the circuit design with the open-circuit output voltage of the lithium iodine power cell being 2.8 V. Delivering a 2.5 V output pulse did not require any special additional circuitry. Decreasing the output below 2.5 V saved some energy but on a proportional basis, not as much as it cost to increase the output above 2.5 V. Increasing the output to between 3.0 and 5.0 V required the use of a voltage doubler and charge pumps which are energy inefficient. Increasing the output to 5.5 V or higher requires the use of a voltage tripler (47–49). The impact of different output settings on battery current drain is shown in Table 19.3. These measurements were obtained from implanted pacemakers capable of providing this information by way of telemetry.

The growing availability of AutoCapture capabilities, first introduced in Europe by St. Jude Medical® in their Microny™ family of single-chamber rate-modulated pacemakers has been expanded to the ventricular channel in the Affinity™ family of dual-chamber pacemakers (50–52). Similar but not identical algorithms have now been introduced by other manufacturers thus reducing the need for periodic capture threshold assessments. However, it does not totally eliminate the need to consider the combined concerns of patient safety and device longevity and periodically assess the event counter diagnostics that accompany this feature. While AutoCapture will protect the patient to

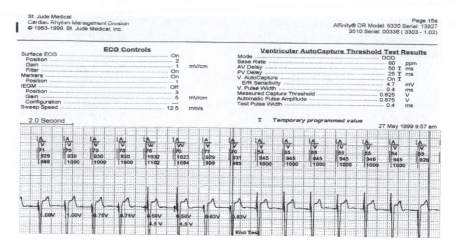

Fig. 19.5 Ventricular AutoCapture Threshold test performed with the Model 3510 Programmer at the time of a routine follow-up visit. The higher output back-up pulse is identified by the second "V" output marker and the much larger stimulus artifact following each loss of capture associated with the primary output pulse. During the test with the programmer, the delivered voltage associated with each pulse is also reported. The measured "up-threshold" is 0.625 V at a 0.4 ms pulse duration in a system that had been implanted 3 months earlier. Based on this result, the automatic pulse amplitude is set to 0.875 V by the AutoCapture algorithm.

a greater degree than a fixed safety margin, it will still have a maximal output and if the capture threshold were to rise to levels higher than the maximal output, the patient will still experience loss of capture. As such, AutoCapture does not eliminate the need for periodic follow-up evaluations although it does enhance patient protection between scheduled visits. To minimize battery current drain yet maintain patient safety, the AutoCapture system automatically adjusts the ventricular output to 0.25 V above the measured capture threshold. This is a working margin, not a safety margin. The only way that this narrow working margin is safe is if the system is able to monitor the presence or absence of capture on a beat-by-beat basis and should noncapture be detected, consistently and reliably deliver a relatively high-out back-up pulse shortly after the diagnosis of noncapture associated with the primary pulse. The back-up pulse provides a safety margin which is much higher than the clinical standard of 2:1. As the usual output is so very low, the overall impact on battery current drain associated with the microprocessor-controlled algorithm is minimal with a significant net increase in pulse generator longevity. The behavior of the system can be visualized during an automatic capture threshold evaluation that can be triggered via the programmer at the time of a follow-up evaluation (Fig. 19.5).

Integral to the automatic capture or capture threshold algorithms is a long-term capture threshold graph displaying the performance of the capture threshold over time (Fig. 19.6). This also allows the physician to identify unexpected threshold rises that may have occurred between the scheduled office visits and, in retrospect, help to understand the impact of multiple different pharmacologic agents and pathophysiologic conditions on capture threshold (40–42,46). An integral part of each office-based follow-up evaluation is to assess the system's performance based on the diagnostic event counters which can be retrieved from the implanted unit.

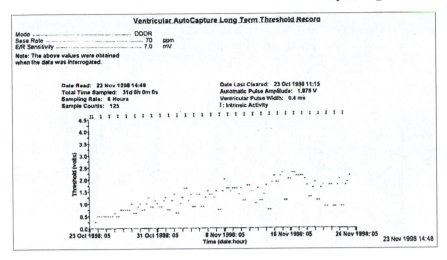

Fig. 19.6 Long-term capture threshold display from an Affinity DR pacemaker implanted 1 month previously. There is marked instability in the threshold due to microinstability. Had the capture threshold been measured at discharge, it would have been 0.5 V and if measured at the 1 month point, it would be 0.75 V implying impressive threshold stability. However, based on this graph, the threshold was actually very unstable yet AutoCapture automatically compensated for these fluctuations as well as identifying their presence.

Sensing

Sensing is the ability of the pacemaker to both detect and respond to intrinsic atrial and/or ventricular depolarizations. While a common shorthand is to discuss the behavior of the pacing system with respect to P wave or R wave sensing, these two complexes are actually the representation of the atrial or ventricular depolarization on the surface ECG. The signal that the pacemaker responds to is the intracardiac electrogram as the wave of depolarization passes by the pacing electrode inside the heart. If this signal were to be recorded, it is often very large with a very rapid deflection corresponding to the intrinsic deflection (53–57). Morphologically, there may not be much difference between the intracardiac atrial and ventricular depolarizations. In those systems that allow for electrogram telemetry, it is recommended that on the first detailed postimplantation evaluation, these electrograms be recorded and included in the patient's record to provide a baseline for future comparison should sensing problems or a change in the sensing threshold develop in the future (Fig. 19.7).

As with the automatic measurement of capture thresholds, systems are being introduced that automatically measure the amplitude of the intrinsic signals minimizing the need to assess the sensing threshold at each follow-up visit. If the implanted system does not have this capability, it will be necessary to evaluate the sensing threshold at the time of the follow-up evaluation. This requires that the patient have an intrinsic rhythm in which ever cardiac chamber sensing is being assessed. If there is not a stable native rhythm, a sensing threshold cannot be determined. If the system is actively pacing on a given channel, it will be necessary to reduce the rate in order to determine if there is intrinsic atrial activity in the dual-chamber mode or intrinsic activity in the appropriate chamber in the single-chamber mode. In dual-chamber pacing, one can try to increase the paced or sensed AV delay to determine if there is

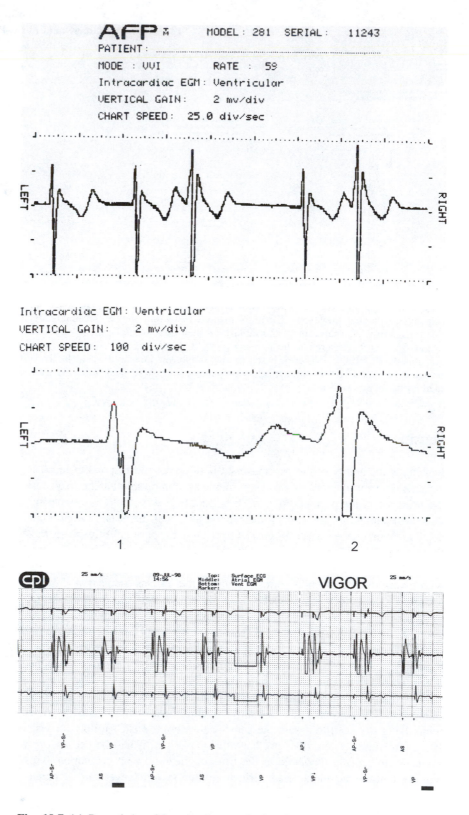

Fig. 19.7 (a) Recorded at 25 mm/s, the ventricular electrograms associated with the sinus QRS and the PVC look very similar in amplitude. Yet, the PVC was sensed properly at 7 mV with loss of sensing occurring at 9 mV, hence a sensing threshold of 7 mV while the sinus QRS was sensed properly at 3.0 mV with a loss of sensing at 3.5 mV.

(continued)

intrinsic ventricular activity as with intact AV nodal conduction. Depending on the system, the allowed AV delay may still be too short resulting in fusion beats. Should that occur, programming the pacemaker to a nontracking mode such as VVI followed by a reduction in the programmed base rate will usually allow the sensing threshold to be assessed. In the absence of an intrinsic rhythm, be this in the atrium or ventricle, a sensing threshold will not be able to be determined.

Two techniques have been used to assess the sensing threshold. One is to record the telemetered electrogram and measure the peak-to-peak amplitude of the resultant signal if this is calibrated (7,8). This may be both misleading and inappropriate if the telemetry system utilizes different filters in its telemetry amplifier in comparison to those which are used in its sensing circuit (58). The sensing circuit tends to use a narrow pass-band filter in an effort to eliminate known but inappropriate signals such as T waves which are relatively low frequency signal (Fig. 19.7). Hence, if the telemetered electrogram shows a prominent T wave associated with the ventricular electrogram, one can be reasonably certain that the filters in the telemetry system differ from those which are integral to the sensing circuit.

The other technique is to progressively reduce the sensitivity setting of the pacemaker. This can be done either manually or using the semiautomatic sensing threshold test that is available in many devices (Fig. 19.8). A loss of sensing will be readily demonstrated by either a loss of the telemetered event marker and/or competition between the native and paced rhythms. When this occurs, the test is terminated and the sensitivity setting is reset to the clinically desired value based on the results of the test. The least sensitive setting of the pacemaker, which is the largest number in terms of millivolts options that can be selected, at which there is consistent stable sensing is the sensing threshold.

The ratio of the sensing threshold divided by the programmed sensitivity defines the sensing safety margin. The recommendations as to setting the sensing safety margin are not as well defined as the capture safety margin. In a patient with known paroxysmal pathologic tachyarrhythmias, one often programs a very sensitive setting independent of the size of the sinus P or R waves because the signal associated with the pathologic arrhythmia often cannot be routinely assessed at a follow-up visit and are commonly significantly smaller than the normal complexes. Too insensitive a setting will preclude adequate detection with either competition or failure to activate special algorithms such as Automatic Mode Switch (59). On the other hand, routinely programming

---

Fig. 19.7 (continued) In addition, the peak-to-peak amplitude of the T wave is between 2.5 and 3.0 mV yet T wave sensing was not present. (**b**) An expanded recording of a single sinus QRS (complex 1) and the PVC (complex 2) at a chart speed of 100 mm/s. Splintering of the sinus ventricular electrogram is seen at this more rapid speed. As soon as there is a reversal in polarity of the intrinsic deflection, the sense amplifier considers the signal to have ended. This accounts for the lower amplitude of the sinus complex in comparison to the PVC. In addition, the slope of the intracardiac T wave is very slow and will be effectively deleted by the filters in the sensing circuit which are different than the filters in the telemetry circuit. (**c**) Simultaneous recording of the surface ECG, atrial and ventricular electrograms, and event markers from a Guidant ® Vigor DDDR pacemaker. The electrograms have been telemetered after being processed by the sensing circuit. Note the diminutive "T" wave on the ventricular EGM due to the filters in the sense amplifier.

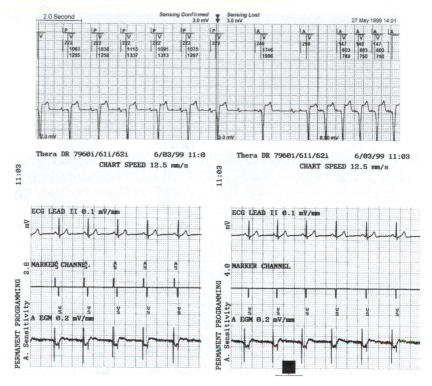

Fig. 19.8 (a) Semiautomatic atrial sensing threshold test with a Trilogy DR + model 2360. Once activated, the system progressively reduces the sensitivity while the rhythm is being monitored in conjunction with telemetered event markers. Although programmed to a base rate of 80 ppm, for the purposes of this test, the base rate was temporarily reduced to 30 ppm. Upon termination of the test by the clinician upon recognition of loss of sensing, the temporary parameters are automatically canceled while the rhythm strip is frozen, centered on the screen, and labeled for printing. The frozen image can be further manipulated prior to printing. In this case, the recording speed was compressed to 12.5 mm/s to include more complexes on the printout. (b) Progressive reduction in atrial sensitivity using telemetered event markers to identify the presence or absence of sensing. The pacemaker is a Medtronic Thera DR which is totally inhibited at the time. One could not determine whether or not sensing is intact from the surface ECG as there is no difference in the rhythm when there is intact atrial sensing at 2.8 mV or loss of atrial sensing at 4.0 mV. However, in the absence of sensing, the patient will have a functional DVI pacemaker during episodes of intermittent AV block. This manual testing is usually performed at a slow chart speed to minimize the use of paper and provide a greater number of complexes in a printout.

the pacemaker to the most sensitive setting that is allowed will predispose to the detection of either physiologically inappropriate signals such as far field signals arising from the opposite chamber (60), repolarization signals or myopotentials causing inappropriate inhibition or triggering depending on the design of the pacemaker (61–63). While the bipolar sensing configuration provides greater immunity to the detection of inappropriate physiologic signals, it is not totally immune to oversensing. If one does have a unipolar system, it is will be important to screen the patient for oversensing. The most common cause being skeletal muscle myopotentials.

When there is no intrinsic signal as in the patient with asystolic complete heart block, it is common to reduce the sensitivity to between 3 and 5 mV on the ventricular channel in an effort to preclude oversensing. The exception is the presence of known premature ectopic beats where an insensitive setting may predispose to undersensing of the premature beats, force competition, and potentially induce a pathologic tachycardia.

In the sensitivity parameter of the pacemaker, the lower the millivolt number, the higher the sensitivity. This number defines the amplitude of the intrinsic signal that can be sensed once it has been processed by the sensing circuit of the pacemaker. At a 2 m V sensitivity setting, the signal, once processed, must be at least 2 mV in amplitude. A 1 mV sensitivity setting means that the signal need only be 1 mV in amplitude. Hence at a 1 mV sensitivity, the system will be more sensitive and able to detect a smaller signal than at the 2 mV setting. If one were to program the sensitivity to 8 mV, the final processed signal will need to be larger than 8 mV for sensing to occur. If the final signal were only 6 mV, it would be detected by the system programmed to both a 1 mV and a 2 mV sensitivity but it would not be recognized at the 8 mV sensitivity setting. Hence, the larger the number with respect to the sensitivity setting, the lower the sensitivity of the system.

Pacing Lead and Battery Status

With time, the energy in the battery will progressively deplete until the battery voltage falls below the manufacturer's predefined level. If this is either not detected or ignored, the battery will continue to deplete until there is virtually no output with the loss of effective pacing. In an effort to minimize the unexpected catastrophic failure of the implanted system due to battery depletion, each manufacturer has incorporated separate markers integral to the design of their pacemaker to provide easily measured clinical clues as to the status of the battery. This is commonly a change in either the basic programmed rate or the magnet rate. Some devices may include a change in pacing mode and/or elimination of one or more special features such as rate modulation and acquisition of event counter data. The behavior of the pacemaker at various levels of battery status is defined by the manufacturer and this information is provided in the technical manual which comes with each device. The rate and other behavior markers identifying the various stages of battery depletion should be prospectively included in the patient's office chart and/or pacemaker chart as sufficient battery depletion to warrant pulse generator replacement will not occur for years.

There are commonly two separate stages with respect to battery depletion. One is the recommended replacement time (RRT), also called elective replacement indicator (ERI) and occurs when the battery voltage, which is different from the output voltage, falls to a manufacturer-defined level. When this stage is identified, one can expect between 3 and 6 months of normal behavior before erratic pacing or total system failure may occur. When recognized, the patient should be electively scheduled for a pulse generator replacement. If battery depletion occurs prematurely or abruptly, the explanted device should be returned to the manufacturer for activation of a warranty credit and to allow a detailed evaluation as to why this occurred. If the RRT stage in the life of

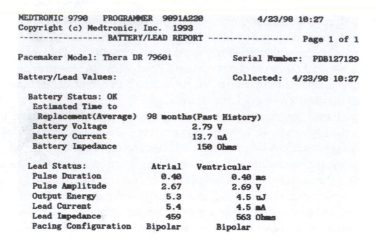

```
MEDTRONIC 9790    PROGRAMMER  9891A220          4/23/98 10:27
Copyright (c) Medtronic, Inc.  1993
---------------- BATTERY/LEAD REPORT ---------------- Page 1 of 1

Pacemaker Model: Thera DR 7960i          Serial Number:  PDB127129

Battery/Lead Values:                     Collected:  4/23/98 10:27

  Battery Status: OK
  Estimated Time to
    Replacement(Average)  98 months(Past History)
  Battery Voltage               2.79 V
  Battery Current               13.7 uA
  Battery Impedance             150 Ohms

  Lead Status:          Atrial    Ventricular
    Pulse Duration       0.40        0.40 ms
    Pulse Amplitude      2.67        2.69 V
    Output Energy        5.3         4.5 uJ
    Lead Current         5.4         4.5 mA
    Lead Impedance       459         563 Ohms
    Pacing Configuration Bipolar    Bipolar
```

Fig. 19.9 Measured data printout from a patient with a Medtronic Thera model 7960I programmed to 2.5 V on both the atrial and ventricular channels. The battery current drain, the lead impedance, and the projected longevity are provided in addition to other data.

the pulse generator is missed, commonly because the patient has been lost to follow-up, the battery voltage will continue to fall until it reaches a stage termed end-of-life (EOL) or end-of-service (EOS). At this point, device function may become erratic and unpredictable. If the system is identified as having entered EOL, it constitutes a relative medical emergency and the patient should be expeditiously admitted to the hospital, particularly if pacemaker dependent, placed in a monitored unit with device replacement scheduled as soon as possible.

Every power source or battery will eventually deplete. It is only a matter of time impacted by the programmed settings of the pacemaker and the degree to which pacing support is required. The effect of pacing rate and output settings on battery current drain can be assessed using the measured data available from many pacemakers. These measurements are made while the pacemaker is in an asynchronous state. If a high output was required on a given channel, the measured battery current drain might be very high but if this channel was basically inhibited by the patient's intrinsic rhythm, the actual impact of this high output on device longevity would be minimal despite the reported battery current drain. At the present time, some implanted systems provide an estimate of device longevity which is based on an assumption of 100% pacing at the present programmed settings (64) (Fig. 19.9). The expectation as to system longevity needs to be modified by the clinician's knowledge of the patient and the degree to which pacing support is actually required and to take this into account, many system report the expected longevity as either "greater than" or a range in terms of months or years. When reporting the range, the shorter duration is the projected longevity presuming 100% pacing at the current settings while the longer duration presumes total inhibition.

The weakest link in the pacing system is the lead. This is an insulated wire which connects the pulse generator to the heart. It is repeatedly flexed, twisted and potentially crushed depending on its actual anatomic course. While some leads have been identified as having an increased incidence of failure, even the best of leads may have a higher incidence of failures if their anatomical course subjects them to an increased level of extrinsic stress (65–67). Given this known behavior, evaluation of lead integrity is an essential part of any detailed follow-up session.

Many available pulse generators provide the ability to measure the resistance or impedance in the lead at the time of pacing and some automatically track this information (Fig. 19.10). This may be tracked over time providing an insight into lead integrity although measurements that are made over a couple of cycles at the time of follow-up evaluation with the patient lying quietly on an examination table may not detect an intermittent problem, particularly if not manifest at the time of the follow-up evaluation. If a problem is suspected but repeated lead impedance measurements are normal, it will be necessary for the patient to perform a variety of provocative maneuvers such a reaching or rotating the arm to stretch the lead in an attempt to unmask a problem while monitoring the ECG, event markers, electrograms, and measured data. It is important to obtain repeated lead impedance measurements as each is made based on the output associated with only one to three forced asynchronous cycles. If the pacing system behavior is normal at the time of these measurements, the measurements will be normal. An over-penetrated chest x-ray may sometimes help identify a problem, particularly if it involves the conductor coil (Fig. 19.11). The insulation, however, is radiolucent and a breach may only be recognized radiographically if there is a concomitant deformity of the conductor wire.

As a general rule, a marked change in the telemetered lead impedance in the absence of a clinically overt pacing system malfunction warrants close follow-up but not necessarily an operative intervention to replace the lead (68–71). If a lead model series is known to have an increased incidence of problems or the patient is pacemaker dependent, it might be prudent to replace the lead on a prophylactic basis even though it was apparently functioning properly. However, if the patient is not dependent on the pacemaker and the system is functioning normally, a manufacturer's advisory should not be taken as a mandate to subject the patient to an operative procedure to replace the suspect device. In this setting, increased surveillance would be warranted. In the presence of overt clinical problems such as a marked capture threshold rise or loss of capture with or without undersensing or oversensing, a dramatic change in the lead impedance measurement from a previously stable will identify the likely source of the problem.

A high impedance above the measurement level allowed by the system implies an open circuit while a low impedance value below the measurement level of system suggests an insulation failure and short circuit. Tracking the lead impedance and potentially displaying this on a graph might facilitate the identification of trends that warrant closer supervision (Fig. 19.10). In the case of a bipolar system, normal behavior can sometimes be restored by

Fig. 19.10 (a) Long-term signal amplitude and lead impedance graph provided by the Guidant Discovery pacing system. These measurements are automatically made by the system on a daily basis. (b) Tabular summary of the same data from the Guidant Discovery pulse generator which was presented in graphic form in (a). The signal amplitude is not measured when the channel is being paced at the time of the measurement. If the channel is being inhibited by a native rhythm at the time of the measurement, no impedance signal is reported. These events are clearly identified in the tabular format.

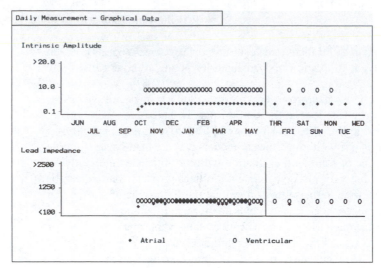

```
Daily Measurement - Graphical Data

Intrinsic Amplitude

>20.0

 10.0                    oooooooooooooooooo oooooooooooo      o  o  o  o

  0.1         .........................................    .  .  .  .  .  .  .

        JUN   AUG   OCT   DEC   FEB   APR      THR   SAT   MON   WED
           JUL   SEP   NOV   JAN   MAR   MAY      FRI   SUN   TUE

Lead Impedance

>2500

 1250

<100         oooooooooooooooooooooooooooooooooooooooo    o  o  o  o  o  o  o

            •  Atrial              O  Ventricular
```

Guidant		DISCOV

27-MAY-99 13

Institution   DALE ISAEFF,M.D.
Patient   JUANITA ____ PF284737   CPI Programmer   004
Model   1274 Serial   403667   2890 Software   2

Daily Measurement - Data Table

	Atrial		Ventricular	
Date	Amplitude (mV)	Impedance (Ω)	Amplitude (mV)	Impedance (Ω)
26-MAY-99	3.4	SENSED	PACED	620
25-MAY-99	>3.5	SENSED	PACED	650
24-MAY-99	>3.5	SENSED	>9.0	650
23-MAY-99	>3.5	SENSED	>9.0	680
22-MAY-99	>3.5	SENSED	>9.0	670
21-MAY-99	>3.5	560	>9.0	670
20-MAY-99	>3.5	SENSED	PACED	670
17-MAY-99	>3.5	560	>9.0	660
10-MAY-99	>3.5	SENSED	>9.0	660
03-MAY-99	>3.5	SENSED	>9.0	660
26-APR-99	>3.5	530	>9.0	660
19-APR-99	>3.5	580	>9.0	660
12-APR-99	>3.5	600	>9.0	650
05-APR-99	>3.5	SENSED	>9.0	650
29-MAR-99	>3.5	560	>9.0	660
22-MAR-99	>3.5	580	>9.0	670
15-MAR-99	>3.5	560	>9.0	660
08-MAR-99	>3.5	550	>9.0	660
01-MAR-99	>3.5	550	>9.0	670
22-FEB-99	>3.5	620	PACED	670
15-FEB-99	>3.5	590	>9.0	670
08-FEB-99	>3.5	600	>9.0	670
01-FEB-99	>3.5	SENSED	>9.0	680
25-JAN-99	>3.5	SENSED	>9.0	680
18-JAN-99	>3.5	640	>9.0	670
11-JAN-99	>3.5	600	>9.0	700
04-JAN-99	>3.5	600	>9.0	680
28-DEC-98	>3.5	590	>9.0	700
21-DEC-98	>3.5	580	>9.0	670
14-DEC-98	>3.5	580	>9.0	700
07-DEC-98	>3.5	SENSED	>9.0	680
30-NOV-98	>3.5	SENSED	>9.0	700
23-NOV-98	>3.5	560	>9.0	700
16-NOV-98	>3.5	590	>9.0	700
09-NOV-98	>3.5	620	>9.0	720
02-NOV-98	>3.5	550	>9.0	700
26-OCT-98	>3.5	SENSED	>9.0	720
19-OCT-98	3.4	SENSED	>9.0	700
12-OCT-98	3.1	SENSED	PACED	670
05-OCT-98	2.0	440	PACED	640

Fig. 19.10 (continued)

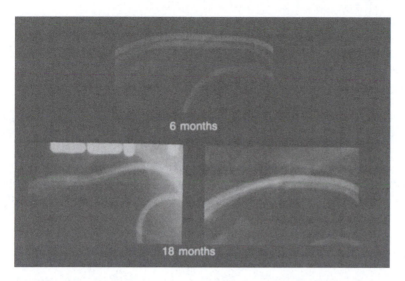

Fig. 19.11 A cone-down view of two leads passing between the inferior margin of the clavicle and the first rib. An x-ray obtained at 6 months postimplant demonstrated totally intact leads. The patient presented at 18 months postimplant with oversensing and a very low telemetered lead impedance ($< 250\ \Omega$) consistent with a breach of the internal insulation of the coaxial bipolar lead. While the insulation is radiolucent, there is a deformity of the conductor coil which is seen best on the view on the right. The lead was subsequently replaced and was able to be extracted. The deformity identified on the chest x-ray corresponded to a visible deformity on the explanted lead and the manufacturer confirmed this to the location of the insulation failure between the proximal and distal conductor coils.

programming the device to the unipolar output and sensing configuration but this should only be considered a temporizing measure. There are many systems that will do this automatically, particularly with repeated out-of-range measurements in the bipolar output configuration. However, programming to the unipolar configuration is not a permanent management option as there is a mechanical problem with the lead and this would be expected to progress over time. As soon as feasible, a definitive correction should be initiated. This usually means replacement of the lead. The chronic malfunctioning lead may be abandoned in place or explanted.

While most pacing system problems, on a statistical basis, involve the lead or the lead-tissue interface, there are cases when the actual problem resides internal to the pulse generator with the lead being mechanically normal. Hence, at the time of an operative intervention, it is important to recheck the sensing and capture thresholds and invasively measure lead impedance using a Pacing System Analyzer before simply replacing the lead. If the initial measurements via the lead are normal, gentle traction while repeating the measurement may unmask a problem with the lead. If a malfunction with the lead is confirmed, the lead should be replaced. If the measurements are normal, even with provocative maneuvers, the physician's attention should be directed to the pulse generator. In this setting, the pacemaker and not the lead should be replaced. If the lead checks out as normal but is suspect based on information provided by the manufacturer or prior noninvasive measurements, it might be prudent to replace both the lead and pulse generator at the time of the operative procedure.

If a patient undergoes an operative procedure to replace a suspect pulse generator or lead, any device or part of the device which is explanted should be returned to the manufacturer for analysis. This will activate the device warranty which is often predicated upon the manufacturer receiving the device back for analysis. Notification of the original manufacturer of the observed problem and returning the explanted device(s), even when another manufacturer's device is used in replacement due to either clinician preference or hospital contract, allow the original manufacturer to determine if there is a systematic problem thus enabling timely intervention and notification of other physicians caring for patients with the same model device. Notification of both the manufacturer and the FDA is also one of the hospital's responsibilities under the Safe Medical Devices Act of 1990 when the observed problem is potentially life-threatening.

Event Counter Diagnostics

The value of retrieving any available event counter diagnostics at the beginning of the follow-up session was mentioned early in this chapter. The full interpretation of this data must await completion of the evaluation of capture and sensing thresholds and any discussion with the patient as to relevant symptoms. The reason is that the event counters are based on the event marker capabilities of the pacemaker. One needs to know that there is a good sensing threshold and a good capture threshold with appropriate safety margins before beginning to interpret the event counter data which provides a very detailed report as to what the pacemaker did over a protracted period of time. It is the physician's responsibility to correlate the behavior of the pacing system as detailed in the event counter diagnostics with the other information which is routinely collected at the time of the follow-up evaluation in an effort to determine if the function of the implanted system is appropriate or inappropriate for the patient.

For example, some years ago, a patient was referred for evaluation of a pacing system that had been implanted over a year previously for sinus node dysfunction following heart transplantation. The pacing system was a single-chamber atrial rate-modulated system and the patient's referring physician wanted to know if the patient continued to need pacing support. The event counter diagnostics reported the total absence of any intrinsic sensed complexes. The entire rhythm, at least according to these counters, was paced and the heart rate distribution was totally consistent with an appropriately programmed sensor, hence AAIR pacing. This information would suggest that the patient still required pacing support. However, the atrial sensing threshold demonstrated consistent loss of sensing. The programmed sensitivity of the pacemaker was 2.0 mV. There was an intrinsic atrial rhythm with a sensing threshold of 1.5 mV. Given the programmed sensitivity of the pacemaker with respect to the sensing threshold, the pacemaker, although capable of sensing, was a functional AOOR system. The pulse generator was behaving properly in that it was performing in accord with its programmed parameters but the settings were not appropriate for the patient. When the sensitivity was increased, normal sensing was established. To evaluate the need for pacing support, the base rate was reduced to 50 ppm, the sensor function disabled, and the patient asked to return in 1 month. During the ensuing month, the pacemaker was totally inhibited and there was a normal heart rate distribution indicating that pacing support was no longer required.

A second patient was seen who had marked sinus node dysfunction and clearly needed pacing support. This was also a rate-modulated device and while rate modulation was enabled, the heart rate histogram reported that virtually all the complexes were atrial-paced ventricular-sensed with less than 1% occurring at rates above the programmed base rate. This would suggest that the sensor was not programmed appropriately. Examination of the patient revealed the residua of a major cerebrovascular accident leaving the patient with a severe hemiplegia and restricted to a bed-to-chair existence. As such, the patient was no longer active and even though rate modulation was enabled, one would not expect any activity-based increase in heart rate. The sensor was functioning properly given the clinical status of the patient. These experiences illustrate a very valuable and recurrent lesson. One should only interpret the event counter data after a comprehensive evaluation of the pacing system combined with a knowledge of the clinical status of the patient.

There are three general classes of event counters that are presently available (25–35). It will not be feasible to discuss each and every event counter from all the manufacturers in this chapter so they will be discussed in general with some illustrations. For additional details as to the capabilities and limitations of the event counter diagnostics in the pacemaker that is implanted, it may be necessary to contact the manufacturer or refer to the technical manual that accompanies each device.

Total System Performance Counter

These are event counters which provide an overview of the behavior or performance of the system over a protracted period of time. The actual time that can be monitored depends on the sampling rate of the counter and the amount of random access memory which had been allocated to the counter by the manufacturer. The data is often presented in either a histogram or a chart format but this does not allow for the temporal separation of different events. A prime example of such an event counter is the "Event Histogram" (Fig. 19.12). In one display, there is the relative percentage distribution of pacing states including atrial sensed-ventricular paced, atrial sensed-ventricular sensed, atrial paced-ventricular sensed, atrial paced-ventricular paced, and premature ventricular events (PVEs). A PVE is a sensed ventricular event or an R wave which is not preceded by atrial activity, this is the pacemaker's definition for a PVC. If automatic mode switch was available, there would also be a column depicting the percent of time which the system functioned in the nontracking (DDI) mode as opposed to the DDD mode. However, when mode switch might have occurred or at what time atrial sensed-ventricular pacing occurred at the maximum tracking rate could not be identified from this histogram.

Another format for this same data is a Heart Rate Histogram showing the relative percentage of atrial paced and atrial sensed events in each rate bin while an event-count chart is also available for those physicians who prefer this format for data presentation.

Similar capabilities are available in the current generation devices from most manufacturers. One should not simply accept the report of the event counter at face value using standard clinical criteria. For example,

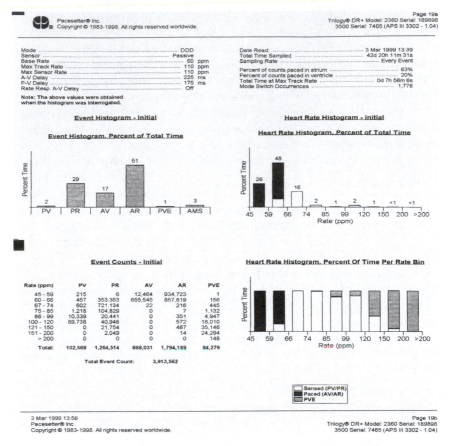

Page 19a
Trilogy® DR+ Model: 2360 Serial: 189898
3500 Serial: 7465 (APS III 3302 - 1.04)

Mode	DDD
Sensor	Passive
Base Rate	60 ppm
Max Track Rate	110 ppm
Max Sensor Rate	110 ppm
A-V Delay	225 ms
P-V Delay	175 ms
Rate Resp A-V Delay	Off

Note: The above values were obtained
when the histogram was interrogated.

Date Read:	3 Mar 1999 13:39
Total Time Sampled:	42d 20h 11m 31s
Sampling Rate	Every Event
Percent of counts paced in atrium	63%
Percent of counts paced in ventricle	20%
Total Time at Max Track Rate	0d 7h 56m 6s
Mode Switch Occurrences	1,776

Event Histogram - Initial

Event Histogram, Percent of Total Time

Heart Rate Histogram - Initial

Heart Rate Histogram, Percent of Total Time

Event Counts - Initial

Rate (ppm)	PV	PR	AV	AR	PVE
45 - 59	215	6	12,464	934,723	1
60 - 66	457	353,353	655,545	857,819	156
67 - 74	602	721,134	22	216	445
75 - 85	1,218	104,829	0	7	1,132
86 - 99	10,339	20,441	0	351	4,947
100 - 120	89,738	40,948	0	572	18,010
121 - 150	0	21,754	0	467	35,146
151 - 200	0	2,049	0	14	24,294
> 200	0	0	0	0	148
Total:	102,569	1,264,514	668,031	1,794,169	84,279

Total Event Count: 3,913,562

Heart Rate Histogram, Percent Of Time Per Rate Bin

Sensed (PV/PR)
Paced (AV/AR)
PVE

Page 19b
Trilogy® DR+ Model: 2360 Serial: 189898
3500 Serial: 7465 (APS III 3302 - 1.04)

Fig. 19.12 Event histogram from a patient implanted with a Trilogy DR+. The indication for pacing was the bradycardia-tachycardia syndrome. Over the past 42 days, the majority of the complexes were in the base rate or sleep rate bins. Rate modulation had not yet been enabled and there were relatively few native atrial rates above 75 bpm. The system functioned in a nontracking mode approximately 3% of the time (AMS bin) with 1,776 mode switch episodes. Based on this event histogram demonstrating the presence of chronotropic incompetence, rate-modulation was enabled.

complexes which are labeled atrial sensed-ventricular sensed (PR) imply an intact atrial rhythm with intact AV nodal conduction. This may not be the case. Significant number of PR and even AR (atrial paced-ventricular sensed) complexes may occur in the presence of complete heart block if there are frequent ventricular ectopic beats that coincidentally occur after a P wave or atrial paced complex.

Similarly, some systems identify an event sensed on the ventricular channel of the pacemaker which is not preceded by an atrial event, either paced or sensed, as a premature ventricular contraction (PVC). PVC's have a very definite implication for the clinician. The pacemaker's definition is far more specific as the pacemaker cannot analyze the morphology of the complex. Hence, nonphysiologic make-break electrical potentials associated with an internal insulation failure or conductor fracture will also be identified as PVCs as will accelerated junctional rhythms or episodes of atrial undersensing but with intact AV nodal conduction. Some systems may also identify runs of ventricular ectopic beats specifically labeling these episodes ventricular tachycardia but an AV nodal reentrant tachycardia would be labeled VT by these systems as the retrograde P wave would coincide with the atrial refractory period of the pacemaker and not be sensed. By the same token, a true PVC occurring coincidentally after a native P wave would be labeled a PR complex implying intact conduction which was not the case. One cannot interpret the event counter data in a vacuum. It must be interpreted in the context of the clinical status of the patient combined with the knowledge that there is an appropriate safety margin for capture and sensing.

Subsystem Performance Counter

These event counters report on the performance of one specific algorithm or subsystem within the overall pacing system. They include but are not limited to a sensor-indicated rate histogram, an automatic mode switch histogram, a long-term capture threshold graph, a high rate episode counter, and a sudden-rate drop response counter. In some cases, the specific events have a date and time stamp. The value of the subsystem performance counter is the detailed information that it provides with respect to the behavior of a specific algorithm or feature of the implanted device. The strength of these counters is also their major limitation, a very focused and limited view of device behavior being restricted to the specific feature which is being monitored. An example is the high rate episode counter from a Medtronic Thera([Medtronic, Inc., Minneapolis, MN] pacemaker (Fig. 19.13). While it provides a date and time stamp for seven high rate episodes along with a graphic depiction of these individual episodes and a single 2.3 s segment of stored atrial electrogram associated with one of the episodes, there is no information provided as to the overall system behavior. The level of detail for the behavior of this specific algorithm would not be feasible within a total system performance counter.

Another subsystem performance counter is the stored electrograms which are triggered by either the patient or activation of a specific algorithm. Stored electrograms, for diagnostic resolution, require a massive amount of memory. One way around this is to use compression algorithms but if the data is compressed to too great a degree, the resultant quality of the data may limit its ability to be interpreted (Fig. 19.14). One can also use this very precise data to determine if the implanted system is responding to a true arrhythmia or some other event such as a far-field R wave thus inappropriately activating a given algorithm such as mode switch. Depending on the capabilities of the implanted device, one can use this information to further adjust the programmed settings.

Time-Based Total System Performance Counter

This is a memory intensive event counter and as such, often holds the smallest amount of information, at least with respect to total duration of monitoring. In a time-based event counter, events are logged as to pacing state and rate with respect to time. When retrieved and displayed, they identify pacemaker behavior relatively precisely with respect to time. This will facilitate an assessment of the pacemaker's response to specific activities and even symptoms if there is a way of storing the pacing system behavior associated with specific events

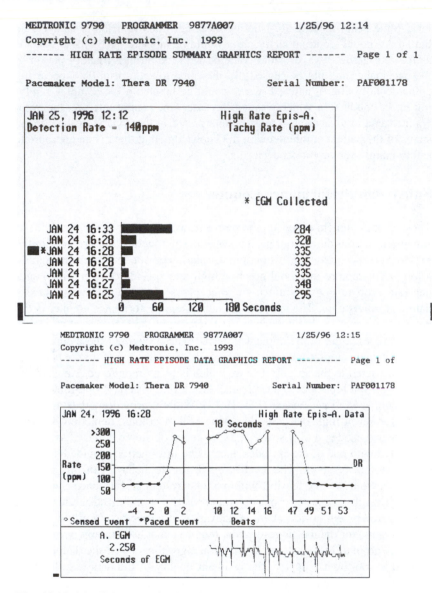

Fig. 19.13 (a) High rate episode subsystem event counter mode switch histogram from a Medtronic Thera. Each recorded episode is identified by time, date, and duration in accord with the allocated memory. (b) Expanded view of one of the high rate episodes detailing the atrial rates (paced or sensed) during the episode. This single counter also provides 2.3 s of stored atrial electrogram clearly identifying the atrial rhythm as atrial flutter.

or symptoms. The display may look very similar to a heart rate trend graphic from a Holter monitor (Fig. 19.15), and in systems with significant random access memory assigned to this event counter, the ability to expand the scale to examine individually recorded events.

Given the amount of memory that is required for this counter, it continuously updates the data by deleting the oldest while adding the newest data. Hence, when the patient is seen and this event counter data is retrieved, the time-based system performance counter may provide relatively detailed time-based

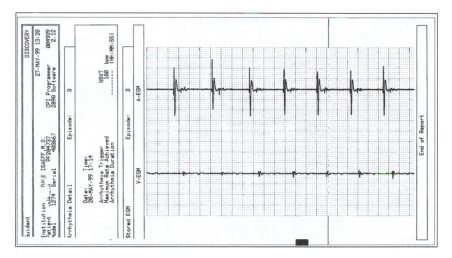

Fig. 19.14 Stored atrial and ventricular electrogram from a patient with a Guidant Discovery pacemaker. Although the system interpreted the atrial rate as a paroxysmal supraventricular tachycardia, the close correlation between the atrial and ventricular rates, the PR interval as measured from the recording, and the normal rate identifies this as a normal rhythm. Hence, atrial sensing of the far field R wave probably accounted for the system's "diagnosis." Knowing this, one can more effectively program the pacemaker and know how to interpret some of its reports.

information over the past 1 h to previous number of days, depending on the sampling rate and allocated memory capacity. To limit the impact on the battery and hence device longevity, some systems such as the stored EGMs from Medtronic require that the duration during which the system monitors the EGM to capture specific events will be programmable with the nominal value being 8 weeks and a maximal programmable value of 24 weeks. St. Jude Medical allows for continuous monitoring or selection of the "freeze mode." In the freeze mode, once the available stored EGMs are filled, the system stops monitoring the electrogram for recording purposes but it will acquire and report the number of triggers that occurred since the counters were last cleared.

On balance, each event counter has its specific strengths and limitations. Having access to all of them simultaneously provides a very effective overview of the system performance since the last evaluation along with specific details as to the behavior of individual special algorithms.

Transtelephonic Monitoring

An integral part of many pacing system follow-up programs is transtelephonic monitoring (TTM) (72–74). This can be initiated by the physician and support staff out of an individual office or provided by a commercial service based on a specific prescription by the physician. Reports of each periodic evaluation are sent to the patient's physician. TTM provides a cost-effective means for frequent monitoring as the implanted device is getting older and there is concern about approaching RRT. It also provides a link between the patient and the physician for those patients who live alone, who are very anxious, or pacemaker dependent.

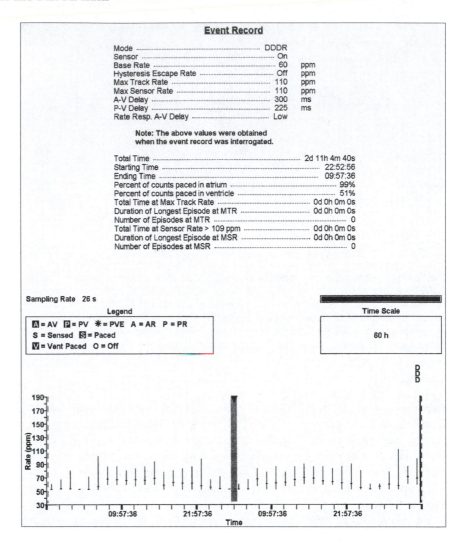

Fig. 19.15 Event record retrieved from a patient with a Pacesetter Trilogy DR + in which sleep mode was enabled. This is a time-based total system performance counter. Set to a sampling rate of 26 s, it provides an overview of the system behavior over the preceding 60 h. The vertical lines represent the minimum and maximum heart rates in each time bin (the overall monitoring period being divided into 40 sub-intervals) with the cross-bar reflecting the mean heart rate. The rhythmic waxing and waning of the base rate documents the normal behavior of the sleep mode. The time scale can be expanded to display individually recorded events, if desired.

The transtelephonic system usually comprises a special transmitter that is acoustically coupled to the telephone when the mouth piece of the telephone is placed over the transmitter. The transmitter is connected to the patient via two electrode cables which can be self-applied although some individuals with severe arthritis or neurologic impairment may require assistance. These are commonly wrist or finger electrodes. The transmitter converts the electrical signal into an auditory signal which is then decoded by a receiver in the physician's office or monitoring station. The receiving unit displays and records the ECG. The pacing intervals are automatically measured and reported. For reimbursement purposes, it is necessary to record 30 s of demand tracing and 30 s of asynchronous behavior (with a magnet placed over the pacemaker). This is then reviewed by a physician who interprets the results of the test with respect to the known behavior of the implanted pacemaker.

These systems commonly identify the pacing stimulus but do not attempt to transmit it via the telephone lines. Rather, it transmits an electronic marker indicating that a pacing stimulus has been detected. The receiver generates a "stimulus artifact" on the ECG to represent the pacing stimulus. If no pacing artifact is actually seen, whether this is due to the low output of the pulse or the specific orientation of the recording system, no stimulus will be displayed on the final ECG. As the recording is a single lead rhythm strip, one does not have the option of examining additional leads. In some cases, it may be difficult to detect an atrial event or even a ventricular event such that one might suspect the patient is asystolic if it was not know that the patient was feeling well and talking to the support staff at a time when the recording was being obtained.

Transtelephonic evaluation is particularly good at identifying markers for battery depletion by measurement of the magnet rate. It is also reasonably good at documenting demand system performance with regard to capture or sensing. There are major limitations including the single lead recording and not being able to adjust rates, other timing intervals and outputs that are an integral part of the office evaluation. For an otherwise stable system, TTM may be needed on a frequent basis while the detailed evaluations are performed much less frequently or on an as-needed basis should symptoms or other concerns arise.

Transtelephonic monitoring commonly provides an emotional umbilical cord between the medical facility and the patient with many elderly patients being comforted by this contact. It is important to counsel the patient that, on occasion, there may be artifacts generated by the telephone lines that raise a concern about a pacing system problem. If these concerns cannot be cleared up by a repeat call, it may be necessary to have the patient come to the office for a detailed evaluation which provides far more information than is presently retrievable via the telephone.

Frequency of Follow-Up Evaluations

The frequency of follow-up and whether this be a detailed in-office "programming" evaluation or a much simpler transtelephonic evaluation should be dictated by the clinical needs of the patient. Often the scheduled frequency is guided by the allowed reimbursement schedule from the Health Care Financing Administration as the majority of paced patients are covered by Medicare, at least in the United States.

The approved Medicare follow-up schedule is detailed in Table 19.4. It is slightly different for dual-chamber and single-chamber devices and whether the pulse generator has a known track record or not. Most of the devices which are being implanted today are relatively new model series and do not have a track record. By the time they do, it is likely that they would have been supplanted by the next generation of device. As such, it is probably reasonable to conclude that while individual manufacturers may have a track record for the overall performance of their systems, their currently released models will not yet have withstood the proverbial test of time.

Table 19.4 Recommended follow-up schedule per HCFA for reimbursement under medicare.

Group I – Devices for which there is not an established track record

Single-chamber pacemakers

1st month – every 2 weeks

2nd through 36th month – every 8 weeks

37th month until RRT – every 4 weeks

Dual-chamber pacemakers

1st month – every 2 weeks

2nd through 6th month – every 4 weeks

7th through 36th month – every 8 weeks

37th month until RRT – every 4 weeks

Group II – Devices for which there is an established track record of good performance

Single-chamber pacemakers

1st month – every 2 weeks

2nd through 48th month – every 12 weeks

49th month through 72nd month – every 8 weeks

73rd month until RRT – every 4 weeks

Dual-chamber pacemakers

1st month – every 2 weeks

2nd through 30th month – every 12 weeks

31st through 48th month – every 8 weeks

49th month until RRT – every 4 weeks

Each physician, based on his or her own experience and commonly modified by individual patient encounters, will develop preferences as to the needed frequency for follow-up (75,76). Our routine is to perform a detailed pacing system evaluation prior to discharge and ask the patient to return approximately 1 month postimplant. Even with steroid-eluting leads which have been very effective in reducing the early rise in capture threshold associated with lead maturation, our tendency is to recommend a relatively high output in the range of 5 V in the absence of AutoCapture. This is commonly higher than the settings which are set in the device by the manufacturer for despite the generally good experience with steroid-eluting leads, there continues to be a low incidence of unexpected threshold rises (44). Presuming that the system is stable, the patient is asked to return about 3 months later which places this visit 4 months postimplantation. At that time, the output is reduced in accord with the desired safety margin for that patient. Another evaluation is performed 6 months after that. The third visit is not quite 1 year postimplantation and if the patient is doing well and clinically stable, the patient is asked to return on either an annual basis, every 6 months or in some cases, every 3 months for a detailed office evaluation which involves everything which had been discussed previously. The elderly confused patient, the patient whose primary care physician is uncomfortable looking at an ECG in case of symptoms, the pacemaker-dependent patient, and the patient who received an investigational pacemaker are all asked to return, at a minimum, on a semiannual basis if it is otherwise stable. If a manufacturer's advisory letter is received concerning a specific model device, the patient may be followed more frequently such as every 3 months. These are the groups that are enrolled in a TTM program early postimplant. The patient who is not pacemaker dependent, who is knowledgeable and without impaired mental capabilities, or whose physician is willing to perform a screening evaluation in the case of symptoms is asked to return for a detailed evaluation on an annual basis. These patients are commonly not enrolled in a TTM program until some years postimplantation or when there are signs of developing battery depletion such as a rising battery impedance.

When transtelephonic follow-up is initiated, it is either on a bimonthly or monthly basis. Bimonthly transtelephonic checks are generally recommended as a less frequent schedule commonly results in some of the patients forgetting how to use the transmitter further complicating these assessments. For the devices which have been implanted for longer than 6 or 7 years, monthly checks are recommended.

Recording Artifacts

The bane of everyone's existence is recording artifacts (77–82). These include but are not limited to the specific dipole or size of the intrinsic pacing stimulus artifact (bipolar or very low output unipolar) making it difficult to detect on a given ECG lead. Other monitoring and recording systems generate a uniform amplitude "pacemaker stimulus" to every high-frequency transient that is seen making it difficult to separate a true pacing stimulus from a pseudostimulus. Pseudostimuli may raise concerns about runaway systems, noncapture, and/or failure to sense (Fig. 19.16) Recording tape or paper speed changes may mimic a change in the paced rate when this is stable while fusion beats may result in a cancellation of electrical forces such that the pacing stimulus may be seen without an apparent evoked potential raising concerns about loss of capture. On a rare occasion, the paced or native depolarization may be absolutely isoelectric in a given lead such that there appears to be loss of capture (Fig. 19.17).

As with a suggested problem based on a transtelephonic evaluation, it is appropriate to carefully evaluate the patient when a single lead recording suggests a problem yet the patient is asymptomatic. This includes examining the rhythm using other lead orientation as well as confirming capture and sensing using the techniques discussed in this chapter.

Provocative Tests

On occasion, the pacing system will appear to be entirely normal as judged by the measured data telemetry, capture threshold, and sensing threshold evaluations yet the patient has reported intermittent symptoms or the pulse generator or lead is the subject of a manufacturer's advisory. At these times, it is appropriate to subject the patient to a variety of provocative tests in an effort to both unmask a problem and reproduce the patient's symptoms. At other times, it is appropriate to screen the patient for specific clinical events that are commonly associated with pacing in an effort to prevent an adverse patient–pacemaker interaction.

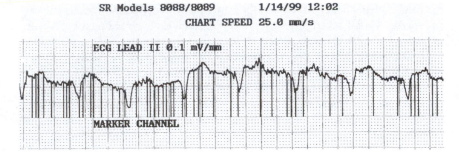

Fig. 19.16 The Medtronic 9790 programmer generates a uniform amplitude "pacemaker" spike in response to any high-frequency transient. Although the paced rhythm can be seen in the background, the multiple pacing stimuli are arising from an unknown source extrinsic to the pacemaker and distorted the recording markedly impeding the pacing system evaluation.

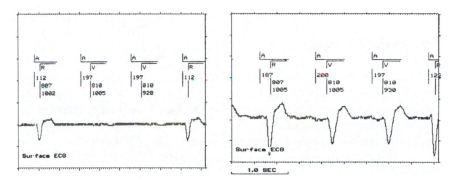

Fig. 19.17 The lead II rhythm strip on the left which was initially monitored had an absolutely isoelectric paced QRS giving the impression of noncapture with impressive asystolic pauses. The patient, however, was asymptomatic and the pulse was stable indicating that there was a heartbeat despite the absence of a visible QRS complex on the ECG. A lead III rhythm strip is shown on the right panel and clearly demonstrates the presence of effective capture associated with the ventricular output.

One of these is myopotential oversensing resulting in either pacemaker inhibition or triggering based on the mode and channel in which sensing is occurring. This is particularly important in the unipolar sensing configuration. Another is the determination as to whether the patient is able to conduct the electrical activity in the heart in a retrograde direction predisposing to an endless loop or pacemaker-mediated tachycardia if the pacemaker is not programmed appropriately. If known, the pacemaker may be specifically programmed to prevent these adverse interactions from occurring.

Myopotential Oversensing

If the pacemaker is programmed to a sufficiently high sensitivity value, it may detect the electrical signal arising from a contiguous skeletal muscle (61–63). In the unipolar sensing configuration with the pulse generator located in the

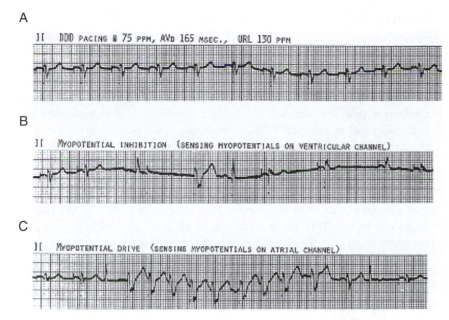

Fig. 19.18 Myopotential oversensing recorded with a standard ECG machine during provocative testing. The top tracing (**a**) shows stable AV pacing in a dual-unipolar DDD pacing system. The middle tracing (**b**) shows oversensing on the ventricular channel with pacing system inhibition demonstrated by programming the ventricular channel to a very sensitive setting. The bottom tracing (**c**) shows myopotential oversensing on the atrial channel unmasked by reducing the ventricular sensitivity so that it no longer saw the myopotential signals. These signals were interpreted as P waves on the atrial channel initiating a burst of atrial-triggered ventricular pacing.

upper chest, the signal most commonly arises from contraction of the pectoral major muscle (Fig. 19.18). For epicardial unipolar systems where the pulse generator is located in an abdominal pocket superficial to the rectus abdominus muscle, the simple act of sitting up from a supine position may trigger myopotential oversensing. This may be a particular issue in dual-chamber unipolar systems where the myopotentials are detected on the more sensitive atrial channel triggering periods of rapid ventricular pacing and depending on the algorithm design, potentially inducing mode switch episodes. In either the bipolar or unipolar sensing configuration, electrical potentials arising in the diaphragm may be detected and transiently impact the behavior of the pacemaker.

A variety of techniques have been used to unmask myopotential sensing. These include tensing the underlying muscle. With the upper chest, this may involve voluntary tightening of it or using the arm which is ipsilateral to the pacemaker implant to reach over and grab the other side of the chest. With an abdominal implant, the patient can be asked to perform a series of sit-ups. If diaphragmatic stimulation is suspected, the patient should be asked to take a deep breath. If the patient had complained of intermittent symptoms, have the patient go through the motions that were being done at the time of the symptoms. This may demonstrate the problem. While this is being done, the ECG potentially with event markers should be monitored.

Retrograde Conduction and Endless Loop Tachycardias

The present generation of pacemakers is not yet capable of differentiating rhythms based on electrogram morphology although this capability has been introduced into some recently released ICDs. As such, whether the atrial depolarization arises from the sinus node, the left atrium, or is a result of backward conduction from the ventricle (retrograde conduction), the pacemaker will treat each event as a proper "P" wave assuming that it occurs during the atrial alert period. In the DDD mode, the P wave will be tracked triggering delivery of a ventricular paced complex at the end of either the sensed AV delay or maximum tracking rate, which ever is longer. If the atrial depolarization is a response to retrograde conduction, the paced ventricular beat may again conduct retrograde, the atrial depolarization is then sensed and triggers another ventricular output. This has the potential to set up an endless loop or macro-reentrant circuit with the pacemaker running at or near its programmed maximum tracking rate. As this would not be a physiologic rhythm, it may cause bothersome symptoms and even contribute to clinical deterioration (83–86). It is imperative that the patient be evaluated to determine if retrograde conduction is present and if it can be sustained. To do this, some physicians have advised programming the pacemaker to the VVI mode while monitoring both the surface ECG along with the telemetered atrial electrogram to determine whether or not retrograde conduction is present. A stable ventricular paced to atrial EGM interval identifies the presence of retrograde conduction where as AV dissociation demonstrates its absence at the time of the evaluation. One prerequisite is that the ventricular paced rate be significantly faster than the intrinsic atrial rate to preclude a brief period of coincidence between the native atrial depolarization rendering the atrial myocardium physiologically refractory when the ventricular paced event occurs.

A second way that this evaluation can be performed is integral to the atrial capture threshold evaluation. The mode must be DDD and the PVARP should be as short as possible. When there is loss of atrial capture (Fig. 19.19), the atrium will not be refractory on a physiologic basis when the ventricular output is delivered. If the patient is capable of conducting in a retrograde manner, an endless loop tachycardia will begin if the patient can both conduct in a retrograde direction and sustain repeated conduction. Then, using the event marker and the recorded ECG, the V to P interval can be measured as can the tachycardia cycle length and hence, rate. In some devices, these intervals are automatically measured and reported on the ECG display screen and can be printed with the ECG. Once this is known, the PVARP can be programmed to a sufficient duration to preclude the future development of an ELT or one of the unique algorithms designed to identify and terminate an ELT, should it occur, could be activated.

Suspect Lead

The weak link in the pacing system is the thin insulated wire connecting the pulse generator to the heart. It is subjected to a multiplicity of extrinsic stresses which may predispose to either a breach in the insulation or fracture of the conductor coil. While this can occur with any pacing lead, there are some which are less than forgiving of these external stresses and have been identified by their manufacturer as having a relatively high incidence of problems

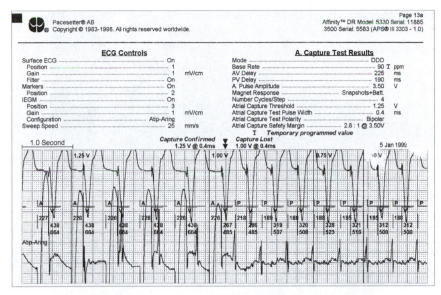

Fig. 19.19 Pacemaker output settings for lowest current drain and maximum longevity induction of an endless loop tachycardia during an atrial capture threshold test in a patient with a Pacesetter Affinity DR pacing system. The automatic PMT detection and termination algorithm recognized the tachycardia and promptly terminated it. Meanwhile, the recording provided details as to the tachycardia interval and the retrograde conduction interval providing guidance as to programming the PVARP.

over the 3–5 years since implantation. In these cases, a safety alert might be sent to all the physicians who had been identified as having either implanted or responsible for monitoring one or more patients with the suspect lead. The manufacturer will commonly provide guidance as to follow-up maneuvers including maneuvers that may be helpful in unmasking an occult problem if not obvious with the patient lying quietly on the examination table. A prime example is the insulation deterioration associated with a number of different model leads from many manufacturers. If everything checks out as being normal on the baseline evaluation, particularly after multiple repeated interrogations, having the patient reach towards the ceiling or rotate and place the arm as far as possible behind his or her back using the arm which is ipsilateral to the implanted pacing system may demonstrate a problem. During these and other maneuvers, the ECG should be monitored along with event markers, electrograms, and lead impedance measurements if the implanted pulse generator provides these capabilities.

On occasion, office-based testing may not be adequate and ancillary tests will be required to complete the evaluation.

Ancillary Testing

Chest X-ray

The chest x-ray is a valuable test to evaluate the position of the lead, subsequent dislodgment, or mechanical disruption of the lead. As such, a baseline x-ray is required for future comparison purposes. It is recommended that an

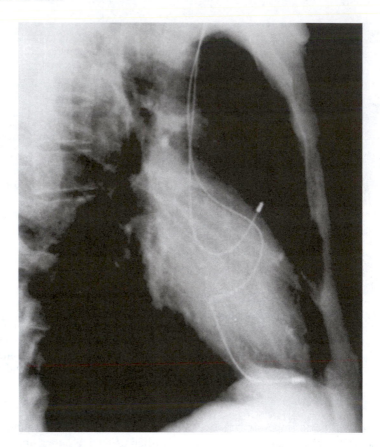

Fig. 19.20 Lateral chest x-ray from a patient with a dual-unipolar DDD pacing system. The course of the ventricular lead is bizarre and attributed to a very pronounced pectus excavatum chest wall deformity. Capture thresholds were excellent, the paced QRS had a LBBB pattern, and a transesophageal echo confirmed that the lead was in the right ventricle.

over-penetrated PA and lateral chest x-ray be obtained prior to the patient's discharge from the hospital. With active fixation leads being used to an increasing degree, it almost does not matter where the lead is located as long as the system is functioning properly (Fig. 19.20). However, one should not reoperate in an effort to treat the chest x-ray showing an unusual location of the lead if the system is otherwise functioning properly. This x-ray provides the baseline for future comparison should problems develop.

In some cases, it is important to periodically repeat the chest x-ray. This is particularly the case with systems which do not have lead impedance telemetry measurements or there is another concern such as a fracture of the retention wire as in the Accufix J lead which will not have any overt electrical manifestations.

Echo-Doppler and Other Measures of Hemodynamics

While this testing need not be done on a routine basis with standard dual-chamber pacing systems, its utility increases in cardiac resynchronization systems. With respect to single-and dual-chamber pacing systems, it can be used to optimize the programmed parameters of the pacemaker with respect

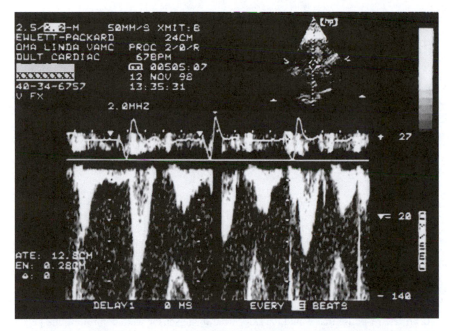

Fig. 19.21 A panel from an echo-Doppler study on a patient with complete heart block and a VVI pacemaker. While the intrinsic sinus activity cannot be seen on this figure, the marked beat-to-beat variation in "stroke volume" recorded in the LV outflow tract confirmed the clinical impression that he would benefit from an upgrade to a dual-chamber pacing system.

to the ideal AV delay or to demonstrating that the patient might benefit from restoration of AV synchrony if a single-chamber pacemaker had been implanted (Fig. 19.21). With CRT systems, it is valuable to optimize both the AV and V-V delays. During this testing, particularly with a dual-chamber pacing system, it will be necessary to make the various measurements of cardiac function at a variety of paced or sensed AV delays in order to determine which might be optimal for the patient.

In addition to echo-Doppler studies, invasive hemodynamic monitoring has been utilized as has radionuclide angiography and noninvasive transthoracic bioimpedance.

Exercise Tolerance Test

It is sometime necessary to perform a formal exercise stress test in an effort to program the rate-modulated features of the pacemaker. This is commonly less than fully optimal as many patients are frightened when asked to walk on the treadmill and tend to hold onto the hand rail. As such, their gate is different from that which they utilize during the course of their normal daily activities. If one is setting up the pacemaker to provide rate-modulated support during their normal activities, it is these activities which should be monitored, not the artificial environment of the exercise lab. Some of the subsystem performance counters such as the Sensor-indicated rate histogram, the prediction model (Fig. 19.22) or exercise test capabilities will facilitate this evaluation eliminating the need for a formal exercise tolerance test and allow the sensor behavior to be monitored and adjusted with the patient performing a normal series of activities.

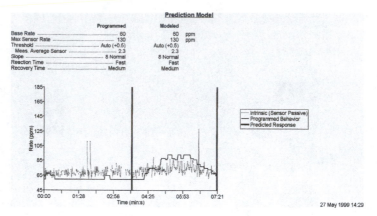

Fig. 19.22 A patient was exercised in an effort to set-up the rate modulated features of his pacemaker as he was identified as having chronotropic incompetence complicating his marked sinus node dysfunction. Rather than using a formal exercise lab, he was taken for a walk in the Clinic corridor and then the Prediction Model of his Trilogy DR + pulse generator was accessed. The period between the two heavy vertical lines represents this exercise. The dotted lines represent the chaotic activity of his atrium during the walk. The sensor had been disengaged (passive) and the thin solid line shows the heart rate response that would have occurred if the sensor were controlling the paced rate at the displayed programmed parameters.

When the exercise test is being performed to evaluate concomitant ischemia, it will be necessary to use an ancillary method for evaluating the presence or absence of ischemia as the baseline ECG will be abnormal with a markedly abnormal ST-T wave. In the presence of both a pace rhythm from the RV apex as well as a spontaneous LBBB, there may be septal perfusion abnormalities detected by a thallium scan even in the absence of atherosclerotic coronary artery disease. The abnormal activation sequence will also cause an abnormal contraction pattern that may impair a stress-echo study.

Ambulatory Electrocardiographic Monitoring

Ambulatory electrocardiographic monitoring in the form of either a Holter monitor or an event recorder is very valuable for detecting frequent symptomatic episodes and determining whether these episodes are related to the pacing system function. They have also been recommended as part of the routine surveillance program as isolated episodes of atrial undersensing or some oversensing which is totally asymptomatic may be detected (87). These do not usually need be addressed if asymptomatic.

If one wishes to obtain an overview of the system behavior, the event counter diagnostics will frequently provide as much if not more information than a Holter monitor, does not impede the individual's ability to pursue their normal activities, is immediately available at the time of a routine follow-up visit, and does not increase the overall expense associated with the patient's care.

Patient Management During a Safety Alert or Recall

Manufacturers are carefully supervised by a number of regulatory authorities. In the United States, it is the Food and Drug Administration while it is HBD in Canada, and MDA in the United Kingdom. There are similar regulatory agencies in Japan, Australia, and other countries. One of the ongoing requirements that all companies must comply with is timely notification of the regulatory authority of both minor and major problems identified in their devices. These are complex devices which are subject to a multiplicity of stresses once they have been implanted. What is remarkable is the overall superb performance of most of the devices. However, if and when a systematic problem is recognized, the clinician who is registered with the manufacturer as either having implanted the pulse generator or as being responsible for following the patient with a particular device will receive either a special technical note describing the behavior or a Safety Alert providing guidelines as to patient management. Hence, if a patient enters a physician's practice with an already implanted pulse generator, it is important that the manufacturer be notified as to who is now responsible for following this patient.

In the setting of a Safety Alert or Advisory, the final decision regarding patient management rests with the clinician. This is why it is so important to know if the patient is pacemaker dependent and the results of prior periodic assessments. The only thing that may need to be done when such a letter is received is to check the patient's record and depending on the identified problem, if the measurements from the device had been retained in the chart allowing confirmation of normal function, no addition testing may be required. The patient might not even need to be called into the office outside of their routine surveillance schedule. In other cases, it would be appropriate to check the system in detail, even more so if prior records are not available or had not been retained. Depending on the device behavior combined with the clinical status of the patient, the required action could range from no change in the routine scheduled follow-up to an increased frequency of evaluation or the prophylactic replacement of the pulse generator or lead.

Should a device malfunction be identified or when a device is explanted in response to a Safety Alert, it is extremely important that the explanted unit be returned to the manufacturer along with copies of any noninvasive or invasive documentation that may be available. This is the only way that the manufacturer has for determining whether or not there really is a problem. In addition, if the clinician is unsure as to the meaning of some of the data that was retrieved from the pacemaker, the technical support engineers that are available 24 h a day, 7 days a week from each of the manufacturers should be contacted. The observed behavior may represent totally normal function of a unique algorithm or functional eccentricity of the specific device which does not warrant an operative intervention.

Documentation

Documentation is essential to the follow-up evaluation. This should include a summary of the physical exam and history, even if limited, along with the results of any testing, programming changes, and the reasons for these changes. The prior evaluations should be reviewed and any changes noted with respect to earlier results such as increases or decreases in capture and sensing thresholds and lead impedance. While changes are expected in the first couple of months postimplantation, a late rise in the capture or sensing threshold may be an earlier marker for a developing lead problem or changes in the underlying myocardial substrate at the electrode–tissue interface.

These records may also be essential for reimbursement purposes and documentation not only that service was actually provided but the full extent of the evaluation. If the records are not available, one might be subject to charges of fraud (88) and at a minimum, have to spend additional time with letter justifying the charges. All of this can be minimized if not avoided by adequate documentation in the medical record.

Detailed records are also essential for patient management as there are few physicians who can recall the exact reasons why they may have prescribed a specific feature in a given patient 5 or 6 years after the fact or in some cases, at the next follow-up visit. In addition, if the physician's judgment is ever called into question during litigation, the documentation as to what was done and potentially why a specific change was made could be critical. Without this, even the appropriate decision may be called into question.

Having completed the evaluation, a final pacemaker prescription is "written." Based on the assessment of the capture and sensing thresholds along with the event counters, the presence or absence of pacemaker dependency, and the underlying indication for pacing, the desired parameters are programmed. Once this is completed, the pacemaker is programmed and a final printout is obtained (Fig. 19.23). Besides placing a copy of this printout in the office record and pacemaker chart, if there are two separate records, a copy is given to the patient. Most patients will not understand the information on the printout, however they are advised to carry it with them along with their pacemaker identification card. Should a problem develop and they are taken to the emergency room of any hospital or see another physician who had not been sent a copy of the follow-up report, they will have the detailed information as to how the pacemaker is presently programmed if questions arise as to how the pacemaker is functioning.

As an aide to the evaluation so that nothing is overlooked, we have developed a worksheet that is then used to generate the final summary note. This is shown in Fig. 19.24. The front side of the sheet has clinical data based on history and the examination while the reverse side has the detailed measurements from the pacing system including capture and sensing thresholds. As noted at the bottom (Fig. 19.24), special information that may impact the follow-up schedule such as unstable threshold, pacemaker dependency, on advisory, and for devices that have been implanted for many years, a indication of their age can be identified.

A separate pacemaker chart is maintained where all the printouts are stored in conjunction with the final report. A copy of the final report is also placed in the hospital chart as our patients are followed in a separate clinic which is based in the hospital. If all the printouts were also included in these records, they would rapidly be congested with information that would not be understood by the noncardiologist. In the pacemaker chart, there is an area for lead and pulse generator information (model and serial number) along with the RRT and EOL behavior of the pacemaker.

St. Jude Medical
Cardiac Rhythm Management Division
© 1983-1999. St. Jude Medical, Inc.

Page 35a
Affinity® DR Model: 5330 Serial: 13927
3510 Serial: 00336 (3303 - 1.02)

Basic Parameters

	Initial		Present	
Mode	DDD	=>	DDDR	
Base Rate	60	=>	70	ppm
Hysteresis Rate	Off		Off	ppm
Rest Rate	Off	=>	55	ppm
Max Track Rate	120		120	ppm
2 : 1 Block Rate	142	=>	135	ppm
AV Delay	170	=>	200	ms
PV Delay	150	=>	170	ms
Rate Resp. AV/ PV Delay	Off		Off	
Shortest AV/ PV Delay	70		70	ms
Ventricular Refractory	250		250	ms
Atrial Refractory	275		275	ms
Ventricular:				
V. AutoCapture	Off	=>	On	
Automatic Pulse Amplitude	*	=>	0.875	V
E/R Sensitivity	*	=>	4.7	mV
V. Pulse Amplitude	3.50	=>	*	V
V. Pulse Width	0.4	=>	0.5	ms
V. Sensitivity	2.0		2.0	mV
V. Pulse Configuration	Bipolar	=>	Unipolar	
V. Sense Configuration	Bipolar		Bipolar	
Atrial:				
A. Pulse Amplitude	3.50	=>	4.00	V
A. Pulse Width	0.4	=>	0.5	ms
A. Sensitivity	0.4		0.4	mV
A. Pulse Configuration	Bipolar		Bipolar	
A. Sense Configuration	Bipolar		Bipolar	
Magnet Response	Battery Test		Battery Test	

Extended Parameters

	Initial		Present	
AutoIntrinsic Conduction Search™	Off	=>	100	ms
Negative AV/PV Hysteresis / Search	Off		Off	ms
Auto Mode Switch	DDI	=>	DDIR	
Atrial Tachycardia Detection Rate	180		180	ppm
Post Vent. Atrial Blanking (PVAB)	100		100	ms
Vent. Safety Standby	On		On	
Vent. Blanking	12	=>	40	ms
PVC Options	+PVARP on PVC	=>	Off	
PMT Options	Auto Detect		Auto Detect	
PMT Detection Rate	110		110	bpm

Sensor Parameters

	Initial		Present	
Sensor	Passive	=>	On	
Max Sensor Rate	110		110	ppm
Threshold	Auto (+0.0)		Auto (+0.0)	
Meas. Average Sensor	2.6		2.6	
Slope	8	=>	Auto (+2)	
Measured Auto Slope	*	=>	9	
Reaction Time	Fast	=>	Medium	
Recovery Time	Medium	=>	Slow	

```
*       Not Applicable
=>      Initial value differs from Present value
T=>     Temporary programmed value
—       Unknown/Invalid values
```

Patient Data

Vent. Lead Type	Unipolar/Bipolar
Atrial Lead Type	Unipolar/Bipolar
Implant Date:	27 May 1999 9:40 am

Patient Information

SS#025-07-5361
A LEAD: MODEL 1388T SN:MJ35157
V LEAD: MODEL 1388T SN:MK49035

IMPLANT PHYS: KEN JUTZY, M.D.
FOLL-UP PHYS: DALE ISAEFF, M.D.

Measured Data

Date Last Programmed	27 May 1999 9:53 am	
Magnet Rate	98.5	ppm
Ventricular:		
Pulse Amplitude	0.7	V
Pulse Current	1.6	mA
Pulse Energy	0.5	µJ
Pulse Charge	1	µC
Lead Impedance	468	Ω
Atrial:		
Pulse Amplitude	4.0	V
Pulse Current	9.8	mA
Pulse Energy	15.2	µJ
Pulse Charge	4	µC
Lead Impedance	408	Ω
Battery Data	(W.G. 9438 - nom. 0.95 Ah)	
Voltage	2.76	V
Current	14	µA
Impedance	<1	kΩ

Test Results

Atrial Capture Threshold	2.25	V
Atrial Capture Test Pulse Width	0.4	ms
Atrial Capture Test Polarity	Bipolar	
Atrial Capture Safety Margin	1.8 : 1 @ 4.00V	
Vent. Capture Threshold	0.75	V
Vent. Capture Test Pulse Width	0.4	ms
Vent. Capture Test Polarity	Bipolar	
P-Wave Amplitude	1.0	mV
Atrial Sense Test Polarity	Bipolar	
Atrial Sense Safety Margin	2.5 : 1 @ 0.40mV	
R-Wave Amplitude	5.0	mV
Vent. Sense Test Polarity	Bipolar	
Vent. Sense Safety Margin	2.5 : 1 @ 2.00mV	
Measured Evoked Response	13.98	mV
Safety Margin	3.0:1@4.7mV	
Measured Lead Polarization	0.39	mV
Safety Margin	12.0:1@4.7mV	
The safety margins are acceptable for AutoCapture.		
Measured Capture Threshold	0.625	V
Automatic Pulse Amplitude	0.875	V
Test Pulse Width	0.4	ms

27 May 1999 10:20 am
St. Jude Medical
Cardiac Rhythm Management Division
© 1983-1999. St. Jude Medical, Inc.

Page 35b
Affinity® DR Model: 5330 Serial: 13927
3510 Serial: 00336 (3303 - 1.02)

Fig. 19.23 Final interrogation and measured data printout obtained at the end of the evaluation.

Role of the Manufacturer's Representative During Follow-Up

The manufacturer's representatives are often superbly knowledgeable about the technical behavior of their devices as well as using the programmer. They can serve as a very effective technical consultant to the physician and staff. However, the responsibility for the patient rests with the physician. The programmed parameters of the pacemaker are, in effect, a pacemaker prescription.

There are two situations in which participation by a manufacturer's representative will play an essential role in the follow-up evaluation. One is to actually perform the assessment but this should only be done under the physician's direction. In this setting, the physician should provide very specific instructions to the individual who is actually using the programmer, be this a nurse, technician, or company representative. For example, it would be appropriate to have this individual evaluate the sensing or capture threshold and then set the pacemaker in accord with the physician's instructions, e.g., set the output to maintain a 2:1 safety margin. The nonphysician performing this test should record hard copy printouts of all test results with appropriate ECG documentation. It then becomes the responsibility of the physician to review these and decide whether or not the interpretation was appropriate and whether copies should be retained in the medical record. Our recommendation is to keep copies of all test results. The programming of other parameters such as AV delay, sensor response, special algorithms such as automatic mode switch, sleep mode, and the like should only be initiated upon the direct instruction of the physician. Who actually "pushes the buttons" is inconsequential.

DUAL CHAMBER
HEART INSTITUTE PACEMAKER CLINIC

Name _____

Date _____

Weight _____ BP _____

Problems Since Last Visit   YES   NO

Chest Pain   ___   ___

Shortness of Breath   ___   ___

Dizziness   ___   ___

Palpitations/Rapid Heart Rate   ___   ___

Edema (ankles/hands)   ___   ___

Pocket (clear)   ___   ___

Daily Pulse Check   ___   ___

Other   ___   ___

Onset/Characteristics (aggravating & relieving factors)/ Course Since Onset/Better, Worse or Unchanged/Effect of Therapy.

_____
_____
_____
_____
_____
_____
_____
_____
_____
_____
_____
_____

Describe _____

Rate _____

_____
_____
_____
_____

	$\bar{s}$	$\bar{c}$			$\bar{s}$	$\bar{c}$
Last Previous Visit, Date			Last Previous Visit, Date			
Rate			Rate			
Rate Interval (msec)			Rate Interval (msec)			
Atrial Pulse Width			Atrial Pulse Width			
Ventricular Pulse Width			Ventricular Pulse Width			
AV Interval			AV Interval			

Manufacturer _____   Implant Date _____

Next Clinic Visit: _____   Next Phone Appt. _____

Rhythm:	NSR	S.T.	AT.FIB.	AT.FLUT.		S.B.
	PVCs	PACs	S.V.T.	Cannot be defined		
	Totally paced Rhythm			Average Rate	/minute	
	Ventricular Aberrancy					

| Type of Pacemaker: | VVI | VVIR | DDDR | DDD | DVI (noncommitted) | |
| | DVI (committed) | | AAI | | | |

| Mode of Pacemaker | VVI | VVIR | DDDR | DDX | VOO | DDI |
| | DVI (noncommitted) | | DVI (committed) | | AAI | VVT |

If **DDD** choose pacing **function** present:

	Atrial pacing	Atrial Synchronus	AAI
		AV sequential	VVI
		Inhibited by intrinsic rhythm	

Atrial sensing:	Normal		Abnormal	☐ Rhythm dominated by pacing, sensing cannot be evaluated
	☐ Undersensing ☐ Oversensing ☐ Myopotential ☐ Present ☐ Absent			
	Normal at_____mv. loss at_____mv.			

| Atrial capture: | Normal | Abnormal | ☐ Does Not Apply |
| | | | ☐ Cannot Define |

Ventricular sensing:	Normal		Abnormal	☐ Rhythm dominated by pacing, sensing cannot be evaluated
	☐ Undersensing ☐ Oversensing ☐ Myopotential ☐ Present ☐ Absent			
	Normal at_____mv. loss at_____mv.			

Ventricular capture:	Pseudopseudofusion QRS	Fusion QRS	Pseudofusion QRS
☐ Normal ☐ Abnormal		☐ One ☐ Occas.	☐ One ☐ Occas.
☐ Cannot define		☐ Int. ☐ Predom.	☐ Int. ☐ Predom.

Hysteresis: _____ bpm.

Magnet Response ☐ Normal ☐ Abnormal ☐ Not evaluated

Threshold Margin Test: ☐ Normal ☐ Abnormal ☐ Incorrectly performed, patient will be contacted again

CONCLUSION: Pacemaker functioning: ☐ Normal ☐ Abnormal
☐ Pacemaker rate is satisfactory
☐ Recommended replacement rate has occurred

CLINIC

Electrograms: P waves = _____mv. R waves = _____mv.

Pulse Wave From Analysis: Normal Abnormal Not performed

Auto Threshold	: **Atrium**		: **Ventricle**	
	: Satisfactory capture	ms v	: Satisfactory capture	ms v
	: Intermittent capture	ms v	: Intermittent capture	ms v
	: Loss of capture	ms v	: Loss of capture	ms v
	:		: :	

| Threshold is: | ☐Stable ☐ Increased ☐ Decreased | ☐Stable ☐ Increased ☐ Decreased |
| | Since_____ | Since_____ |

PROGRAM CHANGES: Please fill out corresponding form.

RTC _____ Phone q _____ CXR: yes no last visit outside facility LLUMC

☐ Unstable threshold ● ☐ Pacer > _____ years ●
☐ Pacer dependent ☐ On advisory

Fig. 19.24 (**a**) Front section of the follow-up worksheet and (**b**) reverse side of the worksheet used in the Pacemaker Clinic at Loma Linda University Medical Center. On a periodic basis, these are reassessed and updated to reflect the evolving capabilities of the devices being utilized.

The second setting in which it is not only appropriate but often essential to have the manufacturer's representative present and assisting during the evaluation is the first few times that a new pulse generator or new programmer is being used. In some cases, a patient will enter the practice with a pacemaker already implanted but which is not routinely being followed by that physician and for which a programmer is not available. In these cases, the follow-up visit must be coordinated with the manufacturer's representative so that the programmer can be provided.

In the ideal world, the manufacturer's representative serves as a technical consultant to the clinician and office or clinic staff. The responsibility for the patient, however, remains with the physician. Even if the physician is not personally performing the pacing system assessment, the physician remains responsible for generating the pacemaker prescription.

Summary

Pacing therapy is no different than other therapeutic modalities. Once initiated, it is essential to periodically evaluate the continued appropriateness of the present pacemaker prescription, the mechanical integrity of the leads, the electrical performance of the pulse generator including battery status, and the overall performance of the pacing system with respect to the patient. The diagnostic capabilities integral to the pacemaker including noninvasive programmability, measured data, event marker and electrogram telemetry, and the ability to monitor the pacing system behavior storing this information in a variety of dedicated event counters until the data can be retrieved have greatly facilitated the clinician's ability to perform these periodic assessments. This can be done in the standard office environment utilizing sophisticated but dedicated computers called pacemaker programmers which are provided by the manufacturers to support their devices. The manufacturers also provide technically knowledgeable individuals both in the field who can come to the physician's office upon the physician's request as well as in the home office to provide technical support to the clinical community facilitating the care of these patients.

References

1. Griffin JC, Schuenemeyer TD, Pacemaker follow-up: An introduction and overview, Clin Prog Pacing Electrophysiol 1983; 1: 30–39.
2. Levine PA, (ed), Proceedings of the Policy Conference of the North American Society of Pacing and Electrophysiology on programmability and pacemaker follow-up programs, Clin Prog Pacing Electrophysiol 1984; 2: 145–191.
3. Castellanet MJ, Garza J, Shaner SP, Messenger JC, Telemetry of programmed and measured data in pacing system evaluation and follow-up, J Electrophysiol 1987; 1: 360–375.
4. Levine PA, Love CJ, Pacemaker diagnostics and evaluation of pacing system malfunction. In Ellenbogen KA, Kay GN, Wilkoff BL, (eds) Clinical Cardiac Pacing (second edition). Philadelphia, W. B. Saunders Publishers, 1999; Chap. 30.
5. Stassen J, Ector H, de Geest H, The underlying heart rhythm in patients with an artificial pacemaker, PACE 1982; 5: 801–807.
6. Levine PA, Why programmability? Indications for and clinical utility of multiparameter programmable pacemakers. Sylmar, CA, Pacesetter Systems, Inc., 1981.
7. Strathmore NF, Mond HG, Noninvasive monitoring and testing of pacemaker function, PACE 1987; 10: 1359–1370.
8. Bernstein AD, Irwin ME, Parsonnet V, et al., Report of NASPE policy conference on antibradycardia pacemaker follow-up: Effectiveness, needs and resources, PACE 1994; 17: 1714–1729.
9. Levine PA, Schuller H, Lindgren A, Pacemaker ECG utilization of pulse generator telemetry – a benefit of space age technology. Siemens Pacesetter, Inc., Sylmar CA, 1988.
10. Kruse I, Markowitz T, Ryden L, Timing markers showing pacemaker behavior to aid in the follow-up of a physiologic pacemaker, PACE; 1983: 6: 801–805.
11. Olson W, McConnel M, Sah R, et al., Pacemaker diagnostic diagrams, PACE 1985; 8: 691–700.
12. Levine PA, Pacemaker diagnostic diagrams (letter), PACE 1986; 9: 250.
13. Furman S, The ECG interpretation channel (editorial), PACE 1990; 13: 225.
14. Olson WH, Goldreyer BA, Goldreyer BN, Computer-generated diagnostic diagrams for pacemaker rhythm analysis and pacing system evaluation, J. Electrocardiol 1987; 1; 376–387.

15. Levine PA, Sholder JA, Duncan JL, Clinical benefits of telemetered electrograms in assessment of DDD function, PACE 1984; 7: 1170–1177.
16. Clarke M, Allen A, Use of telemetered electrograms in the assessment of normal pacemaker function, J Electrophysiol 1987; 1: 388–395.
17. Levine PA, The complementary role of electrogram, event marker and measured data telemetry in the assessment of pacing system function, J Electrophysiol 1987; 1: 404–416.
18. Gladstone PJ, Duxbury GB, Berman ND, Arrhythmia diagnosis by electrogram telemetry: Involvement of dual chamber pacemaker, Chest 1987; 91: 115–116.
19. Marco DD, Gallagher D, Noninvasive measurement of retrograde conduction times in pacemaker patients, PACE 1988; 11: 1673–1678.
20. Hughes HC, Furman S, Brownlee RR, Del Marco C, Simultaneous atrial and ventricular electrogram transmission via a specialized single-lead system, PACE 1984; 7: 1195–1201.
21. Feuer J, Florio J, Shandling AH, Alternate methods for the determination of atrial capture thresholds utilizing the telemetered intracardiac electrogram, PACE 1990; 13: 1254–1260.
22. Sarmiento JJ, Clinical utility of telemetered intracardiac electrograms in diagnosing a design dependent lead malfunction, PACE 1990; 13: 188–195.
23. Nalos PC, Nyitray W, Benefits of intracardiac electrograms and programmable sensing polarity in preventing pacemaker inhibition due to spurious screw-in lead signals, PACE 1990; 13: 1101–1104.
24. Gladstone PJ, Duxbury GB, Berman ND, Arrhythmia diagnosis by electrogram telemetry, involvement of dual chamber pacemakers, Chest 1987; 91: 115–116.
25. Sanders R, Martin R, Frumin H, et al., Data storage and retrieval by implantable pacemakers for diagnostic purposes, PACE 1984: 7: 1228–1233.
26. Levine PA, Lindenberg BS, Diagnostic data: an aid to the follow-up and assessment of the pacing system, J Electrophysiol 1987; 1: 396–403.
27. Hayes DL, Higano ST, Eisinger G, Utility of rate histograms in programming and follow-up of a DDDR pacemaker, Mayo Clin Proc 1989; 64: 495–502.
28. Levine PA, Sholder JA, Florio J, Obtaining maximal benefit from a DDDR pacing system: a reliable yet simple method for programming the sensor parameters of Synchrony. Siemens Pacesetter, Inc., Sylmar, CA, 1989.
29. Levine PA, Utility and clinical benefits of extensive event counter telemetry in the follow-up and management of the rate-modulated pacemaker patient. An introduction to PDx model 3037a software. Siemens Pacesetter, Inc., Sylmar CA, Feb 1992.
30. Newman D, Dorian P, Downar E, et al, Use of telemetry functions in the assessment of implanted antitachycardia device efficiency, Am J Cardiol 1992; 70: 616–622.
31. Stangl K Sichart U, Wirtzfeld A, et al., Holter functions for the enhancement of the diagnostic and therapeutic capabilities of implantable pacemakers. Vitatext, Dieren, The Netherlands, Vitatron Medical 1987; 1–6.
32. Levine PA, Holter and pacemaker diagnostics. In Aubert AE, Ector H, Stroobandt R (eds), Cardiac Pacing and Electrophysiology, A Bridge to the 21st Century. Dordrecht, The Netherlands, Kluwer Academic Publishers, 1994; 309–324.
33. Novak M, Smola M, Kejrova E, Pacemaker built-in Holter counters match up to ambulatory Holter recordings. In Sethi KK (ed) Proceedings of the VIth Asian-Pacific Symposium on Cardiac Pacing and Electrophysiology, Bologna, Italy, Monduzzi Editore S.p.A., 1997; 61–64.
34. Limousin M, Gerous L, Nitzsche R, et al., Value of automatic processing and reliability of stored data in an implanted pacemaker, initial results in 59 patients, PACE 1997; 20: 2893–2898.
35. Machado C, Johnson D, Thacker JR, Duncan JL, Pacemaker patient-triggered event recordings, accuracy, utility and cost for the pacemaker follow-up clinic, PACE 1996; 19: 1813–1818.

36. Ohm OJ, Breivik K, Hammer EA, Hoff PI, Intraoperative electrical measurements during pacemaker implantation, Clin Prog Pacing Electrophysiol 1984; 2: 1–23.
37. Bernstein AD, Parsonnet V, Implications of constant-energy pacing, PACE 1983; 6: 1229–1233.
38. Irnich W, The chronaxie time and its practical importance, PACE 1980; 3: 292–301.
39. Stokes K, Bornzin G, The electrode-biointerface: Stimulation. In Barold SS (ed), Modern Cardiac Pacing. Armonk NY, Futura Publishing Co, 1985; 33–77.
40. Levine PA, Confirmation of atrial capture and determination of atrial capture thresholds in DDD pacing systems, Clin Prog Pacing Electrophysiol 1984; 2: 465–473.
41. Sowton E, Barr I, Physiologic changes in threshold, Ann NY Acad Sci, 1969; 167: 679–685.
42. Preston TA, Fletcher RD, Lucchesi BR, Judge RD, Changes in myocardial threshold. Physiologic and pharmacologic factors in patients with implanted pacemakers, Am Heart J 1967; 74: 235–242.
43. Hayes DL, Effect of drugs and devices on permanent pacemakers, CARDIO 1991; 8: 70–75 (January).
44. Danilovic D, Ohm OH, Pacing threshold trends and variability in modern tined leads assessed using high resolution automatic measurements, conversion of pulse width into voltage thresholds, PACE 1999; 22: 567–587.
45. Syed J, Lau C, Nishimura S, Circadian and unexpected changes in stimulation threshold, PACE 1999; 22: 757.
46. Schuchert A, van Langen H, Michels K, et al., Present day pacemakers for pulse generator exchange: Is 3.5 Volts a sufficient nominal setting for the pulse amplitude? PACE 1996; 1824–1827.
47. Marco D, Pacemaker output settings for lowest current drain and maximum longevity, Reblampa 1995; 8: 159–162.
48. Crossley GH, Gayle D, Simmons TW, et al., Reprogramming pacemakers enhances longevity and is cost-effective, Circulation 1996; 94 (Suppl II): 245–247.
49. Furman S, Hurzeler P, de Caprio V, Cardiac pacing and pacemakers III. Sensing the cardiac electrogram, Am Heart J 1977; 93: 794–801.
50. Clarke M, Liu B, Schuller H, et al., Automatic adjustment of pacemaker stimulation output correlated with continuously monitored capture thresholds, a multicenter study, PACE 1998; 21: 1567–1575.
51. Cameron DA, Hale C, Cusimano RJ, et al., Dual chamber ventricular AutoCapture device, an initial experience, PACE 1999; 22: 854.
52. Nowak B, Kampmann C, Schmid FX, et al., Pacemaker therapy in premature children with high degree AV block, PACE 1998; 21: 2695–2698.
53. Breivik K, Ohm OJ, Engedal H, Long term comparison of unipolar and bipolar pacing and sensing using a new multiprogrammable pacemaker system, PACE 1983; 6: 592–600.
54. Ohm OJ, Demand failures occurring during permanent pacing in patients with serious heart disease, PACE 1980; 3: 44–55.
55. Griffin JC, Finke WL, Analysis of the endocardial electrogram morphology of isolated ventricular beats, PACE 1983; 6: 315.
56. Bricker JT, Ward KA, Zinner A, Gillette PC, Decrease in canine endocardial and epicardial electrogram voltage with exercise: Implications for pacemaker sensing, PACE 1988; 11: 460–464.
57. Frohlig G, Schwerdt H, Schieffer H, et al., Atrial signal variations and pacemaker malsensing during exercise: A study in the time and frequency domain, J Am Coll Cardiol 1988; 11: 806–813.
58. Levine PA, Podrid PJ, Klein MD, Keefe J, Selznick L, Pacemaker sensing: Comparison of signal amplitudes determined by electrogram telemetry and noninvasively measured sensing thresholds, PACE 1989; 12: 1294.

59. Palma EC, Kedarnath V, Vankawalla V, et al., Effect of varying atrial sensitivity, AV interval, and detection algorithm on automatic mode switching, PACE 1996; 19: 1734–1739.

60. Brandt J, Fahraeus T, Schuller H, Far-field QRS complex sensing via the atrial pacemaker lead, I: Mechanism, consequences, differential diagnosis and countermeasures in AAI and VDD/DDD pacing, PACE 1988; 11: 1432–1438.

61. Secemsky SI, Hauser RG, Denes P, Edwards LM, Unipolar sensing abnormalities: incidence and clinical significance of skeletal muscle interference and undersensing in 228 patients, PACE 1982; 5: 10–19.

62. Levine PA, Caplan CH, Klein MD, Brodsky SJ, Ryan TJ, Myopotential inhibition of unipolar lithium pacemakers, Chest 1982; 82: 461–465.

63. Gross JN, Platt S, Ritacco R, Andrews C, Furman S, The clinical relevance of electromyopotential oversensing in current unipolar devices, PACE 1992; 15: 2023–2027.

64. Technical Information Report – Systems used to forecast remaining pacemaker battery service life, Washington, DC, Association for the Advancement of Medical Instrumentation, 1998, Document # AAMI TIR No. 21 - 1998.

65. Jacobs DM, Fink AS, Miller RP, et al., Anatomical and morphological evaluation of pacemaker lead compression, PACE 1993; 16: 434–444.

66. Magney JE, Flynn DM, Parsons JA, et al., Anatomical mechanisms explaining damage to pacemaker leads, defibrillator leads and failure of central venous catheters adjacent to the sternoclavicular junction, PACE 1993; 16: 445–457.

67. Antonelli D, Rosenfeld T, Freedberg NA, et al., Insulation lead failure: Is it a matter of insulation coating, venous approach or both? PACE 1998; 21: 418–421.

68. Ben Zur UM, Platt SB, Gross JN, et al., Direct and telemetered lead impedance PACE 1994; 17: 2004–2007.

69. Danilovic D, Ohm OJ, Pacing impedance variability in tined steroid eluting leads, PACE 1998; 21: 1356–1363.

70. Sharif MN, Wyse DG, Rothschild JM Gillis AM, Changes in lead impedance over time predict lead failure, Am J Cardiol 1998; 82: 600–603.

71. Siegmund JB, Wilson JH, Lattner SE, et al., Impedance of pacemaker leads: Correlation of different methods, PACE 1996; 19: 90–94.

72. Furman S, Pacemaker follow-up in Furman S, Hayes D, Holmes D (eds) A Practice of Cardiac Pacing. Armonk NY, Futura Publishing Company 1993; 571–603.

73. Vincent JA, Cavitt DL, Karpawich PP, Diagnostic and cost-effectiveness of telemonitoring the pediatric pacemaker patient, Pediatric Cardiol 1997; 18: 86–90.

74. Dreifus LS, Zinberg A, Hurzeler P, et al., Transtelephonic monitoring of 25, 919 implanted pacemakers, PACE 1986; 9: 371–378.

75. Greendahl H, Pacemaker follow-up with prolonged intervals in the stable period of 1 to 5 years postimplant, PACE 1996; 19: 1219–1224.

76. Sweeesy MW, Erickson SL, Grago JA, et al., Analysis of the effectiveness of in-office and transtelephonic follow-up in terms of pacemaker system complications, PACE 1994; 17: 2001–2003.

77. Levine PA, Electrocardiography of bipolar single and dual-chamber pacing systems, Herzschrittmacher 1988; 8: 86–90.

78. Lesh MD, Langberg JJ, Griffin JC, et al., Pacemaker generator pseudomalfunction: an artifact of Holter monitoring, PACE 1991; 14: 854–857.

79. Van Gelder LM, Bracke FALE, El Gamal MIH, Fusion or confusion on Holter recordings, PACE 1991; 14: 760–763.

80. Engler RL, Goldberger AL, Bhargava V, Kapelusznik D, Pacemaker spike alternans: An artrifact of digital signal processing, PACE 1982; 5: 748–750.

81. Slack JP, Identification of recording artifact in a dual chamber (DDD) paced rhythm, clues from the electrocardiogram, Clin Prog Pacing Electrophysiol 1984; 2: 384–387.

82. Levine PA, Pacemaker pseudo-malfunction, PACE 1981; 4: 563–565.

83. Levine PA, Selznick L, Prospective management of the patient with retrograde ventriculo-atrial conduction, prevention and management of pacemaker mediated endless loop tachycardias. Sylmar, CA, Pacesetter, Inc., 1990.

84. Limousin M, Bonnet JL, A multi-centric study of 1816 endless loop tachycardia (ELT) responses, PACE 1990; 13: 555.

85. Oseran D, Ausubel K, Klementowicz P, et al., Spontaneous endless loop tachycardia, PACE 1986; 9: 379–381.

86. Levine PA, Postventricular atrial refractory periods and pacemaker mediated tachycardias, Clin Prog Pacing Electrophysiol 1983; 1: 394–401.

87. Famularo MA, Kennedy HL, Ambulatory electrocardiography in the assessment of pacemaker function, Am Heart J 1982; 104: 1086–1094.

88. Saksena S, Clinical practice patterns in implantable rhythm management device therapy: New players and new norms, PACE 1999; 22: 814–815.

Follow-Up of the Patient with an Implanted Cardiac Defibrillator

Ejigayehu Abate and Fred M. Kusumoto

Since the initial development of the implantable defibrillator in the 1970s by Michel Mirowski, and commercial introduction in 1985, national surveys and industry analysts have estimated that more than 160,000 implants have been performed in the United States (1). Multicenter randomized trials have demonstrated the effectiveness of the implantable cardioverter-defibrillator (ICD) for reducing mortality in high-risk patient groups (2,3). It has been estimated that more than 700,000 patients are eligible for an ICD in the United States. The newest generation of ICDs are capable of defibrillation of ventricular fibrillation, pace termination of ventricular tachycardia, single or dual chamber pacing, and cardiac resynchronization therapy (CRT) depending on the model. In addition, ICDs now have multiple additional features including extensive programming options, detailed event histories, and real-time telemetry. Unfortunately, even with the most recent generation of ICDs, adverse clinical events such as inappropriate detection (providing tachycardia therapy when no ventricular arrhythmia was present) and lead failures remain relatively common, approaching 50% in the first 2 years (4,5). In addition, a multicenter study that analyzed terminal events in patients with first-generation ICDs, found that approximately 15% of patients who had sudden death presumed secondary to arrhythmias had ICDs that indicated battery depletion (5,6). Finally during 2005 a number of well publicized recalls for potentially fatal device malfunction caused both the public and physicians to question the reliability of ICD therapy. This chapter reviews the basic follow-up of ICDs, and how to troubleshoot an ICD suspected of malfunction.

Evaluation

Evaluation of the ICD normally occurs in two settings. At the office visit, interval history, physical examination, and baseline interrogation of the ICD are performed (Table 20.1). At times, more detailed information on the ability of the ICD to terminate tachyarrhythmias may be required and noninvasive programmed stimulation is performed in a monitored setting, usually the electrophysiology laboratory.

Table 20.1 Complete office evaluation of ICDs.

Components	Specific points
History	
Symptoms suggestive of arrhythmias?	Palpitations, syncope, dizziness
Symptoms of inappropriate therapy delivery?	Device discharges
Symptoms of depression?	Depression, reduced sense of well-being may be present, particularly in patients who have experienced multiple discharges
Physical examination	
Pocket	Signs of infection
	Twisted leads, which would suggest Twiddler syndrome
	Erosion of the ICD
	Migration of the ICD (downward or to the axilla)
Ipsilateral shoulder	Strength, range of motion
Chest radiograph	6- to 12-month intervals for epicardial patches
	Utility not known for nonthoracotomy leads
Electrocardiography	Probably not required if a biventricular device is not present
Basic device interrogation	See Table 20.2

History and Physical Examination

The history is one of the most important parts of the follow-up of patients with ICDs. Important points to include in the history are summarized in Table 20.1. The patient should be asked about any symptoms suggestive of arrhythmias such as dizziness, syncope, or palpitations. If the patient has an ICD that uses epicardial electrodes, symptoms suggestive of constrictive pericarditis, such as exertional dyspnea, should be sought (7). The patient should also be asked whether he or she had been aware of any device therapies since the last follow-up. During these episodes the circumstances prior to and after the event must be evaluated. Specifically, patients should be asked about the presence or absence of chest pain, whether a rapid heart rate was noted, whether associated syncope or light-headedness was present, and what type of activity the patient was performing prior to the episode. Finally, the physician should inquire about the patient's mental status. Some, but not all, studies have suggested higher rate of anxiety and depression in patients with implanted ICDs (8,9). In particular, devices that fire frequently are associated with a poor sense of well being (10).

On physical examination, the ICD pocket should be inspected carefully. Originally devices were placed in the abdomen because of their large size (240 mg, 145 cm³). Current devices are more than 60% smaller and are now most commonly placed in the pectoral area, either above or below the pectoralis major muscle (4). Regardless of location, the skin overlying the ICD should be examined for erythema, warmth, or other signs of infection; infection occurs in approximately 1–4% of patients (4,11,12). Redundant lead in the shoulder area should be inspected and palpated; excess patient manipulation of redundant lead or Twiddler syndrome has been reported in patients with ICDs (13). The ipsilateral shoulder should be evaluated for range of motion and function. Reduced shoulder function has been reported in the majority of patients with pectoral ICD implants. Fortunately, the problems normally resolved within 1 year after implantation (14).

Routine chest radiography may be useful for identifying problems associated with epicardial patches and transvenous leads (15). Routine chest radiography has less value for nonthoracotomy leads after the first month of implantation unless lead-related problems are suspected, although some have recommended yearly radiographs (16,17). Specific radiographic examples of ICD abnormalities are discussed in Chap. 18. Routine electrocardiography is usually not necessary at follow-up for patients with ICDs but can be useful in specific circumstances, such as identifying the patient with retrograde ventriculoatrial conduction. However, the electrocardiogram is useful for patients with ICDs that are providing CRT pacing therapy to confirm left ventricular capture and to compare QRS morphology to implantation. In addition, continuous ECG monitoring during left ventricular threshold testing can be used to identify changes in ventricular activation patterns that could impact on cardiac resynchronization therapy.

Baseline ICD Interrogation

The essential parts to the baseline ICD interrogation include evaluation of the detection and therapy measurements, real-time measurements, pacing system function, and if present, review of any tachycardia episodes (Table 20.2).

Detection and Therapy Parameters

Detection Parameters: All ICD systems continuously measure bipolar electrograms sensed from two ventricular electrodes. In older devices two separate epicardial rate-sensing leads were used, whereas newer devices use a single endocardial lead that incorporates both sensing/pacing electrodes and shocking electrodes (Fig. 20.1). In endocardial lead systems, two electrodes (tip and ring) can be used (dedicated bipolar design), or one electrode (tip) and the distal shocking coil can be used (integrated bipolar design). The ICD continuously monitors the rate of ventricular electrograms and classifies them into several preset ranges or zones. Malignant ventricular arrhythmias are usually assumed to be present by the ICD when the rate and duration of these electrograms falls within a preprogrammed tachycardia zone. Multiple tachycardia zones can be programmed to allow individualized therapies for tachycardias with relatively lower rates (ventricular tachycardia) and higher rates (ventricular fibrillation). For example, the detection parameters and therapies for an ICD with two tachycardia zones are shown in Fig. 20.2. In this example, if the device detects 12/16 electrograms at a rate greater than 188 bpm it assumes that ventricular fibrillation is present and if the device detects 12/12 electrograms at a rate between 150 and 188 bpm the device assumes that ventricular tachycardia is present. If the ventricular tachycardia detection parameters are met, the ICD is programmed to rapidly pace (using a programmable pacing protocol) in an attempt to terminate the arrhythmia. Pace termination of

Table 20.2 Baseline ICD interrogation.

Components	Considerations
Detection and therapy parameters	
Detection criteria	
Rate/duration	What tachycardia zones are present?
Sudden onset	Programmed on?
Rate stability	Programmed on?
Electrogram width	Programmed on?
Therapies	
Pace termination	Are pacing therapies programmed?
	How many pacing sequences?
	Pacing type: ramp vs. burst
Shocks	What energies are programmed?
	When was the last DFT measurement?
Real-time measurements	
Battery voltage	Is the battery voltage within normal limits?
	If the battery voltage decreases, closer follow-up or ICD replacement may be required
Baseline electrograms	Large R waves
	No baseline noise
Pacing system function	Pacing thresholds
	Are pacing thresholds stable?
	Resistance of the pacing electrodes
	Check the pacing histograms to evaluate whether appropriate pacing therapy is being delivered. Minimize ventricular pacing unless a device with cardiac resynchronization therapy is present
Event history	
Electrograms at detection	
Ventricular fibrillation	Rapid rates, often with signals of varying amplitudes
Ventricular tachycardia	Rapid rate, usually with sudden onset and different EGM morphology than baseline
Atrial fibrillation	Similar EGM morphology to baseline, sudden onset, and irregular signals
Regular supraventricular tachycardia (ST, PSVT, atrial flutter)	Similar EGM morphology to sinus rhythm
	PSVT and atrial flutter have sudden onset; ST has more gradual onset
Noise	Very rapid high-frequency signals
Effects of therapy	Successful treatment?
	Lead impedance if shocked

ventricular tachycardia is frequently associated with fewer symptoms (18). If these two attempts fail, the device will cardiovert the patient with a shock. If the ventricular fibrillation detection parameters are met, the device is programmed to immediately defibrillate the patient. The rate cutoffs, the number of cycles required, and the therapy types and numbers can be individually programmed to provide the most optimum therapy for a specific patient.

Although rate is the primary method that ICDs use to detect malignant ventricular arrhythmias, other arrhythmias, such as atrial fibrillation, atrial flutter, or sinus tachycardia may be associated with ventricular rates that would fall within the rate-detection criteria. Manufacturers have developed additional

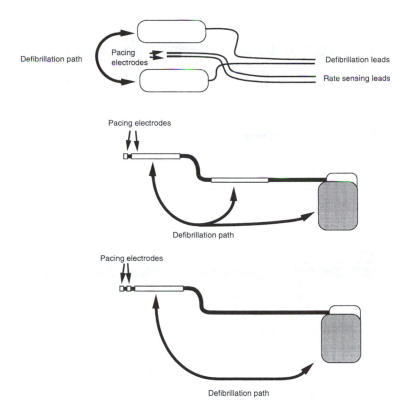

Fig. 20.1 Schematics of three currently available lead systems. *Top*: Traditional epicardial system that utilizes two-rate sensing leads for detection of ventricular arrhythmias and two high-voltage patches that are placed epicardially for defibrillation. *Middle*: Endocardial lead system that uses a distal pacing electrode and a distal shocking coil for detection and pacing (integrated bipolar system). Energy for defibrillation is delivered between the distal and proximal shocking coil electrodes and may also use the defibrillator "can." *Bottom*: Endocardial system that uses two separate electrodes for detection and pacing (dedicated bipolar system). Energy for defibrillation is delivered between the shocking coil electrode and the defibrillator "can."

methods to help discriminate supraventricular tachycardias from ventricular arrhythmias. These programmable options include sudden onset, rate stability, and electrogram width criteria (19–21). It is important to remember that although each of these programmable options increases the specificity of the device and reduces the incidence of inappropriate therapies, programming these options "on" reduces the sensitivity of the ICD for detecting ventricular tachycardia.

To help reduce the chance that an ICD will deliver therapy for sinus tachycardia, most ICDs have *sudden onset criteria* that can be programmed on. If the tachycardia does not start suddenly (often defined by evaluating the prematurity of the first beat of tachycardia), the device will assume sinus tachycardia and withhold therapy. Using sudden onset criteria, the ICD is able to accurately reject more than 95% of episodes of sinus tachycardia. However, using sudden onset criteria, one study found that 0.5% of episodes of ventricular tachycardia were not detected (20).

ICD Model: Gem 7227
Serial Number: PIP110914H

Oct 15, 1999 19:48:01
9962 Software Version 2.0
Copyright (c) Medtronic, Inc. 1997

Parameter Settings Report   Page 1

Detection

	Enable	Interval (Rate)
VF	On	320 ms (188 bpm)
FVT	Off	ms (bpm)
VT	On	400 ms (150 bpm)

Number of Intervals to Detect

	Initial NID	Redetect NID
VF	12/16	9/12
VT	12	12

Sensitivity

Ventricular	0.3 mV

Ventricular SVT Criteria

VT Stability	Off
EGM Width	Off

ICD Model: Gem 7227
Serial Number: PIP110914H

Oct 15, 1999 19:47:48
9962 Software Version 2.0
Copyright (c) Medtronic, Inc. 1997

Parameter Summary Report   Page 1

Therapy	VT 150–188 bpm	VF 188–500 bpm
1	Ramp Pacing	Defib 24 J
2	Burst Pacing	Defib 35 J
3	CV 15 J	Defib 35 J
4	CV 35 J	Defib 35 J
5	CV 35 J	Defib 35 J
6	CV 35 J	Defib 35 J

Brady Pacing

Mode	VVI
Lower Rate	40 ppm

Fig. 20.2 Detection and therapy parameters for an ICD. *Top*: Detection parameters. As programmed the ICD defines ventricular tachycardia (VT) as 12 beats greater than 150 bpm and ventricular fibrillation (VF) as 12 of 16 beats greater than 188 bpm. An optional fast ventricular tachycardia (FVT) zone has not been programmed on. *Bottom*: Therapies for ventricular fibrillation are a first shock at 24 J and subsequent shocks at 35 J. Therapies for ventricular tachycardia are two pacing sequences followed by cardioversion attempts at 15,35,35, and 35 J. Pacing for bradycardia is set at 40 bpm.

To reduce the chance that an ICD will deliver therapy for atrial fibrillation manufacturers have developed a feature called *rate stability*. Although ventricular tachycardia may initially have some R-wave-to-R-wave irregularity, it usually regularizes within 10–20 beats. In atrial fibrillation, R-wave-to-R-wave irregularity continues. If rate stability is programmed on, if a tachycardia fulfills rate criteria, but is noted to have irregular intervals, therapy will be withheld. Rate stability can reduce inappropriate detection of atrial fibrillation but is also associated with underdetection of ventricular tachycardia (20).

The *width of the R waves* sensed by the ICD can also be used to distinguish supraventricular arrhythmias from ventricular arrhythmias (22). Instead of evaluating the electrogram between the tip and a ring electrode or the distal coil electrode, electrograms are obtained between the distal electrode and the more proximally located defibrillation coil or between the distal electrode and the ICD itself. The greater distance between the electrodes allows recording of more far field activity within the heart and makes the electrogram appear more like a surface QRS (Fig. 20.3). Electrogram width can accurately distinguish supraventricular tachycardias from ventricular tachycardias in more than 90%

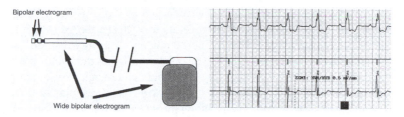

Fig. 20.3 *Left*: Electrograms are usually obtained between two distal electrodes that have relatively close spacing. In addition electrical signals can be measured between a larger distance (wide bipole). *Right*: Signals from the surface ECG (top tracing), close bipolar electrograms (first three electrograms) and wide bipolar electrograms (fourth through sixth electrograms) are shown. Notice that the wide bipolar electrograms have more baseline noise, and that far field activity owing to artial depolarization can be seen.

of cases. However, like sudden onset and rate stability, a small percentage of ventricular tachycardias will not meet the detection criteria, and therapy will be withheld inappropriately (20,21). More sophisticated algorithms evaluate the specific *electrogram morphology* by storing a template during sinus rhythm and comparing the electrogram morphology during tachycardia to the stored template. During ventricular tachycardia the morphology (amplitude, polarity, number, and order of peaks) of the electrogram will generally be different from sinus rhythm due to different ventricular activation patterns. In one study morphology discrimination algorithms alone had sensitivities of 63–78% and specificities of 92–95% (23,24).

The presence of an atrial lead will usually reduce the likelihood of inappropriate therapy (25–28). Each device manufacturer has developed algorithms to use information from the atrial lead to help discriminate atrial from ventricular arrhythmias. In one retrospective study, inappropriate therapy occurred in 22% patients that received single chamber ICDs and only 5% of patients with dual chamber ICDs (26). However, in a prospective randomized study no difference in inappropriate tachyarrhymia therapy was identified between single chamber and dual chamber ICDs (25). Recently the results of the Detect Supraventricular Tachycardia Study have become available (27). In this prospective randomized trial, 400 patients received dual chamber ICDs and were randomized to optimal single or dual chamber tachycardia detection algorithms. For individual patients, the rate of inappropriate detection of supraventriclar tachycardia was 46.5% for single chamber detection algorithms and 32.3% for dual chamber detection algorithms (27).

To reduce the risk of inappropriate withholding of therapy, programmable features such as sudden onset, rate stability, and electrogram width are usually only available for lower rate zones. In addition, manufacturers have developed another programmed feature called *sustained rate duration* (19). If tachycardia persists for a programmable amount of time, the ICD will deliver therapy even if stability or sudden onset criteria have not been met. Sustained rate duration can act as a "safety net," reducing the likelihood of untreated sustained ventricular arrhythmias.

Therapy Types: The therapies for each tachycardia zone should be noted during baseline interrogation. Usually, in the highest rate zone, the patient is defined to have ventricular fibrillation, and shocks only are given. Shocks are delivered by the ICD generating energy by batteries, amplifier, and capacitor, and then delivering the high voltage between two or more specially designed electrodes (Fig. 20.1). In the current generation of ICDs, the generator itself functions as an electrode ("active can"). The amount of energy that the device is programmed to is usually a function of the defibrillation threshold, which is determined at implant and periodically thereafter. In general, shocks are programmed to a value 10 J greater than the defibrillation threshold, so that the heart will be reliably defibrillated, although a recent multicenter study has suggested that lower energies may be equally safe (28,29). Higher energies have the disadvantage of requiring increased time to charge the capacitors and of having more rapid battery depletion.

For the treatment of ventricular tachycardia, pacing protocols are frequently chosen. Pacing has the advantage of terminating the tachycardia with minimal symptoms (18). Even relatively low-energy shocks (1–5 J) are associated with a significant amount of pain. Antitachycardia pacing (ATP) is very effective for terminating ventricular tachycardia. In a large study of more than 20,000 episodes of ventricular tachycardia, ATP was able to terminate ventricular tachycardia in 94% of cases, 5% of episodes were associated with unsuccessful ATP, and in only 1.4% of cases acceleration of ventricular tachycardia was observed (30). Specific pacing protocols for termination of ventricular tachycardia are summarized in Chap. 8.

ATP should be programmed for almost any patient with clinically manifest ventricular tachycardia. In addition, even in patients who receive an ICD after surviving a ventricular fibrillation arrest, ventricular tachycardia is the most common recurrent arrhythmia (31). Recent data has also suggested that antitachycardia pacing therapy may be beneficial in patients that receive ICDs for primary prevention. In a cohort of 93 patients with reduced left ventricular ejection fraction (<0.35) due to either ischemic or nonischemic cardiomyopathy that received ICDs, 39% patients experienced significant ventricular arrhythmias of which two-thirds was ventricular tachycardia (32). Antitachycardia pacing was effective in terminating 86% of the ventricular tachycardia episodes. Traditionally, ATP protocols have been programmed by studying the effects of pacing on arrhythmias induced in the electrophysiology laboratory. In patients without inducible ventricular tachycardia, ATP has usually not been programmed on, because of concerns of acceleration of ventricular tachycardia to a more malignant arrhythmia. Recent studies have suggested that ICD-induced proarrhythmia and acceleration are uncommon, which has led to a trend toward empiric programming of pacing protocols (30–35). The number of pacing trials depends on the hemodynamic stability of the arrhythmia; in most cases two to five ATP trials are tried.

Traditionally antitachycardia pacing has been reserved for slower ventricular tachycardias. Data from several recent trials suggests that pacing therapy may be effective for fast ventricular tachycardias and can reduce the number of ICD shocks (36,37). In one study that evaluated 49 episodes of fast ventricular tachycardia (mean cycle length 286 ms), ATP was effective in terminating 89% of arrhythmias and significantly reduced the number of shocks delivered (35). In the larger Pacing Fast VT Reduces Shock Therapies (PainFREE Rx) trials, ATP was effective in terminating 82–89% of fast ventricular tachycardias (cycle lengths 320–240 ms) with only a 1–4% incidence of acceleration (36,37).

Real-Time Measurements

The latest generation of ICDs allows real-time measurements of several parameters. Most modern ICDs use a lithium silver vanadium oxide battery that provides battery voltages that can be a fairly reliable indicator of remaining capacity. Battery voltages at the elective replacement interval (ERI) vary from device to device because of design differences. Earlier generations of ICDs implanted in the 1980s used lithium silver pentoxide batteries that required evaluation of the battery by first charging the device to form the capacitors, and then repeating the charge cycle and measuring the time required (Ventak C, 1500, 1550, 1600). These devices are not encountered today.

Electrogram morphology during real-time measurements should be noted (Fig. 20.4). The R waves should be large. The R-wave amplitude should be compared to the R wave at implant. Prominent T waves or P waves observed during sinus rhythm suggest the possibility of overcounting. However, the electrograms in ventricular tachycardia or fibrillation are, as a general rule, different from those obtained in sinus rhythm. The baseline should be evaluated for any high-frequency signals; artifacts noted on the electrogram suggest the possibility of lead problems.

Finally, measuring the lead impedance can assess lead integrity. Impedances can be measured at the pacing-sensing electrodes by delivering a pacing pulse and measuring the lead impedance (outlined in the following). Impedance of the high-voltage electrodes traditionally required the delivery of a low-energy shock (approximately 1 J), which was associated with significant pain and the possible induction of ventricular fibrillation. Newer devices allow impedance to be measured across the defibrillation electrodes using a smaller output that cannot be felt by the patient. Changes in impedance have been associated with impending separation between the ICD body and the header (38).

Evaluation of Pacing Function

All ICDs implanted since the 1990s have pacing function. Pacing threshold should be evaluated. (The methodology is similar to that discussed in Chap. 10.) In one study the pacing thresholds of defibrillation leads demonstrated

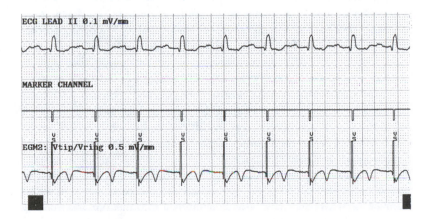

Fig. 20.4 Baseline electrograms from a patient are shown. The R waves on the bipolar electrode (EGM2) are approximately 8 mV. Notice that the T waves are approximately 2 mV. The marker channels show that at baseline the ICD is appropriately counting the R waves (VS) but not the T waves. Chart speed: 25.0 mm/s.

a steady increase over a 1-year follow-up period (39). Similarly, the lead impedance should be evaluated and compared to the value obtained at implant. Pacing lead resistances will vary depending on the design of the lead (integrated bipolar versus dedicated bipolar); measured resistances for a lead should be documented in the patient's chart. Low resistances should arouse suspicion of insulation failure, and high resistances suggest the possibility of conductor failure.

For patients with ICDs that have CRT capabilities, effective CRT therapy must be assessed (Chapter 11). Conversely, for patients with standard ICDs, the device should be carefully evaluated to ensure that minimal if any ventricular pacing is occurring. Several large multicenter studies have confirmed that ventricular pacing is associated with an increased incidence of heart failure. In an analysis of the Multicenter Automatic Defibrillator Implantation Trial (MADIT) II, the presence of > 50% ventricular pacing was associated with almost a two-fold increase in the probability of hospitalization for heart failure or death (40). Similarly, in the Dual Chamber and VVI Implantable Defibrillator (DAVID) Trial, 506 patients were randomized to rate adaptive dual chamber pacing at a basal rate of 70 bpm or the VVI paving mode at a rate of 40 bpm. Death or heart failure hospitalization was significantly higher in patients with dual chamber pacing and right ventricular pacing more than 40% of the time (41).

Evaluation of Tachycardia Episodes

All currently implanted ICDs provide a detailed therapy history. Any therapies that had been delivered since the last follow-up should be carefully evaluated. The electrograms at detection, the delivered therapy, and the effectiveness of therapy should all be noted. The patient's symptoms at the event should also be recorded.

All devices implanted today will provide a summary screen for specific events that required therapy (Fig. 20.5). This summary screen will provide basic information on the arrhythmia detected, therapy provided, and outcome as defined by the device. In addition to this summary screen, the individual electrograms for the episodes are usually available. The onset, rate, and morphology of the electrograms at detection should be carefully evaluated. Ventricular fibrillation usually will have an abrupt onset with very rapid and sometimes irregular ventricular activation (Fig. 20.6). Ventricular tachycardia will have similar characteristics but usually has a slower, more regular rate. In both ventricular fibrillation and ventricular tachycardia the morphology of the electrograms will often be different from that of the electrograms obtained in sinus rhythm because of differences in ventricular activation. Supraventricular tachycardias such as atrial fibrillation or atrial flutter may be difficult to differentiate from ventricular tachycardias; if the electrogram recorded during tachycardia is similar to the electrogram at baseline, supraventricular arrhythmias should be suspected. Unipolar electrograms or electrograms obtained from a wider bipole (tip to proximal defibrillation coil or the defibrillator "can") are available in the latest generation of ICDs, and may provide additional information. The ventricular electrograms in atrial fibrillation will often be irregular. Sinus tachycardia should be considered if a gradual increase in heart rate was observed (Fig. 20.7). Dual chamber ICDs devices allow monitoring of atrial activity (via a separate atrial lead or specially designed floating electrodes located on the defibrillation

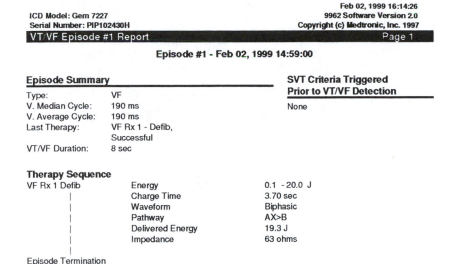

Feb 02, 1999 16:14:26
9962 Software Version 2.0
Copyright (c) Medtronic, Inc. 1997

ICD Model: Gem 7227
Serial Number: PIP102430H

VT/VF Episode #1 Report   Page 1

Episode #1 - Feb 02, 1999 14:59:00

Episode Summary   SVT Criteria Triggered
                                             Prior to VT/VF Detection
Type: VF
V. Median Cycle: 190 ms   None
V. Average Cycle: 190 ms
Last Therapy: VF Rx 1 - Defib,
                     Successful
VT/VF Duration: 8 sec

Therapy Sequence
VF Rx 1 Defib   Energy   0.1 - 20.0 J
     | Charge Time   3.70 sec
     | Waveform   Biphasic
     | Pathway   AX>B
     | Delivered Energy   19.3 J
     | Impedance   63 ohms
     |
Episode Termination

Fig. 20.5 Summary report for an episode of ventricular fibrillation. The duration of the episode was 8 s; 3.7 s were required for the ICD to charge to 20 J. The impedance during the shock was 63 Ω.

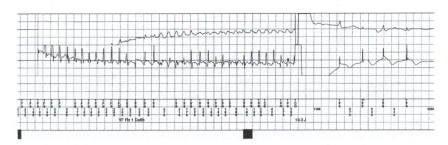

Fig. 20.6 The actual electrograms from the episode summary report in Fig. 17.5. The bipolar electrograms during ventricular fibrillation are relatively large but because of variability some of the electrograms were not sensed by the ICD (signal dropout). This underscores the importance of using a percentage of sensed ventricular depolarizations for detection of ventricular fibrillation. After delivery of energy, the ICD diagnoses "success" because of the slower rate of ventricular activity. CD, cardioversion/defibrillation; CE, end of charge; FD, fibrillation detect; FS, fibrillation sense; VS, normal sense.

lead) and as discussed previously can decrease the likelihood of inappropriate therapies. Noise from myopotentials, T-wave sensing, and P-wave sensing can cause inappropriate ICD discharge, and is discussed more fully in the section on troubleshooting.

The effects of therapy should be evaluated once it is determined that the electrograms and symptoms are consistent with a ventricular tachyarrhythmia. Evaluation of electrograms also provides clues on the effects of therapy. After therapy was given did the patient have return to sinus rhythm or was persistent arrhythmia present? For episodes treated with shocks, the impedance measured during the event should be compared to impedances obtained during shocks at implant. Impedances normally range from 30–80 Ω, depending on lead type

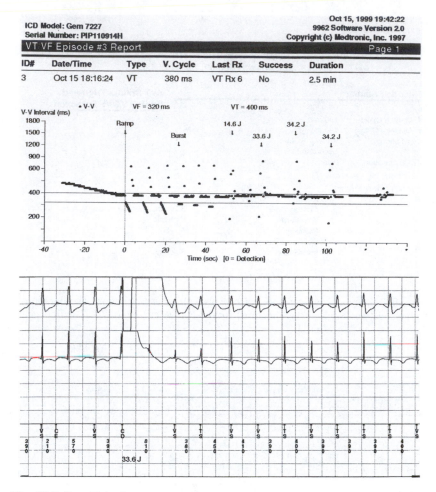

Fig. 20.7 *Top*: Episode report from a patient who received four shocks in rapid succession. In this ICD a rate trend analysis over time is shown. Gradual increase in rate (decrease in the V-V interval) suggests the possibility of sinus tachycardia. *Bottom:* Inspection of the electrograms during delivery of one of the shocks confirms inappropriate therapy for sinus tachycardia. The electrogram morphology during the event was identical to the electrograms obtained during sinus rhythm (not shown).

and position. Lower impedances than those obtained at implant suggest the possibility of insulation break, whereas higher impedances should arouse suspicion of a conductor failure. In addition, the charge time, which is dependent on the amount of energy delivered, should be less than 5–10 s. Similarly, if the episode was treated with ATP, the effectiveness of therapy must be evaluated.

The device counters should be cleared once each tachyarrhythmia event has been fully evaluated. In some ICDs the information can be cleared from the device and downloaded to disk for archiving and future reference.

ICD Monitoring Functions

Some devices provide a significant amount of nonarrhythmia related information for patient management. The current generation of defibrillators uses data from the accelerometer to provide information on patient activity (42,43).

Patient activity data has been shown to correlate with 6-min walk, New York Heart Association heart failure class, and quality-of-life.

Thoracic fluid is associated with decreased impedance between a ventricular lead and the pacing system generator. Two preliminary clinical studies have reported varying results on the clinical utility of thoracic impedance monitoring for predicting hemodynamic status. The Medtronic Impedance Diagnostics in Heart Failure Trial (MID-HeFT) evaluated 33 patients with Class III or IV heart failure due to systolic dysfunction (n = 25) or diastolic dysfunction (n = 8) (44). Thoracic impedance appeared to correlate with pulmonary wedge capillary pressures and importantly impedance decreased by 11% over approximatey 2 weeks prior to hospitalization for heart failure. In contrast, in a cohort study of 115 patients with ICDs that allowed thoracic impedance monitoring, 45 alerts for decreased thoracic impedance were recorded but signs and symptoms of congestive heart failure were present in only 15 cases (45). The investigators reported a sensitivity of 60% and a specificity of 73% for detection of heart failure with intrathoracic impedance. Larger randomized prospective studies are required to determine whether ICDs equipped with hemodynamic sensors are associated with improved outcomes.

Evaluation of the ICD's Ability to Terminate Tachycardia

(Noninvasive Programmed Stimulation)

Although complete interrogation and evaluation in the office will give clues to the function of the defibrillator, particularly if tachycardia episodes can be analyzed, full evaluation of the ability of an ICD to terminate tachycardia requires induction of arrhythmia in a monitored setting. All ICDs implanted since the 1990s have the ability to perform an electrophysiologic test via the device (noninvasive programmed stimulation or NIPS). This important feature allows induction of arrhythmias without requiring the insertion of a temporary multielectrode-pacing catheter.

Ventricular stimulation by NIPS is done using the same protocols that are employed for standard invasive electrophysiologic testing (46). If ventricular tachycardia is induced, the effectiveness of ATP protocols is assessed. At the end of the study the ability of the ICD to detect and treat ventricular fibrillation can be evaluated. Ventricular fibrillation can usually be induced by ultrarapid ventricular pacing (30–50 stimuli/s) or an appropriately timed low-energy shock on the T wave. The defibrillation threshold can be evaluated using the methods outlined in Chap. 8.

The timing and necessity of noninvasive electrophysiologic testing after ICD implantation is controversial, as outlined in the following.

Recommendations for Follow-Up of the ICD Patient

Clinic Visit Timing
The most recent consensus statements from the American College of Cardiology/American Heart Association and the Heart Rhythm Society suggests that devices should be followed at 1- to 4-month intervals, depending on the patient and ICD type (47,48). ICDs generally should also be checked if new cardioactive medications such as amiodarone or sotalol have been started

or if there has been deterioration in clinical condition. Current Medicare guidelines allow ICD follow-up every 90 days. At our institution a wound check is performed 10 days after implant and follow-up is scheduled 1 month and 3 months after implant and at 6-month intervals thereafter with additional evaluation as clinically indicated.

Noninvasive Programmed Stimulation Testing Timing

Although clinic visits provide important information, the efficacy of the ICD for terminating tachyarrhythmias cannot be evaluated unless electrograms from an episode of tachycardia are present. The physician cannot be sure the ICD is functioning optimally, even in the presence of electrograms and historical markers from tachycardia episodes. In the first generation of transvenous ICDs, a gradual rise in defibrillation threshold with time has been described. Although in most cases this rise was relatively small, in approximately 10% of patients the increase was ≥5 J (49–54). Fortunately in the most recent generations of ICDs that use a biphasic waveform and the ICD itself as the anode ("active can"), it appears that defibrillation thresholds decrease over time (49). In a prospective study of 50 patients, defibrillation thresholds were 9.2 ±5.4 J at implant, 8.3 ±5.8 J at discharge, and 6.9 ± 3.6 J at long-term f/u (approximately 1 year). The effect was most prominent in patients with high implant defibrillation thresholds (>15 J) and the investigators postulated that one reason for the findings was "maturation of the pocket."

Unfortunately, implanted leads, both epicardial and endocardial, have a definite failure rate (55–58). In certain leads (Medtronic 6987 and 6921 patch electrodes) the failure rate can approach 30% at 4 years (15). Fractures often occur more than 2 years after implantation, and patients frequently remain asymptomatic. Epicardial patches may develop lead fractures in the lead bodies. Endocardial leads can develop problems at the point of introduction in subclavian leads and at points within the pocket where the large defibrillator presses against redundant leads (56). An endocardial lead system (Medtronic 6936 and 6966) are susceptible to failure due to metal ion oxidation of the middle insulation layer (57). Lead fractures may be associated with ineffective ICD therapy (see the following), but are frequently unsuspected. In a study of approximately 100 patients without spontaneous discharges for greater than 12 months, 1.9% of patients had unexpected lead fractures (59). Lead failure involving the defibrillation coils can sometimes only be detected by performing follow-up electrophysiology testing.

Traditionally, follow-up electrophysiology testing was performed prior to discharge, at 2–3 months, 1 year, and thereafter at yearly intervals (60). Several preliminary studies have questioned the utility of frequent testing in the newest generation of devices (61,62). In a prospective study, Lurie and coworkers randomized 31 patients to either receive or not receive predischarge testing (63). They were unable to detect any differences in clinical outcomes in the two patient groups, and elimination of prehospital discharge testing was associated with a savings of $1,800/patient. Similarly in a cohort of 302 patients, investigators found that predischarge defibrillation testing provided no additional information that would have not been detected with simple ICD interrogation (61). In contrast, other studies have suggested that routine predischarge testing and 2-month evaluation will uncover critical problems in 10–15% of patients, including failure to appropriately sense tachyarrhythmia and lead dislodgment (64,65). One study suggested that patients at high risk for future ICD failure can be identified by the concomitant presence of a permanent pacing system or high (≥15 J) defibrillation thresholds at implant (66). Another study has suggested that routine defibrillation threshold testing may be useful in pediatric patients and patients with congenital heart disease (67). Finally, it has been generally recommended that patients undergo repeated defibrillation threshold testing with changes in antiarrhythmic drugs, particularly with the initiation of amiodarone. Again this may not be required with the currnt generation of ICDs. In a substudy of the Optimal Pharmacolocial Therapy in Cardioverter-Defibrillator (OPTIC) trial, although amiodarone was associated with an increase in defibrillation thresholds the effect size was small (8.53 ± 4.29 J–9.82 ± 5.84 J) (68).

Recommendations for the timing of electrophysiologic follow-up testing of ICDs have not been clearly stated in any of the guidelines. Electrophysiologic follow-up testing should be considered if the patient has been started on new antiarrhythmic drugs (amiodarone or sotalol) or cardiac status has worsened. Current Medicare guidelines allow electrophysiologic follow-up testing when clinically indicated with no time limitations.

Home Monitoring

Transtelephonic monitoring is commonly used for the evaluation of pacing systems (69). During the last several years there have been a number of studies exploring the feasibility and utility of home monitoring of patients with ICDs (70). In the current generation of ICDs patients can use a home monitoring base that can receive information from the ICD (usually wirelessly) and transmit the data to a central location (service center/central server/web site) where the data can in turn be accessed by health professionals or the information is sent directly to the follow-up center. In a study of 271 patients followed for one year, home monitoring data was sent before a routine follow-up visit (71). Clinical information derived from both evaluations was similar in 83% of cases. Particularly concerning was a 14% rate of false negatives (home monitoring suggested normal function while follow-up visit found a clinically relevant problem). Problems with the leads (dislodgment, change in lead thresholds) and misinterpretation of stored tachycardia episodes accounted for approximately 30% of the false negative results. The authors suggested that home monitoring could be used safely if first follow-up visits, patients with intervening hospitalizations, symptoms, tachycardia episodes, or prior lead problems were excluded.

Other Recommendations

The current recommendation is for patients to avoid driving a motor vehicle for at least 3 months and preferably 6 months after the last symptomatic arrhythmic event (72). In a subgroup analysis of 295 patients in the Antiarrhythmics Versus Implantable Defibrillator (AVID) Trial that resumed driving, 8% reported a shock while driving (73). Patients that have ICDs implanted for primary prevention can resume driving once they have recovered from the defibrillator implant. However, it is important to warn patients that the annual risk for defibrillator discharge derived from the large primary prevention trials is approximately 7–8%. Recommendations for driving after pace termination of asymptomatic or minimally symptomatic ventricular tachycardia have not been defined but generally any therapy should trigger a waiting period to determine whether or not significant additional arrhythmias will occur. Patients with defibrillators cannot be certified as commercial drivers (74). Implantable defibrillators can potentially interact with environmental sources of electromagnetic interference, as discussed in Chapter 17 for pacing systems (75–77).

Troubleshooting

Suspected Inappropriate Therapy

The causes for suspected inappropriate therapy (ICD discharge in the absence of symptoms) are summarized in Table 20.3. It is important to remember that approximately 30–40% of patients will be completely asymptomatic with appropriate ICD discharges/therapies for ventricular tachyarrhythmias.

Inappropriate therapy is the most common adverse event associated with ICDs (53). With the first generation of ICDs (Ventak 1500, 1550, inappropriate shocks ranged from 15–25%. Unfortunately, the frequency of inappropriate therapy with the latest generation of devices is probably similar (5). In the Defibrillators in NonIschemic Cardiomyopathy Treatment Evaluation (DEFINITE) Trial, that evaluated the use of ICDs in patients with nonischemic cardiomyopathy, inappropriate therapy was more likely than appropriate therapy (22 versus 18%) (78). A case of an inappropriate shock due to noise oversensing inducing ventricular fibrillation and subsequent death in a patient has been reported (79). Finally it is important to confirm from the device that therapies were in fact delivered; "phantom shocks" are not uncommon, occurring in approximately 6–7% of people (80).

Table 20.3 Causes and treatment options of inappropriate shocks[a].

Possible causes	Incidence (%)	Treatment options
"Phantom" shocks (a shock is perceived but has not been delivered)	6–7	ICD support groups. Counseling
Asymptomatic ventricular arrhythmias	30–40	Often, no changes are necessary
		Consider increasing the time or intervals required for arrhythmia therapy to be delivered.
Supraventricular tachycardia	35–45	Program additional detection criteria (sudden onset, morphology)
		Consider therapy for supraventricular arrhythmias (tachycardia, drugs, or AV node ablation for atrial fibrillation)
		Consider implantation of an atrial lead.
False detection	2–5	Evaluate for possible sources Noise (EMI, lead problems), T-wave or P-wave sensing, or pacemaker stimuli

[a]Shock or antitachycardia pacing in the absence of symptoms.

Causes

Inappropriate therapy can occur in two instances: supraventricular tachycardia that meets the detection criteria for ventricular tachyarrhythmia and false detection in the absence of arrhythmia.

Almost any type of supraventricular tachycardia (atrial fibrillation, atrial flutter, atrial tachycardia, sinus tachycardia) may be associated with a ventricular rate that falls within the detection criteria for an ICD. In one study, approximately 70% of inappropriate therapies are due to supraventricular arrhythmias being misclassified as ventricular arrhythmias requiring therapy (81).

False detection in the absence of tachycardia can occur in a number of situations, which are also listed in Table 20.3. First, if the T wave is of sufficiently large amplitude, T-wave oversensing can occur. In the latest generation of devices that utilize some type of automatic gain, the incidence of T-wave oversensing is approximately 2% (5). Methods for automatic gain control are reviewed in Chap. 8. Second, a small percentage of patients also have an implanted pacing system and double counting of the pacing output stimulus; ventricular depolarization is not uncommon in this situation (82,83). Third, noise detection is a common cause of false detection in the absence of tachycardia. Lead problems such as insulation breaks or conductor fracture can cause high-frequency signals that lead to spurious discharges (Fig. 20.8). Electromagnetic interference from various medical and nonmedical devices is another cause of noise detection. Potential environmental sources of electromagnetic interference are analogous to those reviewed for pacing systems (Chap. 17). However, instead of inhibiting the delivery of a pacing stimulus, signals from the source of interference are counted as ventricular depolarizations and, if frequent enough, lead to delivery of therapy. Finally, algorithms used in ICDs can lead to inappropriate detection. For example, in an older device-lead (Guidant Endotak lead-Ventritex ICD) combination system, noise detection during bradycardia pacing owing to autogain of sensitivity caused inappropriate discharges (82–84).

Evaluation

Usually, with evaluation of electrograms from the suspected episode of inappropriate therapy, the diagnosis is relatively straightforward. As discussed earlier, the electrogram morphology may provide clues whether the tachycardia originated within the ventricle or was supraventricular. In addition, sudden onset of tachycardia makes sinus tachycardia less likely. Conversely, gradual increase in the ventricular rate until it falls within the detection criteria should arouse suspicion of sinus tachycardia, but the reader should remember that ventricular tachycardia might also present in this manner. Noise usually results in very rapid and irregular high-frequency signals. T-wave sensing and double counting of pacing stimuli are often suggested from examination of the electrograms and marker channels. The presence of atrial signals during the tachycardia can provide definitive information on whether an atrial arrhythmia was present during the episode.

Failure or Delay to Deliver Therapy

Causes

Failure or delay to deliver therapy (symptoms without "noticed" therapy) can occur from undersensing, underdetection, and deactivation of the ICD (Table 20.4).

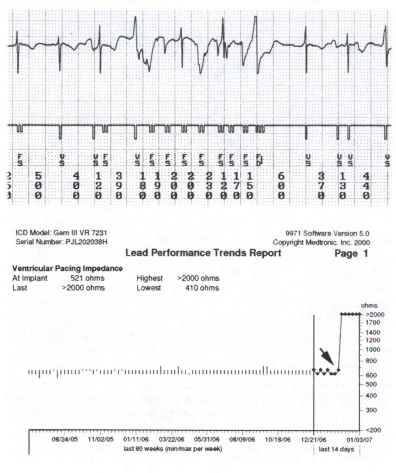

Fig. 20.8 *Top*: Noise detected on the ventricular channel leads to false detection of ventricular fibrillation. *Bottom*: Daily monitoring of lead impedance in the same patient shows a sudden increase in resistance. In this case the patient was notified remotely via a home monitoring system and came to the pacemaker clinic before an inappropriate shock was delivered.

In addition, patients may have transient symptoms owing to ventricular tachycardia that is treated appropriately with ATP.

Undersensing: The amplitude in a ventricular electrogram can vary more than tenfold during a single episode of ventricular fibrillation (Fig. 20.6) (85–87). This variability can lead to "dropout," which can potentially lead to undersensing of ventricular fibrillation. For this reason most ICDs require only a percentage of electrograms to fall within the rate detection criteria. The true incidence of undersensing is not known, but 1% has been forwarded by several investigations (87). Reducing the number or percentage of required signals for detection algorithms can minimize undersensing caused by dropout.

Problems owing to misprogrammed sensitivity are relatively uncommon in the newer generations of ICDs, which incorporate some type of automatic gain control rather than a fixed sensitivity value (as used in pacing systems) (87).

Undersensing occurred more frequently after a shock in earlier generations of ICDs and endocardial leads because of attenuation of the electrogram

Table 20.4 Causes and treatment options for suspected ineffective therapy (Symptoms without therapy).

Possible causes	Incidence (%)	Treatment options
Asymptomatic therapy, or ineffective therapy (antitachycardia pacing)	Unknown	Consider reprogramming the detection criteria to more rapidly provide therapy for ventricular arrhythmias.
		Evaluate effectiveness of antitachycardia pacing electrograms or via NIPS
Undersensing	1	Consider reprogramming sensitivity and observe ICD function in electrophysiology laboratory during NIPS
		Lead status must be evaluated. Lead repositioning may be required
Underdetection	1–10	Review tachycardia rate boundaries and detection rate stability, electrogram morphology may need to be programmed "off")
		Consider therapy for slow ventricular arrhythmia
Deactivation	<1	Reactivate the ICD via the programmer
		Evaluate for possible sources of magnetic fields

(86,87). The decreased amplitude after a shock may be owing to polarization effects or transient cellular injury (Chap. 1) (87,88). In addition, shocks may cause larger signal variability, which increases the risk of dropout. Endocardial leads that used an integrated bipolar design have been reported to be more likely to exhibit postshock signal attenuation. However, increasing the distal tip-to-distal coil distance from 0.6 to 1.2 or 1.8 cm has minimized this problem in the most recent generation of endocardial leads with an integrated bipolar design (88–90).

Finally, lead fracture and insulation break-down have been associated with undersensing. The lead must be carefully evaluated by NIPS, and in some cases operative evaluation is required.

Underdetection: Ventricular tachycardia will not be detected in some cases, even in the presence of adequate sensing. One troublesome cause of under-detection is slow ventricular tachycardia with rates that are lower than the programmed tachycardia detection rate. Patients who receive concomitant antiarrhythmic drugs may be predisposed to this problem owing to slowing of ventricular tachycardia. In one study, 8% of patients who received ICDs developed ventricular tachycardia with rates that had significant overlap with spontaneous sinus rates (89). Similarly, irregularity of the tachycardia, which causes sensed rates to straddle two zones (between sinus rhythm and ventricular tachycardia or between ventricular tachycardia and ventricular fibrillation), may lead to delayed therapy. Another cause of underdetection is programming "on" additional tachycardia detection criteria such as rate stability, sudden onset, or electrogram width. Although each of these features increases the specificity for identifying ventricular tachycardia, they reduce sensitivity for detection of ventricular tachycardia.

Deactivation: All ICDs become temporarily deactivated when exposed to large magnetic fields. Older ICDs manufactured by CPI-Guidant could be deactivated permanently (until reexposed to a magnet for 30 s) by a greater than 30-s exposure to a magnetic field. In addition some currently available ICDs have a feature that will deactivate the device with the application of a magnet. Inadvertant deactivation of ICDs has been reported in both the medical and nonmedical environments.

Evaluation

Evaluation of an ICD suspected of failure to deliver therapy usually requires rapid and judicious evaluation. Any changes in medication should be evaluated closely; amiodarone and other antiarrhythmic drugs may cause slower ventricular tachycardia rates that fall below the programmed tachycardia detection zone. On initial interrogation, the status of the ICD should be checked to confirm that the ICD has not been inadvertently deactivated. The detection parameters of the ICD should be noted, particularly if additional detection criteria have been programmed on. Real-time electrograms should be inspected carefully for the presence of noise. High impedance of the pacing electrodes may suggest the possibility of a lead fracture. A chest radiograph may also show a lead abnormality.

Induction of arrhythmia is required in almost all cases of suspected failure to deliver therapy, in order to evaluate the ability of the ICD to sense ventricular arrhythmias. Both induction of ventricular fibrillation and, if possible, ventricular tachycardia should be performed. Finally, intentional delivery of a subthreshold shock to verify the ability of the ICD to redetect ventricular fibrillation may be required, particularly if an older integrated bipolar endocardial lead is present (90).

Ineffective Therapy

Ineffective therapy during a tachyarrhythmia can obviously have significant consequences and must be treated aggressively. The causes of ineffective ICD therapy are summarized in Table 20.5 and discussed below.

Causes

ICD discharges may fail to terminate tachycardia in several situations. First, change in myocardial substrate, such as worsening cardiomyopathy and myocardial ischemia, may significantly increase the defibrillation threshold (6). Second, antiarrhythmic drugs such as amiodarone and the Na^+ channel blocking drugs (procainamide, quinidine, flecainide) can cause an increase in the defibrillation threshold. Third, in a study of first-generation devices, battery depletion was present in 15% of patients who died with ICDs in place. Finally, failure of the high-voltage electrodes (endocardial coils, epicardial patches) may be associated with ICD failure. The incidence of lead failure can approach 30% in some lead systems.

Table 20.5 Causes and treatment options for failure to provide effective therapy.

Types	Incidence (%)	Possible causes	Evaluation
Defibrillation failure	2–3	Increased defibrillation thresholds (worsening cardiomyopathy, drugs)	ICD interrogation and evaluation with NIPS
		Battery depletion	
		Lead failure or dislodgment	
Antitachycardia pacing failure	5–10	Increased pacing thresholds (drugs, lead dislodgment)	Same as above
		Ineffective pacing protocols	

Failure of ATP protocols to terminate tachycardia is more common. Suboptimal programming of the pacing parameters can be associated with multiple failed attempts for ventricular tachycardia termination. Capture threshold of the pacing electrodes may have increased. Capture threshold may be increased because of medications (Na^+channel blocking agents and amiodarone), and some data suggest that the pacing thresholds for defibrillator leads may progressively increase over time. Some ventricular tachycardias, particularly those present in patients with dilated cardiomyopathy, may be due to increased automaticity. Pacing does not reliably terminate ventricular tachycardia owing to this mechanism. A randomized trial evaluating whether biventricular pacing protocols provide any additional efficacy over right ventricular pacing is in progress (ADVANCE-CRT).

Evaluation

Failure of Discharge to Terminate Tachycardia: On ICD interrogation, the data from the tachycardia episode should be carefully evaluated. The initial electrograms may provide clues to confirm that a tachyarrhythmia was truly present and to help differentiate between atrial and ventricular arrhythmias. The shocking impedance should be checked. A change in the lead impedance should arouse suspicion of lead failure. A chest radiograph should be obtained to evaluate the position of endocardial and epicardial leads. It is not surprising that occasional failures to defibrillate will be observed because defibrillation is a probability function. However, careful testing in the electrophysiology laboratory should be performed in almost all cases of ineffective defibrillation therapy, and reasons for an increase in defibrillation threshold should be aggressively sought. At the electrophysiology laboratory, the leads can be repositioned, new electrodes can be added if necessary, the shocking vector can be changed (for example, taking the superior vena cava coil out of the circuit), and the polarization of the defibrillation pathway can be reversed (Chap. 8).

Failure of Pacing Protocols: In a retrospective review of patients with ICDs and ATP protocols programmed "on" pacing protocols were effective in terminating ventricular arrhythmias in more than 90% of cases (24).

removal of chronically implanted endocardial defibrillator leads may be difficult because of the fibrosis at the shocking coils.

Recalls and Reliability

The reliability of ICDs has come into question in the wake of several well publicized recalls (95). In an analysis of recalls and safety alerts during 1990–2000 52 advisories for pacemakers and ICDs were issued by the Food and Drug Administration. The Food and Drug Administration has defined advisories into four levels (Table 20.7). During the 1990s there were 18 recalls involving ICDs that affected almost 115,000 devices. However, ICDs were generally considered reliable by physicians and the public until 2005 when a death in a young man with hypertrophic cardiomyopathy occurred (95). The cause of ICD failure was an insulation break that caused the device to short and fail to deliver electrical energy to the electrode. The risk of failure was estimated to be 0.1% (96–99). During the same year Medtronic reported a problem of premature battery depletion due to an internal battery short and St. Jude reported memory chip problems due to atmospheric radiation (Table 20.8). In a comprehensive evaluation of the three worldwide registries (Bilitch Registry that monitored 22,786 patients from 1982 to 1993, the Danish Registry, and the UK National Registry), it has been reported that ICD reliability generally improved from initial introduction in the mid 1980s through the late 1990s but unfortunately increased between 2000 and 2005 (96). It is not unexpected that ICD failures will occur, given the quest for smaller and more complex devices. These failures have highlighted the importance of large registries to identify rare but potentially catastrophic problems with implanted cardiac devices and the need for free exchange of information among manufacturers, physicians, and patients.

Once a problem is identified, the response to a recall/ICD advisory can be difficult. In one study involving 17 Canadian medical centers, 2,915 patients with recalled devices were identified, and of these 533 patients had their ICD removed (97). After a short follow-up period (2.8 months), complications occurred in 43 patients (8.1%) including reoperation in

Table 20.7 Food and drug administration enforcement report definitions.

Type	Definition
Class I recall	Reasonable probability that the product will cause serious adverse health consequences or death
Class II recall	Use of the product may cause temporary or medically reversible adverse health consequences or the probability of serious adverse health consequences is remote
Class III recall	The use of the product is not likely to cause adverse health consequences
Notification or safety alert	Communication issued by manufacturer to inform the risk of substantial harm from a medical device. These situations can be of the same importance as class I, class II, or class III recall

Table 20.8 Summary of selected recalls/advisories involving defibrillators.

Company/device	Date	Advisory	Clinical sequelae	Failure rate (%)
Medtronic Marquis	February 2005	Accelerated battery depletion due to an internal battery short	Rapid battery depletion that prevents delivery of effective therapy	0.2
Guidant Ventak Prizm 2 DR, Renewal, Renewal 2	June 2005	Electrical overstress caused by insulation problem within the header	Shorting prevents delivery of effective therapy	Prizm: 0.1 Renewal (2): 0.72–1.8
Guidant Contak Renewal 3, 4	August 2005	Faulty magnetic switch that may "stick" in the closed position	Potential withholding of therapy. Significant battery depletion (up to 45%)	0.01
Guidant Ventak Prizm 2, Vitality, and Vitality 2, Rnewal TR, Renewal TR 2	June 2006	Malfunctioning capacitor from a specific supplier.	Intermittent loss of pacing therapy/telemetry and premature battery depletion	7.6% from the specific lot of 996 devices.
St. Jude Epic, Atlas		Software problem that can occur during delivery of multiple shocks.	ICD may miss a charging cycle or provide a persistent increase in the pacing rate	Unknown. Software needs to be upgraded during ICD interrogation
St. Jude Photon, Atlas	October 2005	Memory chip affected by atmospheric radiation	Temporary loss of pacing function and permanent loss of defibrillation capabilities. The ICD will enter a hardware reset mode that provides VVI pacing at 60 bpm	0.00167

31 patients (5.8%) and death in two patients. In comparison there were three advisory-related device malfunctions (premature battery depletion in Medtronic ICDs) identified during the same period. Remote monitoring may provide an important method for identifying premature battery depletion and certain other types of recalls in a timely fashion and reduce the likelihood of "wholesale" device removal and the attendant complications associated with device revision.

Another issue related to ICD reliability is battery longevity. In a large multicenter trial from seven large centers it was found that only 26% of ICDs and less than 10% of ICDs with rate adaptive or cardiac resynchronization capabilities continued to function 5 years after implantation. Short service life means a significant lifetime risk for complications due to repeated procedures.

Future

ICD therapy has now evolved into a first-line therapy for patients with severe ventricular arrhythmias or at risk for sudden cardiac death. Despite the increased complexity of ICDs, follow-up has actually become more straightforward. Regularly required tasks such as capacitor reforming are now automatically performed by the ICD. Although this trend toward increased automation will continue, even with current and future generations of ICDs, it is clear that problems will continue to arise that will require careful and methodical follow-up by the clinician.

References

1. Bernstein AD, and Parsonnet V. Survey of cardiac pacing and defibrillation in the United States in 1993. *Am J Cardiol* 1996;78:187–196.
2. Moss A, Zareba W, Hall W, Klein H, Wilber DJ, Cannom DS, Daubert JP, Higgins SL, Brown MW, and Andrew ML. Multicenter automatic defibrillator implantation trial II investigators. Prophylactic implantation of a defibrillator in patients with myocardial infarction and reduced ejection faction. *N Eng J Med.* 2002;346:877–883.
3. The AVID investigators. A comparison of antiarrhythmic drug therapy with implantable defibrillators in patients resuscitated from near fatal ventricular arrhythmias. *N Engl J Med* 1997;337:1576–1583.
4. Kadish A, Dyer A, Daubert J, Quigg R, Estes M, Anderson KP, Clarkins H, Hoch D, Goldberger J, Shalaby A, Sanders W, Schaechter A, and Levine J. Prophylactic defibrillator implantation in patients with nonischemic dilated cardiomyopathy. *N Eng J Med* 2004;350:2151–2158.
5. Rosenqvist M, Beyer T, Block M, Dulk KD, Minten J, and Lindemans F. Adverse events with transvenous implantable cardioverterdefibrillators: a prospective multicenter study. *Circulation* 1998;98:663–670.
6. Lehmann MH, Thomas A, Nabih M, Steinman RT, Fromm BS, Shah M, and Norsted SW. Sudden death in recipients of first generation implantable cardioverter defibrillators: analysis of terminal events. *J Interventional Cardiol* 1994;7:487–503.
7. Chevalier P, Moncada E, Canu G, Claudel JP, Bellon C, Kirkorian G, and Touboul P. Symptomatic pericardial disease associated with patch electrodes of the automatic implantable cardioverter defibrillator: an underestimated complication? *Pacing Clin Electrophysiol* 1996;19:2150–2152.
8. Hegel MT, Griegel LE, Black C, Goulden L, and Ozahowski T. Anxiety and depression in patients receiving implanted cardioverter defibrillators: a longitudinal investigation. *Int J Psychiatry Med* 1997;27:27–69.
9. Crow SJ, Collins J, Justic M, Goetz R, and Adler S. Psychopathology following cardioverter defibrillator implantation. *Psychosomatics* 1998;39:305–310.
10. Heller SS, Ormont MA, Lidagoster L, Sciacca RR, and Steinberg S. Psychosocial outcome after ICD implantation: a current perspective. *Pacing Clin Electrophysiol* 1998;21:1207–1215.
11. Hammel D, Scheld HH, Block M, and Breithardt G. Nonthoracotomy defibrillator implantation: a single-center experience with 200 patients. *Ann Thorac Surg* 1994;58:321–327.
12. Schwartzman D, Nallamothu N, Callans DJ, Preminger MW, Gottlieb CD, and Marchlinski FE. Postoperative lead-related complications in patients with nonthoracotomy defibrillation lead systems. *J Am Coll Cardiol* 1995;26:776–786.
13. Robinson LA, Windle JR. Defibrillator twiddler's syndrome. *Ann Thorac Surg* 1994;58:247–249.

14. Korte T, Jung W, Schlippert U, Wolpert C, Esmailzadeh B, Fimmers R, Schmitt O, and Luderitz B. Prospective evaluation of shoulder-related problems in patients with pectoral cardioverter-defibrillator implantation. *Am Heart J* 1998;135:577–583.

15. Brady PA, Friedman PA, and Trusty JM. High failure rate for an epicardial implantable cardioverterdefibrillator lead: implications for long-term follow-up of patients with an implantable cardioverter-defibrillator. *J Am Coll Cardiol* 1998;31:616–621.

16. Gupta A, Zegel HG, and Dravid VS. Value of radiography in diagnosing complications of cardioverter defibrillators implanted without thoracotomy in 437 patients. *Am J Roentgenol* 1997;168:105–108.

17. Drucker EA, Brooks R, Garan H, Sweeney MO, Ruskin JM, McGovern BA, and Miller SW. Malfunction of implantable cardioverter defibrillators placed by a non-thoractomy approach: frequency of malfunction and value of chest radiography in determining cause. *Am J Roentgenol* 1995;165:275–279.

18. Nathan AW. The role of cardioversion therapy in patients with implanted cardioverter defibrillators. *Am Heart J* 1994;127(4 Pt 2):1046–1051.

19. Barold SS, Newby KH, Tomassoni G, Kearney M, Brandon J, and Natale A. Prospective evaluation of new and old criteria to discriminate between supraventricular and ventricular tachycardia in implantable defibrillators. *Pacing Clin Electrophysiol* 1998;21:1347–1355.

20. Swerdlow CD, Chen PS, Kass RM, Allard JR, and Peter CT. Discrimination of ventricular tachycardia from sinus tachycardia and atrial fibrillation in a tiered-therapy cardioverter-defibrillator. *J Am Coll Cardiol* 1994;23:1342–1355.

21. Klingenheben T, Sticherling C, Skupin M, and Hohnloser SH. Intracardiac QRS electrogram width: an arrhythmia detection feature for implantable cardioverter defibrillators: exercise included variation as a base for device programming. *Pacing Clin Electrophysiol* 1998;21:1609–1617.

22. Favale S, Nacci F, Galati A, Accogli M, De Giorgi V, Greco MR, Nastasi M, Pierfelice O, Rossi S, and Gargaro A. Electrogram width parameter analysis in implantable cardioverter defibrillators: influence of body position and electrode configuration. *Pacing Clin Electrophysiol* 2001;24:1732–1738.

23. Theuns DAMJ, Rivero-Ayerza M, Goedhart DM, van der Perk R, and Jordaens LJ. Evalution of morphology discrimination for ventricular tachycardia diagnosis in implantable cardioverter-defibrillators. *Heart Rhythm* 2006;3:1332–1338.

24. Soundarraj D, Thakur RK, Gardiner JC, Khasnis A, and Jongnaransin K. Inappropriate ICD therapy: does device configuration make a difference? *Pacing Clin Electrophysiol* 2006;29:810–815.

25. Theuns DAMJ, Klootwijk APJ, Goedhart DM, and Jordaens LJ. Prevention of inappropriate therapy in implantable cadioverter defibrillators. Results of a prospective, randomized study of tachyarrhythmia detection algorithms. *J Am Coll Cardiol* 2004;44:2362–2367.

26. Purerfellner H, Gillis AM, Holbrook R, and Hettrick DA. Accuracy of atrial tachyarrhythmiadetection in implantable devices with arrhythmia therapies. *Pacing Clin Electrophysiol* 2004;27:983–992.

27. Friedman PA, McClelland RL, Bmlet WR, Acosta H, Kessler D, Munger TM, Kavesh NG, Wood M, Daoud E, Massumi A, Schuger C, Shorofsky S, Wilkoff B, and Glikson M. Dual-chamber versus single-chamber detection enhancements for implantable defibrillator rhythm diagnosis. The detect supraventricular tachycardia study. *Circulation* 2006;113:2871–2879.

28. Marchlinski FE, Flores B, Miller JM, Gottlieb CD, and Hargrove WC 3rd. Relation of the intraoperative defibrillation threshold to successful postoperative defibrillation with an automatic implantable cardioverter defibrillator. *Am J Cardiol* 1988;62:393–398.

29. Neuzner J. Safety margins: lessions from the low energy Endotak trial (LEET). *Am J Cardiol* 1996;78(5A):26–32.

30. Nasir N, Pacifico A, Doyle TK, Earle NR, Hardage ML, and Henry PD. Spontaneous ventricular tachycardia treated by antitachycardia pacing. *Am J Cardiol* 1997;79:820–822.

31. Ruppel R, Schluter CA, Boczar S, Meinertz T, Schluter M, Kuck KH, and Cappato R. Ventricular tachycardia during follow-up in patients resuscitated from ventricular fibrillation: experience from stored electrograms of implantable cardioverter-defibrillators. *J Am Coll Cardiol* 1998;32:1724–1730.

32. Grimm W, Plachta E, Maisch B. Antitachycardia pacing for spontaneous rapid ventricular tachycardia in patients with prophylactic cardioverter-defibrillator therapy. *Pacing Clin Electrophysiol* 2006;29:759–764.

33. Olatidoye AG, Verroneau J, and Kluger J. Mechanisms of syncope in implantable cardioverter-defibrillator recipients who receive device therapies. *Am J Cardiol* 1998;82:1372–1376.

34. Schaumann A, von zur Muhlen F, Herse B, Gonska BD, and Kreuzer H. Empirical versus tested antitachycardia pacing in implantable cardioverter defibrillators. A prospective study including 200 patients. *Circulation* 1998;97:66–74.

35. Jimenez-Candil J, Arenal A, Garcia-Alberola A, Ortiz M, del Castillo S, Fernandez-Portales J, Sanchez-Munoz J, Martinez-Sanchez J, Gonzalez-Torrecilla E, Atienza F, Puchol A, and Almendral J. Fast ventricular tachycardias in patients with implantable cardioverter-defibrillators: efficacy and safety of antitachycardia pacing. A randomized prospective study. *J Am Coll Cardiol* 2005;45:460–461.

36. Wathen MS, Sweeney MO, DeGroot P, Stark AJ, Koehler JL, Chisner MB, Machado C, and Adkisson WO, for the PainFREE Rx Investigators. Shock reduction using antitachycardia pacing for spontaneous ventricular tachycardia in patients with coronary artery disease. *Circulation* 2001;104:796–801.

37. Wathen MS, DeGroot PJ, Sweeney MO, Stark AJ, Otterness MF, Adkisson WO, Canby RC, Khalighi K, Machado C, Rubenstein DS, and Volosin JK, for the PainFREE Rx II Investigators. Prospective randomized multicenter trial of empiric antitachycardia pacing versus shocks for spontaneous rapid ventricular tachycardia in patients with implantable cardioverter-defibrillators. Pain FREE Rx II trial results. *Circulation* 2004;110:2592–2596.

38. Laborderie J, Bordachar P, O'neill MD, and Clementy J. Fluctuation of atrial and ventricular lead impedances heralding subtotal separation of device header and generator in a patient with an implantable cardioverter-defibrillator. *Heart Rhythm.* 2007 Feb;4(2):218–220.

39. Epstein AE, Plumb VJ, Kirkk KA, and Kay GN. Pacing threshold increase in non-thoractomy implantable defibrillator leads: implications for battery longevity and margin of safety. *J Int Cardiac Electrophysiol* 1997;1:131–134.

40. Steinberg JS, Fischer A, Wang P, Schuger C, Daubert J, McNitt S, Andrews M, Brown M, Hall WJ, Zareba W, and Moss AJ; MADIT II Investigators. The clinical implications of cumulative right ventricular pacing in the multicenter automatic defibrillator trial II. *J Cardiovasc Electrophysiol.* 2005 Apr;16(4):359–365.

41. Sharma AD, Rizo-Patron C, Hallstrom AP, O'Neill GP, Rothbart S, Martins JB, Roelke M, Steinberg JS, and Greene HL; DAVID Investigators. Percent right ventricular pacing predicts outcomes in the DAVID trial. *Heart Rhythm.* 2005 Aug;2(8):830–834.

42. Gilliam FR, Kaplan AJ, Black J, Chase KJ, Mullin CM. Changes in Heart Rate Variability, quality of life, and activity in cardiac resynchronization therapy: Results of the HF-HRV Registry. *Pacing Clin Electrophysiol* 2007;30:56–64.

43. Kadhiresen VA, Pastore J, Auricchio A, Sack S, Doelger A, Girouard S, and Spinelli JC. A novel method-the activity log index- for monitoring physical activity of patients with heart failure. *Am J cardiol* 2002;89:1435–1437.

44. Yu CM, Wang L, Chau E, Chan RH, Kong SL, Tang MO, Christensen J, Stadler RW, and Lau CP. Intrathoracic impedance monitoring in patients with heart failure: correlation with fluid status and feasibility of early warning preceding hospitalization. *Circulation* 2005;112:841–848.

45. Ypenburg C, Bax JJ, van der Wall EE, Schalij MJ, and van Erven L. Intrathoracic impedance monitoring to predict decompensated heart faiure. *Am J Cardiol* 2007;99:554–557.

46. Mickelsen S, and Kusumoto FM. Balancing quality and thoroughness with efficiency in invasive cardiac electrophysiology. *Cardiac Electrophysiol Rev* 2000;4:133–136.

47. Gregoratos G, Abrams J, Epstein AE, Freedman RA, Hayes DL, Hatky MA, Kerber RE, Naccarelli GV, Schoenfeld MH, Silka MJ, Winters SL, Gibbons RJ, Antman EM, Alpert JS, Gregoratos G, Hiratzka LF, Faxon DP, Jacobs AK, Fuster V, and Smith SCJ. ACC/AHA/NASPE 2002 Guideline update for implantation of cardiac pacemakers and antiarrhythmia devices: summary article: a report of the American College of Cardiology/American Heart Association Task Force on Practice Guidelines (ACC/AHA/NASPE Committee to Update the 1998 Pacemaker Guidlines). *Circulation* 2002;106:2145–2161.

48. Winters SL, Packer DL, Marchlinski FE, Lazzara R, Cannom DS, Breithardt GE, Wilber DA, Camm AJ, and Ruskin JN. NASPE policy statement. Consensus statement on indications, guidelines for use, and recommendations for follow-up of implantable cardioverter defibrillators. *Pacing Clin Electrophysiol* 2001;24:262–269.

49. Rashba EJ, Olsovsky MR, Shorofsky SR, Kirk MM, Peters RW, and Gold MR. Temporal decline in defibrillation thresholds with an active pectoal lead system. *J Am Coll Cardiol* 2001;38:1150–1155.

50. Venditti FJ, Martin DT, Vassolas G, and Bowen S. Rise in chronic defibrillation thresholds in nonthoractomy implantable defibrillator. *Circulation* 1994;89:216–223.

51. Schwartzman D, Callans DJ, Gottlieb CD, Heo J, and Marchlinski FE. Early postoperative rise in defibrillation threshold in patients with nonthoracotomy defibrillation lead systems: attenuation with biphasic shock waveforms. *J Cardiovasc Electrophysiol* 1996;7:483–493.

52. Olsovsky MR, Pelini MA, Shorofsky SR, and Gold MR. Temporal stability of defibrillation thresholds with an active pectoral lead system. *J Cardiovasc Electrophysiol* 1998;9:240–244.

53. Gold MR, Khalighi K, Kavesh NG, Daly B, Peters RW, and Shorofsky SR. Clinical predictors of transvenous biphasic defibrillation thresholds. *Am J Cardiol* 1997;79:1623–1627.

54. Tokano T, Pelosi F, Flemming M, Horwood L, Souza JJ, Zivin A, Knight BP, Goyal R, Man KC, Morady F, and Strickberger SA. Long-term evaluation of ventricular defibrillation energy requirement. *J Cardiovasc Electrophysiol* 1998;9:916–920.

55. Epstein AE, Kay GN, Plumb VJ, Dailey SM, and Anderson PG. Gross and microscopic pathological changes associated with nonthoracotomy implantable defibrillator leads. *Circulation* 1998;98:1517–1524.

56. Mehta D, Nayak HM, Singson M, Chao S, Pe E, Camunas JL, and Gomes JA. Late complications in patients with pectoral defibrillator implants with transvenous defibrillator lead systems: high incidence of insulation breakdown. *Pacing Clin Electrophysiol.* 1998;21:1893–1900.

57. Hauser RG, Cannom D, Hayes DL, Parsonnet V, Hayes J, Ratliff N 3rd, Epstein AE, Vlay SC, Furman S, Gross J. Long-term structural failure of coaxial polyurethane implantable cardioverter defibrillator leads. *Pacing Clin Electrophysiol* 2002;57:879–882.

58. Lawton JS, Wood MA, Gilligan DM, Stambler BS, Damiano RJ, Jr, and Ellenbogen KA. Implantable transvenous cardioverter defibrillator leads: the dark side. *Pacing Clin Electrophysiol.* 1996;19:1273–1278.

59. Zilo P, Weiss DN, and Luceri RM. Late retesting of system performance in ICD patients without spontaneous shocks. *Pacing Clin Electrophysiol.* 1996;22:197–201.

60. Stanton MS. Follow-up of implantable cardioverter-defibrillator patients. *ACC Curr J Rev* 1995;4:35–37.

61. Bindra PS, Ruskin JN, and Keane D. Usefulness of predischarge defibrillation testing after defibrillator implantation in hospitalized patients. *Am J Cardiol* 2002;90:798–799.

62. Delvecchio A, Trivedia HA, Fisher JD, KimSG, Ferrick KJ, Gross JN, and Palma EC. Value of pre-hospital discharge defibrillation testing in recipients of implantable cardioverter defibrillatos; *Pacing Clin Electrophysiol* 2005;28:S260–S262.

63. Lurie KG, Iskos D, Fetter J, Peterson CA, Collins JM, Shultz JJ, Fahy GI, Sakaguchi S, and Benditt DG. Prehospital discharge defibrillation testing in ICD recipients: a prospective study based on cost analysis. *Pacing Clin Electrophysiol* 1999;22:192–196.

64. Goldberger JJ, Horvath G, Inbar S, and Kadish AH. Utility of predischarge and one-month transvenous implantable defibrillator tests. *Am J Cardiol* 1997;79:822–826.

65. Higgins SL, Rich DH, Haygood JR, Barone J, Greer SL, and Meyer DB. ICD restudy: results and potential benefit from routine pre-discharge and 2-month evaluation. *Pacing Clin Electrophysiol.* 1998;21:410–417.

66. Stanton MS, and Bell GK. Economic outcomes of implantable cardioverter defibrillators. *Circulation* 2000;101:1067–1074.

67. Stepheson EA, Cecchin F, Walsh EP, and Berul CI. Utility of routine follow-up defibrillator threshold testing in congenial heart disease and pediatric populations. *J Cardiovasc Electrophysiol* 2005;16:69–73.

68. Hohnloser SH, Dorian P, Roberts R, Gent M, Israel CW,Fain E, Champagne J, and Connolly SJ. Effect of amiodarone and sotalol on ventricular defibrillation threshold: the optimal pharmacological therapy in cardioverter defibrillator patients (OPTIC) trial. *Circulation* 2006;114:104–109.

69. Kusumoto FM, and Goldschlager N. Cost-effective follow-up of pacing systems. *Electrophysiol Board Rev* 1999 (in press).

70. Fetter JG, Stanton MS, Benditt DG, Trusty J, and Collins J. Transtelephonic monitoring and transmission of stored arrhythmia detection and therapy data from an implantable cardioverter defibrillator. *Pacing Clin Electrophysiol.* 1995;18:1531–1539.

71. Brugada P. What evidence do we have to replace in-hospital implantable cardioverter defibrillator follow-up? *Clin Res Cardiol* 2006;95(Suppl 3):III/3–9.

72. Epstein AE, Baessler CA, Curtis AB, Estes NA 3rd, Gersh BJ, Grubb B, and Mitchell LB. Addendum to "Personal and public safety issues related to arrhythmias that may affect consciouness: implications for regulation and physician recommendations: a medical/scientific statement from the American Heart Association and the North American Society of Pacing and Electrophysiology." Public safety issues in patients with implantable defibrillators. A scientific statement from the American Heart Association and the Heart Rhythm Society. *Circulation.* 2007 Feb 7.

73. Akiyama T, Powell JL, Mitchell LB,, Baessler C. Antiarrhythmics versus Implantable Defibrillators Investigators. Resumption of driving after life-threatening ventricular tachyarrhythmia. *N Engl J Med.* 2001 Aug 9;345(6):391–397.

74. Blumenthal R, Braunstein J, Connolly H, Epstein A, Gersh BJ, and Wittels EH. Cardiovascular advisory panel guidelines for medical examination of commercial motor vehicles drivers. FMCSA-MCP-02–2002. Washington DC: US Department of Transportation, Federal Motor Carrier Safety Administration FMCSA-MCP-02–2002; October 2002.

75. Rosenthal ME, and Paskman C. Noise detection during bradycardia pacing with a hybrid nonthoracotomy implantable cardioverter defibrillator system: incidence and clinical significance. *Pacing Clin Electrophysiol* 1998;21:1380–1386.

76. Seifert T, Block M, Borgreffe M, and Breithardt G. Erroneous discharge of an implantable cardioverter defibrillator caused by an electric razor. *Pacing Clin Electrophysiol* 1995;18:1592–1594.

77. McIvor ME, Reddinger J, Floden E, and Sheppard RC. Study of pacemaker and implantable cardioverter defibrillator triggering by electronic article surveillance devices (SPICED TEAS). *Pacing Clin Electrophysiol* 1998;21:1847–1861.

78. Kadish A, Dryer A, Daubert JP, Quigg R, Estes NA, Anderson KP, Calkins H, Hoch D, Goldberger J, Shalaby A, Saundes WE, Schaechter A, and Levine JH: Defibrillators in nonischemiccardiomyopathy treatment evaluation (DEFINITE) investigators. Prophylactic defibrillator in patients with nonischemic dilated cardiomyopathy. *New Engl J Med* 2004;350:2151–2158.

79. Messali A, Tomas O, Chauvin M, Coumel P, and Leenhardt A. Death due to an implantable cardioverter defibrillator. *J Cardiovasc Electrophysiol* 2004;15:953–956.

80. Prudente LA, Reigle J, Bourguignon C, Haines DE, and DiMarco JP. Psychological indices and phantom shocks in patients with ICD. *J Interv Card Electrophysiol* 2006;15:185–190.

81. Kelly PA, Mann DE, Damle RS, and Reiter MJ. Oversensing during ventricular pacing in patients with a third-generation implantable cardioverter defibrillator. *J Am Coll Cardiol* 1994;23:1531–1534.

82. Nunain SO, Roelke M, Trouton T, Osswalds S, Kim YH, Sosa-Suarez G, Brooks DR, McGovern B, Guy RN, Torchiana DF, Vlahakes GJ, Garan H, and Ruskin JN. Limitations and late complications of third generation automatic cardioverter-defibrillators. *Circulation* 1995;91:2204–2213.

83. Fogoros R, Elson J, and Bonnet C. Actuarial incidence and pattern of occurrence of shocks following implantation of the automatic cardioverter defibrillator. *Pacing Clin Electrophysiol* 1989;11:2014.

84. Credner SC, Klingenheben T, Mauss O, Sticherling C, and Hohnloser SH. Electrical storm in patients with transvenous implantable cardioverter defibrillators: incidence, management, and prognostic implications. *J Am Coll Cardiol* 1998;32:1909–1915.

85. Mann DE, Kelly PA, Damle RS, and Reiter MJ. Undersensing during ventricular tachyarrhythmias in a third generation implantable defibrillator: diagnosis using stored electrograms and correction with programming. *Pacing Clin Electrophysiol* .1994;17:1525–1530.

86. Swerdlow CD, Ahern T, Chen PS, Hwang C, Gang E, Mandel W, Kass Rm, and Peter CT. Underdetection of ventricular tachycardia by algorithms to enhance specificity in a tiered therapy cardioverter-defibrillator. *J Am Coll Cadiol* 1994;24:416–424.

87. Jung W, Manz M, Moosdorf R, Tebbenjohanns J, Pfeiffer D, and Luderitz B. Changes in the amplitude of endocardial electrograms following defibrillator discharge: comparison of two lead systems. *Pacing Clin electrophysiol* 1995;18:2163–2172.

88. Berul CI, Callans DJ, and Schwartzman DS, et al. Comparison of initial detection and redetection of ventricular fibrillation in a transvenous defibrillator system with automatic gain control. *J Am Coll Cardiol* 1995;25:431–436.

89. Herre JM, USA Endotak Investigators. Detection and redetection characteristics of the Endotak C transvenous lead system.

90. Goldberger JJ, Horvath G, Donovan D, Johnson D, Challapalli R, and Kadish AH. Detection of ventricular fibrillation by transvenous defibrillating leads: integrated versus dedicated bipolar sensing. *J Cardiovasc Electrophysiol* 1998;9:677–688.

91. Stevenson WG, Friedman PL, Kucovic D, Sager PT, Saxon LA, and Pavri B. Radiofrequency catheter ablation of ventricular tachycardia after myocardial infarction. *Circulation* 1998;98:308–314.

92. Rothman SA, Hsia HH, Cossu SF, Chmielewski IL, Buxton AE, Miller JM. Radiofrequency catheter ablation of postinfarction ventricular tachycardia: long-term